PRACTICAL DECISION MAKING IN HEALTH CARE ETHICS

Cases and Concepts

PRACTICAL DECISION MAKING IN HEALTH CARE ETHICS

Cases and Concepts

Raymond J. Devettere

Georgetown University Press / Washington, D.C.

Georgetown University Press, Washington, D.C.
© 1995 by Georgetown University Press. All rights reserved.
Printed in the United States of America
10 9 8 7 6 5 4 3 2   1995
THIS VOLUME IS PRINTED ON ACID-FREE ∞ OFFSET BOOK PAPER

Library of Congress Cataloging-in-Publication Data

Devettere, Raymond.
    Practical decision making in health care ethics : cases and
concepts / Raymond Devettere.
        p.   cm.
    Includes indexes.
    1. Medical ethics.   I. Title.
    [DNLM: 1. Decision Making. 2. Ethics, Medical. 3. Resuscitation
Orders.   W 50 D491p]1995
R724.D48   1995
174'.2—dc20
ISBN 0-87840-589-5 (cloth : alk. paper).
ISBN 0-87840-594-1 (paper : alk. paper)   95-6353

For Paula

Epigraph

It is a characteristic of reason to proceed from general principles to particular conclusions. Nonetheless, speculative reason does this one way, and practical reason another. Speculative reason is chiefly concerned with necessary things which cannot be otherwise than they are, and so truth is found without diminution in the particular conclusions just as in the general principles. But practical reason is concerned with things which can be otherwise than they are, and this includes human behavior, and thus, even if there is some force in the general principles, the more you descend to the particular conclusions, the greater is their failure.

Thomas Aquinas, Summa Theologiae,
I II, q. 94, a.4, 13th century

In short, our moral discourse . . . involves the concept of an objectively or absolutely valid moral action-guide, and our moral judgments and decisions claim to be parts or applications of such an action-guide.

William Frankena, "the
principles of morality," 1973

Whereas young people can become proficient in geometry and mathematics, we do not find young people proficient in prudential reasoning. The reason is that prudential reasoning is about particular cases and knowledge about particulars comes from experience.

Aristotle, Nicomachean Ethics,
1142a12-16, 4th century B.C.E.

The argument aims eventually to be strictly deductive . . . (C)learly arguments from such premises can be fully deductive, as theories in politics and economics attest. We should strive for a kind of moral geometry with all the rigor which this name connotes.

John Rawls, A Theory
of Justice, 1971

Contents

Preface

The past few decades have been an era of great interest and accomplishment in the field of health care ethics. It is impossible to acknowledge my indebtedness to all those working in the field whose writings have influenced and instructed me. The writings of several authors, however, have been especially valuable, and they will be mentioned by name in alphabetical order: George Annas, Daniel Callahan, Albert Jonsen, Richard McCormick, and Edmund Pellegrino.

This book originated from notes complementing textbooks in numerous courses in health care ethics taught during the past decade. Although the book presents an alternative to the way these textbooks approach ethics, I want to acknowledge my admiration and appreciation of the contribution these authors have made to the teaching of health care ethics. Especially helpful to me have been the following: Tom Beauchamp and James Childress, *Biomedical Ethics;* Thomas Mappes and Jane Zembaty, *Biomedical Ethics;* Ronald Munson, *Intervention and Reflection: Basic Issues in Medical Ethics;* and Baruch Brody, *Life and Death Decision Making.*

I am also indebted to the many students at Emmanuel College, Boston College, and the New England Baptist Hospital School of Nursing, who provided important feedback while using earlier versions of this book in the past few years. More than anything else, it was teaching students—some of them young, some of them adults with decades of experience as health care professionals—that led to the approach taken in this book. One basic question hovered over many classes: Why should I be ethical? No satisfactory answer emerged in the health care ethics derived from the modern deontological and rule–utilitarian moralities. These theories provided no cogent reason why moral agents should always follow a general rule or a maxim they wanted to be a universal moral law, or a rule designed to achieve the welfare of everyone; they did not tell us why a health care professional or a patient ought to regulate her personal decisions in every situation by the action-guiding principles of autonomy, beneficence, and justice.

The question "Why should I be ethical?" readily finds an answer in an ethics of happiness and fulfillment. Here ethics is simply the effort to discover in each of life's challenges what feelings, habits, and behaviors will give the moral agent the best chance of living a happy and flourishing life. The notions of principles, rules, and rights can play an important role in this ethics, but only to the extent that they help the moral agent to live well. When ethics is viewed as doing what constitutes living well for the person deciding what to do, no reasonable person would think of not being ethical.

This book is not intended to be exhaustive. It does review most of the current topics in health care ethics but does not cover not all of them. However, it provides the reader with an approach, prudential reasoning, that can readily be extended to other issues of great moral concern not treated in the text—issues such as genetics, health care costs and rationing, and the AIDS epidemic.

I am indebted also to fellow members of the Ethics Committee at Newton–Wellesley Hospital for many thoughtful dialogues over the years and to two anonymous readers at Georgetown University Press for their helpful comments on the text.

In order to maintain consistency of vocabulary throughout the book, the translations of Aristotle and Aquinas are my own, but I was aided immensely by several standard translations of their works. Especially helpful for Aristotle was J. Tricot's richly annotated and textually faithful translation entitled *Éthique à Nicomaque* (Paris: J. Vrin, 1983).

Introduction

This book offers an alternative approach to health care ethics. The field is currently dominated by ethical theories centered on obligation and duty. These theories make moral principles the centerpiece: they propose a set of general action-guiding principles and rules that we apply to particular situations to determine what we are obliged to do. Sometimes the principles and rules are derived from ethical theories, sometimes from experience, sometimes from an equilibrium of both theory and experience, but it is always the principles and rules that occupy the central position in these moral philosophies.

The ethics proposed in this book is not an ethics of obligation and duty determined by principles and rules. It is an ethics of personal well-being and fulfillment. These theories make the good life—my good life—the centerpiece: they propose a process of prudential reasoning to determine what habits, feelings, and behaviors in the various situations of life will fulfill the goal we all ultimately share—living a fulfilled and happy life.

The ethics of personal fulfillment and happiness is not a new ethics; most ancient ethical theories were centered on happiness, not obligation. This book was influenced chiefly by one such theory—that of Aristotle. Aristotle (384–322 B.C.E.) grew up in Macedonia but lived most of his life in Athens, although he never enjoyed the privileges of Athenian citizenship. He accomplished an extraordinary amount of scientific and philosophical research during his lifetime and lectured on many topics, including ethics. Some of his lectures on ethics comprise the first major books in our culture devoted exclusively to ethics—the *Nicomachean Ethics* and the *Eudemian Ethics*.

Aristotle's work is impressive because it was the first sustained study of ethics as a discipline and was extraordinarily profound. It has also proven relevant far beyond its original cultural milieu. Sixteen hundred years after Aristotle, for example, Thomas Aquinas (1225–74) embraced Aristotle's approach in ethics and saw no trouble integrating it with his religious faith and Christian theology. Today, seven hundred years later, we may be able to retrieve something of value from the ethics of Aristotle and Aquinas.

This book will attempt such a retrieval in reference to health care ethics. It is not, however, a book pretending to explain the ethics of Aristotle or of Aquinas, nor is it a defense of their ethical positions. Rather, the intention is to capture the fundamental intuition of these ethicists and to approach the moral issues of contemporary health care ethics in their philosophical spirit. This move is motivated by the conviction that ethics is more about the habits, feelings, and behaviors that we need to cultivate and practice in order to live well than it is about our obligations; more about flourishing in life than about duties. Implied in this preference is the idea that fulfilling moral obligations and duties, while necessary, is simply not sufficient to bring happiness and to make any human life a good and noble life.

There are, of course, serious obstacles confronting any attempt to retrieve an older ethics. Some problems are textual: we do not have any original manuscripts, so the texts we do have are not always consistent. Some problems are cultural: one reason why we cannot fully understand older texts is that we do not share the cultural context in which they were produced.

Some problems are linguistic: most people cannot read Aristotle's Greek or Aquinas' Latin and must rely on translations. Translations can be notoriously misleading. For example, H. Rackham's translations of both the *Nicomachean Ethics* and the *Eudemian Ethics* in the Loeb Classical Library editions render Aristotle's key phrase *kata ton orthon logon* as "according to the right principle," thus giving the incorrect impression that the ethics of Aristotle is an ethics of principles in the same way the modern deontological and utilitarian ethics are ethics of action-guiding principles. Aquinas' translation of this phrase as "according to right reason" (*secundum rectam rationem*) is accurate. The point is worth noting because both Aristotle and Aquinas went to extraordinary lengths to show that right reason in ethics is prudential reasoning, a reasoning quite unlike principle-based reasonings.

Finally, some problems are philosophical; philosophers have always differed and undoubtedly will always differ over how we should understand the moral philosophies of Aristotle and Aquinas. There is no definitive interpretation of their doctrines, and sometimes their texts give rise to conflicting positions. Unfortunately, they are not here to explain their ideas to us. In many ways, then, the moral philosopher influenced by the texts of Aristotle and Aquinas is faced with problems similar to those faced by believers seeking to learn from the Bible. The original texts are lost, other texts were copied by hand and the copies introduced errors and editorial variations, the Biblical languages of Hebrew and Greek are unknown to many, and we can never be sure what the author meant or (in some cases) who the author was. Nevertheless, the believer recognizes the value of the Biblical texts and works from them. And the ethicist can do likewise in a retrieval of older philosophical texts.

It is important to note three things about the older ethics of happiness and prudence retrieved in this book. First, the ethics of prudential reasoning is not a moral relativism. It is a normative ethics, and its norm is a moral absolute. According to its norm, only those feelings, habits, and behaviors constituting a life of happiness and fulfillment for the moral agent are morally good. All deliberate feelings and behaviors undermining the agent's flourishing as a good and noble human being are always unreasonable and immoral. Moreover, some absolute concrete claims are compatible with an ethics of prudential reasoning. Thus, as Aristotle noted, the wrongfulness of murder is absolute. No matter how history develops, murder will never be morally acceptable. Murder is, by definition, always the morally unreasonable taking of human life.

Second, the ethics of happiness should not be confused with modern ethical egoisms. In modern versions of egoism the moral agent evaluates behavior only in terms of himself. In the ethics of happiness the moral agent thinks of human existence as interpersonal and social. His happiness and flourishing is inherently entwined with that of others, and thus their happiness and flourishing matters as well. This is why the predominantly self-centered virtues such as temperance and courage are complemented in an ethics of personal fulfillment by other-centered virtues such as love and justice.

Third, Aristotle did not think the ethics of prudential reasoning was relevant for everyone. In an intriguing but seldom noted remark at the beginning of Book VII of the *Nicomachean Ethics,* he acknowledged that certain rare individuals live lives of such heroic virtue that they have no need of prudential reasoning. He also noted that other individuals are so terribly evil—he called them bestial—that they are simply incapable of prudential reasoning. Aristotle was nothing if not a realist.

The ethics in this book is not written in the language of principles, rules, rights, or duties. It is written in the language of prudential reasoning, the deliberation most of us employ to determine how to live fulfilled and happy lives in the situations confronting us. Since prudential reasoning is primarily a reasoning attuned to situations and contexts, the study of cases is important for seeing how prudential reasoning works. The cases in this book are therefore presented as an integral part of the chapters describing treatment options. We do not first learn principles and rules, and then apply them to cases; we first understand something about prudential reasoning and then learn how to do it by working our way through cases involving treatment decisions viewed from the different perspectives of the people involved.

The cases in this book are not imaginary. They were chosen because they actually happened, and in most instances were the subject of highly publicized court battles. These public cases were selected because they are morally interesting and instructive, and because they give the reader the opportunity to learn something of the history of health care ethics in the United States. As new generations of people interested in health care ethics emerge, they can profit from acquaintance with the widely known cases discussed and debated by those already working in the field.

The book also takes positions in these cases, sometimes agreeing and sometimes disagreeing with what was done. It is important to note that these positions are not intended to be authoritative and dogmatic. Rather, they are invitations for dialogue and discussion. Ethics is not science; we are not studying the physical realities we find around and within our bodies. Ethics is the study of what might become reality as the result of our choices, and an interminable self-correcting process of dialogue and debate is needed to figure out what choices will actually help us live good lives in the ever-changing circumstances of history. As slavery was once seen as ethical and then rejected, what seems ethical today may be rejected in the future as unethical by subsequent discussion and debate.

Each case is presented in an extremely simplified way comprised of two stages. The first stage is called *situational awareness.* Here we attempt to discover and identify the pertinent facts and values in the case. We uncover the facts by asking what is happening here, who are the decision makers, what can be done, and what circumstances are relevant. We become aware of the values by asking what features embedded in the situation are good or bad for the people involved and what good and bad will result from our action or inaction.

The second stage is *prudential reasoning*. Here we take the position of each major moral agent in the case—patient, proxy, physician, nurse, attorney, and judge—and ask what each of them could do to live well. The goal in life is living well, living a good life, living happily; moral agents behave morally when they behave so as to achieve this goal. This is what we mean by acting according to right reason.

A final word about the cases. The intent in considering these real, and often tragic, cases and in taking a position on what was or was not done is not to attack the personal integrity of the participants in the original story. We simply want to use the stories, which became public when they entered the legal process or were reported in the press, as examples and to learn from them. *The analyses of the cases are not intended to make any judgment, or to reach any conclusion, about the personal or moral character of any person, living or dead, involved in the cases.*

This book also differs from many texts in moral philosophy by the place it accords the Biblical religious traditions and moral theology. History shows that religion has been a powerful force in shaping ethical attitudes, and it simply cannot be ignored in ethical analysis. Nonetheless, there are reasons for saying ethics also shapes religion. When it comes to deliberating about how to live well—the major focus of ethics—the moral norm of prudential reasoning embraces all human behaviors, including those proposed in the name of religion and theology. The ethics of prudential reasoning, therefore, is relevant, as the texts of Aristotle and Aquinas show so well, both for those who believe in a caring God and for those who do not so believe.

Many people turn to ethics looking for answers. Answers are important, and sometimes we can give them with great confidence. Most of us know the right answer to questions about the morality of slavery, and we also know that most moral philosophers and theologians (including Aristotle and Aquinas) had the wrong answer until a few centuries ago.

In addition to moral answers, however, something else is important— moral awareness. The Bible tells a story—and stories are always important in ethics—about moral awareness. King David once spotted a beautiful woman undressed and bathing, and he wanted her. Her husband was a military commander away on a campaign, so they began an affair. When she became pregnant, David recalled the commander from the front lines, hoping that he would sleep with his wife during his home visit so that the king's paternity could be concealed. The commander declined to go home, and stayed in a military camp during his time away from the front. King David then devised a second strategy to cover his tracks—he arranged for the commander to be sent on a useless suicide mission, where he lost his life. David then took the now-widowed Bethsabee as one of his wives, totally oblivious to the immorality of what he and Bethsabee had done—adultery and murder.

A religious man highly respected by King David, Nathan, was not so oblivious to the immorality. One day he told the king how a rich man had taken the young lamb that a poor man had adopted as a pet and loved dearly, and had slaughtered it for a meal. The king was outraged, and ordered the man apprehended and punished. "But," said Nathan, "you are the man." David then realized the terrible thing he had done. He recognized himself as an adulterer and a murderer, and thereby achieved moral awareness, which is the crucial first step in living a good life.

If this text does no more than raise moral awareness about some of the complex ethical issues of health care, it will serve some purpose.

1

What Is Ethics?

It should be no surprise that ethicists disagree about the answer to this question. The current debates about abortion, nuclear warfare, homosexuality, and euthanasia remind us that ethicists often disagree about ethical matters. We will begin, however, not with the disagreements emerging from the various definitions of ethics, but with the similarities they all share.

DEFINING ETHICS

Despite their differences, most ethical theories include the following features.

Ethics Is About Choices

Here we make but two points, one requiring some explanation, the other needing only a brief statement.

First, ethics is concerned with what we choose to do intentionally or on purpose. Ethics is not concerned with what people do accidently or unintentionally, even if these behaviors cause bad things. If I am getting in a crowded elevator and accidently step on your foot despite trying to be careful, this is not really an ethical matter. Although I may say "I'm sorry," and thus imply that I did something intentionally, in reality I did not intentionally step on your foot, and nothing unethical or immoral was involved.

The situation becomes more complex if I stepped on your foot in the process of pushing and shoving my way into the crowded elevator. Here I would have to admit some degree of ethical responsibility. True, I did not intend to step on your foot, but I did intend to push my way into the crowded elevator, and thereby I did choose behavior known to entail a high risk of stepping on someone's foot in these circumstances.

Tremendous debates have existed for centuries in psychology, philosophy, and legal theory about whether human beings are able to choose freely or whether they are totally determined by biological, psychological, or sociological factors. These debates need not detain us here. We do know, with the wisdom of everyday experience and of a long criminal justice tradition, that we make choices in life and are therefore responsible in some degree for what we do. To deny this is to deny that a jury could ever find a person guilty of a criminal action. Philosophers and scientists may question our ability to make choices, and some have advanced powerful arguments for explaining our behavior in terms of some form of determinism. But these arguments have not yet convinced us to abandon our experience of choice or to abolish a legal system that holds people responsible, and responsibility implies the person need not have done the deed, but chose to do it.

It is important to note that choice embraces what we choose not to do as well as what we choose to do. Choice is about omissions as well as actions. Choosing to do nothing in a situation where we could do something is just as much of a choice as the choice to do something. We are responsible both for what we freely choose to do and for what we freely choose not to do but could do.

Second, although ethics is about choice, not every choice is ethically significant. The only choices of concern in ethics are those giving rise to significant good or bad in the world. Many choices we make in life are too remote from the sphere of good or bad to be of ethical concern. I might very carefully choose what shirt or blouse to wear today, but this choice does not ordinarily give rise to significant good or bad in the world, and so it is not an ethical choice. My choices of what to wear are not usually ethically significant, nor are my choices of dinner, of a new car, of computer software, of a TV program, and the like.

The recognition that ethical choices are concerned with significant good and bad features in life brings us to the second common theme in ethics—the effort to distinguish what is good and bad.

Ethics Is About Evaluation

Ethics inevitably employs determinations and judgments about values. In their simplest form, determinations and judgments about values are differentiations between the good and the bad. Every ethics tells us certain things are morally good and other things are morally bad, and encourages us to choose the good and avoid the bad.

Sometimes the differentiations between good and bad are clear and uncontroversial—nothing bad is involved in the choice of the good, and nothing truly good is involved in the choice of the bad. I take care of my children, for example, or I abuse them. Caring for my children is clearly and simply good; abusing them is clearly and simply bad. Again, I send money to a local charity, or I embezzle money from the local charity. In normal circumstances, contributing to a charity is simply good; stealing from it is simply bad.

Other ethically significant choices, however, are complex in the sense that they involve both good and bad. One and the same action brings about damage and suffering to myself or others, but also brings about some good. Euthanasia destroys a human life, but brings a quick and peaceful end for a suffering patient dying a slow and painful death. The complex ethical choices, those embracing both good and bad, are the actions and omissions that generate the great controversies in ethics.

Some ethicists distinguish two types of evaluation: "good or bad" and "right or wrong." They advocate evaluating actions as right or wrong and all other morally significant factors—persons, intentions, motives, character traits, consequences, and the like—as good or bad.

Although there is some merit to distinguishing evaluations of "good or bad" from "right or wrong," this is not the approach we will adopt in this text. One reason for not using two types of evaluations (good or bad and right or wrong) is that all ethical evaluations can be expressed in the basic terms of good or bad. Doing the right thing is always good, and doing the wrong thing is always bad.

More important, whenever we distinguish between actions and all other relevant moral aspects in ethics, an unfortunate tendency develops. The distinction inclines us to isolate moral actions from other morally important features such as feelings, character traits, and the impact of the actions on ourselves and others. The result is an ethics focused on actions considered by themselves and neglectful of the way feelings, intentions, habits, and personal character affect, and are affected by, our actions. As one important contemporary author, William Frankena, put it in two remarks he made in the opening pages of his widely read book entitled *Ethics*: (1) "We must not let our decision be affected by our emotions . . ." and (2) "the only question we need answer is whether what is proposed is right or wrong; not what will happen to us, what people will think of us, or how we feel about what has happened."

Frankena is typical of many contemporary ethicists—he distinguishes the evaluation of actions from the evaluations of other factors. He proposes two kinds of moral judgment: "judgments of moral obligation," which evaluate actions in terms of right and wrong according to principles, and "judgments of moral value," which evaluate motives, intentions, character traits, and consequences in terms of good or bad. He calls this a "double-aspect conception of morality."

Although Frankena proposed that we should regard the morality of principles and the morality of character traits and the other considerations as complementary, he insisted that the principles are the basic aspect of morality and the other considerations are secondary. The character traits, for example, are viewed as supporting the principles and are understood in light of them.

Frankena tells us that character traits support moral principles four ways. First, they support us in moments of trial when we are tempted to act contrary to the principles. Second, they sustain us when we have to determine what principle it is our duty to follow when two or more principles conflict. Third, they sustain us when we are trying to revise the working rules of actual duty. Fourth, they allow us to recognize excuses and extenuating circumstances when a person did not act according to the principles but at least tried to do the right thing. In other words, the character traits are considered important only when we need help to carry out the obligations indicated by the principles, or need to resolve conflicts between them, or need to revise rules derived from them, or need to excuse or understand others who have failed to follow the principles. The complementariness of the double-aspect morality is not a complementariness of equals; the principles are basic and the character traits play a supporting role.

As will become clear in the course of this chapter, the position developed in this book is contrary to that suggested by the two remarks of Frankena. Since virtue pertains to feelings, virtuous feelings will affect our decisions, and rightly so. Second, in an ethics of the good, the most important question in ethics is precisely what will happen to us if we do, or do not, behave in a certain manner. The only question we need answer in ethics is not whether our actions are right or wrong, but whether our actions, feelings, and character traits are making our lives good lives. Judgments about our actions in an ethics of the good are very much concerned with what happens to us. Actions are good when they help us live well, bad when they undermine our living well.

In an ethics of the good, the virtues and the prudential reasoning needed to establish them in each situation are basic, not the principles. Action-guiding principles enter the picture only when they are helpful, as they often are, in reinforcing the virtues.

Evaluating moral features as good or bad implies, of course, some standard of evaluation. Any ethicist making evaluative judgments about good and bad is employing a criterion or norm. Judgments presuppose standards, and this brings us to our next point—ethical norms.

Ethics Is Normative

Some authors make a distinction between descriptive ethics and normative ethics. This distinction is misleading if it implies that ethics is not normative; that is, if it implies that ethics is a description of what people believe is right or wrong and of how they reason morally. In the long tradition of moral philosophy and ethical theory, ethics has never meant this. Ethics was never understood simply as research into what people actually hold, or how they actually solve moral dilemmas. Ethics was always understood to be normative. It recognized that there were good beliefs, behaviors, and ways of reasoning morally, and that there were bad beliefs, behaviors, and ways of reasoning morally.

It would be better to call the important work done in descriptive ethics moral psychology or moral anthropology, because it is not ethics in the traditional sense. It is moral psychology and not ethics, for example, when the researchers interview people to find out how they reason morally or what their values are. A well-known example of moral psychology is the work of Lawrence Kohlberg and his colleagues, who developed first six, and then seven, stages of moral reasoning from their research on children as they grew into adults.

Another example is the work of Carol Gilligan, who pointed out imbalances in Kohlberg's analyses. Other examples of moral psychology or moral anthropology include programs of values clarification and studies of the moralities actually embraced by people of different racial, sexual, cultural, ethnic, and religious backgrounds. In health care, surveys of what nurses or physicians think is ethical regarding certain options—decisions about the withdrawal of feeding tubes, for example—fit into this category of moral psychology.

The key factor in descriptive ethics is that researchers discover, usually by extensive interviews, what people value or what people think is good or bad. The research is important and no good ethicist would want to be without it, but it is not really ethics in the traditional sense because the work is purely descriptive and empirical. Ethics in the traditional sense always included a normative component. Ethicists strove to determine not simply what people thought was good, but what was good; not simply what people did in fact value but what was truly valuable; not simply how people reasoned morally, but how best to reason morally.

The oldest ethical text we have, the stone tablet recording the code of Hammurabi (now preserved by the Louvre Museum in Paris), is not simply descriptive of what the Babylonians around 1800 B.C.E. thought was morally good or bad behavior; it is a normative code backed by the authority of the king. And Moses did not first interview his people around 1000 B.C.E. to find out what they thought was moral or immoral behavior; he introduced the commandments as God's laws and made them normative. And Aristotle did not accept what many people of his day (around 350 B.C.E.) thought was the way to live and act, but insisted there was a norm for judging the morality of our feelings, habits, and behaviors—and the norm was whether or not they contributed to our living well.

Ethics is not about someone's belief that "x" is good and that "y" is bad. Ethics begins when we ask someone *why* he thinks "x" is good and *why* he thinks "y" is bad. Ethics begins when we begin giving reasons why something is good or bad, and the appeal to the reasons why something is good or bad is an appeal to something normative.

When a person gives reasons why stealing is bad, she is appealing to norms. Perhaps she will say stealing is wrong because it violates God's law, or the natural law, or a person's natural right to his property, or the duty of justice as conceived by Kant, or the greatest happiness principle of Mill. If she is following the older tradition of ethics typified by Aristotle, she may say stealing is ultimately wrong because it threatens to undermine the thief's good life and happiness as both an individual and a social being by violating the virtue of justice, and the virtues are what we need to live well and happily.

Ethicists and moral philosophers disagree on what might serve as the normative basis of moral judgment, but they do not disagree on the need for something normative. The fact that a person believes something is right or wrong is not enough; the moral philosopher insists that those beliefs must be justified by something normative, and that the exploration of what is normative for our behavior is the work of ethics. Ethics is not simply about reality—the positions people actually hold as moral—but about norms, norms that enable us to say (to the extent that it can be said) what positions are morally good and what positions are morally bad.

This point about the normative component of ethics is important because some published work in professional journals associated with health care frequently refers to purely descriptive research into what people think is right or wrong as "ethics." Empirical research in ethics, however, is not ethics or moral philosophy in the traditional sense, unless it also evaluates the findings in terms of something morally normative, be that norm rights, principles, laws, rules, or human fulfillment and happiness. The important normative component in ethics introduces our next topic—reasoning.

Ethics Includes Reasoning

Faced with the challenges of life, we have to figure out what is truly good for ourselves and what is truly bad. The ethical wisdom embedded in our traditions is a rich source for discerning what is good or bad, but it is not enough. Sometimes moral traditions misguide us—our tradition found slavery morally acceptable for centuries but now condemns it. Sometimes, and this is especially true in health care, our moral traditions fail to guide us because our predecessors never experienced or even thought about what we face today.

When responding to the moral questions created by new techniques and technology—ventilators, artificial hearts, transplantation, cardiopulmonary resuscitation, medical feeding, and medically assisted reproductive interventions, for example—we are very much on our own because we are the first generation to encounter these situations. Following moral traditions, the moral responses given by previous generations, while important, simply will not do. Aristotle correctly identified what we do in ethics: "All people seek the good, not the way of their ancestors." This means we have to think and reason about what will achieve a good life, and not simply adopt the ready-made judgments of a moral tradition constituted by our predecessors.

Figuring out what is truly good or bad can be difficult for several reasons. First, some things seem good for us but really are not, and some things seem bad but really are good. The pint of ice cream in the freezer looks good to the overweight person with high cholesterol and heart disease but really is not, and fasting from food and fluids for many hours seems bad if we are hungry and thirsty, but it is really good for us if we are about to undergo surgery.

Second, good things are often mixed with bad things. Surgery often brings life-prolonging benefits, yet it also brings the burdens of risk, pain, and physical mutilation. When the good and bad are inextricably entwined, as they often are in health care situations, reasoning can only figure out how best to enhance one's good life and reduce what undermines it.

Third, our ability to figure out what is good and what is bad is always distorted to some extent by psychological and social biases beyond our control. Our view is always a point of view, the view of a particular person or persons, in a particular place, at a particular time, with a particular history, and in a particular social, cultural, and (perhaps) religious matrix. This means that the conclusions of our moral reasonings are never absolute but always relative in some degree to our historical and psychological perspectives.

It is also helpful to recognize that the reasoning we encounter in ethics appears on three different levels. The first and most immediate level is the *personal* level. Here I find myself faced with a situation where I must not only decide what is good, but actually do or be affected by what I decide. I am the moral agent. For example, I am of advanced years and declining health, and I need a lung biopsy. I have to decide whether or not it would be better for me to allow physicians to attempt cardiopulmonary resuscitation in the event of a cardiac or pulmonary arrest during the biopsy. As the result of my decision, a order not to attempt resuscitation will, or will not, be written for me.

Another example: I am a physician, and a patient suffering from AIDS has asked for medications I know he intends to use for suicide in the future.

I have to decide whether it will be better to write the prescription or to refuse a dying man what he considers a reasonable request.

Figuring out what I will actually decide in a particular situation where I am personally engaged is the kind of reasoning the earlier ethics of Aristotle and Aquinas (an ethics we will retrieve in this book) called *prudence*.

The second level of ethical reasoning is *judgmental*. Here I also find myself considering a particular situation and want to know what will achieve the good in the circumstances, but I am not actually going to do, or be significantly affected by, what I decide. I am not the moral agent. Making ethical judgments on this level is far less personal than practicing prudence because someone else is confronted with the ethical question. In the examples given above, I might be a friend of the person wrestling with the decision about cardiopulmonary resuscitation, or I might be a colleague helping the physician decide whether or not he should give the patient with acquired immune deficiency syndrome (AIDS) access to medications that will probably be used for suicide.

Some ethicists do not make a distinction between the *personal* reasoning of the person actually confronted with the ethical challenge and the *judgmental* reasoning of the person considering the case but not so engaged that she will carry out or be significantly impacted by whatever decision is made. They consider both the personal and judgmental levels of reasoning as instances of moral judgment about what should, or should not, be done. In a sense, this is true. There are important similarities between the personal reasoning about what is good or bad when I am faced with doing and being affected by what I decide and the moral judgments I make about what is good or bad for others to do.

Despite the similarities between these two levels of moral reasoning, however, there are reasons for noting the difference between them. The person faced with making a decision about something she will do or be affected by has an important existential perspective not shared by those judging behaviors they will not actually pursue. Her personal reasoning is a part of her life, her story, her future, and these existential and historical factors introduce an important context not shared by anyone else. She is not looking on as a judge; she is the principal involved in the case.

In the last analysis, the final moral decision rests with the moral agent faced with doing or being affected by what she decides, and her position is unique. This uniqueness is better preserved by distinguishing the personal and the judgmental levels of moral reasoning, a distinction reminiscent of that previously made in theological ethics between following one's conscience even when everyone else's ethical judgments might indicate one should do otherwise.

In this book, we will not really be operating on the personal level of ethical reasoning because you and I are not actually going to carry out, or be affected by, the evaluative decisions we make in the cases we study. When we study the cases we will be operating on the level of judgmental reasoning, not prudence or personal reasoning, just as we do when we try to help friends figure out what is good or bad, or when we review cases in ethics committee meetings at a hospital or nursing home, or when we make moral judgments about particular cases reported in the media, etc.

At the same time, since the personal and judgmental levels are similar, experience in reasoning on the judgmental level will ideally help us to make better personal decisions in our lives when we are actually faced with ethical challenges similar to those we study in this book. These challenges are challenges practically nobody can avoid. Most of us will be making morally significant health care decisions for ourselves and for others, most likely our parents, spouse, or children.

The third level of ethical reasoning is *theoretical*. Here we study carefully and critically what others have written and said about ethics, and we attempt to develop some sort of theoretical account that explains the nature of ethics. If I try to show that biomedical ethics is fundamentally a matter of obligations derived from principles and rules, or if I try to show that biomedical ethics is fundamentally not a matter of obligation but of following our natural inclination to achieve a good life, to live well, I am reasoning on the theoretical level. Also on the theoretical level are the attempts to develop an ethics based on divine law (as found in the Hebrew, Christian, or Islamic traditions) and the attempts to base an ethics on natural law, on natural rights, on the greatest happiness principle, and on the respect for persons principle obliging us to treat every person as an end and not merely as a means.

The theoretical study of the nature of ethics, its concepts, and its language is the work of ethicists—the moral philosophers and moral theologians. They try to explain what ethics is all about and to clarify the thoughts and language we use in our judgments and personal decisions. It is very important and very demanding work, requiring extensive study. There is a large body of important ethical literature stretching from Plato, Aristotle, the Stoics, and early Hebrew and Christian texts, through Cicero and Augustine, Aquinas, Spinoza, Locke, Hume, Kant, Hegel, Bentham, and Mill to the seminal authors of our own century. It all must be understood to some extent if one is to enter the conversation about ethics on the theoretical level.

Although the theoretical study of ethics—moral philosophy and moral theology—seems far removed from our personal ethical reasoning about what to do in a particular situation, it is not. Ethical theory does have an impact on our lives, although its role is often unnoticed until we undertake a serious and critical examination of our moral beliefs. Hence, the academic or theoretical work we do in ethics, no less than the cases we form judgments about, has the same practical goal as does our personal deliberation when we are confronted with a situation where we have to decide what to do. That goal is learning how to live well.

Since this book is not intended for the specialist, the emphasis is not on the theoretical level. Nonetheless, some theoretical background is necessary, and we will present some theoretical considerations in the early chapters of the book. Most of the time, however, we will work on the judgmental level of ethical reasoning. We will try to make our judgmental reasonings as close as possible to the personal reasoning of a moral agent actually engaged in an existential situation by looking at actual cases from the different perspectives of the patient, the proxy, the physicians, the nurses, the attorneys, the administrators, and the judges. In this way, the ethical analysis of each case will approximate the prudential reasoning each of us practices in life as we strive to live well. The work on the theoretical and judgmental levels will enrich our ability to discern and to do what actually will better achieve the good in our lives. All the work we do in ethics—even the theoretical work—has the same attractive goal: achieving personal happiness in our lives.

We turn next to a description of the two kinds of ethics we find in our cultural tradition.

TWO KINDS OF ETHICS

The major ethical theories in our cultural background fall into two general groups. The theories of the first group are related by the emphasis they place on moral obligation or duty. Behavior in accord with our moral obligation is considered morally right; behavior not in accord with our moral obligation is considered morally wrong. Underlying these theories is the assumption that people do not naturally tend and desire to live well. If this assumption is embraced, it makes sense to say that people must be obliged to live well and that the morality of behavior is a morality of duty.

Moralities of obligation are moralities of law, where law is understood as a system of precepts or rules people are obliged to follow. Moralities of law appear in different forms. Some rely on divine law, others on natural law, still others (Kant, for example) on the moral law we give to ourselves. Today the morality of law appears most frequently as an ethics based on principles, rules, and rights, where the principles, rules, and rights are understood as action-guides that we have a moral obligation or duty to observe and respect.

The theories of the second group are related by the emphasis they place on the good of the person performing the action. Behavior making our lives good is considered virtuous, and behavior making our lives bad is considered worthless and a vice. These theories of the good assume that most everyone naturally seeks to live well, and they make this desire for a good life the starting point of ethics. The key notion of modern ethics—obligation—is scarcely present in the theories of this group. It makes little sense to say people are obliged to seek what they already want. Instead of obligation, the key notion in an ethics of the good is virtue. Virtues are the feelings, habits, and behaviors that do in fact create a good life.

The two kinds of ethics, of course, are not totally unrelated. After all, an ethics encouraging people to live up to their obligations implies it is good for them to do so, and an ethics encouraging people to live well implies living up to their obligations. Yet the differences between an ethics of obligation and an ethics of the good are important, and they result in two significantly distinct approaches to ethics. An example from a seminal work that has influenced a number of American ethicists will reveal sharply the difference between an ethics rooted in obligation and duty and an ethics rooted in the good and virtue.

In an important book published in 1930 entitled *The Right and the Good*, W. D. Ross developed what was to become an influential position. First, as

Frankena was to do after him, he distinguished actions that are right from actions that are morally good: ". . .'right act' cannot mean the same as 'act that ought to be done and *also* the same as 'morally good act'." For Ross, it is clear that "'right' does not mean the same as 'morally good'" and that "moral goodness is quite distinct from and independent of rightness."

Once he made this distinction, Ross went a step further: he claimed ethics is primarily concerned with whether or not actions are right, not with whether or not they are morally good. He contrasted his position with that of another prominent philosopher, G. E. Moore. Moore had argued in his *Principia Ethica* (1903) that ethics attempts to answer two distinct questions: (1) What is good in itself (that is, what has intrinsic value) and (2) what kind of actions ought we to perform? Moore claimed that ethics is primarily concerned with what is intrinsically good and not with what actions we ought to perform; Ross held the reverse.

When we understand how Ross focused on the rightness and wrongness of actions and on what "ought" to be done (that is, on obligation), we will not be surprised by his subordination of the morally good to moral obligation and moral duties. We can see this most clearly at the end of his book, where he considered moral motivation. He wondered what motivation for actions would be morally best and offered two candidates: actions motivated by duty and actions motivated by love, one of the major virtues in an ethics of the good. The question was: which actions are morally superior, those done for duty or those done for love?

His conclusion was consistent with his preference for what is right over what is good: "(T)he desire to do one's duty is the morally best motive." He acknowledged that many will question this and argue that actions springing from love are morally superior to actions springing from duty, but he argued that they are wrong. When a genuine sense of duty conflicts with any other motive (even love), the sense of duty takes precedence. And if, Ross told us, both love and duty incline us to one and the same action, our action will be morally better if we act from the motivation of duty rather than the motivation of love: "(W)e are bound to think the man who acts from sense of duty the better man."

This kind of ethics suggests that parents caring for their children act in a morally superior way when they care for them because it is their duty rather than because they love them. It suggests that a partner in a marriage behaves in a morally superior way when he supports his wife because it is his duty rather than because he loves her. It means a physician or nurse acts in a morally superior way when his interaction with patients is motivated by the duties of the clinician–patient relationship rather than by the love of neighbor.

It is precisely this priority of duty over love that separates sharply the moralities of obligation from the moralities of the good. In the ethics of Aristotle and Aquinas retrieved in this text, love is the major virtue whereby we constitute and create our lives as good lives. Aristotle devoted more space to love in the *Nicomachean Ethics* than to any other virtue, and Aquinas made love the crowning virtue of his moral philosophy and theology. There is, then, a kind of fundamental option in health care ethics today—the option between an ethics based on obligation and duty, with its principles, rules, and rights that we must obey and respect, and an ethics based on living well, with its virtues that create a good life.

The ethics of obligation has appeared in many forms in our ethical tradition. We turn next to its major historical manifestations.

HISTORICAL VERSIONS OF THE ETHICS OF OBLIGATION

We can identify five major versions of theories based on obligation. The first two versions originated over 2000 years ago, the remaining three only in the past few centuries.

Divine Law Theories

These influential theories originated in the land known today as Iraq, but known in ancient times as Babylonia and Mesopotamia. Here a nomadic patriarch named Abraham was born and grew up about 4000 years ago. Consistent with the Semitic cultures in this area of Western Asia, Abraham and his people believed that God gives commandments to his people. God's law creates the moral obligations in our lives; human beings are obliged to follow the laws of their creator.

The divine law theories continue today in the Jewish, Christian, and Islamic religious traditions, for these are the three major world religions tracing their lineage to Abraham and his God. Most people in our culture became familiar with the divine law theory when they first heard of the "Ten Commandments," a set of laws Moses promulgated to his people about 3000 years ago. These commandments, along with hundreds of other divine laws, are preserved in the early books of the Hebrew Bible, which many Christians call the Old Testament.

Natural Law Theories

Plato is widely recognized for his efforts to develop an ethics based on metaphysical norms (that is, on other-worldly, transcendent, eternal, unchanging "Ideas" or normative "Forms") that the wise person must grasp in order to know what is good or bad behavior in the particular situations of this temporal and changing world. At the end of his life, however, after wrestling with numerous difficulties about the famous metaphysical Ideas or Forms, Plato began to speak of physical nature in a morally normative way. He began to argue that actions were virtuous if they were "according to nature" and not virtuous if they were "contrary to nature."

In his last work, *The Laws*, Plato had the "Athenian stranger" (undoubtedly Socrates) say that there is an "unwritten law" against incest recognized by everyone. The Athenian stranger then argues that legislators ought to mold public opinion in such a way that people will recognize that this unwritten law should be extended to all sexual behavior that is not "according to nature" (that is, all sexual behavior not appropriate for reproduction in marriage). Homosexuality, fornication, and masturbation were explicitly condemned by Plato, in addition to incest, as being not according to nature. Homosexuality also receives a stronger prohibition: it is not simply not according to nature—it is "contrary to nature," a transgression of nature.

While "according to nature" is not an exact equivalent of "according to natural law," Plato's use of the phrases "unwritten law," "according to nature," and "contrary to nature" are obviously normative. He believed that sexual actions not in accord with nature are immoral and should become the subject of legal prohibitions.

Early Greek Stoicism (a philosophy inaugurated by Zeno, who had studied at Plato's Academy in Athens, more than a half century after Plato's death) also stressed "according to nature" as morally normative. Following Plato, the Greek Stoics did not explicitly speak of natural law, but they did view nature as permeated by a rational order (*logos*), and then concluded that ethics is living and acting "according to rationally ordered nature."

The Stoic influence on ancient thought was immense. Stoicism played a dominant role in the moral thinking of the ancient world until late in the fourth century of the common era, when Christianity replaced it after the Roman emperor made Christianity the official religion of the vast Empire in southern Europe, northern Africa, and the Middle East. Many Stoic ideas continue anonymously in our culture to this day. Most ancient people, for example, believed with Job and Sophocles that bad things happen to good people without reason, and that tragedy can destroy a good life. The Stoics were popular because they assured people that this was not so, that "everything happens for the best" in a universe permeated by rational order.

According to some scholars, these two Stoic notions—the *logos* of nature and acting "according to nature"—were independently developed into "acting according to the natural law" by two important figures, Cicero of Rome and Philo of Alexandria. Both of these major figures may have been influenced by a common source, Antiochus of Ascalon (ca. 130–68 B.C.E.), whose doctrine represented a transformation of the early Stoic "according to nature" to an inchoate notion of "according to the law of nature."

Cicero studied in Greece and wrote extensively on Greek ethics in Latin during the last century before the common era. In his treatments of the Stoics, he sometimes freely translated the "*logos* of nature" as the "law of nature," and "according to nature" as "according to the law of nature." Greek philosophy had almost always distinguished nature and law, *physis* and *nomos* (Plato's remarks in *The Laws* are an exception to this), but Cicero tended to obliterate the distinction. He wrote in his *Laws*: "The highest reason (*logos* in Greek, *ratio* in Latin) implanted in nature is law, which commands what ought to be done, and forbids the opposite." (I,v,18)

Cicero put the moral law into nature and thus presided at the birth of natural law theories. With him, the transition from "according to nature" to "according to the law of nature" and "according to natural law" became reality. His ideas were later developed at length by Roman jurists looking for a theoretical foundation for civil law, by Christian canonists eager to provide a foundation for Church law, and by medieval theologians and philosophers in the developing universities of the twelfth and thirteenth centuries looking for a basis for ethics in reason to complement the biblical basis rooted in divine revelation.

Philo was of Jewish heritage and wrote from Egypt in the first century of the common era. His language was Greek, and his concept of the law of nature as a source of moral obligation may well have been the result of a desire to reconcile his Jewish tradition of living according to the Law of the Torah with the Stoic philosophy of living according to nature. Philo believed that the universal principles of morality, what he called the "archetypes," are derived from the law of nature and known by all, and that the laws formulated in the Torah are more specific statements of these universal principles. His writings influenced a considerable number of his contemporaries, both Jewish and Christian, who were more comfortable thinking and writing in Greek than in Hebrew or Latin.

The natural law concept introduced into Latin ethical thought by Cicero and into Greek ethical thought by Philo exerted a tremendous influence that persists to this day. There are many variations of natural law theory, but they all hold that actions contrary to the natural law are immoral. Natural law, for example, is often cited as a basis for considering homosexual behavior immoral, and Pope Paul VI cited the natural law as the basis for his condemnation of contraception in the 1968 encyclical *Humanae Vitae*.

In the past few centuries, many ethicists have moved away from the claim that our moral obligations arise either from divine law or from natural law. In place of these older theories, they have created several new approaches. The major ones are natural rights, utilitarianism, and a universal moral law we give to ourselves.

Natural Rights

Some ethicists, following political philosophies developed by Thomas Hobbes and John Locke, say our moral obligations come from individual rights possessed by all people. People are thought to have natural or human rights, chiefly the right to life, the right to choose, and the right to property, and our obligation is to respect these rights. These theories of obligation are called "rights-based" theories.

Rights-based theories of moral obligation explain the tendencies to justify ethical judgments on the basis of such rights as the right to die, the right to health care, the right to life, the right to choose, the right to refuse treatment, and so forth. If someone has a right to die, a rights-based theory obliges us to respect that right; if a fetus has a right to life, the theory obliges us to let the fetus live; if a woman has a right to choose abortion, the theory obliges us to let her have it; if a person has a right to health care, the theory obliges someone to provide it.

Utilitarianism

Some ethicists, following Jeremy Bentham and John Stuart Mill, say that our moral obligation arises from what will benefit the most people. We are obliged to act on behalf of the greatest happiness for the greatest number. These theories are called "utilitarian" because our obligation is to use whatever means are useful for achieving the greatest happiness. Although it is misleading to say simply that utilitarianism is a philosophy whereby the end, the greatest happiness for the greatest number, justifies the means, this caricature does help us to grasp in a preliminary way the basic dynamic of the moral theory.

Today, most utilitarian theories are rule utilitarianisms; that is, our moral obligation is to follow the rules that will result in the greatest happiness for the greatest number. For example, most utilitarians accept the rule stating that it is immoral to kill an innocent person intentionally. They argue that I am always obliged to follow this rule even though, at a particular time, intentionally killing an innocent person might actually result in greater good for a greater number than not killing him.

Autonomous Moral Law

By autonomous moral law we mean a moral law that comes neither from God nor from nature, but from ourselves. The Greek roots of "auto-nomous" are "self" and "law." Each ancient Greek city was autonomous (that is, it made its own laws), and this is why the cities were called city-states. In this moral theory of autonomy, we constitute the moral law for ourselves.

This may sound like pure subjectivism or even anarchy, but it is not. The originator of this powerful moral theory, the eighteenth-century German philosopher Immanuel Kant, insisted that any maxim that we propose as a moral law for ourselves must be universally desirable (that is, the maxim must condone the behavior that we would want everyone to do). Hence, if I find myself in a tight spot and need a lie to escape, I might consider giving myself a moral maxim that permits lying. But no moral maxim can condone lying because no reasonable person would want such a maxim to be universal (that is, to be a maxim that would apply always and everywhere).

And why not? Because a universal moral maxim permitting lying would make life impossible. Such a maxim would make it morally right for the bank to lie about the balance in my account, for the airline to lie about the destination of my flight, for the surgeon to lie about my need for surgery, and for the professor to lie about the quality of my work in the course.

Kant's theory is an example of a "deontological" theory of obligation. Deontological theories oblige us to avoid certain actions without exception. The proscribed actions are always immoral regardless of good intentions, of extenuating circumstances, or of the good consequences resulting from the action. The end never justifies the means. Deontological theories, then, are sharply distinguished from utilitarian theories, yet both are theories of obligation.

All these five theories share a common theme. They view ethics as primarily a matter of obligation. Something—perhaps God's law, perhaps the natural law, perhaps another's rights, perhaps the greatest happiness of the greatest number, perhaps the moral law we give to ourselves—requires us to behave a certain way regardless of whether we want to behave in that way. Morality is a matter of obligation, and obligation connotes doing something we have to do, but may not want to do.

MORAL REASONING AND THE THEORIES OF OBLIGATION

The moral reasoning associated with an ethics of obligation tends to manifest two major characteristics: it is both deductive and inductive. We could describe it as *deductive–inductive* reasoning. Although logically we can clearly distinguish deductive and inductive reasonings, in practice most deductive reasonings have an inductive phase and most inductive reasonings have a deductive phase. It is often said, for example, that ancient science was deductive and modern science is inductive. But this is a gross oversimplification. Aristotle's science was very much inductive, despite his description of science in the *Posterior Analytics* as syllogistic; and modern science is very much deductive once it establishes the hypotheses its experiments are designed to confirm or disprove.

In moral theories of obligation, we seldom find purely deductive or purely inductive reasoning. Some theories stress deduction but include induction; some stress induction but include deduction; and some advocate a dialectical balance between deduction and induction whereby the prima facie principles and duties will sometimes dictate a particular judgment and the particular judgments will sometimes modify, revise, or supplement the prima facie principles and duties.

The deductive component begins when we apply one of the general norms—a divine or natural law, or a human right, or an action-guiding moral principle—to a particular situation. By applying the law, right, or principle to the particular situation, we are able to make a moral judgment that reveals our moral obligation in the particular case.

For example, if we begin with a human right as a general norm—the right to life, for example—and apply it to a particular situation involving a feeding tube sustaining the life of a permanently unconscious patient, then we could easily judge that the withdrawal of the tube is unethical because it violates the patient's right to life. This moral judgment would then oblige us to continue the feeding tube.

The inductive component of the deductive–inductive reasoning is what gives rise to the general norms and allows us to modify them. It does this chiefly in two ways. First, from our inherited social practices and rules we can generate general norms and, if necessary, subsequently revise them. The general norms are then applied to future situations. Second, from the judgments we make in particular cases we can develop general principles and rules, then apply them (sometimes in a modified way) to future analogous cases as they occur. This latter form of induction is often called casuistry.

The deductive–inductive model of moral reasoning can be sketched as follows.

Moral theory (e.g., theories of divine law, natural law, rights, etc.)
↓
General norm (e.g., a natural right, or a principle, rule, or law)
↓
Particular case (e.g., whether or not we should treat this baby)
↓
Particular moral judgment (e.g., we are obliged to treat)

If the moral reasoning makes the theory and norms foundational, and then applies the norms to particular cases to determine what we are obliged to do, then it is primarily deductive and the morality is usually described as applied normative ethics. If the moral reasoning stresses the origin of the norms in particular judgments coalescing over time into a common shared morality giving rise to general rules obliging us in analogous cases, then it is primarily inductive and is sometimes called casuistry. If the moral reasoning moves with equal ease from the general norm to the particular and from the particular to the general norm, it is dialectical and sometimes called coherentist. "Coherentism" is a term describing the effort to develop a coherence between the general norms and the particular judgments by constantly adjusting each as experience develops. In practice, however, most coherentists tend toward the path staked out by Frankena; that is, the principles are basic.

The deductive reasoning in the deductive–inductive model is analogous to the reasoning we find in geometry. Certain geometrical axioms are given, and from them we can deduce certain truths about particular figures—circles, triangles, rectangles, etc. The axioms are true by definition, and if they are applied to a particular figure correctly through deductive reasoning, the conclusions about the particular figure will be true. Moralists disagree on where the analogues to the axioms—the principles or laws—come from. Some say they precede and transcend our experience, as in the theories of divine laws or Kantian moral law; others say they come from our cultural experience of a shared morality. Once established, however, they tend to operate deductively; the principles and laws are norms employed to determine what people are obliged to do.

Sometimes the geometrical flavor of contemporary moral theory emerges explicitly. John Rawls, in his landmark book entitled *A Theory of Justice*, wrote:

> The argument aims eventually to be strictly deductive . . . (C)learly arguments from such premises can be fully deductive, as theories in politics and economics attest. We should strive for a kind of moral geometry with all the rigor which this name connotes.

What follows are some extremely simplified examples of deductive moral reasoning in health care ethics using the rights-based and principles-based approach. When you look at these examples, set aside your opinions; that is, pay no attention to whether or not you agree with the conclusions. Focus instead on the structure of the reasonings. Notice how they employ a general principle or a right that everyone is believed to have, and then apply it to a particular situation in order to generate a conclusion. Remember also that we are leaving aside questions about where the general principles or rights originated; it makes no significant difference in these reasonings whether the principles or rights were derived from a transcendent or transcendental source such as divine law or Kant's pure reason, or from shared moral tradition, a common morality we inherited much as we inherit a language.

1. The general principle is that we must always do what will result in the greatest happiness for the greatest number;

   this withdrawal of life-sustaining treatment will bring the greatest happiness for the greatest number;

   therefore this withdrawal is morally justified.

2. The general principle is that we must always treat another person as an end and never merely as a means;

   this cesarean section is treating the woman merely as a means because its sole purpose is to let a resident practice the surgery;

   therefore this surgery is not morally justified.

3. The most fundamental right is the right to life;

   withdrawing nutrition and hydration will cause loss of life by starving the person to death;

   therefore withdrawing nutrition and hydration is not morally justified.

4. The most fundamental right is the right to choose;

   terminating my pregnancy is my choice;

   therefore terminating my pregnancy is morally justified.

5. The basic moral principle in medicine is beneficence—doing good to others;

   this surgery will be good for the patient;

   therefore this surgery is morally justified.

6. The basic moral principle in health care is patient autonomy or patient self-determination;

   this competent dying patient wants me to help him commit suicide;

   therefore assistance in his suicide is morally justified.

If we could deduce the morally right way to act in any particular case by the deductive–inductive model of reasoning, it would be very comforting. Once general rights and principles are accepted, a person faced with a particular dilemma simply gets the facts straight, recalls the established principles and rights, and then follows the rules of deductive reasoning to find the right answer. Only if more than one principle or right is in play or if the principle or right leads to a highly implausible particular judgment does the person have to engage in some creative and imaginative thinking to balance the conflicting principles or rights, or to revise one of them.

In an ethics of the good, the deductive–inductive kind of moral reasoning is not the primary way we reason. As we will see in chapter two, figuring out how to live well is a matter of prudential deliberation and judgment. Its model is not geometry but figuring out, while actually engaged in a goal-oriented process, how to achieve the goal.

CONTRASTING THE ETHICS OF OBLIGATION WITH AN ETHICS OF THE GOOD

The basic idea in an ethics of the good can be expressed in three relatively simple assumptions. First, it is taken as uncontroversial that people do not simply want life, but a good life; that people do not simply want to live, but to live well. Second, it is also taken as uncontroversial that achieving a good life, living well, depends to some extent on the choices we make in life. Finally, it is taken as uncontroversial that intelligent choices, choices that constitute rather than undermine living well, require thought and reasoning. Ethics clarifies the goal we all seek—a good life—and determines, to the extent it can be determined, the choices we need to make to achieve it. Clarifying what truly constitutes a good life and deliberating thoughtfully about how to achieve it in the actual and varied situations confronting us in life constitute the subject matter of ethics in an ethics of the good.

It is important to understand that the good life or living well is not something we should or ought to seek, but something we in fact do seek. A good life is something we all desire—the ultimate and underlying goal of every human being. Nobody in his right mind would strive to live a bad life, to live badly.

It is also important to understand that the good life I seek in this ethics is my own happiness and good. What I seek is my good, a good life for myself. Rightly understood, this is not, as we will see, selfishness. My good is inextricably interwoven with the good of others, especially those who are my family, friends, and members of my communities.

This ethics of the good, no less than the ethics of obligation, is a normative ethics. The norm is a good life, a life of fulfillment and flourishing. The feelings, habits, and behaviors that constitute living well are precisely the feelings, habits, and behaviors that are ethical; those that undermine living well are unethical.

In an ethics of the good, the reasoning is not an effort to deduce moral judgments from rights, principles, or rules. Rather, the person first acknowledges that the overarching goal of life is to live well, and then figures out what will achieve this goal. The feelings, habits, and actions contributing to a good life are called the virtues; those that undermine a good life are worthless and can be called the vices. The deliberation or practical reasoning called prudence does not lead to a moral judgment that I am obliged to obey whether I want to or not, but to a moral decision that I want to execute because the behavior will make my life good.

RETRIEVING THE ETHICS OF THE GOOD

The ethics of the good has not been fashionable for centuries. One reason why it fell out of favor was the difficulty in getting clear about just what constitutes a good life. In this section we need to give a brief account of what we mean by a good life, and also to explain why it is important to include a figure such as Aquinas in our retrieval of the ethics of the good from Aristotle.

In chapter six, we will develop the notion of what constitutes one of us; that is, a notion of what it means to be considered a member of the human population. We will suggest that the notion of "psychic body" is key for understanding when one of us exists. A human body becomes psychic when it becomes aware and a human body ceases to be psychic when it can no longer be aware. A fetal human body becomes one of us when it begins to feel; and a totally unconscious human body ceases to be one of us when it suffers irreversible loss of awareness or feeling.

If we consider each one of us a psychic body, then our question about what constitutes a good life is a question about what is good for a psychic human body. This is, after all, what each of us is, regardless of our age, race, gender, etc.

For purposes of analysis we can distinguish several major natural inclinations each one of us—each psychic body—possesses. Although it is somewhat arbitrary to separate the interwoven strands of any existing psychic body, three important sets of inclinations characterize human psychic bodies.

First, some inclinations are markedly biological in nature, and satisfying them contributes to a good life. Living well means we have adequate food, shelter, health, etc.

Second, some inclinations are markedly psychic in nature, and satisfying them contributes to a good life. Living well means we have satisfying emotional and cognitive lives, and the freedom or liberty to exercise some choice over how we live and what we do.

Third, some inclinations are markedly social in nature, and satisfying them contributes to a good life. Living well means we have healthy interpersonal relationships of love and friendship, contractual agreements with others rooted in justice, and relationships with the political community constituting the society in which we live. Human existence is always a coexistence, an existence with others, and this coexistence is sometimes interpersonal, sometimes contractual, and sometimes communitarian.

Each of us has inclinations to forge relations with loved ones and friends, to enter into agreements with others, and to live in just and peaceful communities that we help to build. The political community is not a social contract we establish for the protection of our individual rights; our very existence is fundamentally communal as well as personal. Building community is building a good life for ourselves because living in a well-ordered society working toward peace and justice contributes significantly to living a good life. Satisfying our inclinations for love, friendship, mutual agreements, and a decent society are very much a part of living well.

In recent decades, we are beginning to realize that our existence is a coexistence in yet another way. Our lives are interwoven with all life on this planet, and we live well when we treat all life well. We are beginning to recognize that the mistreatment of animals and of the environment is something that truly undermines our living well, and is thus something we had best avoid.

There are, of course, disagreements about what constitutes a good life, just as there are disagreements among all the various schools of moralities of obligation. The disagreements over what constitutes a truly good life for human beings in particular situations, however, should not blind us to the widespread agreement about many general features of a good human life. We know health is good; and sickness and suffering are bad. We know adequate nutrition is good, and malnutrition is bad. We know a life with love and friendship is good, and a life without love and friendship is bad. We know societies with checks and balances are better in the long run than societies governed by dictators. We know trials by jury are better than the medieval trials by ordeal. We know a life with adequate resources is good, and a life of poverty is bad. We know slavery is not good, nor torture, nor political or judicial corruption. We know education is good, illiteracy and ignorance are bad. We know war is terrible, and that it is good to make every effort to avoid it. We know reproducing and rearing children in stable and loving relationships is better than other alternatives. We know it is bad when people lie to us, steal from us, break their promises, attack us, and discriminate against us; and we know it is good when people are honest with us, respect our property, keep their promises, support us, and treat us fairly.

The shared view of what constitutes a good life manifests itself very clearly when we reflect on what we try to teach children, perhaps as parents, or as relatives, teachers, coaches, mentors, etc. By word and by example we try to show children how to live a good life, and a great consensus exists on what that good life is. We do not encourage them to lie, steal, or cheat. We do not teach them how to become promiscuous, destructive, or violent. We do try to teach them to be temperate, fair, kind, loving, caring, brave, concerned for others, generous, etc. Why do we teach them these virtues? Because we want them to live a good life, and we know living a good life is, in large measure, living virtuously.

The shared ethics of the good actually maintains its identity in a wide variety of different human lives. It is easily adaptable to different cultures and to different eras. The adaptation of Aristotle by Aquinas is an example of this. The two men lived in two different worlds—fourth century B.C.E. Greece and thirteenth century Europe. Yet Aquinas found Aristotle's ethics relevant and, almost 1600 years after it had been all but forgotten in Europe, Aquinas retrieved Aristotle's ethics of the good.

This is surprising and suggestive, given their very different worldviews. Aquinas believed in a God who created the world, conserves it in being, directs it in his providence, loves the people he created, and saves them from the clutches of evil and sin. Aristotle also spoke of God, and sometimes gods, but his god did not create the world, does not conserve it, does not direct it, does not love or even know people, and does not redeem or save anyone. Aristotle's God or gods are not deities in any religious sense. They neither know nor care about us, and all prayers to them will be unanswered because unheard. In short, Aquinas thought a deep religious faith augmented living well; Aristotle did not.

Moreover, Aquinas accepted the Hebrew Bible as the revealed word of God, a source of truth about the world as well as about God; Aristotle did not. Aquinas believed in a personal life after death, in the immortality of each personal soul destined one day to be rejoined with its resurrected body; Aristotle did not believe in any personal life after death, although his mentor Plato had so believed. Aquinas believed in heaven and hell, states of eternal beatitude and suffering where the good triumph and the bad are punished; Aristotle did not believe in any heaven or hell. Aquinas believed virginity was better than marriage, and lived as a religious friar; Aristotle believed that the virtue of temperance indicated a loving sexual relationship was better than the extremes of either promiscuity or virginity, and lived as a married man. Aquinas rejected all abortion and suicide; Aristotle accepted abortion and suicide in some situations. Aquinas supported the Inquisition and thought it was morally good to execute people with heretical ideas; Aristotle fled Athens at the end of his life in fear that he would be executed for his views, a fate that had befallen Socrates earlier in the century.

What is the significance of emphasizing the different worldviews of Aristotle and Aquinas despite their agreement on an ethic of the good? For one thing, it shows how their differences did not prevent a deep-seated agreement on what they thought constitutes living well; that is, on what constitutes living virtuously. Aquinas' development of prudence and the moral virtues is very Aristotelian; both men agreed that the goal of ethics is to guide us in living a good life, where living a good life is defined in terms of living virtuously. What the example of Aquinas and Aristotle shows is that an ethics of the good life can be shared despite great differences in worldviews.

It also presents something that might be relevant for us today. We live in a multicultural society. Some believe in God; others do not. Some are Christian or Jewish, others are not. Some believe in life after death where the good are rewarded and the bad punished; others do not. Some favor libertarian values that emphasize individual rights; others favor communitarian values that emphasize the common good. Some have ethnic and cultural roots in Europe; others in Africa; still others in Asia. What we need in health care is a common ethics that cuts across religious, political, ethnic, cultural, and social backgrounds, an ethics that respects different worldviews but also accommodates what we all share as human beings. Aquinas, despite the vast differences between his religious and cultural worldview and that of Aristotle, saw how Aristotle's ethics of the good had an appeal that transcends its original cultural matrix. This suggests that an ethics of the good might have important relevance in our multicultural society today.

There are, of course, differences between Aquinas and Aristotle—most notably Aquinas' religious faith—just as there were differences between Aristotle and other ancient Greek theories of the good life developed by the Platonists, Epicureans, and Stoics. These differences, however, should not blind us to the unifying factor these ethical theories of the good share: they are all ethics grounded on our natural desire to live well and based on the conviction that living and doing well is living and behaving virtuously.

This book will approach health care ethics from the perspective of an ethics of the good rather than an ethics of obligation. More specifically, it will rely on Aristotle's ethics of the good, an ethics receiving increasing attention by ethicists today. It will also draw on Aquinas' ethics of the good. This approach is somewhat different from the mainstream of current health care ethics. It is presented as an alternative to the more widely known principle-based and rights-based ethics of our culture. Even if you prefer those ethics of obligation and duty, it is still worthwhile knowing about the other major alternative in our cultural tradition—the ethics of the good.

BIOETHICS TODAY

Contemporary health care ethics is currently dominated by the various modern moralities of obligation. The idea that rights, especially the rights of patients, must be respected is very strong. Stronger still in current bioethics is the idea that both utilitarianism and Kantian deontology, different as these two theories are, somehow generate, or at least defend, a common set of normative principles and rules that we are obliged to follow in practice.

If you are at all familiar with the dominant vocabulary of American bioethics, you are undoubtedly aware that it is an ethics based on principles, most notably the principles of autonomy, beneficence, and justice. People involved in health care, especially physicians and nurses, are expected to apply these general principles to particular situations to determine what they are morally obliged to do. If the principles clash, as they often do, then they must be balanced against each other to determine which one obliges. In the minds of many, health care ethics is synonymous with making moral judgments by applying principles to particular cases.

In chapter fourteen, a chapter devoted to medical research, we will show how this philosophical approach, now called by some "principlism," received a major boost when Congress set up the National Commission for the Protection of Human Subjects in 1974. Congress asked the commission to identify basic ethical principles and to develop ethical guidelines derived from these principles that could be applied to biomedical and behavioral research. In 1978 this commission issued its final report, known as the *Belmont Report*, in which it dutifully identified three basic principles: autonomy, beneficence, and justice. It described a basic ethical principle as a "general judgment that serves as a basic justification for particular prescriptions and evaluations of human actions."

The theoretical background of basing ethics on principles that oblige, however, was established decades before the national commission. It goes back to several prominent moral philosophers who developed the ethics of duty, first elaborated in its modern form by Kant in the eighteenth century, to a high degree. One such influential philosopher was William Ross, whom we have already mentioned. A brief consideration of ethics of obligation, which has influenced several prominent American bioethicists, will help us to understand something of the background of the national commission and of American bioethics.

Unlike Kant, who had proposed that some duties deriving from his single basic principle of morality were so strict that no exceptions could be tolerated, Ross suggested a cluster of prima facie duties. For Ross, the term "prima facie duty" referred to the characteristic of the kinds of action that we would be obliged to perform if the action in the particular case would not be in conflict with another prima facie duty. For example, the prima facie duty of fidelity requires me to keep my promises, but if I had promised to take my son for ice cream at three o'clock and he breaks his arm at two-thirty, then the prima facie duty of beneficence (taking him for medical treatment) overrides the prima facie duty of fidelity that obliges me to keep my promises.

Ross named six basic prima facie duties: beneficence, justice, not injuring others, self-improvement, gratitude, reparation, and fidelity. Today, Ross's prima facie duties, and the exercise of balancing or weighing them when they are in conflict, have reappeared in American bioethics as prima facie principles, most notably the prima facie principles of autonomy, beneficence, nonmaleficence, and justice.

These principles are taken as prima facie binding. This means that they are normative principles and it is our duty to abide by them. However, and this is what makes them prima facie, whenever they conflict we have to balance them against each other to determine which one prevails and becomes our actual obligation in the particular situation. Hence, although these principles are normative (that is, more than rules of thumb), they are not absolute because they can be overruled by other principles and they can be modified and revised in the course of time and experience.

Most of the textbooks on health care ethics published in the last two decades—the books designed to help medical and nursing students learn about health care ethics—have relied chiefly on a handful of basic principles as the basis for moral judgment. The ethics of principles is an ethics of obligation; it is never far from the idea that ethics is about our duties and not about the natural desire to live well.

Despite some similarities, then, an ethics of the good is not ultimately compatible with an ethics of obligation. An ethics of the good assumes that ethics is primarily about our natural inclination to seek what is good for ourselves, and that we can figure out what is ethical by a practical reasoning called prudence, whereas an ethics of obligation assumes that ethics is primarily about our obligations and duties, and that we can figure out what is ethical by a process of deductive–inductive reasoning based on general principles.

Put briefly, an ethics of the good understands morality primarily in terms of what I do to myself, not what I do to others. Its chief concern is with moral agents and their lives, not with actions or their consequences. Its primary evaluation is whether the life I am living is good or bad, not whether my actions are right or wrong according to action-guiding norms such as laws, principles, rules, rights, or duties. An ethics of the good is intensely personal—its primary commitment is taking care of my moral life and well-being. The modern ethics of obligation is more impersonal—its primary commitment is taking care of everybody impartially and equally. In such an ethics, my welfare counts no more, and no less, than the welfare of each and every other person.

We do have to make a fundamental choice, then, between the two approaches. In this text, the choice is to adopt the ethics of the good. Seeking what is good for ourselves is not a matter of obligation, but of natural inclination. Rights, principles, and rules can find a place in an ethics of the good— sometimes it is good for a person to respect another's right or to apply a principle—but these general norms are secondary. They are helpful only to the extent that they help us to achieve a good life for ourselves.

The next chapter will develop the ethics of prudence and the good that we will use in this book.

SUGGESTED READINGS

Two good introductions to the history of ethics are Lawrence Becker and Charlotte Becker, eds., 1992. *A History of Western Ethics*. New York: Garland; and Robert Cavalier, James Gouinlock, and James Sterba, eds. 1989. *Ethics in the History of Western Philosophy*. New York: St. Martin's. The first volume contains selections from the *Encyclopedia of Ethics*, also published by Garland in 1992. For a history of Christian moral theology, see John Mahoney. 1987. *The Making of Moral Theology: A Study of the Roman Catholic Tradition*. Oxford: Oxford University Press.

For William Frankena's influential position, see his 1963. *Ethics*. Englewood Cliffs: Prentice-Hall. The two remarks cited in the text are found on page 2, and his remarks about the basic role of principles in his "double-aspect conception of morality" are found on pages 53–54. For W. D. (William David) Ross's views, see 1988. *The Right and the Good*. Indianapolis: Hackett, pp. 1–11 and 165–66. The quote from John Rawls is from 1971. *A Theory of Justice*. Cambridge: Harvard University Press, p. 121.

For a clear description of the difference between the modern and classical approaches to ethics, see Richard Taylor. 1988. "Ancient Wisdom and Modern Folly," in *Midwest Studies in Philosophy*, vol. 13, *Ethical Theory: Character and Virtue*, ed. Peter A. French, Theodore E. Eehling, and Howard K. Wettstein. Notre Dame: University of Notre Dame Press, pp. 54–63; and Robert Louden. 1992. *Morality and Moral Theory: A Reappraisal and Reaffirmation*. New York: Oxford University Press, especially chapters 1–5.

Plato's view on what is not "according to nature" can be found in his Laws 636C-D, and 838D–839D. For Stoic ethics, see A. A. Long and D. N. Sedley, eds. 1987. *The Hellenistic Philosophers*, vol. 1, *Translation of the Principle Sources with Philosophical Commentary*. Cambridge: Cambridge University Press, sections 56–67.

Examples of typical and thoughtful approaches to developing a health care ethics based on principles include Tom Beauchamp and James Childress. 1994. *Principles of Biomedical Ethics*, fourth ed. New York: Oxford University Press; Thomas Mappes and Jane Zembatty. 1991. *Biomedical Ethics*, third ed. New York: McGraw-Hill; and Ronald Munson. 1992. *Intervention and Reflection: Basic Issues in Medical Ethics*, fourth ed. Belmont, CA: Wadsworth Publishing Company. An interesting theological approach to health care ethics based on principles is developed by Benedict Ashley and Kevin O'Rourke. 1989. *Healthcare Ethics*, third ed. St. Louis: Catholic Health Association. The authors advocate a formal procedure they call "prudential personalism," which bases ethical decisions on a system of fourteen ethical principles derived from a Catholic value system "contained in the Christian Gospel, interpreted by the Church in its life of faith and authoritatively formulated by the Pope and bishops" (p. *xv*).

2

Prudence and Living A Good Life

In this chapter we will examine more fully the major elements in the ethics of the good developed by Aristotle in the fourth century B.C.E. and retrieved by Aquinas in the thirteenth century. We will consider the first principle of this ethics, then its notions of happiness and the virtues, and finally the reasoning it employs—prudence.

THE FIRST PRINCIPLE OF ETHICS: PEOPLE SEEK THEIR GOOD

In the ethics of obligation, the word principle means an action-guide either derived from a moral theory or generalized from widely accepted judgments in a shared moral tradition. Earlier theories of obligation—Kant and Mill are examples—had posited one supreme action-guiding principle, but today most advocates of an ethics of obligation posit a cluster of normative principles and duties that we are obliged to follow. In health care ethics, the most familiar central principles or duties are autonomy, beneficence, and justice.

The first principle in an ethics of the good is not understood this way. It is not an action-guide derived from a moral theory nor generalized from moral judgments widely accepted in a moral tradition. The first principle in an ethics of the good describes the reality of human life that gives rise to ethics in the first place. It is the starting point of the ethics, where it all begins. In an ethics of the good that starting point, that first principle, is simply the goal we all naturally seek—to live well, to live a good life, to achieve fulfillment, to flourish, to be happy while we live. Ethics is grounded on our natural inclination to seek what is good for ourselves. The natural inclination to live well—the natural desire for a good life—is the starting point or first principle of morality.

An ethics of the good begins simply by stating that the good life is what we all desire. It makes no attempt to prove this because there is no way to prove it. We cannot give any reasons for saying each of us strives for what is good for ourselves. We cannot justify or validate this claim because it is the foundation for every justification and validation in morality. It is the self-evident first principle in ethics, and we cannot give reasons for first principles in ethics any more than we can give reasons for first principles in theoretical knowledge.

First principles in philosophy are so called because they really do come first. All efforts to give reasons presuppose the first principles, and therefore the first principles cannot themselves be established by reasons. If we attempted to give reasons for a first principle, we would be presupposing the very thing—the first principle—that we are trying to establish. First principles are a necessary condition for reasoning, and we cannot coherently establish the necessary condition for reasoning by reasoning. The first principle of any reasoning is always logically prior to the reasoning because we cannot reason without it. This is why we cannot give any reasons for (that is, "prove") the existence of any truly first principle in philosophy.

Aristotle was the first philosopher to develop the idea of first principles in both theoretical reasoning (his sciences of nature, mathematics, and theology) and the practical reasoning used in ethics. He insisted that the first principle in theoretical reasoning is the principle of noncontradiction: we cannot think and say that something both is and is not at the same time. We cannot think and say that something is, at this moment, both a circle and not a circle (that is, that something is a "square circle"). So impressed were medieval theologians with the scope and power of this Aristotelian first principle that they acknowledged it taught them something about God: God is all powerful, but God still cannot make a square circle.

All theoretical reasonings depend on the principle of noncontradiction. Without it, our thoughts and language become gibberish, nonsense. Since we cannot prove this principle, it must be self-evident. It is self-evident in this sense: we readily see that if we do not accept it, our language becomes meaningless because contradictory statements could be simultaneously true. Without the principle of noncontradiction, for example, we could claim that two plus two is both four and not four, or that something can both be a circle and not a circle (that is, something could be a square circle).

Moral reasoning also has its first principle, and it is this: people naturally seek their good. We strive for a good life, to live well, to be happy. We cannot give reasons for this principle, but we can say that without it, no authentic ethical reasoning is possible. Just as theoretical reasoning cannot unfold unless we accept its first principle, the principle of noncontradiction, so ethical reasoning cannot unfold unless we accept its first principle, the principle that we naturally seek a good life.

If we ignore the principle of the personal good in ethical reasoning, the result is moral disaster because, without the principle of personal good, we have no reason for being ethical. If ethics is a matter of obligation, and if one of its principles obliges me to do something that is not good for me, then there is no reason why I or any reasonable person would do it. No reasonable person will deliberately do what is not truly good for herself. Accepting the first principle in an ethics of the good means being ethical is always in my self-interest. It provides the one convincing reason why I want to behave morally, even when it is difficult—living morally is what makes my life a good life and brings me happiness.

The personal good, flourishing, fulfillment each of us seeks in life was called happiness by the Greek moralists. The time has come to take a closer look at this important concept.

HAPPINESS

The Greeks had a name for living well; that is, living the good life. They called it *eudaimonia*. The word has no exact equivalent in English but happiness, rightly understood, is the most adequate translation. The good life is a life of happiness. A person lives happily when he flourishes as a human being. The first Greek dictionary, composed over 2000 years ago, defined happiness as living well and doing well. A happy, flourishing life is an intrinsically rewarding life, a life of fulfillment.

What Happiness Is Not

First, we do not equate happiness with feelings of pleasure and the absence of pain. Pleasure may well accompany happiness but this is not necessary and, as is well known, pleasure can mislead us about what is truly good and thus undermine our happiness. And the presence of pain, although unpleasant, does not necessarily indicate that we are doing something bad.

The identification of happiness with feeling pleasure and avoiding pain has a long history going back at least to Epicurus (342?–270 B.C.E.) and his famous cloistered garden outside the walls of Athens. In modern times Thomas Hobbes and Jeremy Bentham, both important political philosophers, were leading proponents of reviving this notion. But feelings of pleasure cannot be equated with happiness understood as what is truly good for ourselves, because pleasure often distracts us and sometimes leads us toward what is not truly good.

Second, we do not equate happiness with the satisfaction of whatever desires a person happens to have. Happiness is not getting what we want but achieving a good life. Sometimes a particular thing we want is not good for us, and getting it will not bring us happiness despite our thinking that it will.

Third, we do not equate happiness with whatever a particular person believes it to be. A person might believe happiness is living promiscuously, and so live this way, but his belief that he is happy does not provide the happiness of which we speak because such a life is not truly good for human beings. The word happiness designates what is truly good for a person, not what the person believes is good or brings happiness. In an ethics of happiness, the simple fact that someone declares he is happy is not enough for us to say he has achieved happiness; it must also be shown that he has achieved what will truly bring happiness—that is, a good life. It is always possible for people to think that they are living fulfilling lives when in fact they are not. People afflicted with Down's syndrome, for example, often seem more happy and content in life than many other people, but no Greek moralist would have said such a life was a good life, something any rational person would deliberately seek.

Happiness and Selfishness

Making personal happiness the starting point and goal of ethics could easily suggest something close to narcissism, egoism, individualism, or a crass "looking out for number one," but it should not. Any understanding of personal happiness implying selfishness is incompatible with a credible morality.

Sensitivity to this threat of egoism or selfishness is at least partly the reason why many modern moral philosophers and theologians have proposed something other than personal happiness as the foundation of ethics—perhaps rights, or principles, or an altruistic Christian life of self-sacrifice. These modern theories are so influential that many people have forgotten the blunt appeal to personal happiness in earlier philosophical and religious ethics.

While the ethics of Aristotle is typical and perhaps the best known ancient morality grounded on personal happiness, his understanding of ethics was not unique in the earlier centuries. Just about every philosopher and religious leader proposed personal happiness as the goal of morality. Consider but two examples, one from Plato (427?–347) and one from the Christian scriptures (ca. 60–ca. 100).

In the beginning of Plato's *The Republic*, a man named Thrasymachus insists there is no good reason for being ethical or just. "The just man is always a loser, my naive Socrates. He always loses out to the unjust" (343D). Socrates disagrees, and insists that the just and ethical person is a winner. He tells the mythical story of Er, a good man killed in battle. On the twelfth day he rose from the dead and reported what he had witnessed in the life after death: evil people were being punished tenfold and good people were being rewarded tenfold. Socrates drew the obvious conclusion—the wise person will choose the ethical life, "for this is how a man will find his greatest happiness" (619B). If we live justly "we shall be friends to the gods and to ourselves both in this life and when we go to claim our rewards, like the victors in the games go forth to gather their prizes" (621C–D). Socrates' point is clear: ethical living is what achieves the best for ourselves—our greatest happiness.

The Christian tradition also insists that living morally is in our best interest. It never tires of reminding us that bad people "will go away to eternal punishment, and the virtuous to eternal life" (Mt 25:46). Christ's teachings were demanding, and his followers often wondered what was in it for them. Sometimes they spoke in blunt terms: "What about us?" he (Peter) said to him. "We have left everything and followed you. What are we to have then?" The response was equally blunt: Jesus told Peter he will "be repaid a hundred times over, and also inherit eternal life" (Mt 19:27–29; cf. Lk 18:28–30). It is undoubtedly difficult for a man to give up home, land, and loved ones to follow Jesus, but he has the assurance that the loss will be balanced by compensation a hundred times greater in this life and then, after death, by eternal life as well. Christian living is constantly presented in the Christian scriptures as the way to gain great happiness for yourself both before and after death.

Socrates willingly gave up his life for the sake of what he saw as the good, and Peter left all to follow Jesus and was eventually killed for his choice. These actions are complex. On the one hand they represent the ultimate self-sacrifice, the greatest act of altruism a human being can make—sacrificing one's life for a good and noble cause. On the other hand, Socrates and Peter performed these actions of great sacrifice convinced that they will in the end gain ten or a hundred times more than they gave up.

The dynamic is clear: invest now, profit later; sow now, reap later; give up a lot, gain much more. Socrates and Peter sacrificed much, but the sacrifices were investments in a far greater happiness. Does this make them selfish and narcissistic? Not according to the ancient philosophical and religious traditions. In these traditions, paradoxical as it seems to us today, living rightly is in our self-interest because it results in the greatest possible personal happiness, yet this self-interest is neither narcissistic nor selfish.

It is well to remember that most people who existed before the past few modern centuries did not have as individualized a notion of each person as we do today. People did not think of themselves as isolated individuals joining together in some sort of social contract to protect their individual rights and freedoms. It was Descartes, the father of modern philosophy, who said in the seventeenth century, "I think, therefore I am"; most people before him said, "I belong to a community, therefore I am." Personal human existence was always a social human existence, an existence intricately integrated with the existence of others in personal and political relationships.

Some philosophers of the twentieth century have tried to recapture this older notion of social existence, and to redress the excessive individualism of modern philosophies and liberal political theories stressing individual rights. Our existence, they tell us, is never singular but always a coexistence. Being human is not the same as being a rock or any other thing. Take away all the rocks in a pile but one, and that remaining rock is every bit the rock it was before the others were removed. Take away all the people in a community but one, and that remaining person is no longer the human being she was before the others were removed. Since human existence is a coexistence, if the existences of others are undermined, so is mine. Human being is social being; my being is a being-with-others.

Once we understand ourselves not as discrete atomic entities related to others by some kind of social contract we decide to embrace but as existentially interconnected with others in the very being we call human being, then the tendency to understand an ethics advocating personal fulfillment and happiness as selfishness is derailed. If my life is always a life-with-others, then my happiness and flourishing is always entwined with the happiness and flourishing of others. If my existence is a coexistence, then it is impossible for me to flourish at the expense of others. Treating them unjustly or insensitively undermines my good as well as their good.

Understood in the framework of its origination, where human beings were thought of as essentially social beings, an ethics of personal happiness is anything but an ethics of selfishness. The happiness of any human being is the happiness of a social being, not of a discrete individual. This is why, for Aristotle, the study of ethics—how I go about making moral decisions— is only a phase in a larger study, a study he called politics.

This can be difficult for the modern mind to understand because the modern approach (whether influenced by the liberal political philosophies extolling individual rights and liberty but neglecting community or by the more conservative political philosophies extolling family and communitarian values but neglecting the important modern values of liberty and self-determination) assumes the dichotomy of self and others, of individual and community, and then opts for one over the other. But it is anachronistic to place the ethics of personal happiness developed by Aquinas or Aristotle in the modern conceptual framework that dichotomizes the individual and her societies, and then to criticize it.

The familiar dichotomies of egoism and altruism and of self and community were, in the forms we experience them, unknown to earlier moralists. They never hesitated to claim that acting for the sake of virtue was acting in our own best interest. Nor did they hesitate to claim that acting for the good of others was also acting in our own best interest. They simply assumed that human beings are political beings, that human existence is always a coexistence with others in communities.

Hence an ethics of the good retrieved from Aristotle and Aquinas is not an ethics of the liberal self striving primarily for his happiness, nor is it an ethics of the communitarian self striving primarily for the common good; it is both. Living well has both individual and communal dimensions. Speaking of my good is also speaking of the common good; speaking of my happiness is also speaking of the happiness of others; speaking of my flourishing is also speaking of the flourishing of my communities.

Happiness Is a Collective Term

We have said that the happiness we speak of in ethics is not simply pleasure, nor is it the satisfaction of whatever desire we happen to have, nor is it whatever we happen to think it is, nor is it anything selfish. What, then, is this personal happiness? What can we say about it?

We can begin by saying happiness in ethics is a collective term describing the right balance and coordination of all the important goods in a person's life. That is why it was described by Aristotle as the "complete" good.

An analogy may help us to understand how a collective term is used. A rope is composed of, let us say, a thousand strands twisted together. The rope is not something added to the strands. We do not have a thousand and one things—the thousand strands and one rope—but the strands constitute the rope. In a similar way, our happiness is not some additional good that comes as the result of achieving other good things in life. It is, rather, the life we call good because it combines successfully all the important elements and strands that constitute the human good. Happiness is not the reward gained after a life has been lived well, but the good life itself.

Aristotle thought human life, and therefore happiness, ended at death, whereas Plato and the Christians thought the life of the soul continued after death and would enjoy additional happiness or unhappiness, depending on the life lived on earth. Regardless of these differences about life after death, however, both traditions understood happiness in a collective sense. Happiness was considered the fulfillment of life and the greatest possible satisfaction of every human yearning for the truly good.

The good things in our lives come from two sources: luck and choice. Under luck we include any good thing we receive apart from our own effort. Some people prefer to speak of "blessings" instead of luck. By luck or blessings we may have inherited good health or happen to live in peaceful times with an abundance of friends and wealth, for example. Good luck and many blessings will certainly contribute to our personal happiness, but they are not the crucial factors. Luck will not by itself bring us the personal happiness envisioned in ethics, and its absence will not preclude this happiness. Something else is much more important.

The more important source of personal happiness is our ability to choose intelligently our actions and reactions in the various situations arising in our lives. We exercise significant, albeit not total, control over what we feel and how we behave, and the choices we make are the primary constituents of our personal happiness or misery. The chosen feelings and actions that enhance our happiness are called virtues, and the chosen feelings and actions that sabotage our happiness are called vices.

The virtues are the feelings, habits, and behaviors in life that constitute our happiness. We achieve our goal—personal happiness or a good life—by being virtuous. An ancient work attributed to Aristotle, the *Magna Moralia*, put it succinctly: "Being happy and happiness consists in living well, and living well consists in living in accord with the virtues."

Seeking happiness is complicated by the fact that good things in life often conflict. We see this in our examples of Socrates who gave up one good, his life, for another good, his integrity, and of Peter who gave up home, family, and eventually his life for what he saw as another good—following Christ. The conflict between good things can take different forms. Sometimes a moral good conflicts with other goods that are not moral. Here the right course of action is clear—the moral good has priority.

Sometimes, however, moral goods themselves conflict. A person with political power must exercise it with justice and fairness, but this can conflict with the love and kindness he feels for his family and friends who need jobs and contracts. The conflicts between goods are the most troublesome dilemmas in ethics, and they abound in health care. It is good to keep people alive, but it is also good to remove feeding tubes from irreversibly unconscious people because the intervention provides no benefit they can experience.

Happiness and Tragedy

Being ethical does not absolutely guarantee happiness in this life. The claim is more modest: living ethically provides the greatest chance of happiness in life. Happiness in life always remains limited by the human condition and by luck. Living and behaving morally will achieve the greatest happiness allowed by the circumstances. It can be undermined by bad luck, the misfortune of living in terrible times or of becoming the victim of violence, illness, deception, etc.

A serious challenge to the idea that living virtuously constitutes happiness comes from all too frequent examples of good people whose lives are haunted by tragedy. Bad things do happen to good people. The tradition knows two general responses to this challenge, depending on what the moralist believes about personal survival after biological death. Aristotle did not believe in life after death, as we have seen, and thus his happiness is a vulnerable happiness always dependent to some extent on luck. It is "fragile," as one moral philosopher puts it, so fragile that in extreme situations happiness may not be possible at all. Aristotle admitted that we cannot say that the virtuous person being tortured is happy. Yet Aristotle firmly held to the conviction that virtuous living offers the greatest chance at the greatest happiness possible in life.

A second response assumes a belief in a personal life after death. This allows a more secure idea of happiness, since the vision of the next life can be so designed as to preclude the destruction of the virtuous person's happiness by tragedy. Socrates and Plato believed in this stronger version of happiness, as we saw in the references from *The Republic* to the tenfold reward awaiting the good in a life after death. Christian philosophers and theologians also embrace this stronger version of happiness. They see the life after death as an eternal life with God that will permanently satisfy every human aspiration and bring perfect happiness to those who have lived well.

There is no way to resolve this difference of opinion about happiness—whether it can occur only in this life and can be undermined by bad luck or whether it can also occur in a life after death where all bad luck can be neutralized. Each person is left with a fundamental option here. One will opt for the view of Aristotle, which was also the view of Abraham, Moses, and Job; another will opt for the view of Socrates, Plato, and the Christians.

For our purposes, it makes no difference which option is embraced, for both are compatible with the ethics we develop in this book. Aquinas has shown us the way here. His ethics is very much a revival of Aristotle's approach, yet he embraced the Christian belief in life after death. The lack of consensus about whether happiness is confined to this life or extends beyond death does not undermine the central thesis in this ethics of the good: ethics is about our personal happiness, what it is, and how we achieve it.

There is, however, one very important, and generally ignored, question facing those believing with Aristotle that this life is all there is. Sometimes people find themselves in a situation where nothing they can choose will result in happiness. None of the options will promote a good life; no chance for any significant happiness exists. If happiness is the goal of life and the criterion for what is ethical and unethical, what happens when nothing the person can do will promote her happiness? If she believes in life after death, of course, there is no problem because the impossibility of happiness in this life is not final; happiness is always possible in the life after death.

But Aristotle did not believe in life after death. What, then, can be said about an ethics of seeking our good when none of the available choices promote a good life? Does the ethics of the good go on a holiday when this tragic situation arises? Suppose, for example, a person is dying of widespread and painful cancer. Realistically, these are his choices: (1) he may choose to remain alert as long as possible, and thus experience great pain; (2) he may choose heavy pain medication, and thus spend his last days so drugged he loses all meaningful contact with reality; or (3) he may choose euthanasia, and thus give up his life. None of these options leads to happiness. Living in pain or in a drugged state is not living a good life, nor is euthanasia, for that ends life. What, then, could an ethics of the good and personal happiness offer in tragic situations when achieving a good life and happiness are no longer possible?

The answer to this question in Aristotle and Aquinas is important. In tragic situations where no choice will lead to happiness, an ethics of the good acknowledges an important corollary: when we can no longer achieve a good life, the best we can do is avoid what is contrary to a good life. In other words, when none of our choices will promote our happiness, when all options are undesirable and unwanted, then we are reduced to choosing the less worse. The ethical aim of our life is to live well and be happy; if living well and happiness are not possible, then all we can do is reduce the bad features in the situation as far as possible. Not choosing the less worse is immoral because it undermines an ethics of the good by promoting more bad than is necessary.

The ethics of the good, then, is understood this way: behavior is moral when we choose what promotes living well or, in tragic situations where living well is no longer possible, when we choose the less worse. Thus Aristotle, in his discussion of battlefield courage, argued that in some situations a soldier has but two choices, and neither promotes his living well. He can stand, fight, and be killed or he can desert his post and become a coward. Neither choice brings happiness; there is no happiness in being killed or in living as a deserter and a coward. The soldier is caught in a tragic situation and can only choose the less worse. Aristotle argued that fighting unto death will, in most circumstances, be less worse than fleeing, and hence deserves to be recognized as a virtue, the virtue of courage.

In the rare and tragic situations when living well is not an option, when the only choices are the choices promoting a life no one would desire, all the good person can do is choose the less bad. The first principle of an ethics of the good, then, was fully stated by Aquinas as: "Happiness or living well is to be sought and promoted, and the bad is to be avoided." Virtuous action is action done for the sake of living well and happily or, when happiness is no longer a realistic option, for the sake of avoiding as far as possible whatever undermines living well and happiness.

The full statement of the first principle of an ethics of the good is especially important for ethics dealing with areas of human life haunted by tragic situations where no available option can really be considered a contribution to the agent's happiness. Military ethics focuses on one such area, health care ethics focuses on another. Sometimes in health care ethics no option available to a patient, proxy, physician, or nurse promotes to any significant degree what Aristotle called happiness.

The hypothetical example of the dying cancer patient is an example of such a case. Nothing he can choose will bring him happiness, but he behaves morally by choosing the least bad option. His moral reasoning might well unfold as follows. Retaining alertness despite the pain may at first be less worse than masking the pain but losing awareness. Then, if the pain intensifies, the reverse may be true, and masking the pain despite the loss of awareness may be less worse than retaining awareness with the pain. At this stage, he then has two choices: live his last days without pain but heavily drugged, or ask his physician to kill him. It is at least arguable, as we will see in the chapter on euthanasia, that medicating patients even to the point of unawareness if necessary is a less worse way of controlling suffering than killing them, even if they ask to be killed.

Happiness and Moral Obligation

It is important to remember that any ethics of the good also contains an ethics of obligation in two ways. First, there is a sense in which we can say that, given the natural inclination to seek happiness in life, then we ought to seek happiness; that is, we ought to seek a fulfilled and flourishing life, a good life. The language of "ought" is a language of obligation. In an ethics of the good, however, the "ought" denotes obligation in a weak sense because happiness is what each of us already desires anyway.

Second, an ethics of the good may well include laws, principles, and rights. In fact, whenever promulgating laws, principles, and rights will help us to live a good life, they are reasonable. Proponents of an ethics of the good can agree with Kant that a moral law requiring us to keep our promises is helpful in most situations; with Bentham that our social welfare programs should do the most good for the greatest number; and with Locke that people have rights to life, liberty, and property. And we can agree with the prevailing principles of American bioethics that capture important values: patient self-determination, beneficence, and justice are very important considerations, and behaving in accord with them preserves the human good in most cases.

The important point, however, is that human well-being or flourishing is the foundation for what is good, not the laws, principles, and rights. What constitutes a good life determines what the laws, principles, and rights will be and when they will be relevant; the laws, principles, and rights do not determine what we have to do to live a good life.

VIRTUE

A key notion in any ethics of the good is virtue. Virtue meant "excellence" in ancient Greek, and the word was used for both living and nonliving things. A machine can be excellent, or a horse, or a human being. Something is excellent when it is well-formed *and* performs well. A machine is excellent if it is well-made and works well; a horse is excellent if it is well-formed and functions well. A flutist is excellent if she is an outstanding flutist and actually plays exceptionally well. A flutist is not excellent if she has mastered the instrument but does not play, nor is she excellent if she has not mastered the instrument but happens to play well in a particular concert. In the *Iliad*, Homer called a soldier excellent only when the man was a courageous fighter and actually did fight courageously. A courageous soldier who does not fight is not excellent, nor is a cowardly soldier who fights courageously only when stimulated by the wine he drank out of fear.

From these examples we can see that excellence is related to a goal. If a thing is so formed and so functions that the goal is achieved, then it is an excellent thing. If the machine, the horse, and the flutist are so formed and so function as to achieve the goals appropriate to the machine, horses, and flutists, we call them and their performances excellent. The goal is the norm for excellence. Only when we know what the machine, horse, and flutist are expected to accomplish can we judge whether their structures and functions are excellent.

As we have explained, the goal of any human life considered as a whole is personal happiness. We say "considered as a whole" because it is not the subsidiary goals that concern us here. These are many and worthwhile, and include, for example, graduation from school, making a good living, developing loving relationships, having a family, being a good clinician, etc. But in ethics it is the overall goal of every human life that concerns us, and this, as we saw in the last section, is personal happiness.

We can now define an excellent or virtuous human being as a person so formed and so functioning as to achieve personal happiness. Simply put, whenever our habits, feelings, and behavior are in fact achieving personal happiness, we call them excellent or virtuous. The virtues are those human qualities that promote personal happiness. Virtues are the feelings, habits, and behaviors constitutive of living well.

The virtuous human qualities, according to Aristotle and Aquinas, are of two kinds: moral and intellectual. The moral virtues pertain to what we choose, and the intellectual virtues pertain to how we think and reason. When we speak of *human* excellence we are mostly concerned with our uniquely human characteristics: our abilities to choose and to reason.

Moral Virtues

Moral virtues are the feelings, habits, and behaviors best suited to achieve personal happiness. The moral virtues pertain to our feelings, to our habits (our character, what kind of person we are), and to our behavior (the actions we choose to do or not to do). The four major moral virtues in Greek ethics are justice, courage, temperance, and love. An excellent person will be a person who (1) *is* habitually just, courageous, temperate, and loving; (2) has just, courageous, temperate, and loving *feelings*; and (3) *behaves* justly, courageously, temperately, and lovingly.

There is no definitive list of the virtues. The four moral virtues just mentioned appear in some form on just about every list and may be considered an invariable core. Considerable variation occurs among different authors, and sometimes within works of the same author, regarding other virtues. Aristotle's works, for example, clearly show the indefinite and open-ended nature of any list of virtues. In book I of his *Rhetoric* he lists seven moral virtues: justice, courage, temperance, magnificence, magnanimity, generosity, and gentleness. The virtue of love is noticeably absent here, but he does define and discuss it at some length in book II of the same work.

The *Eudemian Ethics* includes all the moral virtues of the *Rhetoric* and adds love, respect for self and others, righteous indignation, truthfulness, dignity, and patience.

The *Nicomachean Ethics* has an indefinite list of moral virtues. It includes courage, temperance, generosity, magnificence, magnanimity, truthfulness, wit, gentleness, justice, love, and a few additional virtues for which, Aristotle says, there are no names.

The lack of a definitive list of moral virtues is not a problem in a virtue ethics because the virtues are not going to function the way principles do in an ethics of deductive reasoning. Virtues are not a stock of axioms that we apply to particular situations. They are simply the ways of being and doing that are integral to living a good life (that is, a life in which personal happiness is achieved).

The moral virtues have their beginnings in both nature and nurture. We are not born with them, but we do have a natural disposition or aptitude for them. This natural disposition to virtue is reinforced by parents and by other institutions, especially those that are educational and religious. We begin our road to virtue by being habituated into the moral customs of our families and societies. Only with this moral education in our younger years can we hope to develop prudence and the moral virtues later in life.

Our natural dispositions and cultural habituations become truly moral virtues when we go a step beyond the formation we received in our youth and begin to deliberate personally about what we might do to live well. Once we begin to choose our behavior—choose to be kind, just, loving, courageous, and so forth—we are behaving morally and becoming virtuous.

Then these chosen actions of kindness, justice, love, and courage gradually build up our moral character so we actually become kind, just, loving, and courageous human beings. And the stronger our habitual moral character, the more easily and often we can perform the virtuous actions. A reciprocal dynamic thus occurs whereby our virtuous character and virtuous behavior ever more strongly reinforce each other. And the converse is also unfortunately true. The more we act unjustly, the more we tend to become unjust; and the more unjust we become, the more we tend to act unjustly.

When we speak of virtue, then, we are speaking of habits, feelings, and behavior. We are speaking of who we are and what we feel and do. The morality of happiness is a morality of virtue in that the virtuous feelings, habits, and behavior are what constitute living happily.

An ethics of the good focuses much more on personal feelings and character than do the modern deontological and utilitarian theories, with their focus on deriving moral judgments about particular actions from normative principles or rights. Yet a virtue morality does not confine itself to moral habits and character. It is also a morality of action because the virtuous habits forming the person's moral character are built up by the repetition of virtuous actions. As virtuous actions are repeatedly performed, they become spontaneous and habitual. Hence, in any given situation, it is important to act justly, kindly, patiently, courageously, lovingly, etc., for these actions will strengthen our moral character and help us achieve the overriding goal of life, which is to live well (that is, happily).

Intellectual Virtues

Two intellectual virtues play a major role in Aristotle's philosophy: prudence and wisdom. Prudence is the intellectual virtue needed in ethics, and we will treat it at some length in the next section. Here we will briefly consider wisdom for two reasons. First, we want to contrast prudence with wisdom and, second, we want to show that most modern theories of ethics rely more on what Aristotle called wisdom—the virtue he thought was largely irrelevant to ethics—than on the practical reasoning known as prudence.

Wisdom

What Aristotle called wisdom begins by grasping principles and then argues deductively from them to a conclusion. It is very similar to the reasoning many high school students use in plane geometry, where certain axioms are given with a figure and the student must then find the area or length of a line or the degrees of an angle. Wisdom embraces both the intellectual intuition by which we grasp the axioms and the deductive reasoning (which Aristotle called science) by which we proceed from these principles to reach a true conclusion about the object of our investigation.

Wisdom is the intellectual virtue most suited to the realities we discover around us and for which we are not responsible. According to Aristotle, these realities include three sets of things: the natural phenomena we observe, the numbers and operations of mathematics, and the imperceptible realities such as minds and other beings (including gods) that we do not observe but can nonetheless know. The study of these three sets of beings was called philosophy or wisdom.

The important thing to remember about wisdom so understood is that it does not refer to human action deliberately chosen. It does not refer to what we make or to what we do. It is knowledge about the realities we find around us, and about the categories our minds tell us are needed to explain the changing things around us.

Wisdom is called theoretical because it is the kind of knowledge typical of spectators, not participants. In Greek, the word theory was used to describe the role enjoyed by the invited delegations from neighboring city-states at the athletic contests and games. The visitors did not play in the games; they watched. The theoretician is a spectator, not a player. She looks at what she studies; she does not make it. On the other hand, the person seeking to live a good life is not a spectator, but a player. His knowledge is not theoretical, but practical. He is not primarily concerned with what already is, but with what can be as the result of his choices.

Ethics is not watching; it is playing. It is not theoretical but practical reasoning. Ethics is not about demonstrating truths, but about choosing what we should actually do to enhance our personal happiness in a unique situation with all its particular circumstances and relationships.

Although wisdom or theoretical knowledge, with its deductive approach from axioms and principles and its insistence that all contradictions be removed, is not appropriate to ethics according to Aristotle, this type of thinking, as we noted earlier, has been widely accepted in ethics for a long time. In its most popular form, it consists in setting forth a few rights or principles and then using these rights or principles, and rules derived from them, to justify moral judgments and actions in particular situations.

Prudence

This brings us to the intellectual virtue central to ethics—prudence. Prudence is practical reasoning, the kind of knowledge we need for directing a military operation as it unfolds, for practicing medicine, for playing a flute, or for living our lives. When we are doing things, we are not spectators, and the knowledge we need is not theoretical but practical.

Theoretical knowledge is suited to realities that already exist; practical knowledge is needed for what does not yet exist but can exist if we so choose. Practical reasoning is figuring out what will work. The practical knowledge we need to figure out how to live our lives to achieve personal happiness is prudence.

Figuring out what will truly make our lives good is the major moral task we all face in life. Prudence is the term we will use for this reasoning and, in the next section of this chapter, we will explain more fully what we mean by it. The explanation is derived from the descriptions of prudence we find in Aristotle and Aquinas. Although most modern ethics, both philosophical and religious, neglect or even dismiss prudence, the classical thinkers made it central to their ethics. We will, therefore, consider it in some detail.

PRUDENCE

We have already noted how Aristotle differentiated prudence from wisdom and science in the *Nicomachean Ethics*. The sciences, the study of what is fixed beyond my control, are of little help when I am dealing with what I control by my choices. When I make choices in life, I am not a spectator but a participant, and hence the theoretical knowledge of what Aristotle called science is of limited value. I need ways of knowing that are appropriate for participants. Figuring out what to do to promote living well, to the extent that living well can be achieved, is what Aristotle called *phronesis*.

Following Cicero, the medieval philosophers and theologians translated *phronesis* into Latin by the word *prudentia*. Aquinas' treatment of *prudentia*, for example, captured well Aristotle's special ethical meaning of *phronesis*.

For many reasons that we cannot go into here, later modern European languages lost the ability to express the rich notion of *phronesis* and *prudentia* that we find in the ethics of Aristotle and Aquinas. The words *prudence* in English and French, and *Klugheit* in German, simply do not convey what *phronesis* and *prudentia* meant in the older ethics. In fact, the "prudent" person today is often not the morally noble person characterized by the *phronesis* and *prudentia* of the earlier ethics, but an overly careful person bent on avoiding difficulties in his life. Such "prudence," however, may in fact be unethical. In health care, for example, some physicians, possibly influenced by legal counsel, think it prudent to avoid any behavior that might result in litigation. They never see that such "prudence" could be highly immoral in some circumstances—when it leads to medically unnecessary tests, for example.

Modern authors discussing Aristotle's *phronesis* and Aquinas' *prudentia* therefore shy away from using the misleading English word "prudence." They employ instead phrases such as "practical wisdom," "practical reason," "practical rationality," "moral insight," "intelligence," and "nonscientific deliberation."

There are good reasons for using these phrases, but there are also drawbacks. One drawback is the confusion caused by the use of different English words to translate one Greek or one Latin word with a very definite meaning in ethics. Another is the fact that, in his *Ethics*, Aristotle takes great care to show that *phronesis* is not associated with wisdom, and thus the frequent translation of *phronesis* by "practical wisdom" is misleading. Moreover, Greek has common words for "practical" and "wisdom" (*pratike* and *sophia*), and this suggests that we should translate *phronesis* by another English word.

Despite the problems associated with the word "prudence" in English, we will use the word to translate what Aristotle called *phronesis* and Aquinas called *prudentia*. The complex and rich meaning these authors gave prudence will hopefully emerge in what follows. Prudence or prudential reasoning is, quite simply, how we figure out what choices are most likely conducive to our goal in any given situation. In ethics, prudence is the deliberation we use to determine what will give us the best chance to achieve happiness (that is, to determine what is ethical or morally good). It tells us what to do in order to achieve a good life.

What Prudence Is Not

We begin by saying what prudence is not. It is not, as we explained earlier, a moral judgment deduced from general norms such as principles, rules, or rights. Prudence never reasons this way. It is much more imaginative, narrative, and creative.

This does not mean, however, that any of the conclusions deduced from principles and rules are necessarily wrong or incompatible with those of prudence. In many cases, the conclusions deduced from the ethics of principles and rights are compatible with those generated by an ethics of prudence. But the contrast we are making here between prudential reasoning and principle-based reasoning centers not on conclusions but on the process of arriving at conclusions.

Prudence does not make general principles or rights central, and then proceed by deductive logic to a particular judgment. Recognizing this may leave some people uncomfortable because the logical certitude available with deductive reasoning is not available. Prudence simply does not provide us with the logical comfort we expect in deductive geometry, or in science, or with religious dogma. An ethics of prudence accepts this discomfort and, with Aristotle and Aquinas, acknowledges that, in matters of concrete human behavior, our knowledge is, at best, valid "only for the most part."

Morality is simply not science. Galileo and Newton taught us how to measure physical bodies and how to predict a high tide or an eclipse or a sunrise a thousand years from now, but no historian or psychologist or sociologist or ethicist can measure human choice and predict future human action with such precision. What should make us uneasy in ethics is not that we do not have the certitude we think we have in modern science or thought we had in ancient metaphysics and theology, but that so many people think we have, or should have, such certitude in the field of deliberate and free human conduct.

This does not mean prudence is some form of guessing or little more than a matter of personal beliefs and opinions. We can certainly guess or sincerely believe or have a strong opinion that something is good or bad, and our guess, belief, or opinion might well be correct, but this is not prudence. The judgments of prudence are always supported by reasons. Feelings play an important role, as we shall see, but they do not replace the need for reasons. What we always have to show in an ethics of prudence is why we think something will indeed contribute to what is truly good. This is why, in the second part of this book where we consider concrete ethical issues, we will always insist on reasons to support the ethical judgments we suggest. And the reasons are valid when they show that an action or omission truly contributes to living well.

Adopting an ethics of the good employing prudence as the reasoning that directs our conduct means that we can never say a behavior is morally good or morally bad "because I believe it with all my heart" or "because that is the way I was brought up" or "because this is what civil or religious authorities say." Prudence, the intellectual virtue at the heart of morality, always supports its judgments with reasons why the behavior in question will, or will not, actually contribute to my human good. Aristotle and Aquinas always insisted that acting prudently is, in the last analysis, acting not according to mere beliefs, nor according to how I was brought up, nor according to the dictates of authority, but "according to right reason."

Finally, we should not confuse prudence with a purely instrumental kind of reasoning, a reasoning concerned exclusively with the means needed to achieve a goal and not with the goal itself. In instrumental reasoning, the end and the means are distinguished. Vacationing in the Caribbean is one thing, buying the ticket weeks ahead of time is quite another. The distinction between ends and means in instrumental reasoning becomes very clear when we have a good end and a bad means—we desire money, so we steal it.

In prudence there is no sharp distinction between means and end. The behavior is not simply the means to happiness but happiness itself. The end, happiness, is embedded in the means. Happiness is not distinct from the virtuous activity that achieves it; happiness *is* living virtuously. Prudence is therefore a reasoning about the end as well as about the means. Prudence grasps the complete good of human life as well as the means to achieve it. We totally misunderstand Aristotle and Aquinas if we think their ethics is an instrumental reasoning where "the end justifies any means." In every case, prudence must grasp the end—living well—and show how the means will promote it.

What Prudence Is

Prudence is the deliberation and reasoning in any particular situation that determines what feelings and behaviors will truly promote my good or at least avoid the worse bad. But how does prudence determine what behavior is virtuous and reasonable? How do I decide what behavior makes my life a good life?

Outside of tragic situations, and excluding situations where what I am contemplating is clearly contrary to a good life by definition (murder, for example), Aristotle suggests prudence begins by recognizing that a good life is enhanced by striking a balance between feelings and behaviors that are neither excessive nor deficient.

Some behaviors, for example, contribute in a significant way to the biological aspects of the human good. The primary examples are eating, drinking, exercise, and sex. But if we eat too much or too little, we undermine living well. Just how much and what to eat will vary from person to person, and from circumstance to circumstance, and prudence is needed to figure out how much we should eat in any given situation. I know too much is not good for me, and obviously too little is not good. I also know circumstances play a role—I should not eat anything before major surgery. So I cannot simply say eating is good for me.

What is good for me is eating reasonably, that is, eating well or virtuously. Eating is reasonable when, given the circumstances, it is neither too much nor too little for me. The knowledge I need to figure out how much I should eat is primarily practical, not scientific, and it is circumstantial. This example of practical knowledge in the matter of eating—which Aristotle and Aquinas considered a matter of the moral virtue known as temperance—gives us a preliminary idea of how prudence works. Prudence, recognizing that good behavior is undermined by excess or by defect, endeavors to determine just where on the spectrum between those extremes the behavior promoting my good will fall in the particular circumstances facing me at any given time.

Some situations, for example, call for courage. Courage falls somewhere between behaving cowardly and behaving rashly. Just where it falls depends on the circumstances and my capabilities. In some circumstances the courageous thing is remaining silent or retreating. In other circumstances the courageous thing is speaking out boldly or attacking forcefully. Prudence in matters where courage is an issue is knowing what to do, when to do it, and how to do it.

Consider this: I arrive home and find my house almost fully involved in fire. If I rush in, at considerable risk, to save the turtle I bought this morning for one dollar, I am not acting reasonably. The behavior is not courageous, but rash and foolish. But if I rush in, despite the risk, to save my baby, then it would be appropriate to say I am acting courageously. This is especially so if other factors are present. Perhaps I am an experienced off-duty firefighter and realize, thanks to my training, that the rescue attempt cannot wait for help to arrive and that I can make the rescue now, even without proper equipment.

Courage is somewhere between cowardice and rashness. My prudential reasoning will determine just how to avoid these extremes, given what is at stake, the circumstances, and my abilities.

Prudence not only determines what achieves my good, it is also decisive. It directs me to behave a certain way. This is what distinguishes prudence from what we called judgment. The process of reasoning in prudence and in judgment are similar but, unlike judgment, prudence directs the person doing the reasoning to do, or not to do, something.

The actual practice of prudential reasoning can be difficult at first. There is no clear methodology similar to the deductive method of deducing particular moral judgments from ethical principles. Indeed, some think method is the enemy of the prudential reasoning needed in ethics.

Fortunately, the person practicing prudence in any moral situation does not start from scratch. Before trying to determine what is right in a particular case, she has the benefit of three things. First, every person has a preliminary natural orientation toward a good life. Living things, including human beings, strive not only to live, but to live well. Second, she has received some moral education from parents, from schools, from society, and frequently from religious organizations. This moral education provides a preliminary apprehension of how to go about living a good life. Third, if she is reasonably mature, she has complemented her natural orientation and moral education toward a good life with a personal awareness that living well is the overall goal of life.

When the practitioner of prudence is faced with a challenging concrete situation, these three background features have already provided a preliminary orientation. Now she must determine what behavior will achieve her personal happiness in the situation. Prudence will provide the answer, to the extent it can be provided, so we must examine its features more closely.

The Features of Prudence

Aquinas lists eight features of prudence and three additional secondary virtues associated with it. His list is a compilation of features drawn mostly from Aristotle, but from others as well. It is not intended to be exhaustive. It is a convenient way to organize the chief characteristics of prudence, as long as we do not mistake the list for any kind of highly organized methodology or for any kind of sequence such as we find in manuals telling us how to operate equipment or build something. Prudence is not like that. It is a way of thinking that cannot be considered a science, or a craft, or a technique, but only as the unique and somewhat disorganized process that it is.

The list that follows is, therefore, not to be taken as steps of a method to be followed every time we make a moral decision. It is simply a compilation of features embedded in prudence and largely unnoticed by the prudent person in the process of exercising prudence. Only in an analytical reflection on prudential activity does the list emerge. Not every feature on the list is of equal importance. Some features are rather obvious and simple, others will require some explanation. And some features are debatable. With these remarks in mind, we will take up the eight features of prudence and the three secondary intellectual virtues associated with it.

Memory
We learn from experience, sometimes the hard way, what contributes to our fulfillment and what does not. What happened to us in the past can serve as plausible grounds or "quasiarguments," as Aquinas calls them, for figuring out what we should do in the present.

Understanding
This term requires some comment for a correct appreciation of its meaning. "Apprehension" might be a better translation of the Greek *nous* and the Latin *intellectus* but, since "understanding" is so often used, we will retain it. We will have to be careful, however, how we understand this "understanding." It is a highly technical term with a precise meaning for Aristotle and Aquinas. It refers to the ability to know something directly (that is, without a reasoning process). Aquinas says things known this way are "known *per se*." They are self-evident and obvious. They need no proof, no arguments, no reasons. Aristotle and Aquinas thought this understanding of the self-evident was the way we came to know two kinds of things: (1) the first principles of both

theoretical and practical knowledge and (2) the moral issues in the concrete situations we face in the course of a life.

We have already seen how this understanding of the self-evident grasps the first principle in the practical reasoning of ethics. But in ethics there is a second area where we have to rely on this direct apprehension called understanding—the grasping of moral issues in each concrete situation in life. In some ways, the situation confronting me here and now resembles other situations I have experienced or know others have experienced, but in other ways each situation is unique because it has new ethical features never before encountered by me or anyone else. These new features in the particular situation are just as much a starting point for prudence as is the first principle of the good we seek.

Memory of past situations is of little help here; we need a way to apprehend directly the moral issues in the new situation. The component of prudence called understanding is how we do this. It grasps directly the particular situation with its salient moral features. The situation we experience is something known *per se*; it is a self-evident given. Prudential reasoning thus begins with two starting points grasped by understanding: the first principle (people seek their good) and the moral nuances embedded in the unique particular situation facing me.

Learning from the prudent

In *The Republic* Plato advanced a famous theory: our communities should be run by philosopher-kings who master philosophy and ethics, and then direct the moral lives of the citizens. The philosopher-kings were the ethical experts. In some religious traditions a similar theory exists: the community should be run by theologian-authorities who master theology and ethics, and then direct the moral lives of the believers.

Aristotle and Aquinas proposed a fundamental revision to this model. They still embraced the idea that a special group provided moral direction, but membership in the group is not confined to philosopher-kings or theologian-authorities. Rather, the group is composed of experienced people who have actually achieved a high degree of moral success in their personal lives. The group comprises people who are in fact prudent, or were prudent when they were alive. They are the people who actually live, or did live, good lives. These people are the ethically successful people; we recognize them as noble human beings.

Aristotle called these people the *"phronimoi,"* the people who had mastered *"phronesis;"* Aquinas called them the "experts," the "elders," and the "prudent." We have all met these people in life. They are the people we recognize as being of high moral integrity; they are good, decent, and noble people. Some are rich, but many are poor; some are powerful, but many are weak or even exploited. Some are political or religious leaders, but many are not. We trust and admire these people of high moral integrity, and both Aristotle and Aquinas insisted we should learn from them.

And how do they teach us? Not in a scientific or theoretical way, and not by statements backed by whatever authority they might have. They do not give us principles, rules, laws, and regulations to follow. Nor are the particular behaviors they chose in their lives necessarily the model for what we should choose in our lives. We do not simply imitate their lives and do what they did. Rather, we learn from their ability to deliberate prudently. In the different situations of their lives they were able to figure out the behavior constitutive of a good life. They did this by prudence. So we want to learn from their example, from how they practiced prudence and went about perceiving the right thing to do in their lives.

These good and noble people do not tell me what behavior is right in my situation; they teach me how to perceive the moral dimensions in particular situations and how to figure out what behavior is best suited to achieve happiness. The prudent people serving as role models do not dictate what is the right thing to do; they offer advice and show us how to figure out for ourselves what is the right thing for us. They serve as examples. We want to study how they made virtuous choices in their concrete situations so we can make them in our own.

Shrewdness

This is the ability to grasp very quickly what is the right thing to do. The shrewd person has the ability to hit the mark, to get right to the point, to cut through all the irrelevant factors and see, while on the spot, what is really necessary to achieve the end. Shrewdness quickly grasps what we should start doing now, in this situation, to achieve our goal—a good life.

Reasoning

Reasoning consists in showing how certain feelings and behavior will truly achieve my good in the particular situation. My reasons will, or should, show how the behavior is better suited to my good than the other options available in the circumstances. And if my action causes bad things to happen to me or to others, then I must produce convincing reasons for the bad I cause.

Consideration of consequences

We can call this foresight. Aquinas calls it "providence" because it is a foreseeing or seeing-ahead. We know our actions have consequences and so we look to these consequences and try to discern how they fit into our personal happiness. Prudence acknowledges that we must always consider the consequences of our actions and whether they will bring good things or bad things for ourselves and others.

Consideration of circumstances

Prudence is about individual actions in particular situations, and hence many circumstantial factors are involved. Some of the circumstances are morally significant and should be a part of prudential consideration. Circumstances can sometimes make all the difference in the world. Something considered good in one situation might not be good in other circumstances. Thus, to use Aquinas' example, it is good to treat another person kindly—unless she happens to be a suspicious and cynical person, for then the kindness may very well make her more suspicious, and eventually disturb and upset her.

The ethical person not only does the good thing but does it in the right way and at the right time. Virtue is living well and doing well, and this depends, in large measure, on circumstances. We have to look at all the circumstances to make a good moral decision because the virtuous mean always depends on the circumstances in which the moral agent finds herself.

The major circumstantial factors affecting morality are well known in Greek, Roman, and medieval ethics. They revolve around who is performing the action, what kind of action it is, where it is being done, by what means it is being done, why it is being done, how it is being done, and when it is being done. Cicero and the medieval moralists often summarized these factors as follows: "who, what, where, by what means, why, how, when." Except for the "what," which refers to the action itself, and the "why," which refers to intention and purpose, all these factors are circumstances.

Caution

Moral situations are often not clear-cut. The good is often mixed with the bad. Therefore, we have to be very careful as we make our way through the jungle of moral dilemmas. Caution rules out any kind of dogmatic or fundamentalist approach in ethics. Prudence always tiptoes along, for it recognizes the complexity and contradictory nature of many situations, and knows that no simple answer is possible in difficult and complex cases.

Listing these eight factors characterizing the intellectual virtue of prudence helps us to understand the virtue better. Prudence is a complex intellectual virtue embracing memory, understanding the first principle and concrete situations, learning from the truly prudent, shrewdness, reasoning ability, the consideration both of consequences and of circumstances, and an element of caution.

The Virtues Allied to Prudence

Closely allied to the virtue of prudence are three additional virtues: deliberation, comprehending judgment (*synesis*), and considerate judgment (*gnome*).

Deliberation. Obviously, the prudent person must be able to deliberate well. This means going through a process of searching, and imagining, and thinking through, and calculating what behavior will best achieve the truly good. The prudent person normally does this by talking out the pros and cons to herself and with others. The process is reminiscent of the dialogues Socrates had with others and, as we know from his oration at his trial in the Athenian court, with himself. Deliberation is the ability to gain knowledge by looking at the different sides of an issue in a kind of conversation with oneself.

Comprehending judgment. Two kinds of judgment are allied to prudence. The first kind, comprehending judgment, occurs when I comprehend, understand, and affirm what another moral agent has decided. In other words, I judge his decision good, and would decide on the same thing if I were in his shoes. Aristotle and Aquinas called this *synesis*.

Considerate judgment. The second kind of judgment allied to prudence is considerate judgment. Aristotle and Aquinas called this kind of judgment *gnome*. It occurs when I would not have reached the same decision as the other, but can understand how she decided as she did. I do not agree with the other's decision, but I am considerate of her position.

Considerate judgment is analogous to what Aristotle and Aquinas called "equity" (*epieikeia*). Just as sometimes we allow people to violate valid laws to achieve a greater good in their situation, so sometimes we can accept a decision of others that runs contrary to what we think is virtuous. Considerate judgment sympathizes with the other's plight; it is close to compassion. It is a judgment characterized by leniency and by a kind of forgiving—we forgive the other person who is doing the best he can, but not doing what we think is good in the situation.

When we make moral evaluations of health care issues as a consultant, or as a member of a committee, or as a student, or as an instructor in an ethics course, we are not practicing prudence but judgment. The reasoning in both cases is similar—the judgments are prudential—but the difference between a personal prudential decision (which commits us to action) and the moral judgment about the actions others will perform is significant. We have much more at stake when we decide about our personal conduct than when we judge that of others. It is one thing to be the actual moral agent; it is quite another thing when we are not actually required to do whatever we decide.

As you read the cases in this book, then, you will be engaged in making moral judgments about the decisions of others, not prudential decisions in your own lives. Yet the text will bring you as close to prudential reasoning as possible by looking at health care dilemmas not simply from the perspective of an ethicist, but from the various perspectives of the moral agents involved— the people who have to decide to do something, or to do nothing. We will first consider each situation from the perspective of the patient or of the patient's proxy, and of the providers. Only then will we introduce a more general ethical perspective, the perspective of an ethicist evaluating actions from the position of the person interested in the moral issue but not burdened with the responsibility of carrying it out.

SUGGESTED READINGS

Although the assumption that happiness is the overriding good in life was widespread in ancient Greece, it was not universal. A notable exception was the Cyrenaic school. Influenced by Aristippus, one of Socrates' followers, its members claimed our ultimate good was pleasure, and if we seek happiness, it is only because it gives us pleasure. Unlike the Epicureans, who claimed happiness is pleasure, the Cyrenaics taught that happiness is a means to pleasure. See Terence Irwin. "Aristippus Against Happiness." *Monist* **1991**, *74*, 55–82.

We rely on Aristotle and Aquinas for the development of personal good or happiness as the central theme of ethics. The classical texts are Aristotle's *Nicomachean Ethics*, especially books 1 and 10; the *Eudemian Ethics*, books 1 and 2; the *Rhetoric*, book 1, chapters 6 and 7; and the *Topics*, book 3, chapters 1 and 2.

See also Stephen White. 1992. *Sovereign Virtue: Aristotle on the Relation Between Happiness and Prosperity*. Stanford: Stanford University Press, especially parts 1 and 2; Richard Kraut. 1989. *Aristotle on the Human Good*. Princeton: Princeton University Press, especially chapters 1, 4, and 5; John M. Cooper. 1977. *Reason and Human Good in Aristotle*. Cambridge: Harvard University Press, especially chapters 2 and 3; and Sarah Broadie. 1991. *Ethics with Aristotle.* New York: Oxford University Press, chapters 1 and 7. Three papers in Amelie Oksenberg Rorty, ed. 1980. *Essays on Aristotle's Ethics.* Berkeley: University of California Press, are also helpful: Thomas Nagel's "Aristotle on *Eudaimonia,*" J. L. Ackrill's paper with the same title, and John McDowell's "The Role of *Eudaimonia* in Aristotle's Ethics." See also Mary Hayden, "Rediscovering Eudaimonistic Teleology," *The Monist* **1992,** *75*, 71–83.

See also Julia Annas, "Self-love in Aristotle." *The Southern Journal of Philosophy* **1988,** *27* (supplement), 1–18; John Cooper, "Aristotle on Friendship" in Rorty, *Essays on Aristotle's Ethics,* pp. 301–40; Nancy Sherman. 1989. *The Fabric of Character: Aristotle's Theory of Virtue.* New York: Oxford University Press, chapter 4; Bernard Williams. 1985. *Ethics and the Limits of Philosophy.* Cambridge: Harvard University Press, chapter 3; A. W. Price. 1989. *Love and Friendship in Plato and Aristotle.* New York: Oxford University Press, chapters 4–7; and J. O. Urmson. 1988. *Aristotle's Ethics.* New York: Basil Blackwell, chapters 9 and 10. For a thoughtful article explaining how Aristotle's morality of happiness leads us to choose the less bad when no available option leads to happiness, see Robert Heinaman. "Rationality, *Eudaimonia* and *Kakodaimonia* in Aristotle." *Phronesis* **1993,** *38,* 31–56.

The major texts in Aquinas supporting the Aristotelian view are the *Summa Theologiae,* I II, questions 1–5; the *Summa Contra Gentiles,* book 3; and the *Sententia Libri Ethicorum* (Commentary on the Book of Ethics), his detailed analysis of Aristotle's *Nicomachean Ethics,* recently reprinted as *Commentary on Aristotle's Nicomachean Ethics,* C. I. Litzinger, trans. (Notre Dame: Dumb Ox Books, 1993).

Aquinas' treatment of the parallel between the self-evident first principle of theoretical reasoning (the principle of noncontradiction) and the self-evident first principle of moral reasoning (people seek their good) is found in the *Summa Theologiae,* I II, q. 91, a. 3 and q. 94, a. 3. In q. 94, a. 2 he wrote: "The first principle (*primum principium*) is all seek their good and this leads to the first precept (*primum praeceptum*) which is: do and seek the good, and avoid the bad." For a provocative, and controversial, reading of Aquinas on the first principle of practical reasoning see Germain Grisez. "The First Principle of Practical Reason." *Natural Law Forum* **1965,** *10,* 168–96, reprinted in an abridged form in Anthony Kenny, ed. 1976. *Aquinas: A Collection of Critical Essays.* South Bend: University of Notre Dame Press, pp. 340–82. Aquinas also states that the first principle of human action is reason: "Reason is the *principium primum* of all human actions." *Summa Theologiae,* I II, q. 58, a.2. This is merely another way of making his point. Reason apprehends what is good for us and directs us in achieving it.

Both Aristotle and Aquinas insist that an ethics of seeking our good (that is, our personal happiness) is an ethics advocating an abiding and sincere concern for others. Both insist that we cannot be happy without justice and love. See books 4, 5, 8, and 9 in the *Nicomachean Ethics,* and *Summa Theologiae* I II, qq. 26–29 and II II, qq. 23–27 and 57–63. See also Arthur Madigan, "Eth. Nic. 9:8: Beyond Egoism and Altruism," in John P. Anton and Anthony Preus, eds. 1991. *Aristotle's Ethics.* Albany: State University of New York Press, pp. 73–94; and Mary Hayden. "The Paradox of Aquinas's Altruism: From Self-Love to Love of Others." *Proceedings of the American Catholic Philosophical Association* **1990,** *63,* 72–83.

The classic texts in Aristotle elaborating his doctrine of the intellectual and moral virtues are the *Nicomachean Ethics,* books 2–7, and the *Eudemian Ethics,* books 2 and 3. See also Sherman, *The Fabric of Character,* chapters 1–3; and Broadie, *Ethics With Aristotle,* chapter 4.

The central texts on the virtues in Aquinas are the *Summa Theologiae* I II, q. 49–67 and II II, q. 47–170. Also important is his more technical analysis entitled *De Virtutibus* in Communi (The Virtues in General), one of the Questiones Disputatae (Disputed Questions). See Questiones Disputatae, vol. 2 (Turin: Marietti, 1949), pp. 707–51. Aquinas claims virtuous habits are necessary for three reasons: (1) they give a certain uniformity to our actions, so that we respond habitually in just or loving or courageous ways to individual situations; (2) they enable us to respond promptly by relieving us of the necessity of an elaborate inquiry to figure out what is right every time we are faced with a moral decision; and (3) they enable us to act more easily and with enjoyment, since such actions become second nature thanks to the virtuous habits (De Virtutibus in Communi, a. 1).

Aristotle's development of prudence (phronesis) is set forth in book 6 of the Nicomachean Ethics. See also Pierre Aubenque. 1986. La prudence chez Aristote. Paris: Presses Universitaires de France, pp. 33–152; Norman O. Dahl. 1984. Practical Reason, Aristotle, and Weakness of the Will. Minneapolis: University of Minnesota Press, pp. 3–135; Paul Schuchman. 1980. Aristotle and the Problem of Moral Discernment. Frankfort am Main: Peter D. Lang, chapters 1, 4 and 5; David Wiggins, "Deliberation and Practical Reason," in Rorty, Essays on Aristotle's Ethics, pp. 221–40; Hans-Georg Gadamer. 1991. Truth and Method, second revised edition. New York: Crossroad, pp. 312–24; Martha C. Nussbaum. 1986. The Fragility of Goodness. Cambridge: Cambridge University Press, chapter 10, entitled "Non-scientific deliberation"; Charles Larmore. 1987. Patterns of Moral Complexity. Cambridge: Cambridge University Press, chapter 1, entitled "Moral judgment—an Aristotelian insight."

Aquinas's development of prudence (prudentia) is set forth in the Summa Theologiae, I II, q. 57, a. 4–6, q. 58, and II II, q. 47–56. His discussion of the virtues allied to prudence—deliberation, synesis, and gnome—is found in the Summa Theologiae, II II, q. 51, and follows closely book six, chapters 9–11, of the Nicomachean Ethics. See also Josef Pieper. 1966. The Four Cardinal Virtues. Notre Dame: University of Notre Dame Press, pp. 3–40. For an overview of Aquinas' doctrine of prudence, see Daniel Nelson. 1992. The Priority of Prudence. University Park, PA: Pennsylvania State University Press, especially chapters 2, 3, and 5.

For a helpful confirmation from contemporary cognitive science of the inadequacy of the rule-based ethics inherited from ancient theories of divine and natural law, as well as from the modern Enlightenment theories of principles, rules, and duties, see Mark Johnson. 1993. Moral Imagination: Implications of Cognitive Science for Ethics. Chicago: University of Chicago Press. Johnson describes the "extremely narrow definition" of morality characterizing our culture as follows: "Morality is a set of restrictive rules that are supposed to tell you which acts you may and may not perform, which you have an obligation to perform, and when you can be blamed for what you have done. It is not fundamentally about how to live a good life, or how to live well. Instead, it is only a matter of 'doing the right thing'—the one thing required of you in a given situation" (p. 246). This narrow definition of morality neglects what he calls prudential reasoning, which is "the practical use of reason to determine the most efficient means of attaining the comprehensive human end of happiness or well-being" (p. 247). Johnson's emphasis on imagination, metaphor, and narrative in moral reasoning is comfortably compatible with the older notions of prudence.

3

The Language of Health Care Ethics

We use language in many different ways. Some sentences state facts, others ask questions, still others give commands. Our words may be simple descriptions, or they may change our lives. The man who says "I do" when someone asks him whether he likes ice cream is simply reporting a preference, but the man who says "I do" when asked whether he takes a woman as his wife is, if the consent is mutual, making a marriage.

The meaning of language depends, to a great extent, on what is going on when the language is used. We have to know the "language game," as the philosopher Ludwig Wittgenstein put it, to know what words and sentences mean. For example, normally we think stealing is immoral and shameful, yet we are delighted when a member of our team steals second base.

One important use of language is classifying and distinguishing the realities we encounter. When classifications and distinctions bring order and clarity to the expression of our thoughts, they can be very helpful. Yet classifications and distinctions can become a source of mischief and sometimes mislead us. In health care ethics, this can happen in two ways.

First, some well-established classifications and distinctions are not always suitable for newly developed techniques and technologies, yet we continue to use them. Instead of recognizing the newness and originality of recent developments, we force or "shoehorn" them into traditional classifications and distinctions. This distorts our descriptions of them, and the distortions undermine our moral deliberations and judgments.

The confusion that results from using traditional classifications for new procedures can be seen readily in the following example. When long term nourishment by feeding tubes became a reality not so long ago, there were two ways people could classify it. They could say feeding tubes were (1) a way of feeding people or (2) a medical treatment. Neither classification is really fitting. Inserting nutrition and fluids through a tube running into the stomach through the nasal passages or surgically inserted through the abdominal wall is not what we call feeding in any ordinary meaning of the term. Nor is it a typical medical treatment because it does not provide medicine or medication but what everyone, sick or healthy, needs for life—nutrition and fluids. These techniques are too much like treatment to be classified as feeding, but too much like feeding to be classified as treatment. For purposes of moral deliberation, nourishing people by feeding tubes is better understood and classified as a new category of action.

Worse than the misleading classification of new techniques and technologies is the tendency to substitute distinctions for moral reasoning. For example, some use the distinction between between ordinary treatment and extraordinary treatment to justify a moral judgment. They claim that (1) the refusal of an ordinary treatment such as an antibiotic for an infection is never morally justified, while (2) the refusal of an extraordinary treatment such as an artificial heart is morally justified. This looks like moral reasoning, but it really is not. Proponents have simply made a distinction, the distinction between "ordinary" treatment and "extraordinary" treatment, and then claimed that the former is always morally obligatory but not the latter.

Sometimes poorly classifying a new technique or technology, or substituting a distinction for authentic moral reasoning, is unintentional and harmless. The process looks like legitimate reasoning and is carelessly accepted as such, but no great harm is done because the conclusion happens to be morally sound.

Sometimes, however, poorly classifying things or substituting distinctions for reasoning is not unintentional and harmless. People may deliberately employ poor classifications and substitute distinctions for reasoning in order to avoid authentic discussion about issues on which they have already taken a firm position. They do not use classifications and distinctions to clarify a subject, but to convince an audience.

People tend to do this when their minds are already made up. Ideologues have nothing to gain from careful classifications and thoughtful distinctions in controversial moral matters. Ideologues are not about to change their minds for any reason. They believe there is nothing to figure out—they already have the right answer. If withdrawing a feeding tube undermines their commitment to the right to life, they will classify it as feeding and insist that patients must always be fed. If withholding antibiotics undermines their conception of the value of human life, they will make a distinction between ordinary and extraordinary treatment, call antibiotics "ordinary treatment," and conclude that they cannot be withheld.

All attempts to show these people that using feeding tubes to keep permanently unconscious patients alive for decades is not reasonable, and therefore not morally obligatory, fall on deaf ears. A classification has become an ideology: "Feeding tubes feed, and if we do not feed those who cannot feed themselves, they starve to death, and that is wrong." Similarly, attempts to show that using antibiotics to reverse the pneumonia of a ninety-year-old man dying in discomfort of metastasized cancer is not reasonable, and therefore not morally obligatory, fail. A distinction has become an ideology: "Antibiotics are simple, inexpensive, painless, and ordinary treatment, and we are not according human life its proper value if we fail to use ordinary means to preserve it."

This chapter will first call attention to several distinctions that often cause confusion in the reasoning and debates about health care ethics, and then will note several other distinctions that can be helpful in our prudential reasoning.

DISTINCTIONS THAT CAN MISLEAD

The following distinctions need to be used with exceptional care, or not at all, because their use so often hinders good prudential reasoning.

Actions and Omissions

The distinction between action and omission, doing something and not doing something, is certainly valid. I can take my medicine or not take it; I can treat or not treat a patient.

The distinction between actions and omissions, however, can easily mislead us in ethics. A major problem arises when the distinction is used in situations where the foreseen outcome is not wanted or desired, and a distinction is made between actions and omissions giving rise to the unwanted outcome. For example, the unwanted outcome of removing life-support equipment is the patient's death. Since many people believe that it is immoral to perform an action leading to the patient's death, they think of what will be done as an omission, the omission of technology needed to support life. This enables them to claim that they are not performing an action leading to death; they are simply omitting inappropriate treatment.

Using the action–omission distinction this way obviously twists language in an unacceptable way. The action of removing life-support equipment is just that—an action. It is not an omission. Twisting language this way is objectionable because it undermines moral reasoning. We cannot reason well if our language is distorted.

Using the action–omission distinction this way also camouflages an important moral consideration. The unspoken assumption behind using the action–omission distinction is often the belief that omissions contributing to a death are easier to justify morally than actions contributing to a death. Sometimes this is true, but not always. Omissions can be as immoral as actions. Not doing something we should do is as morally significant as doing something we should not do. Some actions are ethical, and some are not; some omissions are ethical, and some are not. The danger is that making a distinction between actions and omissions can blind us to the fact that omissions can be as immoral as actions. Unless we see this, we will not properly consider ourselves morally responsible for the foreseen bad outcomes that follow our omissions.

In health care ethics, the basic action–omission distinction appears in two widespread formulations: the distinction between withdrawing and withholding treatment, and the distinction between intentionally causing death and letting die (or permitting a person to die). We need to say a few words about each.

Withdrawing and Withholding Treatment

There are two major problems associated with this distinction. First, the distinction between withdrawing and withholding treatment is not always clear. It is not clear, for example, in situations where we stop treatment by withholding the next step. If we interrupt a series of discrete chemotherapy treatments (one today, one tomorrow, etc.), we could say either that we are withdrawing the chemotherapy treatment or that we are withholding the remaining treatments. The same can be said of discrete dialysis treatments. And some have claimed we do not really withdraw medical nutrition—we simply withhold the next drop in the tube or line.

At other times, of course, the distinction between withholding and withdrawing treatment is clear. One example is the distinction between not connecting a patient to a ventilator and disconnecting the ventilator. Even when the distinction is clear, however, it is not really relevant for making a moral judgment. Both withdrawal and withholding are moral in some situations and immoral in others.

Second, the distinction between withholding and withdrawing treatment can distort our moral judgment. A widespread conviction, for example, holds that it is more difficult to justify withdrawing treatment than withholding it. Psychologically, of course, it is more difficult to withdraw than to withhold life-sustaining treatment from a patient, especially when he will die moments after the withdrawal. But this does not mean that it is more difficult to establish the moral justification of withdrawal than to establish the moral justification of withholding.

Actually, withdrawal of treatment is often easier to justify morally than withholding it in the first place. This is so because in questions of withdrawal we have important information that we do not have in cases of withholding, namely, we know how the therapy actually affects the patient's condition. Moral judgments require the best possible information, and we simply have more good information when we are actually using the treatment than when we have not yet tried it. The added information we have from using a treatment puts us in a better position to make a good moral decision about its benefits and burdens.

Failure to acknowledge the advantage we have in making decisions about treatment withdrawal can lead to unfortunate consequences. For example, if providers think it is morally more difficult to justify withdrawing a ventilator than withholding it, they may not begin the ventilation when they are unsure of its medical value for fear that once they started it, they could not stop it. This means a patient who could have benefited from the ventilator will not have the chance to benefit from it. Again, if providers think it is morally more difficult to justify withdrawing a ventilator than withholding it, they may not withdraw a ventilator that they never would have started in the first place if they had known it would be so burdensome. This means a patient who is unreasonably burdened by a ventilator will be left on it.

Intentionally Causing Death and Letting Die

This is the most sensitive variation of the distinction between actions and omissions. From childhood we are taught "Do not kill." Later most of us learn to accept the morality of exceptions, most notably, killing as a last resort in self-defense or killing enemy soldiers in what is traditionally called "just" warfare. And many people also make an exception for the killing in legal executions. But a long tradition of medical ethics going back to the Hippocratic writings condemns the killing of patients by physicians.

There were always challenges to this tradition and today, as we will see in the chapter on euthanasia and assisted suicide, these challenges are stronger than ever in recent history. Nonetheless, the American Medical Association's ethical guidelines continue to say "the physician should not intentionally cause death." What the guidelines mean is clear—the AMA is opposed to physicians giving lethal injections—but the language is misleading. It forces physicians to think of behaviors with a causal impact on a patient's death as if they were not causal in any way. Thus, some describe the action of removing life-support equipment as "letting die" and maintain that the disease, not the life-support removal, is the only cause of death.

Sometimes the distinction between intentionally causing death and letting die (or, to put it another way, between causing death and letting the disease cause death) is clear. If I intentionally give a lethal injection I cause death, and if I do not attempt CPR I am letting the person in cardiac arrest die. But frequently the distinction between intentionally causing death and letting die is not clear because the providers' actions play a definite causal role in patients' deaths. Consider the following behaviors.

1. Physician gives a lethal injection to the patient.
2. Physician assists a patient with suicide.
3. Physician gives a dying patient medication needed for pain relief although the drugs will hasten death.
4. Physician withdraws nutrition and hydration through tubes or lines.
5. Physician withdraws needed life-sustaining equipment.
6. Physician withholds nutrition or life-sustaining treatment.

Behaviors one through five all involve causal impact on the death of the patient. The causal impact is strongest in the first behavior and weakest in the fourth and fifth. Only the sixth behavior makes no causal contribution to death. Withholding nutrition and treatment is the only real case of letting die on the list. In every other situation, the provider's actions have a causal impact on the patient's death.

The distinction between intentionally causing death and letting die is too simplified to serve as a substitute for moral reasoning. It is disingenuous to ignore the causal impact, for example, of withdrawing a ventilator from someone who will die without it. We would have no trouble acknowledging that a stranger walking into an ICU and withdrawing a ventilator causes the patient's death. Yet if a physician withdraws the same ventilator, some want to pretend that the action plays no causal role in the patient's death. They claim that the physician is only "letting the patient die."

What is really happening when a ventilator is removed from a person needing it, of course, is that both the disease *and* the withdrawal are causes of death, but neither alone is a *sufficient* cause of death. For death to occur at this time, the disease must be making it impossible for the patient to live without the ventilator *and* someone must remove or shut off the ventilator. Sound moral analysis will admit that the physician's action has a causal impact on the patient's death at this time, and then go on to ask whether the withdrawal of the ventilator is morally justified in the circumstances.

Paternalism and Autonomy

The distinction between paternalism and autonomy rests on where we place the power of authorizing medical treatment and on how we perceive the relationship between what the physician thinks is good for the patient and what the patient wants. In general, the older medical tradition made physicians the authorities, and made the paramount moral value doing good for, or at least no harm to, patients. This tradition argued that the physician knows more than the patient and has more experience, and that the patient's ability to think clearly and to choose rationally is often undermined by the illness. Hence, it made sense to say that the physician should do what he thought was best for the patient.

The relationship between physician and patient thus resembled the relationship between a wise and caring father and his child. When the physician acts like a caring father toward a patient, who is a beginner or a child in the world of medicine, we call it paternalism. The physician-father knows best and the patient-child is to follow "doctor's orders."

Some claim that the Hippocratic Oath, a cornerstone of medical ethics for centuries, is one of the sources of this medical paternalism. This oath is thought to have originated around the fourth century B.C.E. among a group of Greek speaking people, the Pythagoreans, who flourished for a time in southern Italy, then a part of the Greek world. These followers of Pythagoras (known to every high school student as the discoverer of the geometric theorem that bears his name) formed a distinct social group with shared religious, philosophical, and moral beliefs. Most people of that era did not share those beliefs, and thus the Hippocratic Oath represents the views of a small and somewhat idiosyncratic group in the classical world.

The physician taking the oath says he will take measures "for the benefit of the sick according to my ability and judgment." This does suggest medical paternalism, especially since there is no mention of any judgment by the patient. And the oath also says that the physician will not provide lethal drugs to patients requesting them, or give an abortifacient to a woman, but these prohibitions were probably not so much paternalistic as important moral values for the Pythagorean physician, who would have accepted the strong belief of his group in the interconnection and value of all life, human as well as animal.

Perhaps an even stronger source of medical paternalism in the tradition was the realization that the power of medical knowledge should be used for good and not for harm. Many people were horrified by the thought that physicians would use their expertise for evil—to devise more exquisite techniques of torture, for example. So the tradition insisted that the physician should always act for the patient's good and do what he thought was best for the patient.

In most cases, the physician knew better than the patient what was good for the patient. From this the tradition concluded that, if he really cared about his patient, he should simply do what was best for the patient. If this meant doing things without the patient's knowledge and consent, so be it. The important thing was to do what was good for the patient, and the physician was the authority in determining this. The physician was like a parent, responsible for the well-being of the patient, and must act accordingly. This commitment to paternal beneficence, to the good of the patient, was one of the great moral values of traditional medicine.

Recently, however, all forms of paternalism in our culture have been widely criticized. In the past few centuries, various philosophies have arisen that locate the source of decision-making more and more in the individual rather than in political or religious authority.

Examples of this trend are many and well-known. The Lutheran Reformation in Christianity, for example, let each individual read and interpret the Bible rather than have church authorities interpret it for her. The powerful political theory of John Locke made the right to liberty one of the three basic natural rights, and his theory is a major source of the right to choose and the right to privacy we hear so much about today. The influential moral philosophy of Immanuel Kant held that the moral law comes not from God, nor from the law of nature, but from ourselves—we are morally autonomous. The popular philosophy called utilitarianism, developed extensively in the nineteenth century by John Stuart Mill, tended to place but one limitation on human freedom: we are not free to do things that will harm others. Finally, various existentialist philosophies, beginning with Kierkegaard and Nietzsche in the past century, held that choosing and willing, rather than thinking and knowing, is the hallmark of human existence. Kierkegaard urged individuals to move beyond ethics to a religious stage; Nietzsche saw only decadence in existing European morality, and encouraged individuals to exercise a will-to-power that would inaugurate a transvaluation of all values.

Major trends such as these, different as they are from each other, all reinforce a central notion, namely, the important value of self-determination and personal choice.

Medical paternalism was bound to run into difficulties with the many modern philosophies and theologies of individual choice. The major value is no longer what someone else, even a caring physician, thinks is good, but what the patient thinks is good, and what the patient chooses. Beneficence remains an important value—no patient in his right mind wants anything bad done to him—but the autonomy of the patient has become a crucial value as well. In the language of those who conceive of ethics as a matter of principles, the principle of autonomy has emerged and, in some cases, has come to dominate the principle of beneficence in health care ethics.

The beneficence supporting traditional medical paternalism meant doing good for the patient in a medical sense; that is, it meant trying to achieve a good clinical outcome. It did not really take into account the patient's personal commitments that might actually conflict with good clinical care. A classic example of this is the treatment of a Jehovah's Witness when blood is needed. The physician may know the unconscious patient in the operating room will die without a transfusion, and is thus driven by beneficence to give it, but the patient may have insisted for religious reasons that blood not be given. In this case, most ethicists, and several important legal decisions, say that respect for the autonomy of the patient should take priority over the beneficence of the physician trying to save the patient's life.

Autonomy, self-determination, and respect for persons are important notions in medical ethics. Sometimes, as we just saw, they can clash with the older idea that the doctor should do what is good for her patient. This leads some to think that we must make a choice between medical paternalism and beneficence, on the one hand, and patient autonomy and self-determination on the other. Almost always, when the choice is presented this way, it is the paternalism that is rejected.

Now things are changing again. In the past few years, ethicists have been moving away from the language of autonomy as they recognize that patients, especially very sick or elderly patients, are really not that autonomous. Moreover, some patients and proxies have misused autonomy and self-determination to demand medically inappropriate treatments. This places physicians in a difficult position. No physician wants to order inappropriate medical treatments simply because his patient or the patient's proxy wants them.

The choice forced by the distinction between paternalism and autonomy, however, is not helpful, and that is why the distinction is best avoided. Both paternalism and patient self-determination reflect important values in a rich ethic of health care. The driving force of paternalism is doing good for the patient, and the driving force of self-determination is the recognition that patients remain persons who cannot be disenfranchised of the responsibility and freedom to make important personal choices in life.

There is no need to distinguish between paternalism and autonomy, and to prefer one over the other. Given the physician's experience and knowledge, and a lack of the same in most patients, and given the impact of disease making it difficult for patients to remain in control of their lives, a paternalistic (or maternal) attitude has its place in medicine and health care. And, given the importance of respecting the personal commitments of patients who see the world differently from the physician, autonomy or self-determination also has its place.

The ideal will be to maintain the best of both paternalism and self-determination, and the most promising way to do this is to have the physician and the patient share the decision-making. This avoids having the physician behave like a father with his child. It also avoids reducing the physician to a hired hand ordered around by a patient autonomously authorizing his or her medical treatment in such a way that the physician no longer exercises professional judgment, but simply carries out the patient's decisions.

It is important to avoid considering the physician's paternalism morally suspect and the patient's autonomous decisions morally acceptable. It is not this simple. In some situations paternalism can be justified, and in some situations the decision of the patient is simply immoral. The fact that a patient exercises her right to choose what will be done to her body does not thereby justify the morality of what she chooses. It is not enough to say: "This is what the patient wants; therefore, this is the right thing to do." The test of the right thing to do is whether what is done achieves the truly good, not whether the patient autonomously chooses it. Important as autonomy or self-determination is, it is not a criterion of what is morally right.

Ordinary and Extraordinary Means of Preserving Life

This distinction has been losing the popularity it once enjoyed. It originated several centuries ago in Roman Catholic moral theology and, when medical treatments were much simpler, it served a useful purpose. It has been kept alive by a number of landmark court cases where judges described respirators and tubal feeding as extraordinary, and then used that description in justifying withdrawal. The New Jersey Supreme Court, for example, described Karen Quinlan's respirator as extraordinary treatment, and the Massachusetts Supreme Court found that Joseph Saikewicz's chemotherapy and Paul Brophy's tubal feeding were extraordinary. These courts then allowed medical personnel to honor requests of proxies to forego the life-sustaining treatments.

The fundamental idea behind the distinction between ordinary and extraordinary treatment is this: although human life is an important value, ethics does not require people to use extraordinary means to preserve it. Hence, if a patient chooses to forego extraordinary treatment, providers withholding or withdrawing that treatment are acting morally even if death follows. On the other hand, the patient's decision to forego "ordinary" treatment is not morally justified.

There are several problems with this approach. The first is now familiar: the temptation to rely on a distinction instead of moral deliberation and reasoning to determine what is morally good behavior.

The second problem centers on just what we are to consider extraordinary life-sustaining treatment. Those supporting the value of the distinction speak of treatment that is very expensive, or unusual, or very painful, or very risky, or highly technological. Sometimes it is easy to use these notions. Most everyone would agree that a heart transplant is, at least at the present time, extraordinary. But in many other situations the distinction is simply not clear. The courts have considered respirators extraordinary but many people would consider a respirator in an operating room, or in an intensive care unit, quite ordinary. And the courts have considered long term use of a feeding tube for an unconscious person not expected to recover an extraordinary treatment, but many people consider nutrition supplied by a simple tube an ordinary means of nutritional support.

Since there is no way to provide a satisfactory definition of extraordinary treatment in modern medicine, the distinction is not helpful and, in fact, can be misleading. If used instead of moral reasoning, for example, it would require us to give ordinary antibiotics to fight the pneumonia of an elderly dialysis patient on a ventilator and dying of painful cancer. The distinction between ordinary and extraordinary means of preserving life, no less than the others we have considered, is no substitute for the prudential reasoning and moral reflection we need to determine what achieves the human good in any situation.

Futile Treatment and Effective Treatment

Futile treatment was not a problem until recently. When physicians were the sole decision makers there was no futile treatment—if the physician thought a treatment was futile, he would never provide it. The recent upsurge of patient autonomy and self-determination has created the problem of futile treatment. At first this trend toward patient autonomy and self-determination centered on the patient's right to refuse treatments, but now the other side is beginning to show itself. Patients or their proxies are demanding treatment, and sometimes the providers are convinced the treatment they demand is futile or useless.

This presents a problem for providers. If they honor the patient's request for treatment they believe is inappropriate, they act contrary to their professional judgment. Sometimes they can transfer the patient to other providers, but sometimes they cannot, and this leaves them in a difficult position. Parents, for example, have demanded painful treatments for their children that providers believed were medically useless. This is upsetting for providers because they are being asked to do something that causes suffering for their patient, but which they perceive as providing no benefit.

To resolve this difficulty, some now propose a new distinction: futile treatment and effective treatment. They would like to use the distinction to justify morally a physician's refusal to supply inappropriate medical treatments demanded by a patient or a proxy. The idea is simple: once the treatment is deemed futile, providers have no obligation to provide it even if the patient or proxy wants it. In fact, some argue that there is a moral obligation not to provide treatment defined as futile. The main effect of the judgment of futility, then, is to limit the autonomy of patients by allowing them to authorize only effective treatment. Once physicians determine a treatment is futile, they no longer have the obligation to provide or continue it, and they do not need the consent of the patient to withdraw or withhold it.

One example of this thinking can be seen in some recent policies about providing cardiopulmonary resuscitation (CPR) in hospitals. Some new policies allow writing a "do-not-resuscitate" (DNR) order without the patient's consent if the physician believes resuscitation efforts would be futile. This is a new development; hitherto, most hospital policies required consent from the patient or proxy before the DNR order could be written. This development reflects the new idea that providers can define futile treatment and then unilaterally withhold or withdraw it.

At first glance this approach seems reasonable because, at least in some cases, the distinction between effective and futile treatment is quite clear and does suggest a basis for moral judgment. Treatment of people on life support who have suffered whole brain death, for example, is obviously futile. And so is periodontal surgery to prevent the loss of teeth ten years from now when the patient is dying. But these are the easy cases, where the futility is clear.

In most cases the distinction between futile and effective treatment is not so clear. This is primarily because the notion of futility is so complex it is useless, much as the confusing notion of extraordinary rendered the ordinary–extraordinary distinction useless. Suppose, for example, the probability of a painful treatment's success is "one in a thousand." Providers may consider it futile to provide such a treatment, but a desperate mother may think one in a thousand is a worthwhile chance for her baby. Again, suppose the respirator is merely preserving an irreversible vegetative state. Providers may consider the treatment futile, but the proxy may consider the treatment effective because it is still preserving human life. We will consider such a case—the Wanglie story—in a later chapter.

We can see from this that the judgment of futility is often not a clear and objective judgment, and that many factors other than medical effectiveness are involved. The distinction between effective and futile treatment is too controversial to serve as the basis of ethical judgments. The distinction should not become a substitute for thoughtful moral deliberation, no more than should the other distinctions we have considered. Providers may well conclude a treatment is futile, but that alone is not enough to justify its removal. Other relevant values and circumstances must be considered.

Direct and Indirect Results

Our actions invariably have many results that we might call consequences, outcomes, or effects. Some of these consequences are unforeseen and unexpected, and these are not morally relevant. The foreseen consequences, however, are morally relevant. We recognize that some of these effects are good and thus desirable, while others are not good and thus undesirable. When a provider gives chemotherapy, for example, the desired effect is the shrinkage of the tumor and the undesirable effects include hair loss and nausea. One and the same action causes both good and bad effects.

In the language of medicine, we sometimes speak of the secondary effects as "side effects." Thus hair loss is a side effect of chemotherapy, an effect alongside the main effect. In the language of some moral philosophies and theologies, we find the term "double effect" used to describe situations where our action gives rise to two effects, one good and the other bad. The desired good effect is considered the direct result of our behavior, while the undesired bad effect is considered the indirect result of our behavior.

The distinction between two results (one called direct because it is desired and good, the other called indirect because it is undesired and not good) has given rise to what is called the "principle of the double effect." However, while this principle is clear and helpful in some scenarios, it is currently the source of great debate both within and beyond the Roman Catholic moral theology that originally generated it. Its fundamental intuition is laudable; it recognizes that the moral world is sometimes an ambiguous place, and that we can morally justify some behaviors despite the bad effects they cause. The use of the principle of double effect, however, often undermines, as does the employment of any moral principle, sound moral deliberation and reasoning.

The classic moral example behind the principle of the double effect is found in Aquinas' analysis of killing in self-defense. As a Christian, he accepted the biblical injunction: Thou shalt not kill. But, he argued, if a criminal makes a life-threatening attack on me, I may use force, even lethal force if necessary, to save my life. My action will have two effects: the direct and good effect of saving my life, and the indirect and bad effect of killing a human being. I can justify the killing, however, because it was not directly intended. I intended to save my life, not to kill someone. The death is an unfortunate, unwanted, and unavoidable bad effect of the same action that saved my life.

Actions with double—perhaps it would be better to say multiple—effects abound in health care. The surgeon removing an appendix, the endodontist doing a root canal, and the nurse starting an intravenous (IV) treatment are all performing actions with multiple results, some good and some bad. The direct effect of the surgery is the removal of an infected appendix, the indirect effect is the pain and trauma to the body. The medical goals are good, but other results—pain, scarring, trauma, etc.—are bad.

From this we can see that the notions of direct and indirect results are grounded on intention. The direct results are the effects we intend; the indirect effects are those we know will occur but do not really intend and actually regret. In self-defense, for example, what we intend is saving our lives, not the death of the attacker, although we know very well when we resort to lethal force to stop him that he will die. And in doing surgery, we intend the removal of the infected gall bladder, not the pain and trauma, although we know very well when we operate that we will cause pain and trauma to the body.

It is important to realize, of course, that we are responsible for all the known effects, indirect as well as direct, of our actions. We are responsible for the attacker's death, and the surgeon is responsible for the bad things like pain and trauma that accompany any surgery. Just because they are side effects or indirect effects does not mean they fall outside the moral sphere.

In moral evaluation, then, the effort to describe something as a direct rather than indirect effect, as something I intend rather than as something I foresaw but did not intend, is not ultimately crucial. Rather, what we have to determine is whether what we are going to do is reasonable, and reasonableness will depend to a great extent on all the expected consequences, both intended and unintended, of our behavior. Aquinas seems to have realized this. Apart from mentioning two effects in his example of self-defense, he never developed what was to be known later as the principle of double effect.

Prudential reasoning considers all the significant effects of our actions, and gains little by dividing them into direct and indirect. In practice, this means prudence looks at the whole picture, considers the complex mixture of good and bad that is involved in the process, and then determines the most reasonable thing to do, given the circumstances and the consequences we think will follow our behavior.

There is, however, a valuable insight captured in the famous principle of the double effect. It recognizes that our actions often have bad as well as good effects, and it justifies our performing such actions when the reasons for acting override the bad we cause. The famous principle, although not really helpful in an ethics of prudence and not used by Aristotle and Aquinas, is a principle of moral realism. It reminds us that if we are not prepared to do bad things for good reasons, then ever more terrible bad things will multiply in life. And it reminds us we need justifying reasons to compensate for the bad we know will follow from the good we are trying to do.

Immoral and Intrinsically Immoral

Some ethicists advocate a distinction between what we might call the simply immoral and the intrinsically immoral or the intrinsically evil. They argue that some actions are immoral by their very nature. It is impossible to think that such actions could ever be ethical. To understand their point, it is helpful to analyze moral behavior into several components:

1. the actual physical action that is performed,
2. the intention of the agent in performing the action,
3. the circumstances in which the action is performed, and
4. the consequences resulting from the action.

The idea behind the notion of intrinsically immoral actions is that some physical actions are immoral regardless of the agent's intention, the circumstances, or the consequences. Other actions may also be immoral but their immorality depends on the intention, the circumstances, or the consequences. In other words, intrinsically immoral actions are always and everywhere immoral—there are no exceptions.

Once the notion of intrinsically immoral actions is accepted, the ethicist invariably proposes a set of moral laws or rules forbidding these actions always and everywhere. The laws or rules allow no exceptions, no matter what the intentions, circumstances, or consequences. Actions that are not intrinsically immoral, on the other hand, may or may not be immoral, depending on the circumstances and consequences, and no moral laws or rules forbidding them can be absolute—exceptions are always possible.

What actions do ethicists propose as intrinsically evil? The list, as you might expect, varies, but many ethicists promoting the notion of intrinsically immoral actions include lying, suicide, contraception, sterilization, abortion, extramarital sex, and masturbation. Killing another human being is not proposed as intrinsically immoral because it is morally justified in some situations—war and self-defense, for example. However, some ethicists consider killing the innocent intrinsically immoral, and its prohibition a moral absolute.

Ethicists holding certain actions always and everywhere immoral, and promulgating moral rules that never allow exceptions, are known today as "deontologists." Deontologists are convinced that there must be some concrete moral absolutes, otherwise morality will quickly degenerate into a situation ethics where the appeal to extenuating circumstances or to consequences, as the utilitarians advocate, will soon be used to justify the worst evils.

The current idea that some actions are intrinsically immoral developed from two major sources. The first is a movement that began in the fourteenth century within Roman Catholic moral theology, and the second is the influential moral philosophy developed by Immanuel Kant in the eighteenth century.

Catholic Theology
As ancient writings from the early Fathers and Augustine attest, a strain of moral rigor was present in Catholic moral theology from the beginning. The doctrine of intrinsically immoral or intrinsically evil actions, however, was not formally developed until the fourteenth century. It grew out of a moral problem that fascinated the medieval theologians—the status of the Ten Commandments. They wondered whether there could be exceptions to God's laws prohibiting killing, adultery, and stealing. If killing is against God's law, how could God tell Abraham to kill his son Isaac? If adultery is against God's law, how could God tell Hosea to sleep with a prostitute? And if stealing is against God's law, how could God condone the theft of Egyptian property as the Hebrews left Egypt in the Exodus?

The creative efforts employed by theologians to explain actions in violation of the Ten Commandments, yet commanded or at least approved by God, need not detain us here. The solution of one relatively unknown fourteenth century theologian, however, is of interest. Durand of Saint Pourcain, (Durandus in Latin), claimed that God could not dispense from the commandments forbidding adultery and stealing because the "matter" forbidden by these commandments has the character of evil or immorality "*intrinsically*." Adultery and stealing are intrinsically immoral.

According to Durand, killing is not intrinsically immoral, and therefore God could order Abraham to kill Isaac. But he could not have ordered Hosea to have intercourse with a prostitute nor the Hebrews to steal from the Egyptians because these actions are intrinsically immoral. How, then, did Durand resolve the biblical accounts of Hosea's sexual liaison with the prostitute and the Hebrews' theft of Egyptian property? By what critics consider a weak argument. He claimed God, the Lord of all, gave the prostitute to Hosea as his wife, so He was not really ordering him to commit adultery or to fornicate with her; and he claimed that God gave the Egyptian property to the Hebrews, so they really were not stealing it when they took it. If you accept this explanation, then you can say that God was not making exceptions to his commandments forbidding the intrinsically immoral actions of adultery and stealing.

It is important to remark, however, that Aquinas, who lived the century before Durand, never held that any physical actions, considered by themselves without any reference to circumstances, could be intrinsically immoral. He did hold, as did Aristotle, that some actions are immoral "*secundum se*," that is, they are immoral "by definition" in that the words used to describe them denote a moral judgment as well as a simple description. Actions so defined are actions described in such a way that a moral judgment is imbedded in the description. Aquinas and Aristotle both claimed, for example, that deliberate homicide was always immoral, and Aquinas would agree that God could never command anyone to commit homicide. But homicide is not an action defined in simple physical terms; a judgment is embedded in the word homicide. Homicide means a killing that should not happen. God could never command people to commit a homicide but He could and, according to the Hebrew Bible, did command people to kill.

As the Middle Ages ended, theologians tended to lose interest in reconciling the Biblical accounts approving killing, adultery, and stealing with God's commandments, but the idea of intrinsically immoral physical actions remained, and the list began to grow. Although later theologians tended to exclude stealing from the list of intrinsically immoral actions—if you were starving you could steal food as a last resort—they added other actions, among them lying, suicide, and various sexual sins.

By the nineteenth century, many of the manuals used to train seminarians had adopted a list of intrinsically immoral actions, and by the twentieth century the moral theology of intrinsically immoral actions had found its way into important papal documents. In *Casti Connubii*, the 1930 encyclical forbidding contraception, for example, Pope Pius XI wrote:

The conjugal act is of its very nature designed for the procreation of offspring; and therefore those who in performing it deliberately deprive it of its natural power and efficacy, act against nature and do something which is shameful and *intrinsically immoral*. (#54, emphasis added.)

Since then, several important official documents of the Roman Catholic church have insisted that a number of other physical actions, most notably abortion, sterilization, homosexual behavior, and masturbation, are also intrinsically immoral. The theology of intrinsically immoral actions continued in the 1993 encyclical of Pope John Paul II entitled *Splendor Veritatis*.

The adoption of this ethics of intrinsically immoral actions by the leaders of the Catholic Church has had a major impact on health care ethics in the United States, where many hospitals are under Catholic auspices. It explains why the ethical directives imposed by the American bishops on these facilities forbid all abortions, even for ectopic pregnancies; all vasectomies, tubal ligations, and medical interventions for contraception, regardless of the circumstances; and all masturbation, even to obtain sperm for fertility diagnosis or for reproductive assistance within marriage by such acceptable procedures as artificial insemination or the transfer of gametes (sperm and ova) to the fallopian tubes (GIFT).

Kant

The second major source of the current idea that some actions are intrinsically immoral (that is, always and everywhere immoral regardless of the agent's motive, the circumstances, or the consequences) is the extremely influential moral philosophy of Immanuel Kant. Kant's basic moral principle was a general imperative that reason imposes on all of us. He called this principle the "categorical imperative." It is an imperative because it commands and obliges us; it is categorical because it is absolute and generates absolute moral norms.

Kant almost always described the categorical imperative in terms of the moral obligations or duties that it generates. Some of these moral duties are positive, some negative. Some of the negative duties are "strict" or "perfect," and these are the ones that interest us. According to Kant, the strict negative duties oblige us to avoid certain actions always and everywhere. Strict negative duties define a class of actions that are always wrong; they can never be morally justified under any circumstances. Why not? Because every attempt to consider any violation of a strict negative duty as moral results in a contradiction. Since Kantian morality cannot tolerate contradictions, these actions are *necessarily* immoral.

Suicide is the paradigm example. The categorical imperative generates moral duties toward myself, among them a strict negative duty never to harm myself. Any moral maxim allowing suicide obviously contradicts the duty never to harm myself. Hence, no moral maxim permitting suicide is possible. Suicide is always immoral.

Kant did not describe violations of strict negative duties as intrinsically immoral, but his doctrine of strict negative duties, duties whose every violation would constitute a contradiction at the heart of morality, was certainly analogous to the medieval doctrine. The doctrine generates a list of actions that are universally and necessarily immoral. No good intention, no circumstances or consequences, could ever morally justify performing one of these actions.

And what physical actions were necessarily immoral for Kant? His list included, in addition to suicide, mutilation of the body, drunkenness, gluttony, contraception, homosexual behavior, extramarital sex, masturbation, bestiality, and lying. Kant's list bears an uncanny resemblance to the list of intrinsically immoral actions developed by the Catholic theologians, but Kant was not a Catholic, and he was not arguing from a theological position. His moral absolutes, he claimed, are deduced from what he called "pure practical reason." By pure practical reason Kant meant a reasoning concerned with behavior (the practical) based on necessary and universal principles unaffected by circumstances, history, or change (the pure).

Kant's inclusion of so many sexual actions in his list of necessarily immoral actions is based on the view expressed in his *Metaphysics of Morals* (Part II, section 7) that sexual actions are intended by nature for the preservation of the species. Our duty, if we choose to engage in sex, is to preserve the race, and corresponding to this is a strict negative duty not to act contrary to this purpose. Any moral maxim permitting masturbation, contraception, homosexuality, and bestiality would contradict this strict negative duty, and hence these actions are necessarily immoral. Even extramarital reproductive sex was necessarily immoral for Kant, since he believed that reproduction should occur only in marriage.

Kant's insistence that certain actions such as contraception, lying, homosexuality, and masturbation are necessarily immoral did not, any more than the theological and papal proposals that these actions are intrinsically immoral, go without challenge. One critic of Kant brought up a disturbing example involving lying. If lying is necessarily immoral, if the maxim forbidding lies always holds regardless of the circumstances, then we run into strange situations where behaving morally promotes immorality. Suppose, the critic said, someone is pursuing my friend with the intent to kill him, and he is hiding in my house. If the would-be murderer asks me if my friend is hiding in my house, what reasonable person would think it immoral if, unable to avoid answering the question, I lied to save my friend's life?

In his *Lectures on Ethics* (ca. 1780), Kant had toyed with the idea of distinguishing falsehood from lying and had suggested that deceiving a person who had no right to know the truth was a falsehood and not a lie. However, in the essay entitled *On the Supposed Right to Lie from Altruistic Motives*, published in 1797 to answer this very critic, he made no such distinction and insisted on the absolute prohibition against lying. Regardless of the circumstances and the terrible consequences that follow when the murderer tracks down my friend after I tell the truth, Kant held that I must tell the truth if I cannot avoid answering the question. The moral law simply forbids all lying; there are no exceptions. Lying is always immoral.

Today many ethicists claiming allegiance to moral principles and rules grounded in Kant's moral philosophy simply ignore many of the strict negative duties his theory generates. It is not unusual to see those who consider themselves Kantians in theory accepting, in some situations, the morality of contraception, organ donation from the living (which involves mutilation), abortion, masturbation (for in vitro fertilization and artificial insemination, for example), and even physician-assisted suicide, yet Kant condemned all these actions as *necessarily* immoral because they contradict the strict negative duties generated by the supreme moral principle of the Kantian moral theory—the categorical imperative.

One might be tempted to say that this is not important and that, after all, those retrieving Aristotle also reject some of his moral positions. This is certainly true—nobody retrieving the ethics of Aristotle would agree with his positions on any number of issues. Aquinas did not accept Aristotle's approval of infanticide, and no one retrieving Aristotle today accepts his position on slavery. But there is a major difference between the moral theories of Aristotle and Kant. Aristotle's theory allows a self-correcting process of reevaluation for all actions; Kant's theory does not allow any reevaluation of necessarily immoral actions deduced from the categorical imperative.

Aristotle's theory is based on right reason and the human good, and the rejection of slavery is simply a question of learning to see how slavery is morally unreasonable because it is contrary to the human good. New moral evaluations occur easily within a moral theory founded on the human good. They do not undermine the foundation of the theory. The prudential reasoning and judgments in Aristotle's theory do not give us necessary conclusions valid for always and everywhere. They produce only our best efforts at the time and in the circumstances to say what will promote our good. Prudential judgments in future times and other circumstances may produce other conclusions. Circumstances are always a factor in prudential judgments about good and bad, and circumstances can vary from time to time as well as from place to place. Hence Aristotle's theory allows the historical development of moral evaluations. Aristotle thought infanticide did not undermine the human good, but prudence could easily move him to hold the opposite today.

Kant's doctrine of strict negative moral duties, however, allows no such development. Any theory holding that certain physical actions are necessarily immoral cannot allow any of these actions ever to become morally acceptable. Once actions such as killing oneself, sterilization, or homosexual behavior are defined as contrary to strict negative duties, no circumstances now or in the future can reverse their immorality. Kant's moral theory is rooted in a categorical imperative that transcends history, and allowing exceptions to a strict negative duty as history unfolds would undermine the theory itself.

Kant seemed aware of this problem, and did raise questions about some of the strict negative duties. He asked, for example, whether it would really be suicide if a person going mad killed himself lest, in his madness, he harm others. But he did not show how such a suicide could be morally justified as an exception to the strict duties we owe ourselves. He raised the question of possible exceptions to the universal maxim against suicide, but did not elaborate on how any exceptions to the universal moral maxim proscribing suicide could be possible.

Moral philosophers studying Kant are also aware of the problem created by defining violations of strict negative duties as always immoral. They have proposed various solutions to it, solutions sometimes reminiscent of the creative efforts employed by medieval theologians to reconcile God's command-ments with God's commands directing certain biblical heroes to kill the inno-cent, to fornicate, and to steal. Many health care ethicists appealing to Kant for support of their positions, however, seem unaware of the philosophical problem. It is truly curious to see some ethical writings on health care justify abortion, contraception, sterilization, and physician-assisted suicide by an appeal to the Kantian principle of autonomy, when what Kant called the Law of Autonomy condemns these actions as always and everywhere immoral.

Many Kantians clearly have difficulty with Kant's notion of strict negative duties and the necessarily immoral actions these duties denote, just as many theologians within the Catholic tradition have difficulty with the notions of intrinsically evil and intrinsically immoral actions. These difficulties alone suggest that the distinction between the simply immoral and intrinsically immoral is problematic. A more important reason for not using the distinction, however, is its incompatibility with an ethics of prudential deliberation and judgment. And, of course, the whole idea of intrinsically or necessarily im-moral actions is foreign to the prudential reasoning of Aristotle and Aquinas.

HELPFUL DISTINCTIONS

We turn now to a set of distinctions that can help us. These distinctions are not faultless, but they can nonetheless serve a useful purpose in moral reason-ing about health care issues.

Reasonable and Unreasonable

This will be a key distinction in our analysis. In moral matters the reasonable thing to do or not do will be the ethical thing to do or not do. The norm in the ethics of the good is reason. What is according to reason is ethical. What is unreasonable is unethical. There is never a situation where the ethical thing to do is unreasonable or the reasonable thing to do is unethical. As Aquinas put it: "Reason is the first principle (*primum principium*) of all human actions." Of course, we have to explain what according to reason means in this context. What, indeed, is reasonable in moral matters?

Put simply, the reasonable is whatever achieves what is truly good for us in the circumstances. If we are deliberately doing something that truly promotes living well, then we are acting reasonably. If we deliberately pursue a course of action opposed to our good, then we are not acting reasonably. Since our good is personal happiness, we can also say that the reasonable is whatever achieves our happiness in the circumstances, and the unreasonable is what undermines it. In practical matters, what is reasonable is determined, to the extent we can determine it, by the reasoning we have been calling prudence.

As we have already pointed out, it is not always easy to determine what is the reasonable or ethical thing to do in a particular situation. We have to acknowledge this and admit that ethics is not a science with definitive answers for every particular case. Moreover, health care ethics usually involves an added complexity, namely, most decisions involve at least two major moral agents: (1) the patient (or her proxy or proxies) and (2) the primary physician (and often several other providers as well).

In a time when the physician made the treatment choices on the basis of what he thought was good for the patient, he was the major (and often the only) moral agent. Today we recognize the patient (or proxy) as a major moral agent along with the physician. This plurality of moral agents adds a tremendous complication to many ethical situations in health care. Physician and patient may not reach the same conclusions about what is good.

In health care, therefore, moral agents not only have to figure out what to do about treatment but, since treatment is a joint effort involving a patient and a number of providers, what to do when there is disagreement on ethical matters among the several moral agents involved. What is the most ethical way to proceed when the physician and patient (or proxy) do not agree on what is the ethical way to proceed? This is an especially difficult problem for providers when they think that patients or proxies are not making reasonable and right decisions about life-sustaining treatment.

Nonetheless, despite the practical difficulties, the norm of ethics remains what is according to reason, where what is according to reason is understood as what will truly achieve the good, or at least avoid the worse, in the situation. If there is a moral conflict between patient and providers, it can only be resolved by figuring out what is reasonable in the circumstances. Hence, the distinction between reasonable and unreasonable is crucial and universal; it is no less than the distinction between the ethical and the unethical, the moral and the immoral.

Prudence and Judgment

Much of the literature on ethics fails to recognize the difference between prudence and moral judgment. As we saw in chapters one and two, prudence is the moral reasoning employed by a moral agent, that is, a person actually enmeshed in a situation and faced with deciding what to do or not do. It is the moral reasoning you and I employ when we are faced with a decision that we will have to carry out. Prudence tells us what to do in the actual situation in order to achieve our good.

Moral judgment, on the other hand, is the moral reasoning we employ when we are reviewing situations where we are not actually involved. Here we are not the moral agent. We are not going to do what we decide is the right thing to do, but we are making judgments about how we think the people actually involved will promote living well.

As was already noted, this means that the work we do in this book is not, strictly speaking, the work of prudence. We will be making moral judgments. However, the way we will go about making moral judgments about particular cases and the way we practice personal prudence are very similar, and thus what we said about prudence in the first chapters will apply also to the moral judgments we will make in later chapters. The two are so related that work in making moral judgments will enhance prudence, just as a highly developed prudence in our personal lives will enhance our ability to make good moral judgments about the situations confronting others.

In the later chapters where we examine particular cases, we will strengthen the similarity between prudence and moral judgment by considering each case from the perspectives of the various moral agents—patients, proxies, physicians, nurses, attorneys, administrators, judges, etc. This will make our moral judgments as close to prudence as possible, for we will ask what we would do if we were the patient, the proxy, the physician, etc., in the particular situation.

Descriptive Language and Evaluative Language

People often confuse description and evaluation when they speak and write about ethical matters. This is understandable because a purely descriptive natural language simply does not exist. The language we speak in life is always biased in some degree. Words, phrases, and sentences are always colored by social, historical, and personal perspectives.

Earlier in this century, some philosophers tried to escape the bias inherent in natural languages by developing a purely formal language using letters of the alphabet to stand for propositions. If you wanted to develop a logical argument, you would first make your language a series of propositions, and then use the letter "p" for the first proposition, "q" for the second, and so forth. Then you would join the propositions together in one of several clearly defined ways indicated by symbols. The idea was to develop a language of logical elegance and clarity, and to encourage people to "watch their p's and q's"; that is, to think and speak in a clearly defined and logical way. The result was a language that was mathematical in its precision and logic, but so narrow and impoverished that it was of little use in life. For this and other reasons the project was abandoned by everyone except specialists interested in its mathematical and logical features.

The desire for a purely descriptive language also arose in modern philosophy of science. Philosophers tried mightily to speak of pure facts in science. They attempted to show how the scientists' belief in the facts meant science was objective and represented things as they truly are, not as what we think they are.

Today, most philosophers of science acknowledge that there are no pure facts, that everything we perceive as fact is theory-laden, that facts cannot be perceived without a theoretical background that will, among other things, indicate what will be counted as a fact. Galileo saw moons circling Jupiter in 1610 and considered it a fact; his adversaries, whose biblical and Ptolemaic conceptions of the universe did not allow such facts, did not consider it a fact. And the fact that the shortest distance between two stars is not a straight line is not a fact for someone convinced that the axioms of Euclidean geometry apply to vast distances in real space. And the fact that minutes and hours pass slower on stars moving faster relative to our solar system is not a fact for someone convinced that the Newtonian concept of absolute time holds for all velocities, even velocities approaching the speed of light.

A purely descriptive or purely factual language is not really possible in the natural languages used in science, nor in the language of ethics. Nonetheless, we do need to strive in ethical reflection for language that is not overloaded with conceptual and evaluative biases. If we are going to talk intelligently about ethical issues we need to use language that, while admittedly not completely descriptive and factual, is essentially so. In ethics, we need to contrast this essentially descriptive language with language that is significantly evaluative. To do this we have to learn how to recognize language that looks descriptive but actually smuggles in moral judgments. Consider the following sentences.

1. John killed Jack.
2. John murdered Jack.

The structures of the two sentences are similar. They have the same "A did something to B" format, and both subjects and objects are identical. The verbs also share the same meaning—they indicate lethal actions. But from an ethical point of view the sentences are very dissimilar. The first is fundamentally descriptive. It describes an action—an action that causes death—but it does not evaluate that action. It does not tell us whether the killing was legal or illegal, moral or immoral. Perhaps Jack stumbled drunk onto a busy high speed road on a rainy night and John, despite driving carefully, struck and killed him. Perhaps John and Jack were soldiers fighting opposite each other in a war, and John fired the weapon that killed Jack. The first sentence tells us something bad happened, but does not tell us whether that something was moral or immoral. "John killed Jack" is an essentially descriptive sentence.

The second sentence is more than descriptive; it makes a moral judgment. Murder is a particular kind of killing. In law it is illegal killing and in morality it is immoral killing. The second sentence is essentially an evaluation, although it retains a descriptive component. It speaks not just of a killing, but of a killing that is illegal and immoral. When I say "John murdered Jack" I am saying (a) John killed Jack and (b) the killing was immoral and illegal. Unlike the first sentence, which describes an action without making a moral or legal judgment, the second sentence both describes an action and makes a moral and legal judgment. "John murdered Jack" is essentially a moral and legal evaluation; it is not a simple description.

The distinction between description and moral evaluation is important in discourse about controversial moral issues. Descriptive language enables people to deliberate and to discuss the issue, and then to move toward a thoughtful moral judgment. Evaluative language subverts moral deliberation and discussion about controversial issues by introducing moral judgments prematurely. True deliberation and discussion becomes impossible when the moral judgments are already made—we are not really deliberating when we have already made up our minds. When there are moral dilemmas or disagreements about what is moral, then people, regardless of their personal commitments, must step back from their evaluative language and use descriptive language to talk about the issue. Otherwise they are preaching to each other, or shouting at each other.

The importance of the distinction between descriptive and evaluative language is relatively easy to see in the example we gave, yet it is often confused in practice. In discussions about abortion, for example, opponents of it sometimes use the language of "murder" and "killing babies." In effect, this ends the moral discussion before it begins because everyone considers murder and deliberately killing babies immoral. The language of murder and killing babies is not a language of description—it is a language of moral evaluation.

On the other hand, advocates of choice in abortion sometimes describe abortion in terms of rights—the right to reproductive freedom, the right to privacy, the right to choose, etc. This also ends the moral discussion before it begins because most everyone favors personal rights and freedom for themselves. The language of rights and freedom is not a language of description, but a language of moral evaluation.

Another example where evaluative language occurs prematurely is in discussions about withdrawing life-sustaining treatments from seriously defective newborns with poor prognosis. On one side are people so dedicated to the infant's right to life that they view withdrawing life-sustaining treatment as killing babies. On the other side are people so sensitive to the burdens of invasive treatment with little benefit for the infant that they view providing it as child abuse. Both descriptions are loaded with moral evaluations, and thus hinder sound moral deliberation and judgment.

When we talk about controversial subjects such as abortion and treatment withdrawals from infants, we need a clear and morally neutral description of what happens. We need a language describing abortion as the termination of a pregnancy or, more exactly, as the destruction of a fetus. And we need to discuss what treatments are promoting what is truly good for the infant, and what treatments are not. Only then can we reason morally to determine whether or not we have adequate reasons for destroying a human fetus or withdrawing life-sustaining treatments from the child.

Intelligent discourse about the morality of any action subject to sincere and serious disagreement has to begin with relatively neutral descriptive language. Reflections on health care issues in the following chapters attempt to avoid heavily loaded evaluative language in favor of essentially descriptive language. Providing a good description, however, is not an easy task. As we pointed out, no description is completely neutral or clean from an evaluative standpoint. But some expressions are more prejudicial than others, and these we must try to avoid. Keeping the distinction between description and evaluation in mind can help us do this.

Bad and Immoral

Some theologians have recently introduced a distinction between what they call "premoral evil" (or nonmoral evil, or ontic evil) and moral evil. Premoral evil is anything harmful and damaging to life, especially human life. Moral evil is anything harmful and damaging to life arising from morally unreasonable human choice. Instead of using the language of premoral and moral evil, we will distinguish the bad and the immoral. We will call premoral evil (or nonmoral evil or ontic evil) bad, and we will call moral evil immoral or unethical.

The bad is not, of itself, immoral. It is simply bad, something we prefer not to happen. Sometimes these bad things arise from the dynamics of nature, perhaps a violent storm causes death or a virus makes me sick. Sometimes these bad things come from human behavior; perhaps someone accidently steps on my foot or perhaps someone intentionally does something causing me pain, but has a good reason. The bad things caused (1) by nature, or (2) by unintentional human behavior, or (3) by intentional human behavior with adequate reasons are not immoral. They are simply bad, and it is unfortunate that we have to deal with them in life.

Only the bad caused by intentional human behavior without adequate reasons is immoral. The immoral embraces only the bad things done (a) intentionally and (b) without a sufficient reason. Intentional actions or omissions giving rise to bad things without good reasons are what we mean by immoral or unethical behavior.

An obstetrician performing a cesarean section causes pain and damage to the woman's body, and these are bad things. If the surgery is done for a good reason—to prevent injury to the baby, for example—the action is morally reasonable. But if the surgery is not done for a good reason—if it is done chiefly for the convenience of the obstetrician, for example—then the surgery is not reasonable, the pain and damage are immoral, and the obstetrician behaves in an unethical way.

We are constantly doing things intentionally that cause bad things in our own lives as well as in the lives of others. We cannot live in the world without hurting people. Sometimes the soldier has to fight the enemy, sometimes the judge has to sentence a criminal, sometimes the dentist has to drill a tooth, sometimes a person has to break off a relationship, sometimes a parent has to say no, sometimes an employer has to fire an employee, and so forth. These actions all cause other people grief, but they are not immoral or unethical if the agents have sufficient reasons balancing the bad things they cause.

Only if we do not have sufficient reasons for causing bad things is our behavior unreasonable and immoral. Intentional behavior giving rise to bad things without sufficient reason is immoral because I can never achieve a truly good life by causing needless pain and suffering, or by damaging or destroying life unnecessarily.

The distinction between the bad and the immoral is a useful distinction. There are times when doing good things will cause bad things—injury, pain, and even death. The distinction between the bad and the immoral allows us to recognize that intentionally engaging in behavior that gives rise to bad things such as suffering and even death is not necessarily immoral. Morality centers on whether or not the suffering and death we cause are reasonable; that is, whether or not there are adequate reasons for doing or not doing whatever brings about the suffering or the death.

The ultimate moral issue is not whether someone suffers or even dies because suffering and dying, while bad, are not immoral. The ultimate moral issue arising from deliberate behavior giving rise to bad things is whether or not there are overriding reasons for allowing or causing the bad outcomes to occur. If we have overriding reasons for the suffering, injury, or death we cause, then we are acting according to reason and in a moral way; if not, we are acting unreasonably and in an immoral way.

Put simply, doing bad things to ourselves, to others, or to the environmental web of life we share with all the living becomes immoral if (1) done deliberately and (2) without a sufficient reason.

Removing nutrition, withholding life-sustaining treatment, destroying fetuses, and the like all involve insults to life. The ethical person will not bring them about . . . unless she concludes from her moral deliberation that she has substantial overriding reasons to do so. Morally good people strive never to cause any bad things; in fact, they try to prevent them whenever possible, but sometimes they cannot achieve a good life without damaging or even destroying life.

This suggests a practical guideline: Whenever what we are going to do, or not going to do but could do, will result in the bad (that is, will give rise to suffering or damage to life), then we will avoid the behavior unless there are overriding reasons not to avoid it. And the greater the bad, the stronger the overriding reasons have to be.

Although ethics is primarily a positive endeavor—it shows us the feelings, habits, and behaviors promoting happiness in our lives—a great deal of effort in ethics is devoted to becoming aware of the bad things arising from our intentional behavior, and to figuring out whether we have sufficient reasons for causing or allowing them to happen. This side of ethics is especially important in health care ethics, where much of what providers might do, or not do, causes pain, suffering, and even the risk of death in patients.

It is well to remember, however, that an ethics devoted only to avoiding the bad would be an impoverished ethics. An adequate health care ethics encourages us to promote the good whenever possible. It encourages us to behave with kindness, compassion, caring, justice, love, honesty, and the like, for this is how we live well and happily.

The purpose of this chapter is to simplify our work later on when we consider various topics in health care ethics. By taking these steps to clarify language, and to set aside some popular but potentially misleading distinctions, we sidestep a number of confusions haunting many recent discussions of ethical issues in health care.

We turn next to a topic of primary importance in health care ethics: Who decides what to do and how do they go about making their decisions?

SUGGESTED READINGS

Deciding to Forego Life-Sustaining Treatment (1983), a report of the President's Commission for the Study of Ethical Problems in Medicine and Biomedical and Behavioral Research (hereafter the "President's Commission"), noted that four distinctions (actions versus omissions leading to death, withholding versus withdrawing treatment, intended versus unintended but foreseeable consequences, and ordinary versus extraordinary treatment) are "inherently unclear" and that using them "is often so mechanical that it neither illuminates an actual case nor provides an ethically persuasive argument" (pp. 60–90).

The report also states, however, that variations of the distinction "intentionally cause death—let die," although often "conceptually unclear and of dubious moral importance," are useful in persuading people to accept sound decisions that would otherwise meet unwarranted resistance" (p. 71). There are strong reasons for disagreeing with this position. Good ethics is undermined by the use of unclear distinctions, and convincing someone to accept a sound decision by deliberately using unclear distinctions suggests manipulation, if not deception. See Raymond J. Devettere. "Reconceptualizing the Euthanasia Debate." *Law, Medicine & Health Care* **1989**, *17*, 145–55.

The moral value of the "ordinary—extraordinary" and "withhold—withdraw" distinctions is also challenged in the report of the Hastings Center entitled *Guidelines on the Termination of Life-Sustaining Treatment and the Care of the Dying*, pp. 5ff. The 1980 *Declaration on Euthanasia* issued by the Roman Catholic Church acknowledged that the "ordinary—extraordinary" distinction is "perhaps less clear" than it once was because it is imprecise and because of the rapid progress in treatment interventions. This document is printed as Appendix C in *Deciding to Forego Life-Sustaining Treatment* (1983).

Early legal decisions accepted the "ordinary—extraordinary" distinction (cf. *Matter of Quinlan*, 70 NJ 10 [1976] and *Superintendent of Belchertown State School v. Saikewicz*, 373 Mass 728, 738, 743–44 [1977]), but some more recent decisions either reject it or relegate it to a very minor place in the decision-making process. See, for example, *Matter of Conroy*, 98 NJ 371–72 (1985).

The distinction between "futility" and what could be called "utility" (that is, what would be effective treatment) is now the subject of intense debate. Daniel Callahan. "Medical Futility, Medical Necessity: The Problem Without a Name." *Hastings Center Report* **1991**, *21* (July), 30–35, frames the issue well. See also Robert Truog, A. S. Brett, and J. Frader. "The Problem with Futility." *NEJM* **1992**, *326*, 1560–64; Robert Truog. "Beyond Futility." *Journal of Clinical Ethics* **1992**, *3*, 143–45; and Stuart Youngner. "Who Defines Futility?" *JAMA* **1988**, *260*, 2094–95. Also helpful is a collection of seven articles on medical futility in *Law, Medicine & Health Care* **1992**, *20*, 307–39 and another collection of articles on futility in a special section of the *Cambridge Quarterly of Healthcare Ethics* **1993**, *2*, 142–227.

The direct–indirect distinction has been well-known in moral theology for centuries. Thomas Aquinas distinguished direct and indirect voluntary behavior in the *Summa Theologiae* I–II, q. 6, a. 3 and q. 77, a. 7, but his distinction is not the same as that used today. According to Aquinas, if I choose to steer the ship against the rocks, I *directly* cause the shipwreck, but if I decline to steer the drifting ship away from the rocks when I could and should have done so, then I *indirectly* cause the shipwreck. Later theologians, however, used the direct–indirect distinction in a different sense, usually in conjunction with the principle of double effect. Here, "direct" referred to the intended effect of the action and "indirect" to the unintended but foreseen effect. See Bruno Schuller, "Direct Killing/Indirect Killing" and Albert Di Ianni, "The Direct/Indirect Distinction in Morals," both in Charles Curran and Richard McCormick, ed. 1979. *Readings in Moral Theology No. 1*. New York: Paulist Press, pp. 138–57 and 215–43; and Richard McCormick, "Searching for the Consistent Ethic of Life," in Joseph Selling, ed. 1988. *Personalist Morals*. Leuven: Leuven University Press, pp. 135–46. A version of this essay also appeared as a symposium paper entitled "The Consistent Ethic of Life: Is There an Historical Soft Underbelly?" in Thomas Fuechtmann, ed. 1988. *Consistent Ethic of Life*. Kansas City: Sheed & Ward, pp. 96–122.

John Dedek has provided a good introduction to the development of the doctrine of intrinsically immoral actions in several articles. See his "Moral Absolutes in the Predecessors of St. Thomas," *Theological Studies* **1977**, *38*, 654–80; "Intrinsically

Evil Acts: An Historical Study of the Mind of St. Thomas," *Thomist* **1979**, 43, 385–13; and "Intrinsically Evil Acts: The Emergence of a Doctrine," *Recherches de Theologie Ancienne et Medievale* **1983**, 50, 191–226. See also Josef Fuchs. 1984. *Christian Ethics in a Secular Arena*, trans. Bernard Hoose and Brian McNeil. Washington: Georgetown University Press, chapter 5, entitled, "An Ongoing Discussion in Christian Ethics: Intrinsically Evil Acts?"; and Charles Curran, ed. 1968. *Absolutes in Moral Theology?* Washington: Corpus, especially Curran's own essay, "Absolute Norms and Medical Ethics," pp. 108–53.

Aristotle's examples of feelings and actions that are immoral by definition, and therefore beyond the scope of prudential reasoning in particular situations, are the feelings of spite, shamelessness, and envy; and the actions of adultery, theft, and homicide. See the *Nicomachean Ethics* 1107a9–26. It is important to note the importance of feelings in an ethics of the good life. Feelings of spite, shamelessness, and envy do not promote my well-being; they do not make me happy. They are, therefore, always immoral by definition.

One of the best recent introductions to Kant's complex and seminal ethical theory is Roger Sullivan. 1989. *Immanuel Kant's Moral Theory*. Cambridge: Cambridge University Press. As Sullivan points out, Kant had a very dim view of human sexuality. The sexually sensual and the erotic were simply lust in his mind, a manifestation of our animal appetites. Only the preservation of the race in marriage justified engaging in sexual behavior. Kant is not even clear on whether married couples could have intercourse when pregnancy is impossible, but he does suggest that sex in such circumstances, something "certainly unallowed," might be allowed "to prevent some greater transgression (as an indulgence)." See Kant, *The Metaphysics of Morals* in Kant. 1983. *Ethical Philosophy*, trans. James Ellington. Indianapolis: Hackett, p. 87. Kant's ethic of duty runs throughout this work.

Kant is especially vehement in his condemnation of homosexuality and masturbation, which he considers both contrary to reason (the moral law) and contrary to nature as well, and contraception, which is contrary to the purpose of our sexual organs. According to him, these actions degrade us below the level of animals which, he said, avoid any of these behaviors. He thought masturbation, homosexuality, and contraception were actually worse than suicide. At least suicide, he says, requires courage, and where there is courage there can be some respect. But in masturbation, homosexuality, and contraception there is no courage, merely a "weak surrender to animal pleasure." See above the *The Metaphysics of Morals*, pp. 85–88, and 1963. *Lectures on Ethics*. trans. Louis Infield. New York: Harper Torchbooks, pp. 162–71. After reading Kant's dim view of sexual behavior and of marriage ("It is by marriage that woman becomes free; man loses his freedom in it," cited by Sullivan, *Kant's Moral Theory*, p. 355), learning he was a lifelong bachelor comes as no surprise.

The idea that ethics is doing what is reasonable recalls Aquinas' remark that "reason is the first principle of all human action," found in the *Summa Theologiae* I II, q. 58, a. 2. For both Aquinas and Aristotle, the ethical is what they repeatedly claim is according to right reason, and it clear from the contexts that the right reason is prudential reasoning or prudence. This does not contradict the idea that my personal good is the first principle of ethics, because my good and reason are understood in terms of each other. The morally reasonable is what achieves my good, and whatever achieves my good is the morally reasonable. Hence to say my good or happiness is the first principle of ethics, or to say behaving according to reason is the first principle of ethics, is to say the same thing in two different ways.

It should again be noted that some translations of Aristotle and Aquinas tran
their respective phrases *kata ton orthon logon* and *secundum rectam rationem* in
misleading way as "according to the right principle" or "according to the right
rule," thus suggesting (incorrectly) that Aristotle and Aquinas advocated a principle-based or rule-based morality much like we find in an ethics of obligation
today. These phrases should be translated as "according to right reason," and
the context makes it clear that the right reason for ethics is prudential reason,
not deductive reason relying on laws, principles, or rules.

The distinction between description and evaluation in natural language is actually
much more complicated than it appears, as J. L. Austin. 1975. *How to Do Things
with Words*, second edition. Cambridge: Harvard University Press, reminds us.
See especially lectures XI and XII.

For background to the distinction between the bad and the immoral, see Louis Janssens.
"Ontic Evil and Moral Evil." *Louvain Studies* **1972,** 4, 115–56, reprinted in Curran
and McCormick. 1979. *Readings in Moral Theology*, No. 1. New York: Paulist, pp.
40–93. Josef Fuchs speaks of "premoral evil" in *Personal Responsibility and Christian
Morality*. Washington: Georgetown University Press, 1983, pp. 136–39, while
Richard McCormick prefers "nonmoral evil" in "Notes on Moral Theology."
Theological Studies **1976,** 37, 76–78. See also Bernard Hoose. 1987. *Proportionalism.*
Washington: Georgetown University Press, especially chapter 2.

ɔlth Care Decisions

Decisions about health care are complex. Various people have legitimate claims to making decisions about health care, and one of them, the patient, may be so affected by medical problems that making good decisions is unlikely or impossible. Moreover, many medical interventions involve moral as well as medical deliberations, and ethical concerns further complicate the decision-making. In the first section of the chapter, we will examine the complexity inherent in making health care decisions.

In the second part, we will consider the capacity of the patient to make decisions, how it is determined, and what constitutes it. Next, we will examine informed consent, the most distinctive feature of health care decision making. Then, we will consider the various advance directives that a patient can make to retain authority if he should lose the capacity to make decisions. Finally, we will discuss the Patient Self-Determination Act.

COMPLEXITY OF HEALTH CARE DECISIONS

The complexity arises from three main sources: (1) both the physician and the patient are involved in making decisions, and they may disagree about the proper medical treatment; (2) the patient's ability to make decisions may be lost or limited; and (3) health care decisions often involve important moral issues, and good clinical decisions are not always good moral decisions.

Disagreements Between Physician and Patient

As was noted in chapter 3, for a long time it was taken for granted that the physician should make the decisions about treatment. This is known as medical paternalism. When it was operative, there were seldom disagreements between physician and patient because the physician made the decisions unilaterally. More recently, some have reacted to this paternalism by proposing the principle of patient autonomy or patient self-determination, and by encouraging patients' rights. This movement makes the patient the primary decision maker. It also sets the stage for conflict because physicians cannot abdicate their responsibility for the medical treatment they provide, or can provide, for their patient.

We now recognize that neither medical paternalism nor patient autonomy provide the best in health care decisions. Medical paternalism, however well motivated, disenfranchises the patient. On the other hand, patient autonomy, however well grounded in a person's right to choose what happens to him, disenfranchises the physician.

Today a new conception of health care decision-making is gaining credence, one that avoids the extremes of both paternalism and autonomy. This new conception, supported by the President's Commission reports entitled *Making Health Care Decisions* and *Deciding to Forego Life-Sustaining Treatment*, is called "shared decision making." It envisions the patient and the physician deciding together how care can be managed best. It tries to combine the best of both worlds—the physician's expertise and the patient's values. The process of making the decision becomes a shared process, a partnership between the patient and the physician. In shared decision making, the answer to the question "who decides?" is "the patient *and* the physician."

Shared decision making in any field, however, is a complex phenomenon. Sometimes it runs smoothly, but the potential for conflict is always present. The physician may want something done, but the patient refuses. And the patient may want something done, but the physician refuses, perhaps because it is not good medical practice, or illegal, or unethical. Even in shared decision making, then, each participant retains autonomy. Patients can always refuse the proposed medical intervention, and physicians can always refuse to practice bad medicine or to behave immorally.

Although the center of the shared decision-making process is the patient–physician relationship, the sharing in the decisions often extends to a wider circle, and this complicates matters even more. On the patient's side, family members frequently play a major role in the health care decisions. On the physician's side, other providers are frequently consulted and may share directly in the decision.

Limitations Affecting the Patient's Ability to Make Health Care Decisions

There are four major ways a patient's role in making effective health care decisions can be limited or lost. First, the patient's capacity to make, or to make known, her decisions may be lost or diminished. She may become unconscious, or be conscious but so overwhelmed by medication, disease, pain, or confusion that she is not really capable of making decisions or, if she can make them, of communicating them to the physicians. If a patient loses the capacity to make or to communicate decisions, a proxy or surrogate will normally step in and try to speak for the patient. We will consider decision making by proxies or surrogates in the next chapter. If a patient retains decision-making capacity, but it has been diminished by age or illness, enabling him to play an appropriate role in the decision making can become very challenging for the physicians, nurses, and family.

Second, when a person becomes a patient he enters an environment where other people are also making decisions about his care. Not only physicians but nurses, other providers, and the institution itself have a say in what they do because they are responsible for their actions. At times, their disagreement will limit the patient's ability to make an effective decision.

Sometimes this conflict can be resolved by communication and negotiation, but occasionally the disagreement persists. For example, a patient imminently dying from widespread cancer may insist on cardiopulmonary resuscitation when he suffers the expected arrest, but the physicians and nurses responsible for performing the CPR may be convinced that attempting resuscitation is medically inappropriate and not want to do it. If they are convinced that it would be medically and morally wrong for them to attempt resuscitation, they cannot do it in good conscience. If the patient insists on resuscitation efforts, their only alternative is to transfer the patient to other providers. In practice, however, this may not be possible at the moment. Thus, it is not inconceivable that providers will have to tell the patient that they will not attempt resuscitation if the arrest occurs while he is under their care. The providers' refusal of treatment limits the patient's ability to make an effective decision about his treatment.

Third, as we will see, the law sometimes restricts a patient's ability to make effective decisions about health care. By "law" we mean two things: legislation and the court decisions constituting the tradition of case law. Thus, a patient may want a physician to kill her by a lethal overdose, but the law forbids it, so the physician refuses. And the single mother of young children may want to refuse a blood transfusion for religious reasons, but a court may overrule her decision lest the children lose their only parent.

Finally, much of health care in the United States is not paid for by the patient, but by third-party payers, most notably Medicare, the Veterans Administration, the military health care system, Medicaid welfare programs, and various private health insurance plans and health maintenance organizations (HMOs). Any of these payers can effectively restrict the patient's ability to make effective decisions about a particular treatment by refusing to fund it when the patient has no other way to pay for it. If an insurance company declines to pay for the surgery a patient wants, this will override the patient's decision, and the physician's as well, if the patient cannot afford to pay for the surgery himself or is unable to find another funding source.

Potential Conflict Between Clinical and Ethical Goals

Almost every health care decision has two goals. One goal is to decide what will be good health care for the patient. This is often an enormously complicated question—it is not always easy to know what is good patient care. We are tempted to say that good patient care is treating to cure disease and preserve life, and this is true is most cases, but not always. Sometimes good care consists in declining or discontinuing treatment because the interventions cause more burdens than any possible benefits they could provide. When this happens the goal is not cure but comfort, not mindless preservation of life, but recognition of medicine's inherent limitations.

The second goal is to decide what will be morally good for the patient and for the providers. Health care decisions are seldom simply about treatment; morality almost always intrudes. This is so because most treatments have risks and harmful side effects, and the need for reasons to justify causing these bad features is a main concern of ethics. Patients and physicians have to decide not only what is good medical care, but what is ethical care, given the circumstances.

The clinical and moral goals sometimes conflict because clinical practice is not identical with clinical ethics. The goal of clinical practice is the good considered as good clinical outcome; the goal of clinical ethics is the good considered as good ethical outcome. The right clinical decision is often the right moral decision, but not always. Transplanting black-market kidneys bought from desperate and impoverished people, for example, might be the best clinical outcome for patients needing the kidneys but, from an ethical point of view, good reasons exist for saying that the implantation of black-market kidneys is immoral. The potential clash between clinical and ethical goals is one more reason why making health care decisions can become so complex.

These, then, are some of the factors that give rise to the complexity inherent in decisions about health care. Next, we turn to an examination of the most essential condition that must be present before a patient can make a health care decision—capacity. By decision-making capacity we mean the ability to make thoughtful and voluntary decisions about health care. Decision-making capacity is a major issue when patients participate in decision making because the dysfunction that makes them patients may very well also limit or undermine their ability to make important decisions. Determining whether or not a patient has decision-making capacity is one of the more important, and difficult, challenges facing physicians and nurses.

DECISION-MAKING CAPACITY

Decision-making capacity in health care is the ability to make reasonable decisions about what to do when confronted with disease, injury, and pain. In a general sense, providers as well as patients need to have decision-making capacity, but we will consider this capacity only in patients. We presume the physicians and other providers have the capacity to make decisions.

Many authors use the word "competence" or "competent" to describe what we are calling decision-making capacity. Using competence to indicate decision-making capacity could be misleading because competence has long been used in a precise legal sense. Our legal system normally assumes an adult is competent unless a court has ruled otherwise. Obviously, then, the legal meaning of competence and what we mean by decision-making capacity are not the same. Many adult patients not declared incompetent by a court do not have the capacity to make decisions about their health care.

Clear examples of patients without the capacity to make informed and voluntary decisions include children, the unconscious, many with mental illness, etc. In many cases, however, the lack of capacity is not so clear. Although it is wise to begin by presuming conscious adults have decision-making capacity, we know that some of them do not have it, and that others will have to make decisions for them. Physicians have the difficult task of determining whether or not their patients have decision-making capacity. This determination is a serious matter because, once a physician determines a patient is incapable of making decisions about his health care, she in effect disenfranchises him of his prerogative to make what could be very important decisions about his life. We need, therefore, a clear understanding of this decision-making capacity.

Capacity is the ability to do something specific; it is related to a particular task. A blind person lacks the capacity to drive a car, but not to hear a symphony. In health care, our interest is chiefly in the capacity or ability of patients to perform a particular task—to make their health care decisions. This capacity for making health care decisions is very specific. Some patients may have the capacity for making health care decisions but not for making other decisions—decisions about their finances, for example. Some patients may retain the capacity to make health care decisions despite psychiatric disorders or organic mental disabilities that leave them confused about other things. And some patients may have the capacity to make some treatment decisions but not others, or the capacity to make treatment decisions at some times but not all the time.

The capacity for making health care decisions has three aspects, and all three must be present for us to say that the patient has decision-making capacity.

1. *Understanding.* Decision-making capacity means a patient can understand relevant information about the disease, the treatment options, and the recommendations of the physician. It also means he is able to communicate with providers.
2. *Evaluation.* Decision-making capacity means a patient has some framework of values that will enable him to judge whether a particular health care decision will accomplish what he considers good for himself.
3. *Reasoning.* Decision-making capacity means a patient can deliberate and reason about how all available courses of action will likely affect him. This implies he can grasp cause–effect relationships, notions of probability and percentages, and the basic form of "if X, then Y" reasonings.

A question that frequently arises is whether or not a patient can be "partially" capable of making a health care decision; that is, whether or not there are degrees of capacity. Experience certainly suggests that there are degrees of capacity. A person's capacity for decision-making could diminish for any number of reasons, and yet not be totally lost. This suggests that we could say some people have a "partial capacity" for making health care decisions.

This may seem like a wise move, but in practice it is not. For practical reasons, it is important to draw a sharp line between decision-making capacity and incapacity. Capacity is an either–or situation: either the patient has decision-making capacity for this situation, or she does not have it.

If we did not draw a sharp line between capacity and incapacity, we could never determine just who has the final responsibility for making the decision about the patient's care—the patient or the proxy. If the patient is capable, the patient has final responsibility for deciding; if the patient is not capable, the proxy has the final responsibility. If we embrace the notion of "partial capacity," the physician would be placed in an untenable position. She would not know whether to accept the decisions of the patient with "partial capacity" or those of the proxy. Only by making a sharp dividing line between capacity and incapacity can we determine who ultimately decides— the patient or the patient's proxy.

Capacity is thus a threshold notion, and a patient is on one side or the other. We cannot think of someone as straddling the threshold between capacity and incapacity. The physician determines whether a particular patient has, or does not have, the capacity to make a particular decision at a particular time.

The major question emerging from considering capacity a threshold notion is just how diminished any of the three aspects of capacity (understanding, evaluating, and reasoning) must be before a patient has crossed the threshold from capacity to incapacity. Ultimately this determination is, as the President's Commission noted, a matter of personal judgment based on common sense. And as we will see in the next chapter, the physician has the responsibility of making this judgment about his or her patient.

However, physicians should not judge patients incapable of making decisions simply because they make a decision that is idiosyncratic or at variance with what the physician thinks is best. For example, a few people routinely refuse blood for religious reasons. Their decision to refuse a treatment almost everyone else considers reasonable is not a reason for their physicians to conclude they have lost the capacity for making health care decisions. In other words, a decision most would consider unreasonable does not automatically mean the person making it lacks capacity. People with capacity can make unreasonable decisions, and they can make mistakes. Conversely, people can make reasonable decisions, yet not have decision-making capacity. We cannot use the outcome of the decision process, the decision itself, as evidence that the person has, or does not have, decision-making capacity.

On the other hand, when patients decide on something that physicians and other providers think is unnecessarily dangerous or obviously unreasonable given the circumstances, it is certainly a warning flag. Physicians concerned about their patient's well-being will be moved to probe deeper into the decision-making process and to question the person's capacity. The more harmful the decision, the more carefully the physician will investigate the issue of capacity when the decision appears unreasonable. An unreasonable decision is not a reason for saying the person does not have capacity, but it is a reason for investigating more carefully the presumption of capacity.

Perhaps the easiest case where providers can accept what they consider an unreasonable decision is when the decision is based on tenets of a sincerely held religious faith. Most everyone considers a patient's commitment to a recognized religious faith an appeal that outweighs all other reasons for using life-saving treatment. Thus many physicians and nurses would consider the refusal of blood in the face of death by a practicing Jehovah's Witness an unreasonable decision from a medical perspective, but not something that they should question because it is based on a sincerely held religious faith.

It is more difficult for physicians and nurses to accept other appeals that patients might use to justify their refusal of reasonable treatment necessary to preserve life. Sometimes paternalistic intervention may be appropriate, sometimes not, and usually only those on the scene can make the right decision. Imagine, for example, a man with a history of heart attacks suddenly having symptoms of another attack as he plays golf. His golfing partners are concerned and want to call an ambulance, but he refuses because he wants to finish the hole. He has not lost the capacity to make a health care decision, although he is certainly making a stupid one. Imagine also that a physician is playing with him, and he knows that a serious situation is developing. One hopes the physician would act in a paternalistic way, ignore the man's refusal to summon paramedics, and take the necessary steps to save his life. Refusing medical help for a life-threatening heart attack in order to finish playing a hole in golf simply does not carry the same weight as refusing life-saving treatment for religious reasons.

When a patient with decision-making capacity makes an unusual decision for reasons the providers believe are trivial, they must respond with a great deal of what we have called prudence. If the patient persists in his position, they must decide whether it is ethical for them to respect the decision, to override it, or to withdraw from the case. Withdrawing from the case is preferable to overriding a patient's request, but withdrawal is not always possible. When no other physician is available and willing to accept responsibility for the care of the patient, an attending physician cannot abandon a patient. This presents, as we saw in the example of the patient dying with cancer who wants resuscitation attempted, a difficult situation for the providers.

In summary, then, we want to remember the following key points about capacity:

1. We begin by presuming conscious adult patients have the capacity to make health care decisions. This assumption ceases when there is evidence that the capacity does not exist, and the physician determines that it is indeed lacking.
2. The capacity for making health care decisions has three aspects: (1) the ability to understand and communicate, (2) the ability to deliberate and reason about alternative courses of action, and (3) the ability to evaluate what is good.
3. Capacity is a threshold notion. It must be determined that a patient either has, or does not have, decision-making capacity for a particular option at a particular time. However, capacity may come and go, and capacity may exist for some decisions, but not for others.
4. An unreasonable decision does not by itself indicate decision-making incapacity, nor does a reasonable decision indicate capacity. However, an obviously unreasonable decision, especially when serious harm will result, should trigger a more extensive probing into the question of the patient's capacity.

One of the most important things a patient with decision-making capacity does is give informed consent for medical interventions. We turn now to an examination of this important concept.

INFORMED CONSENT

Informed consent is a major feature of twentieth century health care. Most of us encounter it for the first time when we need some kind of surgical or medical intervention. A health care provider, usually the physician, explains the medical problem to us, the various options we have, a recommended treatment to correct the problem, and the risks involved in the interventions. We then sign a form indicating our consent for the procedure.

Many patients and providers alike confuse the signing of this form with the reality of giving informed consent. Patients often think they are giving consent by signing the form, and providers often think they are getting informed consent by having it signed. Actually, informed consent has little to do with signing a form. We should think of the signed form as the documentation of informed consent, something we need for the records, but not the informed consent itself.

Informed consent is a personal exchange between physician and patient. The physician provides information so the patient becomes "informed," and the patient then "consents" to the proposed treatment. This interaction between physician and patient constitutes the reality of informed consent. The signed form is the record that this interaction did indeed occur, but it is not the informed consent itself.

Where did the notion of informed consent originate? Undoubtedly its origins are as old as medicine. People got sick, knew that physicians might be able to alleviate the illness, and turned to them for help. This seeking of medical aid implied the afflicted person was somewhat informed about what physicians do and was willing to have it done to them. Moreover, we can easily suppose that many physicians said something to their patients about what they thought was the problem, and what they were going to do about it, before they intervened. We have no historical evidence to suggest that physicians routinely invaded people's lives and forced treatment on them every time they became sick. People knew something about treatments and sought out persons skilled in providing them. This is a long way from the doctrine of informed consent as we now know it, but it does remind us that many patients were getting some information and giving something of consent long before "informed consent" became the popular doctrine it is today.

The modern doctrine of informed consent emerged from several developments over the past few centuries. The modern liberal philosophy of personal rights and liberties certainly provided an important philosophical background. More recently, there has been an understandable reaction to the institutionalization of medicine in hospitals. Informed consent was not as necessary when physicians visited homes. Patients had more control in their homes than they do in hospitals, and they knew more about the traditional remedies than they know about the advanced life-prolonging techniques and technologies associated with modern hospitals.

The most important source of today's doctrine of informed consent, however, is not philosophical or sociological, but legal. Informed consent as we know it today originated in the courts. Several landmark decisions played a key role in making informed consent a fact of life in health care, and reviewing these decisions will help us to understand more clearly the meaning of informed consent.

The Legal History of Informed Consent

We will consider four of the landmark legal decisions that shaped the doctrine of informed consent into the reality so familiar to us today.

The Schloendorff decision (New York, 1914)

Mrs. Schloendorff had steadfastly insisted, despite her physician's recommendation, that she did not want surgery to remove a fibroid tumor. She did agree that he could administer ether and perform an abdominal examination to determine whether or not it was malignant. The physician was so concerned about the tumor that he removed it while she was under the anesthesia.

She sued for damages but did not prevail because no serious harm ensued. However, Justice Cardozo's decision contains one of the most quoted sentences in the legal history of informed consent:

> Every human being of adult years and sound mind has a right to determine what shall be done with his own body; and a surgeon who performs an operation without his patient's consent commits an assault, for which he is liable in damages.

This was not the first time the key word "consent" appeared in court decisions about medical treatment. Almost a decade earlier, decisions in two cases (*Mohr v. Williams*, 1905, and *Pratt v. Davis*, 1905, affirmed 1906) stated that a citizen's first right, the right to himself, forbids physicians and surgeons from violating his bodily integrity without his consent. But the Schloendorff decision attracted considerable attention. Justice Cardozo was a well-known jurist and his language was clear, even eloquent. Most of all, it was ominous: it spoke of an operation without consent as an "assault," and said the surgeon was liable for damages.

The Schloendorff decision made people more aware of the legal requirement for consent, but this was still a long way from informed consent. Although the decision called for consent, it said nothing about *informed* consent. Consent can be uninformed or misinformed (perhaps we could say "disinformed," as in "disinformation"). Consent is uninformed when the patient consents to a procedure without receiving enough information to know what will happen to him, or, if he did receive information, did not understand it. Consent is misinformed when the patient has been misled about what will happen. The notion of *informed* consent did not appear until a California case more than forty years after the Schloendorff decision.

The Salgo decision (California, 1957)

Mr. Salgo had consented to a translumbar aortography, a diagnostic procedure intended to locate the cause of the chronic pain in his leg. The procedure involved the injection of a dye to give the pictures greater clarity. Unfortunately, the procedure caused paralysis in his legs. He sued the Stanford University hospital. His attorneys initially argued that the physicians were negligent in doing the procedure. Later, they added the argument that the physicians had failed to provide their client with information about the risks of the diagnostic procedure.

The trial court ruled in favor of Stanford University, and Mr. Salgo's attorneys appealed. The California Court of Appeals reversed the lower court's decision. In the ruling favoring the patient, the court used, for the first time in a major legal decision, the now well-known phrase "informed consent."

The story of how these famous words "informed consent" appeared in the decision is of interest. The judge writing the decision was struggling with two important values. He wanted to protect the right of patients to know what might happen to them in medical procedures. He also wanted to respect the discretion of physicians and enable them to use their best judgment when they discuss the risks of a procedure with patients. Obviously, if the physicians describe in great detail every possible bad outcome or side effect or risk associated with a procedure, some patients will be so frightened they will decline truly beneficial interventions.

One organization very interested in protecting the right of physicians to use discretion in telling patients about risks associated with surgery was the American College of Surgeons. It submitted an *amicus curiae* (friend of the court) brief to the judge in which it argued that, although physicians did need to disclose all the facts, they also needed to use discretion when discussing risks. The College of Surgeons, of course, was hoping the judge would not find the physicians had acted improperly when they failed to tell Martin Salgo about the risk of paralysis.

The court of appeals did not agree—it decided in favor of Mr. Salgo. And in an ironic twist, the judge writing the opinion in favor of the patient used the language of the *amicus curiae* brief submitted to support the physicians. In so doing, the phrase "informed consent" literally jumped into the everyday language of health care. The famous words in the Salgo decision, words first found in the brief submitted to the court by the College of Surgeons, are:

> . . . (I)n discussing the element of risk a certain amount of discretion must be employed consistent with the full disclosure of facts necessary to an informed consent.

The decision recognized that physicians must use discretion in telling patients about risks lest they frighten them, but said this discretion cannot undermine the patient's need to know the facts. If patients do not know the facts, including facts about risks, they cannot give *informed* consent to the procedure. Mr. Salgo's consent was not truly informed because he had not received all the facts about the risks. The court found the patient's need to know outweighed the physician's effort to be discreet.

This decision made it clear that consent to a medical procedure is not enough. The consent must be informed; that is, physicians must fully disclose the facts. Any recourse by the physician to discretion is strictly limited to what will not undermine this disclosure of the facts necessary to give an informed consent. It is not an exaggeration to say that informed consent, as we know it today, was born in California in 1957.

Of course, like any neonate, the legal doctrine of informed consent was not yet mature. Other cases would follow, and their findings would contribute to its development. We will mention two of these cases. The first one is considered by many to be almost as important as *Schloendorff* and *Salgo*.

The Canterbury decision (District of Columbia, 1972)

In 1959, nineteen year old Jerry Canterbury was suffering from back pain. After a myelogram his surgeon told him he would need surgery to correct a suspected ruptured disk. On the day after the surgery, Mr. Canterbury slipped off the bed while trying to urinate. He became paralyzed from the waist down.

Emergency surgery that night reversed some of the paralysis but left him dependent on crutches and with chronic urologic problems. He sued the hospital and the surgeon, but the judge in the district court ordered a directed verdict: he told the jury it must find in favor of the hospital and physician. Attorneys for Canterbury appealed. The U.S. Court of Appeals sent the case back to district court and ordered a full trial where a jury could hear the evidence and make its own decision. In an ironic twist, the subsequent jury trial also resulted in a decision exonerating the hospital and the surgeon.

What is important for the legal history of informed consent, however, was the position taken by the court of appeals when it sent the case back to the lower court for trial. One of the charges against the surgeon was that he had failed to inform the patient of the risk of paralysis. The court had to acknowledge that it was not clear whether the surgery or the fall had caused the paralysis, but it insisted that this uncertainty did not change the fact that the surgeon might have failed in his duty to disclose the risk. The court then set forth some "first principles" to guide physicians in telling patients about available treatments and their associated risks. Four of those principles provide a richer understanding of informed consent.

1. The "root premise" that every human being has a right to determine what shall be done with his or her body means the person needs whatever information is necessary to make an intelligent decision. The physician has a duty to disclose the information a patient needs for an intelligent decision, even if the patient does not ask for it.
2. The physician's duty to disclose information about all the options and their risks is not something the medical profession itself determines. There is a difference between treatment and disclosure. The standards of the medical profession determine what is appropriate treatment. But the medical profession does not determine what is the appropriate disclosure about medical treatment. This is determined by the more general standard of what is "reasonable under the circumstances."
3. The question of what is "reasonable under the circumstances" is a tricky one. Ideally, the physician must disclose whatever the particular patient would find relevant to his decision. In practice, however, this is a difficult standard because it is impossible for physicians to know what each individual patient would consider relevant to his decision.

Hence the standard of disclosure is more general; it is what a "reasonable person" in the patient's position would consider relevant in deciding whether to give or to withhold consent for treatment.

4. There are two exceptions to the duty to disclose: first, emergencies where treatment is needed and circumstances do not allow disclosure; second, rare situations where disclosure would present a threat to the patient's well-being because of the adverse reactions it would cause.

The Canterbury decision clearly set forth what we now recognize as the two crucial aspects of informed consent. It insisted on *consent* because the patients have the right to control what providers do to their bodies, and it insisted on *information* because patients cannot make intelligent decisions unless they know all the options and the associated risks. If patients are going to consent intelligently they require information, and it is the responsibility of physicians to furnish it. And the standard of how much information has to be disclosed is not determined by what the physician thinks is relevant, but by the "reasonable person" standard, that is, by what a reasonable person in the patient's position would consider relevant.

All this seems so simple today, but the philosophy supporting informed consent is not the philosophy we find in the influential Hippocratic Oath. The Hippocratic tradition encouraged the physician to do whatever he thought was best for the patient. Informed consent, on the other hand, empowers a patient to accept what she thinks is best, and this may not be what the physician, a nurse, or even a judge thinks is best. Informed consent can, therefore, sometimes collide with the medical beneficence advocated in the Hippocratic tradition.

Before we leave the legal history of informed consent, we will look at a case where a court acknowledged the prerogative of a patient with decision-making capacity to decide against life-saving surgery when her daughter, her physicians, and the court all thought her decision was wrong.

The Candura decision (Massachusetts, 1978)

Mrs. Candura had gangrene in her leg, and her physicians recommended amputation without delay. She was properly informed and consented to the surgery, but then she changed her mind. Her daughter went to probate court, asking to be appointed her mother's guardian with the authority to give consent for the surgery. The probate court granted her request, but the guardian *ad litem*, the person designated by the court to speak for Mrs. Candura's interests in the case, appealed the daughter's appointment as guardian.

The Court of Appeals reversed the probate court action. It said that the daughter cannot be the guardian and give consent for the surgery because there is no evidence that her mother is incompetent. The court acknowledged that most people would regard Mrs. Candura's refusal of the life-sustaining surgery as unfortunate. Nonetheless, it is an informed decision (the court said "it is not the uninformed decision of a person incapable of appreciating the nature and consequences of her act") and this informed refusal of treatment must be honored. If it were not, then physicians would be forcing treatment on her without her consent. In short, the "law protects her right to make her own decision to accept or reject treatment, whether that decision is wise or unwise."

This case shows the important reverse side of informed consent. The legal doctrine means patients must be informed so they can consent to treatment but also so they can refuse treatment. The ability to give consent implies the ability to withhold consent. When people have decision-making capacity, their decisions must be respected. Family members may consider the decision unwise and irrational, but that is not grounds for overriding their wishes. As the court wisely stated: "the irrationality of her decision does not justify a conclusion that Mrs. Candura is incompetent in the legal sense." Nor, we might add, does an irrational decision necessarily mean a person is without decision-making capacity in the ethical sense.

The Ethics of Informed Consent

The legal background of informed consent sets forth the two major elements of the informed consent doctrine: information and consent. We will now consider these elements in a wider moral context.

Information

What information must the physician disclose and discuss, and what information must the patient be able to understand and discuss, for the consent to treatment to be an informed consent?

1. Physicians will tell patients their medical diagnosis, and the prognosis if nothing is done. In other words, physicians must be sure their patients understand what is wrong and what will happen if it is not treated.

2. Physicians will tell patients about all the medically accepted treatment options for their condition, as well as the risks, burdens, and benefits associated with each. There is a temptation for physicians to neglect disclosure of the burdens because they are naturally reluctant to discuss comprehensively the burdens and possible side effects of interventions that they feel the patient really needs. Yet the patient needs this information if her consent is going to be truly informed. The requirement that physicians disclose all medically accepted treatments also means that the physician may have to provide information about treatments he does not favor or cannot provide.

3. Physicians will also recommend a treatment plan and give the reasons why they think it is best for the patient. One of the physicians' roles is giving professional advice, and patients rightly expect this. Often a patient will ask: "What would you do in my situation?" or "What do you think is best?" The responses to these kinds of questions allow an important conversation to take place, and provide the basis for a truly shared decision. It is not really adequate for a physician to do no more than lay out the options and let the patient decide; she must participate with the patient in the decision, and this means informing him of her opinion if she has one.

Consent

Consent requires a certain degree of freedom. If you point a gun at the cashier and tell him to hand over the money in the cash register, most likely he will give you the money. Obviously, we would not say he truly consented to giving you the money; he decided to give it to you because he was threatened by the gun and fearful of getting shot. We can truly consent to something only when we have significant freedom to accept or reject it. This means consent in health care must not be forced, coerced, or manipulated.

1. Treatment is *forced* when it is given without consent to a patient capable of giving informed consent. In this day and age of informed consent, it might seem forced treatment is a thing of the past, and to a great extent this is true. But subtle forms of forced treatment can still happen. Suppose a hospice patient wants his Do Not Resuscitate order followed in the operating room. During the subsequent operation, he suffers cardiopulmonary arrest. If the physicians attempt resuscitation, they are forcing treatment on him against his will, and this is unethical. If the surgeons had operated on Mrs. Candura against her wishes, that would have been another example of forced treatment.

2. Treatment is *coerced* when it is given to a patient who gives consent but not freely. The person is under so much pressure to give consent that the consent is not freely given. Usually the coercion is accomplished by some kind of threat, as when the cashier was threatened by the gun. Coercion is rare in health care, but it sometimes occurs. A husband might threaten to leave his wife unless she has an abortion, for example. She may consent to the procedure, and the providers may think her consent is voluntary, but if the threats are what make her seek the abortion, then she is not truly consenting to it. Her consent is coerced. Again, nursing home personnel may threaten to discharge an elderly welfare patient who needs time-consuming spoon feeding unless he consents to a gastrostomy tube for nutrition. He may agree to the surgery, but his consent is coerced, not voluntary.

A rare kind of coercion occurs when civil authorities put pressure on people to accept medical interventions. Thus a judge may tell a woman who irresponsibly reproduces every year and so neglects and abuses her babies that a state agency must find foster homes for them, that she has a choice between a prison sentence or sterilization. If she gives consent for medical procedures to sterilize her in order to stay out of prison, her consent is not voluntary but coerced. This does not mean, however, that this coercion is necessarily immoral. Some ethicists would argue that it is not immoral to give a woman with a history of frequent pregnancies and convictions of child abuse a choice between serving time or sterilization; others would disagree.

It is important to distinguish between threats and information about adverse consequences. Providers may certainly tell, indeed many times must tell, patients about unpleasant things that will happen if they don't accept treatment. But this is providing information, not threatening patients, as long as no effort is made to coerce the patient to give consent to a procedure.

3. Treatment is the result of *manipulation* when some technique is used to get the patient to give consent. There are many ways to manipulate people. Some are trivial and can be ignored, but some are not trivial and are clearly immoral. Giving a little encouragement to a person hesitating to have a needed but difficult procedure is not the kind of manipulation that causes ethical concerns. But there are less savory ways of manipulating people.

Suppose the physician really thinks the patient ought to have the risky procedure and tries to get consent by saying "Don't worry, most people come through this with no problem" when 40 percent of the people suffer serious consequences or die as the result of the intervention. Strictly speaking, what the physician said was true (60 percent is "most" people), but presenting the information this way can be manipulative. If the patient knew 40 percent of the people had serious problems or died as a result of the intervention, he may have withheld consent.

Again, suppose the resident in anesthesia has administered numerous spinal block anesthesias in recent months, but has had no opportunity to administer general anesthesia. She understandably wants more experience with general anesthesia and tries to get her patients to accept it. She spends extra time telling them how safe general anesthesia is for healthy people, and tells them in great detail of the risks associated with spinal blocks. This can easily become a form of manipulation. She is slanting the preoperative conference in an effort to have patients accept general anesthesia; she is trying to manipulate them, and this is unethical.

Psychological manipulation is also possible. There are ways to make people feel bad, or guilty, or upset if they do not follow what you want them to do. Consider the following: A person has given informed consent for surgery. All the preparations are made. He is prepped, the operating room is ready, and the anesthesiologists, nurses, and surgeon are standing by. It is a busy hospital, and the schedules are always tight. Moreover, the administration is making every effort to achieve maximum utilization of the facilities. Then, on the way to the operating room, the patient says he has changed his mind.

The nurses and residents immediately tell him what a terrible disruption this will cause in everybody's schedule, and how it will waste valuable operating room time. They do everything they can to make him feel guilty for waiting so long to change his mind, for not living up to his agreement when he gave informed consent, etc. In brief, they are trying to manipulate him so he will agree to the surgery. Without question, his action has caused a major problem and, if there is no good reason for it, they have reason for being upset. But this does not justify the manipulation.

Ethical Significance of Informed Consent

Informed consent fits very well into the ethical framework advanced in the earlier chapters. This framework views ethics as the way each person seeks his or her good. Each moral agent desires a good life, and whatever behavior contributes to a truly good life is morally reasonable. This ethics places a great premium on the individual figuring out what is truly good in her situation. The ethical person engages in what may be described as either "deliberative reason" or "rational deliberation," to use Aristotle's phrases, and then does what she has decided is good, that is, what she has concluded will achieve her good. Prudence is the intellectual virtue whereby a person "orders" herself to behave in a certain way because that behavior is seen as what will be good.

All this obviously points to the values underlying informed consent. The ethics of personal responsibility requires the moral agent to deliberate, to figure out how best to achieve happiness in what is often a very confusing situation. This stress on personal deliberation, on practical rather than pure reasoning, on the existential rather than the metaphysical, on the prudence of each moral agent rather than principles, on personal decision rather than authoritarian direction, is strongly reinforced by the doctrine of informed consent.

Documentation of Informed Consent

Informed consent is a process involving two major players, the patient and the physician. Normally the patient does not have all the necessary information, so the physician must disclose it. The patient must understand the information, evaluate the impact of the treatment options on his life, deliberate about those options, and then decide to consent or not consent to a course of action. From a moral point of view we have informed consent when this process occurs. Thus informed consent may exist even though the informed consent form is not signed. And, conversely, informed consent may not exist even though the form is signed. This happens when information was not adequately disclosed, or when it was adequately disclosed but not sufficiently understood, or when the consent was forced, coerced, or manipulated.

In our society, however, it is extremely important that the process of informed consent be properly documented. It is important to have a record of the informed consent process. Moreover, the documentation requirement can actually encourage the important shared decision-making process, and remind everyone of its seriousness.

EXCEPTIONS TO INFORMED CONSENT

There are times when medical interventions without the patient's informed consent are ethical. One obvious instance occurs when the patient does not have the capacity to give informed consent. In these situations a proxy will be making the decisions and giving the informed consent. Proxy decision making on behalf of patients without decision-making capacity will be the subject of the next chapter.

For patients with decision-making capacity, there are four major exceptions to the legal and ethical requirement for informed consent before medical interventions are begun.

Legal requirements
Sometimes laws or military directives require health care interventions. Examples here include the law of a country requiring immunizations for public health reasons, or a military order requiring immunizations or drugs to protect the health of military personnel and to maintain an effective fighting force.

Emergencies
In most emergencies there is no time to disclose the necessary information for an informed consent. Here the providers simply act according to what they think will be in the best interests of the patient. These situations fre-

quently happen in hospital emergency rooms and when emergency medical personnel arrive on the scene of an accident or sudden illness.

The emergency exception to informed consent is often quite obvious, but not always so. Consider the following situation. A hospitalized dying patient, with an order not to be resuscitated if respiratory or cardiac arrest occurs, is being transported by ambulance to a nearby facility for a treatment the hospital cannot provide. The patient has not been discharged from the hospital and he will be returned in a few hours. During the transport a cardiac arrest occurs. The ambulance crew are trained in CPR and instructed to begin emergency CPR whenever they are called to the scene of an arrest. Despite knowing the patient has given informed consent for the Do Not Resuscitate order, the ambulance crew attempts resuscitation. In effect, they are forcing treatment on a patient who knew an arrest was a real possibility, and who had made it clear that he did not want resuscitation attempted.

Ambulance personnel will sometimes claim it is ethical for them to attempt resuscitation in such circumstances. They claim emergency personnel must always treat in an emergency, and that an arrest is an emergency. Moreover, their employer's protocols probably require them to treat all people having arrests. This is excellent general advice—the primary response of emergency personnel is to treat if they can.

But attempting resuscitation in these circumstances raises several questions. First, is this really an emergency? The fact that a patient has an order to withhold resuscitation indicates, in most cases, that an arrest is not unexpected. The patient is in the ambulance for routine transportation and not because of an emergency. Second, how can it be plausibly argued that attempting resuscitation for a patient who has declined it is morally justified? If the arrest had occurred at the hospital an hour earlier, no attempt to resuscitate the patient would have been made, and everyone would have thought not attempting resuscitation was the morally right response for this patient. It is difficult to say withholding CPR is no longer the morally right thing to do simply because the patient is being transported in an ambulance for treatment elsewhere.

This example suggests that some interventions made without informed consent under the heading of an emergency are arguably neither emergencies nor in the best interests of the patients. A few states have begun to recognize the problems inherent in this kind of "emergency" resuscitation, and they are taking steps to introduce legal measures to protect patients from unwanted CPR by emergency medical technicians (EMTs) and paramedics.

Waivers

Sometimes patients with decision-making capacity waive their prerogative to give informed consent. They might choose not to be informed of the diagnosis, or of the prognosis, or of the risks. They may even not want to make any decisions about treatment, preferring to leave that in the hands of the physician or another person, perhaps a family member. From a moral point of view, there is no problem with patients waiving their option to give informed consent.

If the patient waives informed consent and expects the physician to make the decisions, however, a difficult situation ensues. In the present cultural climate, many physicians will hesitate to accept a patient's wish that she (the physician) make the treatment decisions without obtaining informed consent for the different interventions where it is customary. So strong is the legal and social climate in favor of informed consent that many physicians are uncomfortable working without it, and they will often seek an appropriate proxy to give informed consent and to sign the form.

A patient's waiver is a complex phenomenon. The patient certainly is morally justified in choosing to waive receiving information or giving consent, but it is less certain that he can waive the physician's responsibility to disclose information and obtain consent before providing treatment. In effect, the patient's waiver is requesting the physician not to disclose information and not to obtain consent before treatment, and the physician may well be unhappy with this arrangement. Moreover, the waiver undermines the ideal of shared decision making by putting the whole burden on the physician.

At times, however, the waiver allowing a physician to treat without informed consent may be morally appropriate. A physician who has known her patient for many years might accept a waiver as the patient, declining with age, becomes less and less able to understand what is going on. Accepting the patient's waiver in these circumstances is more likely to be appropriate when the patient has no immediate family and when the appropriate treatment remains straightforward. Even in these cases, however, a prudent physician may be more comfortable designating a proxy to share the health care decisions.

If a person other than the physician is to make the decisions under the waiver, then the situation is not quite so problematic. It is easy to imagine, for example, an elderly person asking the physician to discuss treatments with a son or daughter, and to accept whatever this person decides. Once the physician is certain her patient wants to proceed this way, there is no moral objection to following the patient's wishes. The major responsibility of the physician will then be to supply the family member with all the information needed for informed consent to the interventions.

Therapeutic Privilege

This is a rather controversial exception to obtaining informed consent from a patient with decision-making capacity. The idea is that giving people the truth about their unfortunate diagnosis, and expecting them to make an agonizing choice to give or withhold consent for burdensome treatment with an uncertain outcome, might devastate them. Physicians and family sometimes fear that the disturbing information and the need for a decision in a tragic situation will cause the patient to become upset, depressed, or emotionally unresponsive, and these negative reactions will make his condition worse. As a result, withholding the bad news might seem to be the right thing to do.

When patients are never told of their unfortunate diagnoses, however, an intolerable situation often develops. Treatments are given, and providers and friends have to perform a dance of pretending—pretending that the illness is only temporary, pretending that the patient "will soon be fine."

Although it may seem that this is the merciful thing to do, most often it is not. There is no evidence that informing patients of their situation when the diagnosis and prognosis are not good is more dangerous to them than pretending everything is fine. Moreover, there are several good reasons for avoiding the dance of pretending. First, it often does not work. People soon begin to sense they are seriously ill and getting worse. And people also sense others are not being honest with them.

Second, it forces the physicians and nurses to live a lie. They know the truth, but are expected to conceal it from the patient. This is especially difficult when patients ask pointed questions about their status and when the providers do not agree with the concealment in the first place. Sometimes nurses have to deal with the pointed questions of a patient whom the physician had declined to inform about the serious nature of the illness. Sometimes physicians have to care for patients whose families insist that the patient could not cope with the diagnosis. This undermines the relationship of trust that should exist between providers and patients.

Third, it denies the patient the opportunity to tidy up relations with loved ones and friends and to prepare for death. For many patients, this is an important process.

For these reasons, the appeal to therapeutic privilege is rarely justified. One situation where we might be inclined to invoke it involves the medical care of people from other cultures without a strong tradition of individual rights, autonomy, and personal freedom, and with a strong tradition of medical paternalism. People from these cultures might even become hopelessly confused, especially if they are older, when they fall ill in this country and are confronted with the unfamiliar process of informed consent.

Another situation where therapeutic privilege might be justified centers on patients with a history of psychiatric problems. These cases require very delicate judgment calls, and great sensitivity is required lest the physician prematurely disenfranchise patients of a say in what happens to them.

In general, there is widespread agreement that therapeutic privilege should be an extremely rare exception to informed consent and that sufficient information, no matter how terrible, ought to be provided so the patient can participate meaningfully in the decision-making process. The disclosure may be difficult for the physician and upsetting for the patient, but this is often less harmful than the efforts at concealment. Concealing the truth disenfranchises patients by preventing them from making their own decisions. Taking this power away from people is a serious step indeed, and the major reason why therapeutic privilege should be so rarely invoked.

ADVANCE DIRECTIVES

Many of us will one day lose our capacity to make health care decisions. When that happens our primary physician will turn to a proxy for decisions about our treatment. Someone else will be giving informed consent for our surgery or ventilator or feeding tube.

If the proxy does not know what treatments we would have wanted, then he may be inclined to give consent for anything that might help to keep us alive. And once life-sustaining therapies are being used, the proxy may find it difficult to request their withdrawal if they become unreasonable. It is not easy to request treatment withdrawals when the result is death.

And if the proxy does request withdrawal of life-sustaining treatment, providers may hesitate to remove it from us unless they have strong evidence that we had previously indicated we did not want the particular therapies. This is so because some state courts, most notably those in Missouri and New York, have insisted that life-sustaining treatment cannot be withdrawn from unconscious patients unless clear and convincing evidence exists that the patient had previously indicated he did not want the specific intervention.

In other words, when we lose our capacity to make decisions, we lose a great deal of control over what happens to us. And it is quite possible that things will be done to us that we would not want done to us.

We can keep some control over what will happen to us in the event we lose our decision-making capacity by making advance directives. Advance directives are our instructions for health care that will become effective if we ever lose our decision-making capacity.

We can set up advance directives two ways: (1) we can prepare written directions about how we want to be treated if certain conditions afflict us, and (2) we can designate someone to report our instructions or, if we didn't give instructions, to make decisions for us. In other words, we can write out how we want to be treated and we can choose someone to speak for us. We will call the instructions for treatment *treatment directives* and the instructions designating who is to speak for us *proxy designations*.

Treatment Directives

There are two kinds of written treatment directives, living wills and medical care directives. Many people call all written directives living wills, but they are not really the same thing. The major differences between the living will and the more generic medical care directive are: (1) the living will is a formal legal document, and the medical care directive is not; and (2) the living will usually designates only unwanted treatments, while the medical care directive almost always includes treatments the person wants. It is helpful, then, to think of a living will as a special type of medical care directive.

Living wills
Strictly speaking, a living will is a legal document similar to the legal will that directs the disposal of our property after death. In the 1960s two groups, the Euthanasia Society of America and Concern for Dying, advocated legal recognition of a will that would allow people to set forth their wishes to have life-support systems withheld or removed in certain situations. For a few years all attempts to pass legislation recognizing such a will failed.

Then the great publicity surrounding the efforts of a New Jersey father to have the respirator removed from his severely brain-damaged and permanently unconscious daughter attracted national attention. The patient was Karen Quinlan and her landmark case will be considered later. The well-known story of Karen Quinlan, more than anything else in the 1970s, made people aware of the new life-support systems being developed and how they could keep the vital functions of a human body going long after there was any hope of significant recovery.

Legalization of living wills followed soon after the Quinlan case. In 1976 California became the first state to recognize them by what it called the Natural Death Act. In the next year, efforts to introduce legal living wills were made in forty-two states, and were successful in seven. Today over forty states have some form of legal living will. The laws vary from state to state. Most states insist on some strict conditions that must be met before the living will can be accepted as valid and then executed. Some states, for example, allow only terminally ill people to make them and may require a waiting period after they have been informed of such a diagnosis. Other states nullify the will if the person becomes pregnant. The conditions are designed to prevent abuse. Unfortunately, they also severely limit the value of the document as an advance directive.

Without question, living will laws represented an important first step in respecting a person's desires not to be treated in ways he would consider unreasonable. But they were only a first step, and today we can see their inadequacies.

1. Many living will laws allow only terminally ill patients, or people whose death is expected within a short time, to make these wills. This leaves everyone else without a means of making advance decisions about treatment.
2. The directives are narrow in that they apply only to treatments people do not want and ignore what treatments they might desire.
3. The language is often vague, using such hard-to-define terms as "heroic measures" or "meaningful quality of life."
4. Most laws providing for living wills do not legislate any penalties if providers choose to ignore them.
5. Providers, especially those working in an emergency situation, have to worry about whether the document really was the person's legal living will. It is always possible that the person had executed it but was thinking of cancelling it, or that the person had executed a more recent living will, or that the document is a forgery.

Efforts are being made, with some success, to overcome the deficiencies of living will laws. At the same time, there has been a movement toward a better type of advance directive, the medical care directive.

Medical care directives

A medical care directive is a written instruction indicating the care people want if they should ever become incapacitated. The directive is more broad than a living will because (1) anyone capable of informed consent can make one—the person does not have to be terminally or seriously ill, as the laws governing living wills often require; (2) the directions are for providing treatment as well as foregoing it; and (3) the language describing the medical problems that might develop, and the treatments that might be employed, is more concrete and complete than the language found in most living wills.

A typical medical care directive will consider three things: what medical problems might occur, what treatments are available, and what treatments I want. The section on what I want can be further nuanced; perhaps I want some care no matter what, or the same care on a trial basis with the understanding it will be withdrawn if it becomes unreasonable. And in some cases I might be undecided about what I would want and state this, leaving the decision up to a proxy.

The kinds of medical problems most often included in a medical care directive are:

1. being in a vegetative state or in a coma with little or no hope of regaining awareness;
2. suffering brain damage or any disease that leaves me totally and permanently incoherent and confused all the time;
3. having any condition, especially a painful one, that is expected to bring death in the next year or so regardless of whether treatments are provided.

The major types of treatment most often mentioned in a medical care directive are major surgery, dialysis, providing air by mechanical devices (ventilators and respirators), providing nourishment by tubes or lines, blood transfusions, antibiotics, and cardiopulmonary resuscitation.

Medical care directives are especially important in states such as Massachusetts, where living wills are not legally recognized. At the very least, they help the physician and proxy decision maker to know what the now incapacitated person would have wanted in the circumstances. As we will see in the next chapter, this puts the proxy in a better position to make good decisions.

Medical care directives have two major advantages for patients. First, they extend the patient's prerogative of informed consent beyond the loss of capacity. Second, they protect the patient from treatments that make little or no sense and that practically no person really wants, but which might be given if no advance directives exist.

Some patients, for example, lost all awareness years ago and live on in a persistent vegetative state. They will never again recover any awareness. Most people do not want to be kept alive this way, yet thousands of people are because they left no advance directives. Without evidence that they explicitly said they would not want the life-sustaining interventions, some state courts and some physicians will not honor a proxy's decision to withdraw the life-sustaining treatment.

While medical care directives are an improvement over legal living wills, they also have their weaknesses. First, it is impossible to anticipate every medical problem that might happen, so the instructions we leave may not be helpful, and they may even mislead those caring for us. Second, people often change their minds as time goes on, and the directives of last year might not reflect the desires of this year. The person functioning as our proxy might be aware of our latest wishes, and thus be trapped between honoring our written directives and doing what is more consistent with our later wishes. Third, many people attempting to compose advance directives become bewildered as they think about all the different kinds of medical situations and treatment options available for each. The task overwhelms them and, if they manage to produce a document at all, it is poorly done.

There is a more serious practical problem as well. The medical care directive is really an extensive and extended informed consent document. It usually covers a whole series of hypothetical medical problems and a host of possible treatments. The average patient will need hours of instruction to understand adequately the various diagnoses, prognoses, risks, benefits, costs, alternative treatments, etc., that are involved in informed consent. Someone has to provide the information leading to advance directives. Normally the physician would be explaining the treatments, risks, side effects, expected benefits, etc., but few physicians have the time to provide all the necessary information and to discuss the many possible situations covered in a medical care directive. And if they had the time, few physicians would be inclined to do it, knowing that almost all the time would be wasted because so many of the problems and treatment options—unfortunately, we cannot be sure which ones—will never be a real issue for the particular patient.

This has led many to suggest a second kind of advance directive—the designation of a proxy or surrogate who will make decisions for us if ever we cannot.

Proxy Designations

The second type of advance directive, the proxy designation, allows us to designate a person who will make the decisions about withholding and withdrawing our treatments, or who will give informed consent for treatment, if we ever become incapacitated. We can distinguish two general kinds of proxy designations: the durable power of attorney and the more general health care proxy designation.

Durable power of attorney

The law allows us to give another person the "power of attorney." This power allows the designated person to carry out certain functions on our behalf. If we are going to be away for an extended time, for example, we can give someone the power of attorney to sign checks to pay our bills. Although the power of attorney usually applies to our property, it could also apply to our person, that is, we could designate a person to make certain decisions about our personal matters as well as about our property. This would seem to make the power of attorney procedure a natural basis for appointing someone to make health care decisions on our behalf if we should ever become incapacitated. Paradoxically, however, this is not the case; the ordinary power of attorney lapses when the person granting the power becomes incapacitated, and this is precisely when we would need the designated attorney to make health care decisions.

One way to prevent the power of attorney from lapsing when the person granting it becomes incapacitated is to authorize a *durable* power of attorney.

The durable power of attorney retains its power when the person granting it loses capacity. All states recognize the durable power of attorney, and most allow it or a similar procedure for the purpose of designating someone to make personal health care decisions for us if we should be unable to make the decision ourselves. Some states have even instituted a durable power of attorney law designed explicitly for health care matters.

Health care proxy designation

The durable power of attorney is not the only way to designate a proxy decision maker for health care. A simple written directive designating the person you want to make decisions for you is most often all that is needed. This is because your physician is the person who will have to find the appropriate proxy for you and, except for extraordinary circumstances, the physician will obviously be relieved to know you have already designated the person he should consult when you can no longer make decisions for yourself.

Some states, however, have formalized the designation of a proxy or surrogate decision maker by passing laws designed to strengthen the power of such a proxy idea. In July 1990 New York enacted a health care proxy law, and Massachusetts followed in December 1990. A brief review of the Massachusetts law will give us a good idea of recent developments in the trend to formalize the designation of a proxy or surrogate in a legal way.

The *Massachusetts Health Care Proxy Act* (HCPA) allows an adult with decision-making capacity to designate another adult as his "agent" to make health care decisions on his behalf in the future. The authority of the agent does not become effective until the attending physician determines the patient has lost the capacity to make decisions and to give informed consent. The physician must notify the patient orally and in writing of this determination (unless the patient is unconsciousness or otherwise unable to comprehend) and must enter the determination of incapacity in the patient's medical record.

The designation of the health care agent must be in writing, but there is no required legal form. To be legally recognized, however, the form must clearly identify the agent and indicate that the person intends to have the agent make health care decisions on his behalf. The form must be signed by the person designating the agent and by two witnesses other than the designated agent or any alternate agents who might be named. The witnesses verify that the person was over 18, had the capacity to designate an agent, and did it voluntarily.

The form must be dated, and it is revoked automatically if the person makes another proxy designation at a later date. It is also automatically revoked by divorce or legal separation, if the agent is the person's spouse. And the person may choose to revoke it at any time orally or in writing or by some action such as crossing it out or tearing it up.

Once the physician has formally determined that the patient has lost the capacity to make health care decisions, the designated proxy in Massachusetts can make any decisions, including decisions to withhold or withdraw life-sustaining treatment, unless the person had restricted the agent's authority on the proxy designation form.

However, the patient, despite being considered incapable of making decisions by the physician, may always veto any of his agent's decisions, unless a court has ruled that the patient is incompetent.

If the physician later determines the person has regained capacity, the proxy loses the authority to make the decisions, but regains it if the physician subsequently determines the patient is again incapable of making the decisions. Physicians may, for ethical or religious reasons, choose not to comply with the agent's decisions, but they will then arrange to transfer the care of the patient to another physician or, if this fails, to seek relief in court. Physicians also enjoy immunity from criminal and civil liability if they carry out in good faith the decisions made by the agents properly designated by the Massachusetts HCPA. And, if there is good cause, a physician can always challenge the agent's decisions in court.

This kind of law can be a big help in reinforcing the moral responsibility we have to help others take care of us if we ever lose the capacity to make decisions. In effect, the laws extend our powers of decision making and of informed consent into a time when we may be incapable of making decisions. We may expect these laws to become more refined as time goes on, and to be accepted in more and more states. We can also expect new developments in this direction. Some states, for example, are fashioning laws that would designate an agent for incapacitated patients who did not make such a designation themselves and do not have a court-appointed guardian. The proposed laws would empower a spouse, adult children, parents, siblings, even close friends, to act as proxies for those who failed to designate a proxy before they lost capacity.

Since December 1991, there has been a federal law supporting advance directives. It is called the Patient Self-Determination Act (PSDA) and we will conclude this chapter with a brief consideration of it.

THE PATIENT SELF-DETERMINATION ACT

In December 1991 the first federal statute on treatment directives and proxy designations went into effect. The law applies to all hospitals, nursing homes, hospices, health maintenance organizations, and home health agencies receiving Medicare or Medicaid funds. Since almost all these institutions do receive these federal funds, the law is almost universal in scope.

The act requires these institutions to provide written information to each adult patient about the right to make health care decisions, to refuse treatment, and to write advance directives for use if the person should ever become incapacitated. The law encourages, but does not require, adults to make both treatment directives and proxy designations.

This statute provides an excellent opportunity for people to think about advance directives and to make some provision for them. Only if people make some kind of advance directives can we avoid the guessing game that often transpires when providers, family, and friends do not know what a patient would want, and it is too late to ask. To this end, the statute encourages community education programs to increase the general public's awareness of advance directives and to urge people to formulate them. This is one of the more important aspects of the act because it will help to create a general social attitude encouraging advance directives.

Only time will tell how successful the Patient Self-Determination Act will be. One weakness lies in the process itself. The information about the right to make decisions and formulate advance directives is provided upon admission to the hospital or nursing home, or upon enrollment in the health maintenance organization. As we all know, clerical personnel, not physicians or other health care providers, take care of the formalities of admission to a clinic or of enrollment in an HMO. The danger is that the very important matter of treatment directives may become separated from dialogue with the physician and become lost in the admissions or enrollment processes.

Formulating advance directives is really a kind of informed consent for future treatment as well as a decision to forego certain treatments. These consents and treatment refusals are serious matters, and the decisions are best shared with the attending physician. If the act encourages people to discuss, with their physicians, their wishes about the more common forms of medical treatments available for serious problems that may arise, then it will be a great success.

Not everybody is happy with the PSDA legislation. Some pro-life groups opposed it, perhaps fearing it would lead to euthanasia. Some people agreed with the idea of treatment directives, but felt it was not a good idea to have a federal law intruding into the area of personal health care decisions. Others felt the legislation should have made physicians, rather than institutions, responsible for providing the information because physicians are the people primarily responsible for treating patients according to their wishes.

ETHICAL REFLECTIONS

Informed consent, advance directives, state health care proxy laws, and the federal Patient Self-Determination Act fit very well with the ethical perspective outlined earlier. This ethics is a morality of the good understood as the good we achieve for ourselves by the moral choices we make in life. Advance directives are an expansion of this ethics into future situations that might happen to us. We imagine what could happen to us, and we indicate what we think our moral response in these situations would be. Our advance directives extend our decision-making into a future when we might no longer be able to make prudential decisions in our lives.

Treatment directives are important for another reason—making them is a virtuous thing to do. They prevent our physician, other providers, and our loved ones from being left in the predicament of trying to figure out how we would want to be treated if we ever lose the capacity to decide. Doing something good for others for their sake is what we call the virtue of love.

Making advance directives also manifests the virtues of courage and justice. It takes courage to deal with our disintegration and death, and arranging to forego unreasonable treatment exhibits justice. Spending money for treatments a person would not want is a terrible waste of resources.

In an ethics where the goal is the good life, rightly understood, of the persons behaving as moral agents, the personal responsibility of persons for their own well-being is obvious. In an ethics whose norm is "according to right reason," treatment directives make a lot of sense. The morally good behavior is always the reasonable behavior designed to achieve the good. Without advance directives the unreasonable is often done, and the good is not achieved.

Good ethics encourages people to make advance directives carefully. Perhaps the best way to do this is by making an advance directive that combines treatment directives with a proxy designation. We might call this the *combined advance directive*.

The combined advance directive has two parts. In one part we consider what might happen in the future and how we want to be treated, and then indicate this in writing to help others know our wishes if it should happen that we are no longer able to communicate them. In the other part we appoint a proxy (and, if possible, an alternate in case the proxy is not available) and grant the proxy the general authority to decide whether to provide, withhold, or withdraw treatment and medical nutrition subject to whatever limitations, if any, we indicate on the form designating the proxy.

The key to any advance directive is clarity. The underlying assumption is that providing all possible treatment all the time is, in this era of modern technology and medical technique, simply not reasonable or moral. So advance directives are decisions about treatment—what to provide and what to forego, and who is to make decisions when I no longer can. But these directives need to be concrete. It is not enough to appoint a proxy; I have to make sure my proxy knows my thoughts about life, suffering, and death, and about treatments I would find reasonable.

The combined advance directive brings together the best of treatment directives and of proxy appointments. It gives my directions in some degree of detail, but it also designates a person for making decisions. This is important because I cannot anticipate every possible aspect of future events in my written directives, and a proxy is very helpful in resolving difficulties of interpretation and in dealing with complications unforeseen by me. The proxy is also someone whom the physician and other providers can communicate with when communication with me is impossible.

The combined advance directive, of course, is not a perfect solution to this difficult problem of extending informed consent and patient decision-making beyond the loss of capacity. Many of the problems associated with treatment directives and proxy designations still haunt the combined directive. Moreover, a conflict may develop between my written directives and what my appointed proxy thinks I would want in a particular set of circumstances. For example, my proxy may conclude that I did not really intend my directive to be followed in the unanticipated situation that actually developed. The proxy may also have reasons for thinking I was changing my mind about some of the treatment directives.

It is not easy to sort things out when my treatment directives and the proxy's opinion of what I would now want are in conflict. I can reduce the problem somewhat if I include in my combined directive some instructions on how I would want such a conflict resolved. I could say that my proxy has the final say, or I could say that the treatment directives should prevail in the event of a conflict. Without such a provision in the combined directive, providers and others will be in a real quandary when these conflicts occur. Seeking relief in the courts is a last resort in health care because the adversarial atmosphere of the courts is not really the place for personal health care decisions, but sometimes there is no alternative.

Advance directives and the recent Patient Self-Determination Act remind us of the important role proxies play in health care decision-making. The next chapter considers the matter of proxy decision making and explains how a proxy makes health care decisions for others.

SUGGESTED READINGS

A good introduction to the notion of decision-making capacity is found in two reports of the President's Commission. See 1982. *Making Health Care Decisions*, volume one. U.S. Government Printing Office, pp. 55–62; and 1983. *Deciding to Forego Life-Sustaining Treatment*. U.S. Government Printing Office, p. 45. Also helpful is the American Hospital Association report entitled *Values in Conflict: Resolving Ethical Issues in Hospital Care*. 1985. Chicago: AHA, pp. 9–12. See also: Paul Appelbaum and Thomas Grisso. "Assessing Patients' Capacities to Consent to Treatment." *NEJM* **1988,** *319,* 1635–38; Bernard Lo. "Assessing Decision-Making Capacity." *Law, Medicine & Health Care* **1990,** *18,* 193–201; James Drane. "Competency to Give an Informed Consent: A Model for Making Clinical Assessments." *JAMA* **1984,** *252,* 925–27; Mary Cutter and Earl Shelp, eds. 1991. *Competency: A Study of Informal Competency Determinations in Primary Care*. Dordrecht: Kluwer Academic Publishers; and E. Haavi Morreim. "Impairments and Impediments in Patients' Decision Making: Reframing the Competence Question." *Journal of Clinical Ethics* **1993,** *4,* 294–307.

An excellent source for the history of informed consent is Ruth Faden and Tom Beauchamp. 1986. *A History and Theory of Informed Consent*. New York: Oxford University Press. For a complete overview of informed consent from the important legal perspective, see Fay Rozovsky. 1990. *Consent to Treatment: A Practical Guide*, second edition. Boston: Little, Brown and Company. See also Franz Ingelfinger. "Informed (But Uneducated) Consent." *NEJM* **1972,** *287,* 466; Eugene Laforet. "The Fiction of Informed Consent." *JAMA* **1976,** *235,* 1579–85; Charles Lidz and Allen Meisel, "What We Do and Do Not Know about Informed Consent." *JAMA* **1981,** *246,* 2473–77; Charles Lidz et al., "Informed Consent and the Structure of Medical Care," in *Making Health Care Decisions*, volume two, pp. 317–410; Gerald Dworkin, "Autonomy and Informed Consent," in *Making Health Care Decisions*, volume three, pp. 63–81; and the series of articles in the special section entitled "Informed Consent in Medical Practice," *Journal of Clinical Ethics* 5 (1994): 189–223 and 243–266.

The citations for the landmark legal decisions shaping informed consent are: *Schloendorff v. Society of New York Hospital*, 211 N.Y. 125 (1914); *Salgo v. Leland Stanford Jr. University Board of Trustees*, 317 P.2d 170 (1957); *Canterbury v. Spence*, 464 F.2d 772 (1972); and *Lane v. Candura*, 376 N.E.2d, 1232 (1978).

For advance directives, see George Annas. "The Health Care Proxy and the Living Will." *NEJM* **1991,** *324,* 1210–13; Linda Emanuel et al. "Advance Directives for Medical Care—a Case for Greater Use." *NEJM* **1991,** *324,* 889–95; Nancy King. 1991. *Making Sense of Advance Directives*. Boston: Kluwer Academic Publishers; Linda Emanuel and Ezekiel Emanuel. "The Medical Directive: A New Comprehensive Advance Care Document." *JAMA* **1989,** *261,* 3288–93; Ezekiel Emanuel and Linda Emanuel. "Living Wills: Past, Present, and Future." *Journal of Clinical Ethics* **1990,** *1,* 9–19; Judith Areen. "Advance Directives under State Law and Judicial Decisions." *Law, Medicine & Health Care* **1991,** *19,* 91–100; and Linda Emanuel. "Advance Directives: What Have We Learned So Far?" *Journal of Clinical Ethics* **1993,** *4,* 8–16.

Commentaries on the Patient Self-Determination Act include: John La Puma. "Advance Directives on Admission: Clinical Implications and Analysis of the Patient Self-Determination Act of 1990." *JAMA* **1991,** *266,* 402–05; Susan Wolf et al. "Sources of Concern about the Patient Self-Determination Act." *NEJM* **1991,** *325,* 1666–71; Elizabeth McCloskey. "The Patient Self-Determination Act." *Kennedy Institute of Ethics Journal* **1991,** *1,* 163–69; Charles Sabatino. "Surely the Wizard Will Help Us, Toto? Implementing the Patient Self-Determination Act." *Hastings Center Report* **1993,** *23* (January–February), 12–16; Mathy Mezey and Beth Latimer. "The Patient Self-Determination Act: An Early Look at Implementation." *Hastings Center Report* **1993,** *23* (January–February), 16–20; Joanne Lynn and Joan Teno. "After the Patient Self-Determination Act: The Need for Empirical Research on Formal Advance Directives." *Hastings Center Report* **1993,** *23* (January–February), 20–24; Elizabeth McClosky. "Between Isolation and Intrusion: The Patient Self-Determination Act." *Law, Medicine & Health Care* **1991,** *19,* 80–82; and Jeremy Sugarman et al. "The Cost of Ethics Legislation: A Look at the Patient Self-Determination Act." *Kennedy Institute of Ethics Journal* **1993,** *3,* 387–399. See also the special supplement entitled "Practicing the PSDA." *Hastings Center Report* **1991,** *21* (September–October), S1–S16.

5

Deciding for Others

Many patients do not have the capacity to make health care decisions. Some, children and those with congenital mental impairments, never had decision-making capacity. Others once had it, but lost it due to various medical or psychological problems. Since patients without decision-making capacity can no longer make decisions to receive or to refuse treatment, other people will make the treatment decisions and give consent on their behalf. The person making these decisions is called a *proxy* or a *surrogate*.

In the previous chapter, we defined the three essential elements of decision-making capacity. They were: (1) the ability to understand and communicate relevant information, (2) the possession of a framework of values providing a context for particular value judgments, and (3) the ability to reason about different outcomes, risks, and chances of success. If any one of these three elements is absent to a significant degree, then the person does not have decision-making capacity.

The responsibility of determining the absence of the capacity to make health care decisions rests with the physician. This is so because, apart from exceptional circumstances such as emergencies, a physician cannot treat a patient without voluntary and informed consent, and consent is valid only if the person has the capacity to give it.

Although the physician determines when a patient lacks decision-making capacity, the determination is not normally based on medical criteria or on a psychiatric consultation. The determination of incapacity is a practical judgment that any mature person, who knows the patient, can make. It is a judgment made by a medical professional, but it is not a medical or professional judgment. The exception to this is mental illness. When mental illness has been diagnosed, medical expertise and psychiatric consultations are often needed to determine whether or not the patient has decision-making capacity.

Sometimes a person lacks all decision-making capacity. This is the case, for example, with unconscious patients or young children. Sometimes, however, a person lacks decision-making capacity in a more limited sense. A patient may have the capacity to make decisions about some treatments but not about others, or to make decisions at this time but not at another time. Hence, what the physician must determine is whether or not the patient has the capacity to decide about a particular treatment at a particular time.

It is also the responsibility of the physician to identify the appropriate proxy when his patient lacks decision-making capacity. Sometimes this is a simple matter. The patient may have already designated a proxy, or supportive family members may be available. When a patient has not designated a proxy, or when family members are not available, the physician's task of identifying the appropriate proxy can be difficult.

When the physician is working with a proxy, he must be aware of any conflict of interest, or of any emotional baggage, that could distort the proxy's decisions. For example, some children, anxious to preserve an inheritance, might decline life-sustaining treatment for an elderly parent suffering from a stroke because they know it can lead to years of expensive care in a nursing home. Again, some children, feeling guilty about neglecting a parent for years, might insist on "doing everything" when the treatment is burdensome and of no real benefit to their parent. The physician's primary clinical responsiblity is always the care of the patient, and he will reject the unreasonable requests of proxies.

BECOMING A PROXY

A person can become a proxy, and make health care decisions for an incapacitated patient, in several ways.

Patient-Designated Proxy

The best way of becoming a proxy is to be designated by the patient before decision-making capacity was lost. When patients have chosen their proxies, it makes everything much easier for the physician as well as for everyone else. If the patient loses capacity, they simply turn to the designated proxy for treatment decisions and informed consent.

In many cases, however, patients have not selected a proxy, and the physician of an incapacitated patient must find the person or persons with whom the shared decision-making will occur, and who will give informed consent whenever it is required for treatment interventions.

Family Members As Proxies

If the patient has supportive and capable family members, identifying a proxy is normally a relatively simple matter for the physician. A spouse is usually the proxy for a mate, a child or children are usually appropriate for a widowed parent, and parents are the proxies of first choice for their minor children.

There is growing recognition, however, that in many families, even loving families, people often do not really have a good idea of their loved one's treatment preferences. Caring about someone and living with her for years does not guarantee that we would know what she wants if she became incapacitated. Many people in families retain a significant degree of privacy about certain areas of their lives, including how they might want to be treated when ill. Adult children may not really know what their aging parents want, and some spouses may not really know what their partner wants.

We cannot, therefore, always assume that members of a family know the wishes of an incapacitated family member. Perhaps they do know, perhaps they do not. This is why physicians cannot simply accept a family member's decisions for a loved one who once had decision-making capacity. Physicians need to ask family members *why* they believe an intervention is something their loved one would, or would not, want. When family members say "She would not want a feeding tube" or "He did not want to be kept alive by machines," physicians do well to ask such questions as: "What did your mother or your father ever say or do that makes you think she or he would, or would not, want the feeding tube or the life-support equipment?"

Significant Others As Proxies

It is always possible that someone outside the family has a better idea of what the patient wants. If this is so, then this person would be in a better position to act as proxy for the patient. Of course, this could easily generate a very volatile situation if the family members object. Unfortunately, if their objections are successful, it could mean a patient will be denied the proxy best suited to report what he wanted.

The typical situation where a "significant other" would make a better proxy than a family member occurs when the patient no longer lives with family and has established a close and enduring relationship with another person, but never married him or her. No simple formula exists for determining when this "significant other" is a better proxy than a family member. It is yet another area where prudence is a valuable resource.

People from the pastoral care and social work support systems, and other members of the health care team, can sometimes provide information of great help to the physician in identifying a "significant other" as the appropriate proxy. The idea is to designate as proxy a person who knows and cares about the patient, is aware of the patient's desires, is available, and is willing to become informed about the diagnosis, the prognosis, the available treatments, and the side effects and risks of treatments. If a patient has had no meaningful contact with his family for decades, it makes no sense to think a family member is the most suitable proxy.

Court-Appointed Proxies

Problems can arise over the designation of a proxy for any number of reasons. Perhaps there is no family or significant other available, or the family is available, but hopelessly divided over what should be done. Perhaps a proxy is requesting something clearly inappropriate for a patient.

Sometimes the physician and social workers can resolve the difficulty, but at other times they must fall back on the last resort, and seek a court-appointed guardian. If a court does appoint a guardian to make health care decisions, the guardian's decisions have priority over those of any other proxy. If the physician or the family disagrees with the court-appointed guardian's decisions, they cannot overrule him, but they can challenge the decision in court.

Once the matter of designating a proxy lands in the courts, the process often becomes complicated, especially if the decision involves withholding or withdrawing life-sustaining treatment. Courts rely on an adversarial process— that is, people present arguments both pro and con. And instead of a simple procedure to appoint a guardian with the power of making a decision, the legal process often extends to the treatment issue itself, and thus turns the case into a whole new question. We can see how this happens by looking at a recent case that went to the Massachusetts Supreme Court.

Jane Doe was a thirty-three year old patient suffering from Canavan's disease, a disease causing irreversible deterioration of the central nervous system. She had been diagnosed in infancy as severely mentally retarded and placed in a state institution, where she had been a patient for the past thirty years. Her responses to stimuli did not indicate any awareness. To keep her alive, physicians had inserted a nasogastric feeding tube. Now they wanted to replace this tube with a gastrostomy tube surgically implanted into her stomach. Unlike the nasogastric tube, the gastrostomy tube requires surgery, and hence the physicians needed informed consent before they could insert it.

Since Jane Doe did not have decision-making capacity, the state institution asked her parents to give consent for the surgery to insert the feeding tube. When they refused, the institution went to court seeking the appointment of a guardian who would give the informed consent for the surgery.

The court first tried to appoint the parents guardians of their daughter, but they again refused. The court then appointed three people to represent Jane Doe: (1) a lawyer to represent her legal interests, (2) a guardian of her person, and (3) a guardian *ad litem*. (A guardian *ad litem* is a guardian for a particular case. The word *lis*, *litis* in Latin meant a legal action; it is the root of the English word "litigation." A guardian *ad litem*'s authority is limited to the duration of the case, whereas the guardian for the person has the authority to make decisions on behalf of the person for as long as the guardianship remains in effect.)

The guardian of her person, with the consent of her parents, declined to give consent for the surgery to implant the gastrostomy tube. Then he, again with the consent of her parents, made a new request—he asked to have the nasogastric feeding tube removed. This, of course, would result in Jane Doe's death within two weeks. The guardian *ad litem* also agreed that the withdrawal of the feeding tube was appropriate. The judge then issued an order allowing the removal of the nasogastric tube.

However, the third court-appointed person representing Jane Doe, the lawyer representing her legal interests, did not think that the nasogastric feeding tube should be withdrawn. He appealed the judge's decision, and the case went to the state supreme court. Eventually the state supreme court rejected his appeal and affirmed the decision of the lower court: the feeding tube could be removed.

The case shows how court procedures tend to become adversarial proceedings, pitting people against each other. The appointment of two or more guardians sets the stage for disagreements. It also shows how an original issue (in this case, whether the nasogastric feeding tube should be replaced by a less troublesome gastrostomy feeding tube) can be displaced by another issue (in this case, whether the nasogastric feeding tube should be withdrawn and not be replaced by a gastrostomy tube). The court-appointed guardians, once they became involved in the case, focused on this issue, and thereby changed the nature of the case. What began as effort to obtain informed consent for surgical insertion of a feeding tube became a debate about feeding tubes, and culminated in court order allowing physicians to forego using feeding tubes.

This does not imply that the guardians acted in a morally questionable way. As we will see in the chapter on medical nutrition and hydration, there are situations where withdrawal of feeding tubes is morally justified, and there are good reasons for saying that this was one of them. What the case does show, however, is how recourse to the courts for the purpose of appointing a proxy, though sometimes necessary, can lead to unexpected developments.

Judges As Proxies

The case of Jane Doe also shows how judges slide into the role of proxy decision makers. In effect, the judge in the Jane Doe case, originally asked only to appoint a guardian to give consent for a simple surgery, eventually became involved in supporting a decision to withdraw the nasogastric feeding tube and to withhold a gastrostomy tube. Sometimes judges become even more deeply involved in cases and actually take on the role of proxies themselves, as the following example shows.

Physicians at New England Medical Center in Massachusetts thought a "Do Not Resuscitate" (DNR) order would be in the best interests of a seriously ill child. The child, abandoned by its mother, had been placed in the legal custody of the Department of Social Services (DSS). DSS would not consent to the DNR order, so the medical center took the case to court. The court appointed a guardian *ad litem*. He sided with the DSS and refused consent for the DNR order. The medical center then asked the juvenile court judge to allow the DNR order.

On October 9, 1982, the judge issued an order allowing the medical center to enter the DNR order in the medical record. The child's lawyer and the guardian *ad litem* appealed the order.

While the appeal was pending, the child's condition improved to the point where the physicians believed that resuscitation efforts should be made if cardiopulmonary arrest occurred. The medical center then asked the juvenile court judge for permission to revoke the DNR order. Despite the fact that, at this time, all parties—the DSS, the child's attorney, the guardian *ad litem*, and the physicians at the medical center—believed that the child should not have a DNR order, the judge refused to cancel it. He found that, if competent, the child still would not want to be resuscitated.

On appeal, the Massachusetts Supreme Court agreed with the juvenile court judge. Thus, against the wishes of the guardian *ad litem* and of the physicians, the DNR order stood. The judges became, in effect, the proxy decision makers for the child. They overruled every other interested party and ordered that nobody could attempt resuscitation if the child arrested.

A more recent example of judges assuming the role of proxies arose in the same state. The DSS had legal custody of a child known as Beth, although her mother retained physical custody. Several months after her birth, as the result of an automobile accident, Beth became comatose, and then lapsed into a persistent vegetative state. The director of the Pediatric Intensive Care Unit at the Baystate Medical Center, where she was a ventilator-dependent patient, believed attempting to resuscitate her in the event of an arrest was medically inappropriate, and he asked the district court to authorize a DNR order.

The judge found that, if competent, Beth would choose not to be resuscitated and issued an order allowing the center to withhold resuscitation. The guardian *ad litem* appealed the order, arguing that resuscitation is no burden for an unconscious child and might keep her alive. The supreme court rejected his argument and affirmed the decision of the lower court judge.

It is important to note that in both these cases the parents had failed to exercise parental responsibilities for their children, and that the state had assumed legal custody of them. Still, the courts could have simply appointed a guardian to serve as proxy in place of the parents. But the judges in these cases played a more active and decisive role—they overruled guardians, and thus became the actual decision makers.

In these examples, the judges made decisions to refuse medical treatment for incapacitated patients. But judges can also order treatment as well, even against the wishes of adults with decision-making capacity. Courts in Florida and Massachusetts, for example, have indicated that the state's interest in protecting the well-being of young children could lead them to order their parents to accept blood transfusions, even though the parents were refusing blood for religious reasons. And courts have ordered, as we shall see, surgery on women with decision-making capacity against their wishes in efforts to save their fetus.

STANDARDS FOR MAKING PROXY DECISIONS

When proxies make health care decisions for other people, they need to rely on some kind of standards to guide their judgments. The two widely recognized standards in health care ethics are called *substituted judgment* and *best interests*. Both these standards are patient-centered. In cases of substituted judgment, the wishes of the patient prevail; in cases of best interests, the benefit to the patient prevails.

Sometimes, however, neither of these standards applies, and the proxy will have to rely on a third standard, what we will call the *reasonable treatment* standard. This standard is provider-centered; the proxy determines what is reasonable treatment in the circumstances.

Substituted judgment is the preferred standard, and the proxy will use it whenever possible. Only if the proxy cannot use substituted judgment will she turn to the best interests standard. And only if neither substituted judgment nor the best interests standard is appropriate will the proxy turn to the reasonable treatment standard.

The Substituted Judgment Standard

Substituted judgment is a rather awkward term, but its meaning is simple. The "judgment" in substituted judgment is the judgment of the patient. All the proxy does is step in as a substitute for the patient and report the patient's wishes to the physician. When using the substituted judgment standard, the proxy is like a substitute teacher who steps in and uses the lesson plan the assigned teacher had already developed. The substitute teacher does not really make the plan for the day, nor does the proxy using substituted judgment really make the treatment decisions. Just as the substitute teacher carries out the lesson plan chosen earlier by the regular teacher, so the proxy using substituted judgment carries out the treatment plan chosen earlier by the patient.

This means the proxy must know how the person wants to be treated if she becomes an incapacitated patient. There are three ways a proxy can know this:

1. The patient could have explicitly told the proxy, orally or in written advance directives, what she wants done;
2. The patient could have implicitly made clear what she wants, perhaps by offhand comments about how silly it is to keep unconscious people alive on machines for months, etc.
3. The patient could have revealed enough about her thinking and values so the proxy knows what she wants, even though the matter was never discussed or even mentioned. This is an extremely weak basis for substituted judgment, but may be valid in some cases. The spouse in a happy marriage where the couple was open and communicated well with each other, for example, may be in a position to rely on it.

The proxy's role in substituted judgment is, therefore, a limited one. The proxy does not really make the decision; he communicates the decision of the patient. In substituted judgment, the proxy reports to the physician what the patient wants. Substituted judgment works very well when patients have discussed in a clear and explicit way their wishes about future treatment with their proxies. Proxies find it more difficult to use substituted judgment when they have to rely on patients' comments and on their familiarity with the person and the person's attitude toward life, sickness, and death. This is why treatment directives and communication with the person who will act as proxy are so vital.

Proxies can use substituted judgment only when they know what the patient would have wanted. The substituted judgment standard cannot be used when proxies have to make decisions for babies or young children, or for adults who never had capacity or, if they did once have it, never revealed enough for the proxy to know what they wanted.

Although this explanation of substituted judgment reflects the standard use of the term in health care ethics, we should note that the phrase is sometimes used in an idiosyncratic way. Some court decisions, and this includes a long history of decisions in Massachusetts, use the phrase "substituted judgment" for decisions to withhold or withdraw treatment from incapacitated people who never had capacity (babies or adults with severe congenital mental deficiencies), or who had it but never made clear what they wanted before they lost it. These courts claim the treatment is something that these people would have declined if they were capable of declining treatment, and they call this hypothetical construct substituted judgment.

This is not really a good use of the substituted judgment standard because there is no evidence to support the claim that we know what such people would have decided if they were able to decide. Some justices are aware of this problem. When the Massachusetts Supreme Court used substituted judgment in the case of Beth that we discussed above, Justice Nolan recognized the problem and wrote a strong objection:

> . . . the court again has approved application of the doctrine of substituted judgment when there is not a *soupçon* of evidence to support it. The trial judge did not have a smidgen of evidence on which to conclude that if this child who is now about five and one half years old were competent to decide, she would elect certain death to a life with no cognitive ability. The route by which the court arrives at its conclusion is a cruel charade which is being perpetuated whenever we are faced with a life and death decision of an incompetent person.

Why do some court decisions allowing the withdrawal or withholding of life-sustaining treatment insist that substituted judgment is the standard for making the decision, even when the patient never had the capacity to make health care decisions? Two reasons comes to mind.

First, the courts recognize a serious obligation to preserve human life, especially vulnerable human life, and thus some judges are uncomfortable with decisions to stop treatments that are preserving life. It is difficult for these judges to give up the obligation to preserve life and if they do, they want the patient, and not anyone else, to make the decision. If the patient never had decision-making capacity, the best these judges can do is claim that the patient would have decided to forego treatment if he could have decided to forego treatment.

Second, the law supports rights of self-determination and privacy, including, as we saw in our discussion of informed consent, the right of people to refuse treatment. And the courts do not think these rights are lost just because a person is not able to assert them. The courts are careful about rights, and some judges can accept letting the life-sustaining treatment be withheld or withdrawn only if they can construe the case as one in which the patient would, if he could, exercise his right to refuse treatment.

Although the efforts of these courts to justify the withholding or withdrawal of inappropriate treatment are laudable, their use of substituted judgment to conjecture what patients who never had capacity would have wanted if they did have capacity is not helpful. In fact, it causes unnecessary confusion. It would be better if these courts could refrain from viewing every decision to withdraw treatment from an incapacitated patient as a form of substituted judgment, and acknowledge that the second criterion of proxy decision-making, best interests, is legally relevant.

The Best Interests Standard

The best interests standard is what the proxy falls back on when the patient's wishes are not known and the substituted judgment standard cannot be used. The "interests" in best interests are the interests of the patient, what will benefit the patient. Often the patient will derive benefit from treatment, but sometimes treatment is more of a burden than a benefit. In such cases, the treatment would not be in the best interests of the patient.

The benefit in question is a net benefit—that is, what will be in the best interests of the patient, all things considered. Best interests does not refer to the benefit of a specific treatment. Suppose a proxy was making a decision for a terminally ill person with periodontal disease. Gum surgery, an uncomfortable procedure, will obviously be a benefit by curing the gum disease but, when everything is considered, it is not in the patient's best interests. The gum disease will not cause distress or tooth loss for another decade, and the person is not expected to live more than a year. We have a similar case when people in pain are clearly dying and then contract pneumonia. Using antibiotics will produce a benefit—the curing of pneumonia—but this treatment may not be in the best interests of these dying patients, all things considered.

The word "best" in best interests is somewhat misleading and could be confusing. It does not mean that the proxy must provide the absolutely best treatment for the patient. If the patient needs surgery, for example, the proxy need not seek the best surgeon in the world for the operation, or seek to place the person in the best medical center in the country. The word "best" in best interests simply means that the proxy should decide on the basis of what he thinks is good for the particular patient—that is, what he thinks will truly benefit him.

Both the substituted judgment and the best interests standards can be overridden in some rare situations. In a triage situation, for example, a provider may decide to withhold or remove treatment in order to provide it for another with a better chance of survival, even though the first patient wanted the treatment, or it is in her best interests to have it. And a national health service may put limits on certain treatments that will place them beyond the reach of most citizens, despite the fact that some patients would want the treatment or that it would be in their best interests to receive it.

The Reasonable Treatment Standard

Sometimes neither the substituted judgment nor the best interests standard is applicable. We cannot use substituted judgment if the patient never gave any indication of what was wanted. And we cannot use best interests if the patient has no interests, and sometimes we do not use it when the patient has interests. Two situations where a proxy cannot rely either on substituted judgment (the patients never expressed their wishes) or on best interests are: (1) some permanently unconscious patients and (2) some incapacitated dying patients kept on life support to preserve organs for transplantation. In the first case, the proxy may decide to withdraw life-sustaining treatment; in the second, she may decide to continue it. In neither case can the proxy's decision be based on substituted judgment (the patients never indicated what was wanted) or, as we will see, best interests. Hence we need our third standard, the "reasonable treatment" standard. To see why this is so, we will look at these situations more closely.

Permanently unconscious patients

Patients in a permanent coma or in a persistent vegetative state no longer have any interests in the usual sense of the word. They are beyond experiencing anything, and therefore beyond all burdens and benefits. It truly makes no difference to them whether they live or die. Their family and friends, and their society, may still have interests in what happens to them, but these patients have no interests. Nothing we do to or for them is a burden or a benefit. Life-support systems and surgeries are neither benefits nor burdens for them because they do not, and never again will, feel anything.

Some ethicists argue that the permanently unaware patient does have interests, or at least has one interest, the interest in living. They say that we can speak of the interests of a permanently unconscious person just as we speak of the interests of a deceased person who left instructions in a will about the disposition of personal property. The executor of the estate respects those wishes and, as we say, looks out for the interests of the deceased.

The interests we speak of in reference to the deceased, however, are not the same as the interests designated in the best interests standard. The interests in reference to the deceased refer to their earlier wishes, and thus relate to the substituted judgment standard, not to the best interests standard. The interests in the best interests standard refer not to what the patient wanted, but to what is beneficial for the patient.

Imagine this situation: A ventilator dependent patient has been in a persistent vegetative state (PVS) for years, and the proxy now wants to withdraw the life-support systems. Since the patient never gave any indication of how he wanted to be treated if he ever permanently lost consciousness, the proxy cannot use substituted judgment. Nor can she use the best interests standard, because permanently unconscious patients have no interests. Nothing matters to them. Yet it is at least arguable, and more likely reasonably certain, that the proxy is morally justified in seeking withdrawal of life-sustaining treatment from a PVS patient.

But what standard guides the proxy's decision? In such a case, the proxy falls back on what we are calling the reasonable treatment standard. The proxy requests the withdrawal of life-sustaining treatment because there is no cogent reason to treat, and many reasons not to treat, permanently unconscious patients year after year. Treatment of PVS patients is not reasonable because it is of no possible benefit to the patient, withdrawing it is of no burden to the patient, and providing the treatment is a considerable burden for others.

Sometimes the reasonable treatment standard is appropriate even when we do know what the patient would have wanted. Imagine this situation: A person once told his proxy that he wants major heart surgery if he ever needs it. Many years ago, he lapsed into a persistent vegetative state. Now he needs the heart surgery. Should the proxy, using the substituted judgment standard, try to arrange for the heart surgery? Or could the proxy ignore the patient's wishes and decline to seek the surgery? It is at least arguable, and more likely reasonably certain, that we should not perform major heart surgery on a person in a persistent vegetative state.

But what is the basis of this judgment? It is not substituted judgment—the patient said he wanted the heart surgery. And it is not best interests—the permanently unconscious patient has no interests. The standard guiding the proxy's decision can only be what we are calling the reasonable treatment standard. And in this kind of case, the reasonable treatment standard of proxy decision-making actually overrules the substituted judgment standard.

Incapacitated organ donors

The reasonable treatment standard may also be invoked in a second kind of situation involving conscious but incapacitated patients. Consider the following. A young child on life-support systems is dying, and the parents and providers have reached the conclusion that withdrawing the life support is in the best interests of the child.

The parents are also ardent supporters of organ transplantation, and would now like to donate the organs of their child after death. It may be that the best chance for successful transplantation will be to keep the child alive on life-support equipment for several days until the recipients of the organs can be located, brought to the hospital of the dying child, and prepared for the surgery. Suppose also that the child can be medicated to prevent suffering while kept alive on the life-support equipment.

If we do decide to continue the life support to preserve the organs, the decision is not based on substituted judgment—a proxy cannot use this standard for a baby. Nor is it based on best interests—we have already said that withdrawal of the treatment is in the best interests of the child. Hence, neither substituted judgment nor best interests can justify the parents' decision to continue the life support keeping the child's organs healthy for transplantation. Quite simply, the baby's life is not being preserved for its benefit, but for the benefit of the organ recipients. Is this ethical?

Once again, the appropriate standard guiding the proxies' decision is the reasonable treatment standard. If it is reasonable, the proxies may decide to continue treatment even when it is no longer in the child's best interests. Given the shortage of infant organs, it is at least arguably reasonable to continue the life-sustaining treatment for a few days, provided we have reason to believe that the prolonged treatment is not causing the baby any suffering.

In summary, then, when patients do not have decision-making capacity, a proxy will decide for them. The proxy normally bases his decision on one of three standards. First, the proxy tries to use the substituted judgment standard and report what the patient wants. If this is not possible, the proxy turns to the second standard—best interests—and tries to decide what is in the best interests of this particular patient. If the patient has left no indication of her wishes and has no interests because of the permanent loss of all awareness, the proxy can only decide on the basis of our third standard—what is reasonable treatment in the circumstances.

The substituted judgment and best interests standards are now widely understood and accepted in health care ethics, and they are easily compatible with the ethics of right reason that we are developing. Our third standard, reasonable treatment, normally used only when the other two are not applicable, is not so widely recognized, although there is growing awareness that neither substituted judgment nor best interests are relevant in all cases of deciding for others, as our examples showed.

In most cases of deciding for others, the standards just outlined can be applied in a straightforward way. Deciding for some classes of patients, however, can be a real challenge. We will now look at three such groups: older children, the mentally ill, and patients from other cultures.

DECIDING FOR OLDER CHILDREN

The task of making health care decisions for neonates and young children, while often difficult because it is so hard to know what is the right thing to do, is fairly straightforward. Since the young children never had decision-making capacity and do not have it now, the decisions made on their behalf, usually by their parents, are based on the best interests standard.

Deciding for children becomes much more complicated when the children are older and have some grasp of the information and some ability to give consent, yet still lack the maturity of an adult. These children are not yet fully capable of making mature decisions, but are not far from it, and may actually have the capacity to make some decisions. The situation is further complicated because the medical needs and the problems they face after puberty are often the kind of problems many children would not want their parents to know of—pregnancy, sexually transmitted diseases, drug abuse, etc. The desire of some minors to prevent their parents from knowing about their problems makes it impossible for physicians to consider their parents as appropriate proxies.

In trying to sort out the conflicting issues surrounding the medical treatment of older children, a brief historical comment may be helpful. Until recently, our common law tradition, along with our ethical heritage, viewed parents as having almost total control over their minor children. Children were not thought to have rights of their own. Parents made all the decisions affecting the children, including health care decisions, until the minor became an adult or established an independent life. For a long time, the age of becoming an adult was twenty-one, but since the federal voting age was lowered to eighteen in 1971, most legislatures now consider eighteen the age a child becomes an adult.

The idea that parents had almost total control over their children slowly broke down in recent centuries. One major factor in the breakdown occurred in the 19th century, when a heightened awareness of the exploitation of children emerged. Parents had always used their children as laborers to work long hours tilling the land and tending the animals. With the rise of industrialization, however, the sight of children working long hours in the miserable nineteenth century factories led to laws designed to protect and promote children's welfare. In some cases, these laws prevented parents from doing what they wanted to do with their children—sending them off to work in factories.

The movement to protect children and improve their welfare did not, of course, immediately enhance their self-determination. The laws restricted what their parents could demand of them, but did not give the children more room for decision making. This came much later, and not without considerable social upheaval and family stress. At the present time, however, our society has arrived at the point where most people agree that older minors should play a major role in significant decisions affecting their lives, including decisions about their medical treatment.

On the other hand, parents still retain a considerable interest in providing for their children, especially those not yet eighteen. And most children under eighteen can still benefit from parental guidance, especially when they are ill and major medical decisions need to be made. The tricky question with a teenage minor, then, is how the real but limited capacity for self-determination in the not yet mature child can be harmonized with legitimate parental concerns and important parental guidance. This is the kind of question not susceptible to a definitive answer; all we can hope to do is grope toward some kind of response.

We will first show how studies on the cognitive development of children suggest strongly that the absolute minimum age necessary for a child to have the capacity to make health care decisions is about twelve. Before this age parents or another proxy must make the decisions because the child lacks the cognitive development to do it. Then we will examine how parents or a proxy should be involved in making decisions for minors twelve and older. We will see how in some cases it may be morally appropriate for the parents or proxy to have nothing to do with the decision, while in other cases it is morally appropriate that they will share in, and perhaps actually make, the health care decision.

The Minimum Age for Minors to Make Health Care Decisions

The first thing to determine is when an older minor has developed sufficient capacity to understand, to evaluate, to reason about the medical realities confronting her, and to consent freely to proposed interventions. In other words, when does a child develop the capacity to make health care decisions?

The answer, of course, will vary from child to child. Some mature very quickly, others take a slower route. Yet developmental studies of normal children show definite stages of advancing toward maturity in understanding, evaluating, reasoning, and consenting. These studies indicate that most children younger than twelve have not yet developed decision-making capacity, that children between twelve and fourteen are in a kind of transition period, and that children fifteen and older may well have enough capacity to make major health care decisions on their own. This is not to say making such decisions on their own is the ideal; obviously, most children under eighteen could benefit from the assistance of loving and caring parents.

Some suggest that minors suffering from chronic illness for many years achieve an understanding and an ability to make decisions about their treatment long before other children. This seems to be so for older minors, but the reverse may be true for younger children, in whom the illness may retard mental and moral development.

It is important to determine when minors achieve the capacity to make their health care decisions because we want to avoid two situations: we do not want to ignore their decisions if they truly have the capacity to make them, and we do not want to accept their decisions if they really do not have the capacity to make them. In other words, we do not want to disenfranchise a child capable of deciding, and we do not want to force decision making on a child not yet ready for it.

To determine when the health care decisions of a minor are valid, we must examine his capacity to make such decisions. In the previous chapter, we identified three elements of capacity: understanding, evaluation, and reasoning.

Understanding. Studies of normal children suggest that a child's understanding of illness is closely related to the developmental stages of cognitive development first outlined in some detail by Jean Piaget decades ago. In this developmental schema, children do not really begin to understand illness, let alone prognoses and the impact of various treatments that might cure or mitigate the illness, until sometime after the age of eleven. Then this realistic understanding of illness will grow over the next few years.

Evaluation. A child's appreciation of what is good and bad also grows in developmental stages. Here the basic work was done by Lawrence Kohlberg, who continued Piaget's work in the relationship between cognitive and moral development. The developmental studies of Piaget, Kohlberg, and others elaborating on their work strongly suggest that mature moral judgments cannot be made until about the age of twelve. Although Kohlberg's work has been criticized, with some reason, because it emphasized the moral development of boys as they grew into men and thus slighted the moral development of girls as they grew into women, his conclusions about when children begin to make moral judgments—be they based on what is perceived as the male orientation to fairness and justice or on what is perceived as the female orientation to relationships and caring—remain widely accepted.

This does not mean mature moral judgments *are* made at this age; only that the minor has the capacity to make them. Both Piaget and Kohlberg insisted on what we all know: achieving a mature cognitive development does not mean moral maturity necessarily follows. People cannot make moral decisions without advanced cognitive development, but this cognitive development does not guarantee that they will make morally mature decisions.

Reasoning. In Piaget's schema, formal reasoning also begins around the age of twelve, when the advanced level of cognitive development that enables adolescents to reason abstractly occurs. At this stage, the child can consider various possibilities, form hypotheses and deduce conclusions from them, and then test these conclusions against experience. Moreover, a child at this stage of cognitive development can reason simultaneously about the alternative treatments and about the risks associated with each. As was pointed out in the last chapter, this is the level of reasoning a person must achieve, at least in rudimentary form, before we can say that he has the capacity to make health care decisions and to give informed consent.

From the developmental studies pioneered by Piaget and Kohlberg, then, it seems clear that children below the age of twelve simply do not have the capacity to make heath care decisions and to give informed consent. Their parents, or some other proxy, must do it for them.

This leaves us with the problems associated with minors in the twelve to eighteen age group. This is the difficult gray area because children this age are achieving the cognitive development allowing them to understand, evaluate, and reason in a mature way, but this maturity is obviously not fully developed, and it will vary significantly from child to child. The difficult question now is: What role do parents play in the health care decisions of this group of children?

Limitations On the Parental Role in Decisions Affecting Older (12–18) Minors

Children from twelve to eighteen are still considered minors, and therefore the assumption is that they are still subject to their parents. However, there are many situations where parents no longer have the authority to make health care decisions for their older minor children, and the children decide for themselves.

Emancipated minors

Emancipated minors have been recognized in law for years, and the recognition seems morally sound. Emancipated minors are no longer subject to parental control. In general, an emancipated minor can make her own health care decisions and give informed consent for medical interventions. Emancipated minors are usually no longer living at home and are supporting themselves. Marriage is an action that emancipates a minor, even if the marriage is followed by divorce and the minor returns to the parental home. Entry into military service also emancipates a minor. A college student under 18 living at college is in an ambiguous situation if the parents are still supporting him financially, but there is a general tendency to consider a college student not living at home emancipated and capable of giving informed consent. A high school student at a boarding school, however, is generally not considered emancipated, and thus parents are the ones to give consent for his medical treatment.

A minor child who has run away from home presents another ambiguous situation, but it seems reasonable to consider him sufficiently emancipated to give informed consent, especially if the runaway teenager does not want the parents involved in the situation, which is often the case. It would also seem appropriate to consider a minor who has become a parent emancipated. Since parents give consent for the treatment of their child, they should be able to give consent for their own treatment even if they are still minors.

Minor treatment statutes

Many states have laws allowing minors above a certain age—which varies from state to state—to give consent for some medical treatment without notifying their parents. The need to treat venereal disease was the problem behind many of these laws. Obviously, many minors would not want their parents to know that they had contracted a sexually transmitted disease, and they would not be inclined to seek treatment if the physicians had to contact their parents to obtain consent for treatment. Without treatment, however, not only would the infected minors suffer, but very likely some of them might spread the disease and create a public health problem. Hence, accepting consent from minors for treatment of sexually transmitted diseases became legally acceptable in many states.

A second situation often covered by these minor treatment statutes is drug abuse. It is easy to understand why many minors would not want their parents to know they have a drug problem, so accepting consent for treatment from the minors themselves also makes sense.

A third situation often covered by these statutes is prenatal care. Many states have laws permitting pregnant minors to give consent for appropriate health care during pregnancy without parental approval or notification.

Contraception

As we will note in the chapter on reproduction, a series of Supreme Court cases has found that restrictions on contraception violate the constitutional right to privacy. In 1965 *Griswold v. Connecticut* allowed access to contraception for married couples. In 1972 *Eisenstadt v. Baird*, a case originating in Massachusetts, allowed access to contraception for unmarried adults; and in 1977 *Carey v. Population Services International*, a case originating in New York, allowed access to contraception for unmarried minors. These interpretations of the Constitution allow sexually active unmarried minors to give consent for contraceptive medical interventions such as anovulant pills, diaphragms, and Norplant without parental notification.

Allowing minors access to contraceptive medical interventions is, of course, a highly charged controversy in our society at this time. On one side, people argue such access is for the good of the sexually active minor and of society because it prevents unwanted pregnancy. On the other side, people argue such access encourages immature sexual relationships, undermines the legitimate concern parents have for their children, and weakens society in general by seeming to encourage widespread sexual activity outside the social structure of marriage and the family. There are thoughtful and caring people on both sides of this debate.

There is not much debate, however, about contraceptive sterilization. These surgeries raise a host of more serious questions because they are very difficult to reverse, and the sterilized minor might well want children at a later date. Many, if not most, people consider the surgical sterilization of minors at their request morally objectionable. Most physicians, of course, would refuse to perform these surgeries on teenagers, and with good reason, since there is no justification for these radical contraceptive interventions at an early age.

Abortion

In 1973 the Supreme Court extended the notion of privacy to abortion in the first two trimesters of pregnancy in *Roe v. Wade* and *Doe v. Bolton*. The women in these cases were adults, so the question of whether a pregnant minor could give informed consent for an abortion was not specifically addressed by the court at that time.

Massachusetts then passed a law requiring both parents, if they were available, to give consent before their daughter under 18 could have an abortion. In *Bellotti v. Baird* (1979), the Supreme Court struck down this law, thereby allowing minors to give consent for their abortions. The opinion required states that considered pregnant minors too immature to give authentic informed consent for abortion to arrange an alternative procedure that would not force the minor girl to seek parental consent for her abortion.

One such alternative procedure exists in Massachusetts and in some other states. A minor seeking an abortion without parental consent must appear before a judge. He or she then determines whether the minor has the capacity to give informed consent for the abortion. If the judge finds the minor has the capacity, then she can give consent for her abortion. If the judge finds she does not have the capacity, then the court must decide whether the abortion is in her best interests. If the court so finds, it can issue an order allowing the abortion. In practice, judges in Massachusetts almost invariably find the pregnant minor has the capacity to give consent for the abortion.

The legal developments allowing minors to give consent for treatment of sexually transmitted diseases and drug problems, and for medical interventions to prevent or terminate pregnancy, have encouraged a trend whereby older minors are considered to have the capacity to make health care decisions for other medical problems as well. This trend implies that they also have the capacity to withhold consent for treatment that their parents may want them to have. The assumption that parents make all the decisions for their minor children has given way to the recognition that older minors are able to make many of their health care decisions.

From an ethical point of view, there are both good and bad features in this trend allowing minors to make their own decisions. The major good feature centers on recognizing the increasing capacity of a maturing minor to assume responsibility for his life. The maturing minor has to form some kind of life plan and make decisions that will determine what kind of adult he will become. It is impossible to do this if parents make all the important decisions until age eighteen, and then the minor suddenly assumes decision-making responsibility. Rather, the process of maturity requires a more gradual transition from a child subject to parental control to a young adult responsible for his decisions. Older minors naturally desire to assume more and more control over their lives, and are actually able to do so successfully to a considerable degree.

Yet the value of self-determination for minors is less than it is for adults, primarily because the decisions teenagers make are limited by their lack of experience and maturity. Good decision making comes only with time, practice, and experience, and the minor simply has not had enough of these. Hence the notions of autonomy and self-determination, so popular in contemporary health care ethics, are of limited value when the patient is a minor.

There are good reasons for allowing minors to give consent for treatment involving health problems associated with sexuality and drugs if they do not want their parents to know of their problems. But this does not mean it is a good idea for them to make all their health care decisions. In many other cases it is in the self-interest of the minor to have parental consultation and guidance in making health care decisions. And, if teenagers have a trusting and open relation with their parents, they might well benefit from parental help in making decisions about the medical issues surrounding sexuality and drugs as well.

A major bad feature of the trend to accept health care decisions from minors without parental consent is the seldom noticed impact it has on the legitimate interests of parents to care for their children. Most parents care about their children, and often know them and their needs better than the children know themselves. This parental caring and interest in the child's welfare does not end as soon as the child develops a minimally adequate decision-making capacity, but continues long afterward. The fact that this parental interest can be distorted, and that some parents try to run their children's lives, should not blind us to the legitimate parental interest and caring that continues through the teenage years, and often beyond.

Once this is acknowledged, the determination that a minor has developed decision-making capacity does not imply that he should exercise it without parental involvement. In some situations—venereal disease, for example—it may be reasonable not to confide in parents, but in many other health care situations the minor will benefit greatly from the involvement of caring parents. Hence, there are many situations where good ethics suggests the participation of parents in the medical decision making affecting their minor children, even though these children may have achieved sufficient decision-making capacity to be able to make the decisions on their own.

There is an additional reason for encouraging parental involvement in the health care decisions of minors whenever possible: the legitimate interest of parents in their family. Parents, and other children in the family as well, may be affected by the health care decision of a minor, and therefore the parents should have some say in what goes on. The parents, for example, may be paying for the treatment, or the proposed treatment may adversely affect the other children in the family, whom the parents have a responsibility to protect. Whenever the minor's treatment impacts on important family interests, the parents have a legitimate interest in participating actively in the decision making.

Making decisions for children when they are between twelve and eighteen, then, is a very complicated matter if they are not emancipated or if they are seeking one of the special forms of treatment where parental notification would create more burdens than benefits. It calls for a great deal of prudential insight. The following comments may provide a general moral orientation.

First, parents are the usual proxies for children without the capacity to make health care decisions. Sometimes, however, it may be necessary for the courts to appoint a guardian or proxy because the parents' behavior disqualifies them from making medical decisions for their children.

Second, when parents make decisions for older minors, they use the familiar standards of substituted judgment and best interests, but in a qualified way. Substituted judgment cannot be used unless the child is an older minor and has indicated some preferences about how he wants to be treated. Since few minors actually do this, the best interests standard is usually the relevant standard, but it has to be qualified somewhat. Best interests of the sick child is not the only concern for parents; they must also consider the decision in light of the best interests of others in the family, especially other children.

Third, when children begin to achieve some capacity to understand and to consent voluntarily to medical treatment, parents should include them in the decision-making process to the extent it is possible. Parents and physicians treat children with respect by sharing information with them and by letting them participate in the decision-making process to the extent they are able to do so. Before children are sufficiently mature to give true consent for treatment, they are able to "assent" to the decisions being made in their best interests, and physicians and parents should seek this assent.

Fourth, when minors have achieved decision-making capacity, parents should still play a role in the decision making unless it would be not be helpful, as may be the case with medical problems caused by sexual activity or drug abuse. Just how strong this parental role should be will depend on the circumstances and the maturity of the minor. The ideal will be a shared decision making between the parents, the minor, and the physician, but this is often not feasible.

Fifth, it sometimes happens that responsible parents want to make an informed refusal of routine treatment for their children. The classic example of this involves families who are practicing Jehovah's Witnesses. This religious group believes that the Bible forbids blood transfusions. Parents, however, may not refuse consent for normal life-saving treatments for their children. If they do, providers may appeal to the state child protective agencies or directly to the courts. The courts tend to respond in one of two ways: either they issue an order for the treatment, or they temporarily remove the child from the parents' custody and appoint a guardian to give consent for it. The basis of the courts' reactions are state child abuse laws, which consider the withholding of necessary medical treatment from a child a form of child abuse and neglect. A state supreme court decision known as *Prince v. Massachusetts* made the important point that a parent may become a martyr for his religious beliefs, but "he is not free to make a martyr of his child."

DECIDING FOR THE MENTALLY ILL

Mental illness can be a terrible tragedy affecting not only the patient but the family and society as well. Many mentally ill people cannot care for themselves, and they may be a danger to themselves or others. Frequently, proxies must make health care decisions for them.

Making health care decisions for the mentally ill opens up a number of legal and moral dilemmas. Some of the troubling questions are: Is it moral to place the mentally ill in institutions against their will simply because they might harm themselves or others? Is it moral to force treatment on them, most especially drugs or surgery or shock treatments, against their will? Is their informed consent for treatment truly voluntary if we have made it clear to them that they will be confined to an institution if they do not accept treatment?

Mental illness is not a clearly defined term. It covers a wide range of dysfunction from the severe to the relatively mild, and the categories used by the American Psychiatric Association are so general that physicians have considerable leeway in diagnosing patients' behaviors. This makes it all the more important to consider the ethical implications of how proxies make treatment decisions for those diagnosed as mentally ill.

We will consider but three issues in this complicated field. First, the relation of mental illness and decision-making capacity; second, decisions to commit or restrain the mentally ill against their wishes; and third, decisions to treat the mentally ill against their will.

Mental Illness and Decision-Making Capacity

A widespread misconception assumes that all mentally ill people are incompetent and have lost the capacity to make health care decisions. This is simply not true. As we pointed out in the last chapter, people are legally competent unless found incompetent by a judge. Most mentally ill people have not been found incompetent by a judge, and hence remain legally competent.

Also, many mentally ill people retain decision-making capacity. Some mental illnesses do not override decision-making capacity or, if they do, it is only temporary, and periods of capacity remain wherein the patient is able to make decisions about treatment. Moreover, capacity, as we pointed out in the last chapter, is task specific, and a mental illness that destroys a patient's capacity to make some decisions does not necessarily destroy the capacity to make all health care decisions.

It is unwise, then, to assume that all mentally ill people have lost the ability to make their health care decisions. Rather, the decision-making capacity of people diagnosed as mentally ill should be determined the same way it is determined for the physically ill; that is, the physician will ascertain whether the patient is able to understand the important facts, to evaluate the illness and possible treatments in light of a framework of values, to reason about the impact that the various treatment options may have, and to give consent freely. Undoubtedly, some mentally ill patients, as some physically ill patients, have lost the capacity to make health care decisions. But other mentally ill patients, as other physically ill patients, retain the capacity to give truly informed consent.

It is true, however, that mental illness often does affect the capacity to make health care decisions and to give voluntary consent for treatment. The illness can undermine any of the three aspects of decision-making capacity: understanding, evaluation, and reasoning. In some forms of schizophrenia, for example, a person may have a fixed belief that medications are really poisons, or that health care providers are part of a plot to trap and imprison him. These beliefs interfere with his ability to understand the diagnosis and the true risks of various treatment options.

In other forms of mental illness—severe depression, for example—the person's ability to evaluate a course of action can be lost because the illness weakens the person's ability to care about any of the goals and projects in life that provide a framework for value judgments. And some manic stages of bipolar illness can distort the reasoning process by introducing a totally unrealistic picture of what can be done.

While mental illness can attack the specific cognitive and volitional abilities needed to make health care decisions, it does not always do so and, if it does, does not always permanently destroy those abilities. Hence the physician must assess each patient carefully to determine decision-making capacity and, if it has been lost, to determine whether it might return. The important thing is to avoid thinking that once a person has been diagnosed as mentally ill, a proxy must make all the treatment decisions from that point onward. This kind of thinking all too easily disenfranchises a human being who retains the capacity to make decisions about his treatment.

Deciding to Commit or to Restrain the Mentally Ill

In recent decades, the number of hospitalized mentally ill people has dropped significantly, from more than half a million in 1955 to a little more than 100,000 now. Many factors prompted this decline; among them are the development of drugs that control or reduce the dangerous or antisocial symptoms of patients, and the growing awareness that patients have liberty interests and should not be hospitalized unless absolutely necessary. In addition, some institutions housing the mentally ill were wretched places, partly because so many patients acted out in the era before psychotropic drugs were widely used, and partly because so many people had become frustrated with the exasperating nature of mental illness that society was content at times simply to "warehouse" patients so it could live in peace. And finally, there was a cost factor. Many of the mental health institutions were state hospitals, and few taxpayers wanted to spend a lot of money on caring for those whom they perceived as hopeless and unproductive members of society.

The deinstitutionalization of mentally ill people has resulted in fewer long-term mentally ill inpatients. Still, decisions by proxies to commit mentally ill persons must be made, and the decisions are both morally and legally difficult. Involuntary confinement is a direct attack on personal liberty. The involuntary confinement is not really a treatment, but a detention. Depriving a human being of the freedom to live in society is a major restriction on his life, and we need a strong reason for doing it.

Two reasons are usually given when a proxy decides to commit a mentally ill patient against his will: he is a danger to others, or he is a danger to himself. We will examine the strength of these reasons.

Danger to others
Certainly, some mentally ill people are dangerous to others, and their erratic behavior can be a source of great fear. But the "danger to others" reason for involuntary commitment has to be put in perspective. We have to remember that many people not mentally ill are dangerous to others—violent crimes are a fact of life—yet we do not detain people simply because there is some reason to believe that they might be a danger to others. If anyone proposed locking up every person who might commit a violent crime, we would be shocked at this proposed violation of personal freedom without cause and due process. People who might commit violent crimes have to be left alone unless they actually commit those crimes. Yet the attitude toward the mentally ill is often quite different. Many think that they should be confined when there is some reason to believe they might be a danger to others. It is this attitude that must be questioned, lest the important constitutional right of liberty and the moral value of freedom be prematurely compromised.

Moreover, the commitment of all mentally ill persons who might harm others will obviously be an injustice to some of them. Suppose, for example, there is an 80 percent chance that patients with a certain diagnosis will harm other people if left free in society. For some, this percentage would be sufficiently high to justify involuntary commitment in order to prevent the violence.

But think of this: If we force involuntary commitment on one hundred people with this diagnosis, then we are confining twenty people who, if left free, will never harm anyone. In order to justify morally confining one hundred people with an 80 percent chance of harming others, we will also have to justify forcing twenty people into confinement who did not harm anyone and will not harm anyone if they are left in society. This is obviously a question of justice, and an ethical dimension of involuntary commitment seldom considered when a decision is made to commit a mentally ill person because it is thought that she might be a danger to others.

The same factors have to be considered when there is a question of restraining hospitalized persons, either by physical restraints restricting their movements or by confining them to a secluded place other than their normal inpatient space. This is also a serious deprivation of freedom, and can be justified only in emergencies or where providers are convinced that harm to others will actually occur.

So, while it is certainly possible to justify involuntary confinement of mentally ill people on the grounds that they are a danger to others, it is not, in the absence of a history of violence, an easy case to make. It is very difficult to predict who will be violent if left in society, and very hard to justify restraining or confining people simply because they might be violent. In order to protect personal rights and avoid injustice to the innocent, society has to leave free many people who might commit violent crime. For the same reasons, society has to leave free many mentally ill people who might be dangerous. The fact that some mentally ill people actually will commit violent actions does not justify confining every mentally ill person who might commit violent actions, anymore than the fact some people will commit violent crime justifies confining everyone who might commit violent crime.

Danger to self

The second reason proxies use for the decision to commit mentally ill patients against their will is to protect them from harming, or even killing, themselves. Now, some mentally ill people certainly are a danger to themselves but, again, the moral reasoning justifying the commitment on the basis of the patient's best interest is complicated.

First, consider the mentally ill person with the capacity to make health care decisions, including the specific decision about commitment to a mental health institution. Suppose his family and physicians have reason to believe that the person is a danger to himself—does that belief justify their committing or restraining him against his will? We might be tempted to reason this way: The person is mentally ill and a danger to himself, therefore confinement in a hospital is the best place for him.

Such reasoning is rooted in the laudable desire to protect the mentally ill person, but it is seriously flawed. If an adult has the capacity to make decisions about hospitalization, there is no sound reason for violating his liberty and confining him to an institution against his will simply because others think that he is a danger to himself. It would be a great tragedy if such an adult was not confined and restrained, and then harmed or even destroyed himself, but it would be a greater tragedy if we committed to institutions, as a matter of course, competent people with decision-making capacity against their will. Forced confinement of sick people who retain decision-making capacity is a major violation of their personal liberty and dignity. Just as hospitals cannot force physically sick people to become patients or to remain in the institution against their will, neither can hospitals force mentally sick people to become patients or to remain in the institution against their will, as long as the mentally sick people retain the capacity to decide for themselves about hospitalization.

The mentally ill person may well be a danger to himself, but this is not enough of a reason to confine him involuntarily if he still has the capacity to make his own decision about hospitalization. And if perchance the mentally ill person is in the hospital, but retains the capacity to make decisions about the hospitalization and wants to leave, it is not morally justified to prevent the discharge. Confining a competent human being with decision-making capacity against his will is a most serious move, and the possibility that he is a "danger to himself" is seldom a strong enough reason to justify it.

Second, consider the mentally ill person who is a danger to herself, and who lacks the capacity to make health care decisions. In this case, a proxy will make the decision whether or not to commit the patient. For a mentally ill person who never had decision-making capacity, or once had it but left no advance indications of what she wanted, the proxy will use the best interests standard when deciding about commitment.

But for a mentally ill person without decision-making capacity who had, during a previous period of capacity, formulated advance directives or given clear indication of her wishes, the proxy will use the substituted judgment standard for the decision. And if the mentally ill person had indicated, during a previous period of lucidity when she had decision-making capacity, that she would not want confinement, the substituted judgment standard now constrains the proxy to decide against confinement, despite the possibility that she may harm herself.

Hence, it is entirely possible that sound moral judgment directs a proxy to decline confinement for a mentally ill patient without decision-making capacity who is a danger to herself. This judgment is not a comfortable one, but the alternative is even more uncomfortable: confining someone who had, by advance directives, made it clear that she did not want the confinement. This is little more than imprisoning an innocent person against her will.

In some cases, however, prudential reasoning can justify, by way of exception, confining a mentally ill person to prevent her harming herself despite her advance directives against it. One such case is when the mentally ill person is actually behaving in a self-destructive way. Perhaps she is engaged in violence against herself; or perhaps she is refusing to eat.

The confinement of the mentally ill against their previous wishes expressed during earlier periods of decision-making capacity is easiest to justify when the confinement is brief and temporary. If they have become so agitated or upset that they have lost the capacity to understand, evaluate, or reason, and now pose a danger to themselves, it would seem morally justified to confine or restrain them involuntarily if they are expected to regain soon the capacity to make decisions for themselves. In some ways, this resembles the "protective custody" used by some police departments to care for an inebriated citizen for a few hours. The police consider such a person a danger to himself and vulnerable to harm from others, so they confine the inebriated person in protective custody until his ability to take care of himself returns.

To sum up, there is seldom justification for the involuntary confinement of a patient suffering from any illness—mental or physical—if the person has decision-making capacity or, if he does not now have this capacity, once had it and had made it clear that he did not want confinement. Exceptions to this will be rare. One exception occurs when it is known with certainty that the person is a serious danger to others; another occurs when the person is actually engaged in harming himself, or is in imminent danger of being harmed by others. The fact that a person might be a danger to himself, however, is not itself a sufficient reason to confine him against his present or previous wishes. Drug addicts are a danger to themselves, but this does not justify forcing them into institutions against their will. Many smokers are endangering their health, yet no one advocates confining them so they cannot obtain cigarettes.

And if a proxy does decide to institutionalize a mentally ill person on the basis of his being a danger to others, it is well to remember that the decision is not really a medical one, despite the fact that the person is confined to a medical facility rather than a prison. The confinement of the socially dangerous mentally ill person is not primarily for the benefit of the ill person, but for the protection of innocent third parties. It is a decision primarily motivated by what is good for others, not by what is good for the sick person. The police power enjoyed by every society, and not medical benefit, is the source of the authority whereby those proven dangerous to others are confined against their will.

Deciding to Treat the Mentally Ill

Treatment is not the same as confinement. The reason for confinement is usually to provide treatment, but this is not always the case—sometimes people are confined because they are truly dangerous. And putting somebody in restraints or in seclusion is not really a treatment, but a step taken to protect the patient from harming himself or others. This is why we consider the treatment of the mentally ill as something different from confinement or the use of restraints.

In general, questions about treating the mentally ill can be resolved the same way questions about treating the physically ill are resolved. If mentally ill patients retain the capacity to make decisions about treatment, normally these decisions will be followed just as they would be followed for physically ill patients with decision-making capacity. And if mentally ill patients have lost the capacity to make decisions, then a proxy will make the treatment decisions based on substituted judgment, best interests, or the reasonable treatment standard.

Yet making decisions regarding treatment for the mentally ill can become rather complicated, as it does in the following situations.

Treatment for the involuntarily confined

For a long time, no one questioned treating involuntarily confined mentally ill patients without their consent. People simply assumed that the treatment was appropriate. If there was a good reason to hospitalize the mentally ill person over his objections in the first place, then there must be, it was thought, good reasons for providing treatments over his objections as well. Thus shock treatments, psychosurgery, or drugs were often used without any effort to determine the involuntarily confined patient's capacity to give informed consent.

Some years ago, however, several legal challenges to this assumption were mounted. In a Massachusetts case that began in federal district court as *Rogers v. Okin* (1979) and was decided by the U.S. Supreme Court as *Mills v. Rogers* (1982), the Supreme Court acknowledged that mentally ill patients can refuse treatment, specifically psychotropic drugs, even if they are involuntarily hospitalized, provided they have not lost decision-making capacity and do not pose a serious threat of physical harm to themselves or to others.

From an ethical point of view, the U.S. Supreme Court's awareness that some people involuntarily confined to mental health institutions retain the capacity to make treatment decisions is sound. The person was involuntarily committed because there was reason to believe he was a danger to society or to himself, not because he had lost decision-making capacity. An involuntarily confined patient may not have lost decision-making capacity or, if he had lost it at the time of involuntary confinement, may have regained it subsequently. Unless it has been specifically determined that the involuntarily confined patient does not have the capacity to make health care decisions, his prerogative to give or withhold informed consent must be respected. If the involuntarily confined patient with capacity refuses consent for an intervention, it cannot be forced upon him, unless extenuating circumstances are present.

Forced treatment on the incapacitated patient

Sometimes an incapacitated patient, without advance directives, refuses treatments that the proxy and physicians believe are in his best interests. The proxy's first reaction in these situations may be to ignore the patient's objections, and to give consent for psychotropic drugs, psychosurgery, or shock treatments. After all, the objections are from a mentally ill patient without decision-making capacity, and therefore cannot be taken as authentic.

But there is an additional feature in these cases that is not present in most other proxy decisions, and it complicates the moral reflection. Unlike a proxy decision made for infants, or for the unconscious, or for the compliant adult, the mentally ill patient will often challenge the treatment, sometimes strenuously. And frequently the objections are based on the patient's personal experience—the patient may have received the treatment or drugs before, and thus knows firsthand how unpleasant the side effects can be.

Forcing treatment on patients when they resist it can cause them so much additional distress that what would have been in their best interests may no longer be a net benefit for them. For example, it could be in the best interests of an incapacitated patient to receive psychotropic drugs, but forcing those drugs on the patient over his objections may cause so much additional upset that the treatment will no longer be in his best interests. Even if patients left advance directives for the treatment, but now, in their incapacitated state, are strenuously objecting to it, their present objections may sometimes carry more weight than their previous directives and wishes.

One exception to this occurs when the unwanted treatment is the only alternative to unwanted confinement. In recent decades, more and more incapacitated mentally ill people are not confined to institutions. They are living in society, and some of them are being treated despite their objections. The central legal and moral argument used to justify treating these patients against their wishes is that the alternative—involuntary commitment—would be worse for them.

From a moral point of view, if the incapacitated mentally ill person is truly a danger to others, this argument has some merit. Involuntary medication would not seem as bad as involuntary confinement, and may be justified if it controls the social danger with fewer bad effects in the patient's life than involuntary confinement. If we can forcibly confine the dangerous mentally ill to protect others, it is reasonable to say we can forcibly treat them outside of the institution unless, of course, the side effects of treatment are so severe they outweigh the disadvantages of confinement.

If the incapacitated mentally ill person is not dangerous, however, and the treatment decision is not based on public safety, but on the best interests of the patient, then, as we noted above, we have to consider carefully how the patient's objections may undermine any good the forced treatment might bring. To show how tricky the question of providing beneficial treatment for the incapacitated mentally ill may become, consider the following story.

Richard Roe III, the son of Richard Roe, Jr., was a young mentally ill adult living in Massachusetts. He had been a bright and popular student, twice elected vice-president of his class in public junior high school. He then transferred to a residential preparatory school where, in his freshman year, he began to drink heavily, smoke marijuana, and take LSD. When his academic performance and personal life deteriorated, he was expelled. He returned to the public high school, but dropped out before graduation. During this time he displayed violent behavior toward his sister and threatened to kill his mother. After police charged him with receiving stolen property, he was committed to a state hospital. He was diagnosed as suffering from chronic undifferentiated schizophrenia.

He was treated and released. After his release he resided at home, where he displayed bizarre behavior. He insisted on wearing a fur coat on the hottest days, and stood for prolonged periods with a glass poised at his lips. He refused all treatment or therapy.

On February 19, 1980, when he was twenty-one, he was back at the state hospital after police picked him up for attempted robbery, and assault and battery. While hospitalized, he had to be restrained after an unprovoked attack on another patient. He was now diagnosed as suffering from paranoid schizophrenia, and treatment with psychotropic medication was recommended. He again refused treatment, and the hospital did not force it upon him.

As the hospital prepared to discharge him on April 18, 1980, his father asked the probate court to appoint him the guardian of his son. The court first appointed him temporary guardian and then in July, after more hearings and a finding that Richard Roe III was legally incompetent, made him permanent guardian. The guardianship gave the father the authority to make treatment decisions for his mentally ill son.

Richard, however, did not want treatment, so his guardian *ad litem*, the person appointed by the court to protect Richard's interests during the case, challenged the father's authority to treat his legally incompetent son against his wishes. The court then restrained the father from ordering treatment so the case could be appealed.

The guardian *ad litem* did not object to the appointment of the father as legal guardian, but he did object to the father having the authority to give consent for drugs his son did not want, and this was the challenge the court had to resolve. The case eventually went to the state supreme court. The major issue of interest to us is: can the parent of a mentally ill adult child lacking decision-making capacity give consent for treatment against the wishes of that child? Granted, the treatment is thought to be in the best interests of the incapacitated patient, but can it be forced on him against his wishes?

As we pointed out above, this is a tricky moral question. Normally, good ethics says that, if an incapacitated patient has not given some indication of his wishes while he had decision-making capacity, then the proxy should make treatment decisions based on what he thinks is in the best interests of the patient. If, on the other hand, the patient once had capacity and had indicated at that time what he wanted, then, of course, the substituted judgment standard becomes the basis of the decision and the proxy should decide in accord with the prior wishes of the patient.

The proxy or guardian for Richard Roe III would, therefore, proceed as follows. He would first consider whether Richard previously indicated his wishes about treatment. In this case, Richard's prior wishes were clear—he had a history of refusing treatment. But can we take those refusals at face value, or were they the wishes of a schizophrenic person already bereft of decision-making capacity?

If Richard did have decision-making capacity when he earlier objected to treatment, then the proxy would have reason to use the substituted judgment standard and to refuse the medications on the basis that the previous decisions were an indication of what Richard would want now. But if he had reason to think Richard did not have decision-making capacity when he previously refused treatments, then the proper standard for the proxy to use is best interests. And there is every reason to believe the treatments are in Richard's best interests.

Let us assume mental illness had already destroyed Richard's capacity to make health care decisions when he previously refused treatments. If this is the case, the proxy will not use these refusals as a basis for substituted judgment, and he will think of giving consent for the pyschotropic drugs on the basis of what is in the best interests of Richard.

But there is a major problem here—Richard is objecting to the treatment and, as we pointed out above, these very objections can undermine the benefits he would otherwise receive from the treatment. The distress of the forced treatments could cancel the benefits the treatments would otherwise provide. Hence, the final moral judgment of the proxy might be: it is more reasonable, given the person's objections to the treatment, to forego it because the burdens of forced treatment will outweigh its benefits.

What did the Massachusetts Supreme Court decide? It said that the guardian of an incompetent adult outpatient should not have the authority to give consent for psychotropic medication over the patient's objections. It went on to say that a judge could order the treatments if he found that the patient would have wanted them if he were competent. In other words, the guardian of an incompetent mental patient in Massachusetts has no authority to give consent for treatments the patient refuses, but the guardian could ask a court to order the treatments, and the court could so order if the judge thought the patient would have accepted them if he were competent.

The important ethical point in this case is the court's recognition that making treatment decisions for the incompetent mentally ill, whose prior wishes may be unreliable because of the mental illness, is not a simple case of relying on the best interests standard. The psychotropic drugs may well be in the best interests of the paranoid schizophrenic patient, but if the patient objects to them, these objections must be taken seriously. Forcing treatments on a person, even an incompetent mentally ill person, is something that undermines his human dignity and can easily undermine the human dignity of the providers. It is not enough to say that we can override the patient's objections because he is "crazy." He may well be mentally ill and have lost decision-making capacity, but he is still a human being with awareness and values, no matter how distorted his perceptions and judgments may be.

On the other hand, paternalism in the care of the incompetent mentally ill is more easily justified than it is for those not mentally ill. This makes it difficult for proxies and providers to withhold beneficial treatment when the patient refusing treatment is mentally ill. It is distressing to withhold helpful treatment when the patient refusing it is known to be mentally ill. The inclination is almost always to disregard the objections of these patients and to provide the treatments.

What, then, can we say about the ethics of providing treatment for mentally ill people without decision-making capacity when they object? Only that the situation is ambiguous, and that the moral deliberation in each case requires most careful prudential reasoning. Proxies must be ever aware that the objections of the patient may well undermine the otherwise beneficial treatment, and that forcing treatment on unwilling human beings creates a situation that can easily undermine respect for them and the self-respect of the provider as well.

Yet there may be times when a limited paternalism can be defended and the proxy can approve the treatments over the patient's objections. Some mentally ill patients, for example, may object to the medication as part of a

game when, in fact, they really are not objecting to it. Other
patients may object to treatment when they are agitated and need it,
acknowledge that they welcome the drugs that quiet them down.

Manipulating the patient with capacity

When we discussed informed consent in the last chapter, we pointed out that
the consent must be voluntary; that is, the patient cannot be manipulated,
coerced, or forced to accept the treatment. The shadow of manipulation sometimes haunts treatment decisions affecting the mentally ill. Suppose, for example, the mentally ill outpatient with decision-making capacity is given a choice:
either accept the psychotropic drugs or be committed to a hospital for the
mentally ill. If she really does not want the drugs but consents to the treatment
to avoid confinement, is the consent truly voluntary?

Again, suppose a hospitalized mentally ill patient is given a choice: either
accept the psychotropic drugs or be confined in a secluded room. If he really
does not want the drugs but consents to them to avoid being confined, is the
consent truly voluntary?

In effect, the providers have already made a major decision affecting the
mentally ill patients in these cases. They have decided that the patients will
either accept treatment or be confined. This does not give the patient much
room to maneuver, nor does it put the patient in a good position to give truly
voluntary consent. It is very close to manipulation. But for reasons of social
good, and perhaps for the good of the patient, it may sometimes be justified
for providers or the courts to make these kinds of decisions. Manipulating
patients to get consent for treatment is normally unethical, but it may be
reasonable in some cases where mental illness is involved. If patients are
restricted to a choice between treatment and confinement, however, it would
seem every effort should be made to avoid presenting the confinement as
punitive. Rather, it should be presented as a necessary last resort if the patient
will not accept treatment compatible with his freedom.

DECIDING FOR PATIENTS OF ANOTHER CULTURE

An interesting moral dilemma arises with patients, usually elderly, from another culture where attitudes of patient self-determination and informed consent do not play the important roles they do in our culture. When these people
become ill in our country, their children will often step forward and begin to
make decisions for them, even when the parents are not incapacitated. The
children may point out that medicine is paternalistic in their parent's country,
that older people do not expect to be told about their diagnosis and prognosis,
and that the responsibility of the physician and family is simply to do what
they think is best. They may further insist that the older people will be
totally confused if they are fully informed and then asked to make their
own decisions. Moreover, a language problem often exists, preventing the
physician from communicating directly with the patient.

The ethical question here centers on whether the physician can go along
with the children and (1) not tell the patient what is wrong and (2) decide with
the children what will be done, even though the parent is not incapacitated and

ght to give informed consent. If we invoke our standard
d consent and insist that the diagnosis and prognosis
rom patients, then the physician could not accept proxy
hildren as long as the patient still had decision-making

ethics attuned to circumstances and dedicated to doing
e human good, it is possible to justify a limited form of
paternalism in this kind of situation. For it is true that
en raised in cultures where the major decisions in life
..., ...isions, where medicine is paternalistic, and where children do
decide what is best for their parents when they reach a certain age. The
children in these situations are, therefore, asking nothing more than to have
their parents treated as they would be treated in their own country. In some
cases at least, it would seem morally justified for the physician caring for
these patients, in what is for them a foreign country, to respect their cultural
heritage. A practical strategy in these situations is to ask the patient to waive
informed consent and to let the children make the decisions.

FINAL REFLECTIONS ON DECIDING FOR OTHERS

In general, the three standards of proxy decision making (substituted judgment, best interests, and what we have called "reasonable treatment") reflect
an ethics of right reason. They are reasonable ways to achieve the human
good as best we can in situations where the patient is incapacitated. Before
ending this chapter, however, two remarks are in order. First, the substituted
judgment and best interest standards of proxy decision making do not absolve
the proxy of his or her responsibility to act reasonably and morally. Second,
you and I will live a better moral life if we appoint a proxy while we are still
able to do so, and if we communicate what we want done in the event we
one day lose the capacity to make our health care decisions. We will say a
word about each of these remarks.

Limitations of Substituted Judgment and Best Interests

The substituted judgment and best interests criteria of proxy decision making
are most often all we need to justify morally the treatment decisions one
person makes on behalf of another. They are not, however, the ultimate
criterion of what is morally right or wrong. They are important standards,
but they are limited because they are patient-centered. The proxy is communicating the patient's decision, if there is one, or deciding what is in the patient's
best interests. We can never forget, however, that the proxy is a moral agent
and therefore responsible for what she does.

In most cases, the proxy acts ethically when she uses the substituted
judgment standard or, if that is not possible, the best interests standard.
Sometimes, however, this is not so. There are cases, rare to be sure, where
a proxy will decline to follow the substituted judgment and best interests
standards for ethical reasons of her own.

A proxy is morally justified in overriding the substituted judgment standard whenever the patient left treatment instructions that the proxy considers clearly immoral or unreasonable. For example, a patient may have left instructions that an order not to attempt resuscitation never be written for him, and now he is permanently unconscious and dying of widespread cancer. There are good moral reasons for saying a proxy could give consent for the DNR order in such circumstances.

A proxy is also morally justified in overriding the best interests standard whenever what is in the best interests of the patient is clearly immoral or unreasonable. For example, it may be in the best interests of the patient to have a kidney transplant, but the only way to get one is from a black market that pays desperate poor people to sell one of their kidneys. Transplanting the black market kidney would be in a patient's best interests, but the proxy may well refuse to give consent on the grounds that using black market kidneys is unethical.

Both substituted judgment and best interests are standards centered exclusively on the patient, but sound moral decisions about the patient may embrace other factors as well. The interests of others (especially of the family, of the providers, and of society itself) are sometimes not negligible and have to be factored into the decision about how incapacitated patients are treated. The doctrine of triage in emergency situations, a doctrine that allows withholding treatment from some so it can be provided for others with a better chance of survival, is a reminder of how treatment decisions are not always focused on a single patient.

Therefore, although substituted judgment and best interests are important criteria and very helpful to a proxy making decisions for another person, the proxy still has a moral responsibility to act morally in his or her role as proxy. The ultimate moral criterion of the proxy's action remains right reason, and sometimes this means that she will not follow the patient's instructions or will not decide according to what is in the patient's best interests. A proxy is not a puppet but a moral agent in her own right, and the morality of virtue encourages her always to seek her good, even when acting as proxy for someone else.

The Moral Responsibility to Designate a Proxy

The difficulties our families and physicians may encounter if we become incapacitated without leaving instructions about who will be our proxy and how we want to be treated suggest that it is morally good for us, in a spirit of kindness and love, to help them by designating a proxy and discussing with that person how we would like to be treated if we ever lose capacity. Appointing a proxy who knows us well, and who has the authority to make decisions on our behalf, will make things much easier for our families and for the people caring for us. It will relieve them of the burden of trying to figure out who should decide and what treatments should be provided.

Aristotle reminded us that we study ethics not simply to know what is virtuous, but to do it. The study of proxy decision making, then, encourages each of us to designate a proxy and to make advance directives. These actions are virtuous because they help us to achieve what is good for ourselves by extending our wishes into a time when we may no longer have capacity, and by making it easier for others who someday may have to make decisions for us.

In the ethics of virtue that we are developing in this book, we would not say that we have a moral obligation to appoint a proxy and to make advance directives. In a morality of the human good, it is enough to remind a reasonable person that these actions are noble and virtuous, and that noble and virtuous actions are what make a life a good life.

SUGGESTED READINGS

A very helpful book on the topic of this chapter is Allen Buchanan and Dan Brock. 1989. *Deciding for Others: The Ethics of Surrogate Decision Making*. Cambridge University Press. Also helpful is 1992. *When Others Must Choose: Deciding for Patients Without Capacity*. New York: New York State Task Force on Life and Law; Part IV of the President's Commission report *Making Health Care Decisions*, entitled "Decisionmaking Incapacity"; Ezekiel Emmanuel and Linda Emmanuel. "Proxy Decision Making for Incompetent Patients: An Ethical and Empirical Analysis." *JAMA* **1992,** *267,* 2067–71; John Hardwig. "What About the Family?" *Hastings Center Report* **1990,** 20 (March–April), 5–10 and "The Problem of Proxies with Interests of Their Own: Toward a Better Theory of Proxy Decisions." *Journal of Clinical Ethics* **1993,** 4, 20–27; Carson Strong. "Patients Should Not Always Come First in Treatment Decisions." *Journal of Clinical Ethics* **1993,** 4, 63–65; Rebecca Dresser and John Robertson. "Quality of Life and Non-Treatment Decisions for Incompetent Patients: A Critique of the Orthodox Approach." *Law, Medicine & Health Care* **1989,** 17, 234–44. See also the nine articles in the special supplement entitled "Practicing the PSDA." *Hastings Center Report* **1991,** 21 (September–October), S1–S15.

The legal citation for the story of Jane Doe is *In re Jane Doe* 583 N.E. 2d 1263 (1992). Two very insightful commentaries on the case are Alexander Capron. "Substituting Our Judgment." *Hastings Center Report* **1992,** 22 (March–April), 58–59; and Susan Martyn. "Substituted Judgment, Best Interests, and the Need for Best Respect." *Cambridge Quarterly of Healthcare Ethics* **1994,** 3, 195–208. The case where the judges in effect ordered resuscitation by refusing to cancel the DNR order for the child is *Custody of a Minor (No. 1)*, 385 Mass. 697 (1982). The story of Beth is taken from *Care and Protection of Beth* 587 N.E.2d, 1377 (1992).

For the important legal background of making decisions for minors, see James Morrissey et al. 1986. *Consent and Confidentiality in the Health Care of Children and Adolescents*. New York: Free Press, especially chapters 1–3; and Angela Holder. 1985. *Legal Issues in Pediatrics and Adolescent Medicine*, second edition. New Haven: Yale University Press, chapters 5–10. Both books consider the ethical as well as the legal dimensions of making decisions for minors. Rozovsky, *Consent to Treatment*, chapter 5, is also very helpful.

For the seminal work in the moral development of the child, see Jean Piaget. 1965. *The Moral Judgment of the Child*, M. Gabain, trans. New York: Free Press. The English translation was first published in 1932. For an introduction to Kohlberg's research see Lawrence Kohlberg. 1981. *The Philosophy of Moral Development*, volume 1. San Francisco: Harper & Row, and "Moral Stages and Moralization: The Cognitive-Developmental Approach." in Thomas Lickona, ed. 1976, *Moral Development and Behavior*. New York: Holt, Rinehart and Winston, pp. 31–53.

The best known work identifying the sexual bias in Kohlberg's early research is Carol Gilligan. 1982. *In a Different Voice: Psychological Theory and Women's Development*. Cambridge: Harvard University Press.

Helpful texts on deciding for minors include Sanford Leiken. "Minors' Assent or Dissent to Medical Treatment." In the President's Commission Report entitled *Making Health Care Decisions*, volume 3, pp. 175–91; Buchanan and Brock, *Deciding for Others*, chapter 5; and Tomas Silber, "Ethical Considerations in the Medical Care of Adolescents and Their Parents." *Pediatric Annals* **1981**, *10*, 408–10.

The legal citations for the paragraphs on contraception and abortion are: *Griswold v. Connecticut*, 381 U.S. 479 (1965); *Eisenstadt v. Baird*, 405 U.S. 438 (1972); *Carey v. Population Services International*, 431 U.S. 678 (1977); *Roe v. Wade*, 410 U.S. 113 (1973); *Doe v. Bolton*, 410 U.S. 179 (1973); and *Bellotti v. Baird*, 424 U.S. 952 (1976) and 443 U.S. 622 (1979). The case cited in reference to parents not making martyrs of their children is *Prince v. Massachusetts*, 321 U.S. 158 (1944).

Three important cases allowing involuntarily confined mentally ill people to refuse treatment if they have decision-making capacity and are not dangerous are *Rennie v. Kline*, 720 F.2d 266 (3d Cir. 1983); *Rogers v. Okin*, 738 F.2d 1 (1st Cir. 1984); and *Rivers v. Katz*, 495 N.E.2d 337 (1986). In *Rivers*, the supreme court of New York (the Court of Appeals) required physicians to establish legal incompetence before they can treat involuntarily confined patients against their will. In *Rogers* (a Massachusetts case) the first circuit also ruled judicial intervention was necessary if the patient was objecting; in *Rennie* (a New Jersey case) the third circuit required safeguards but did not insist on judicial review. Case law continues to develop in this difficult area. The story of Richard Roe is taken from *In the Matter of Guardianship of Roe*, III, 421 N.E.2d 40 (1981).

For discussion about making decisions for the mentally ill, see Clarence Sundram. "Informed Consent for Major Medical Treatment of Mentally Disabled People: A New Approach." *NEJM* **1988**, *318*, 1368–73. Sundram's article reports that volunteer committees in New York are making treatment choices and giving informed consent for some categories of mentally ill people who do not have family proxies. See also Thomas Finucaner et al. "Establishing Medical Directives with Demented Patients: A Pilot Study." *Journal of Clinical Ethics* **1993**, *4*, 51–54; Erich Loewy. "Treatment Decisions in the Mentally Impaired: Limiting but Not Abandoning Treatment." *NEJM* **1987**, *317*, 1465–69; Nancy Rhoden. "The Presumption for Treatment: Has It Been Justified?" *Law, Medicine & Health Care* **1985**, *13*, 65–67; Thomas Gurtheil and Paul Appelbaum. "The Substituted Judgment Approach: Its Difficulties and Paradoxes in Mental Health Settings." *Law, Medicine & Health Care* **1985**, *13*, 61–64; Michael Irwin et al. "Psychotic Patients' Understanding of Informed Consent." *American Journal of Psychiatry* **1985**, *142*, 1351–54. Also helpful is the special section containing six articles on making decisions for persons with mental retardation in the *Cambridge Quarterly of Healthcare Ethics* **1994**, *3*, 174–235; and Rozovsky, *Consent to Treatment*, chapter 6.

6

Determining Life and Death

Knowing exactly when one of us begins and ends would be very helpful in health care ethics. Our ethical judgments about fertilization in laboratories, freezing and splitting embryos, research on embryos and fetuses, transplanting fetal tissue, and abortion are shaped by our views on when an embryo or a fetus becomes one of us. And our ethical judgments about retrieving organs and withdrawing life-sustaining treatment from human bodies lacking the capability for sensation are shaped by our views on when one of us dies.

Unfortunately, neither biology, biochemistry, genetics, neurology, nor any other science can tell us exactly when we begin or end our earthly existence. All we can do is select a stage in the development of human life as the beginning of one of us, and another stage in the subsequent deterioration of human life as the end of one of us. Determinations of the beginning and of the end of human existence are not facts but interpretations of facts.

These interpretations are difficult for two reasons. First, despite great progress in the past few decades, we are still learning the physiological facts of life and death. Second, interpretations always reflect our previously embraced, and often never analyzed, frameworks of meaning and value—that is, our prejudices.

Nonetheless, interpret the facts we must, since determining when a new one of us begins and when one of us dies is of utmost importance for ethics, law, and public policy. It matters a great deal whether a fetus is or is not one of us if we are thinking of destroying it. It matters whether an embryo is one of us if we are thinking of freezing it or using it for research. It matters whether a body with no brain function is one of us if we are thinking of keeping it alive or of removing the heart for transplantation.

Determining the beginning and the end of one of us is an interdisciplinary effort. We need science to provide the facts, and we need philosophy to interpret those facts. It is not enough to know that an embryo is human life with forty-six chromosomes and a specific genetic code to say it is one of us— a brain-dead patient on life-support equipment is similarly composed. And it is not enough to know someone's heart and lungs have permanently ceased to function to say she is dead; she may still be living thanks to a heart–lung machine or transplant. We have to know the facts, but we also have to interpret the facts to determine when one of us begins and when one of us ends.

The stages in the development of human life currently proposed as markers for the beginning of a new one of us are (1) fertilization, (2) implantation (completed by the fourteenth day), (3) appearance of the "primitive streak" (the band on the embryonic disk that begins to appear about the fifteenth day and marks the longitudinal axis of the embryo), (4) fetal "brain life," (thought to begin about the eighth week), (5) viability (once considered to occur about the beginning of the third trimester, but now somewhat earlier), (6) birth, and (7) the end of infancy.

The confusing, and frequently disputed, current public policy in the United States tends to an interpretation whereby one of us begins somewhere between viability and the expulsion or extraction of the living fetus from the uterus. U.S. Supreme Court decisions allow states to make third trimester abortions illegal, unless they are needed to preserve the woman's life. However, an illegal third trimester abortion is not considered murder unless the fetus is removed alive and then destroyed. This approach leads to a confusing notion: deliberately destroying a third trimester fetus in the uterus is not killing one of us, but deliberately destroying a third trimester fetus outside the uterus is killing one of us.

The stages of biological deterioration proposed as markers for the end of one of us, which is death, are (1) the permanent loss of cardiopulmonary functions, (2) the permanent loss of all brain functions, including the functions of the brain stem, and (3) the permanent loss of the higher brain functions necessary for awareness and feeling. The present public policy in the United States reflects interpretations whereby we are dead once we have suffered the permanent loss of cardiopulmonary functions, or of all brain functions, or of both. The permanent loss of the higher brain functions associated with awareness is not considered a sign of death.

Many proposals for determining the beginning and the end of one of us run into serious difficulty for one of two reasons. Either they are reductionist (reducing the problem to scientific facts) or they introduce nonscientific ideas such as soul, mind, self, selfhood, person, personhood, bearer of rights, etc.

The problem with the reductionist interpretations is that many of us think, with some reason, that we are something more than what science observes. And the problem with the nonscientific ideas is the impossibility of verifying them, and hence people can deny them or use them in different ways, often with hidden agendas. If you are familiar with the history of philosophy, you know that "soul" did not mean the same for Plato as it did for Aristotle, that "mind" did not mean the same for Hume as it did for Hegel, that "self" did not mean the same for Locke as it does for Ricoeur, that "person" did not mean the same for Reid as it did for Strawson.

Later in the chapter we will develop positions on the beginning and the end of one of us that will reflect an attempt to avoid both a reductionist position and a position employing ideas that cannot be verified. Before we outline our positions on the beginning and on the end of one of us, however, we will examine the major concepts of human life and death in our culture, and the criteria used to determine when one of us begins and when one of us dies.

In doing this, it will be helpful to keep in mind the important distinction between concepts and criteria. Concepts are how we think and talk about things. You and I can think and talk about disease, health, life, death, etc., in a meaningful way because our minds and language are sufficiently developed to handle the concepts of disease, health, life, and death.

Criteria, on the other hand, are the observable facts verifying the reality of what we are thinking and talking about—they tell us something is indeed the case. Suppose we are talking about infection, for example. We have a concept of infection—we know what infections are and can describe them. But the concept of infection does not tell us that this leg or this arm is actually infected. The criteria do this, and the criteria by which we determine an infection is present are the symptoms: fever, tenderness, inflammation, white cell count, etc.

When we turn to determining when one of us begins and ends, the concepts are not the problem. We already share them—we know what life and death are. If someone says there was an accident in which four people lived and two died, we know what that means. What we want to know are the criteria—how we can tell when a new one of us has begun or when one of us has died? When we ask "How do I know something is one of us?" or "How do I know one of us is dead?" we are asking for criteria. The criteria are the signs indicating that something is indeed one of us or that someone once one of us is no longer one of us.

The concepts and criteria of life and death, however, are not the whole story. Concepts and criteria are embedded in conceptual frameworks, and we need to know something about the presupposed conceptual frameworks if we are to understand the concepts and criteria of life and death.

THE CLASSICAL CONCEPTUAL FRAMEWORK

Until recently, discussions about the beginning and end of human existence would have presupposed some knowledge of how the classical theologians and philosophers conceived of "man." We would have considered their "philosophy of man," their views on the nature of "man," and what they thought marked his beginning and his end.

Today, we would like to find a better term than "man" when we discuss these ideas of classical philosophy. Some suggest "person," but person is a troublesome term. People do not agree on what it means to be a person. Moreover, the modern notion of person did not exist in Greek philosophy, and it played only an inchoate role in medieval thought. For want of a better term, we will employ phrases such as "one of us" or "each of us," phrases we have already been using, to describe what the classical philosophers were talking about when they wrote about "man."

We will look briefly at the classical theologies and philosophies describing what we are, and their views on when each of us begins and ends. It is important to do this because so many features of their thought are still operative in our culture today.

The Mystery Religions; Socrates and Plato

The very earliest philosophers (sixth century B.C.E.) considered us as nothing more than our material bodies. But some of the "mystery" religions (not the civil religion dedicated to Zeus, Athena, and the other gods and goddesses, but the religious beliefs and rituals some ancient people held in private) suggested that we were something more than our bodies. The mystery religions usually called this "something more" a "soul," and some of them included doctrines about the soul leaving the body at death and then coming back into another body. The doctrine of the soul gained influence in the second half of the sixth century with the emergence of a scholarly and religious group in southern Italy—the Greek-speaking Pythagoreans.

Although the mystery religions and the Pythagoreans did not survive, some of their ideas did. Two major philosophers, Socrates (470–399 B.C.E.) and Plato (427–347 B.C.E.), were influenced by them. According to their theory, each of us is a composite of body and soul. The body is material and biological, but the soul is neither material nor biological. Because the soul is immaterial, it cannot be seen, or touched, or observed in any way. Nor does it have a beginning or an end—it is eternal. The soul animates the body— keeps it alive and provides for its growth and movement—and enables the human being to know things and make choices. The immaterial soul enables us to know the things that are not of this material world, things such as numbers and other mathematical notions, as well as universal and unchanging ideas such as justice, courage, etc. And it allows us to escape some of the determinism of the material world in which we are enmeshed, to make choices, and thereby to have some control over our lives.

In this Socratic–Platonic conceptual model, the soul had no beginning; it always was. Its existence is eternal. Each of us begins when the preexisting immaterial soul enters the human body, and we die when the soul departs from this body. Since the soul animates the body, the self-movement of the body indicates the soul is present, and the lack of movement indicates it has escaped. In general terms, then, the criterion of human life was the spontaneous movement of a human body, and the criterion of human death was the permanent cessation of that spontaneous movement.

So powerful was this Socratic–Platonic model of the material body–immaterial soul that many early Christian thinkers adopted it. The Christians did make one important change—they rejected the eternal preexistence of the soul and said, instead, that God created a human soul for each of us at some point in our fetal development. However, the Christians retained, as we will see, the same material body–immaterial soul duality. They explained the beginning of life as the infusion of an immaterial rational soul into the human body, and the end of that life as the departure of the soul from the body.

Aristotle

Plato did not try to determine when the soul came into a developing fetus, but his pupil Aristotle (384–322 B.C.E.) did. Although Aristotle rejected many of Plato's ideas about the soul, including its preexistence and its survival after death in any personal way, he retained the basic concept of an immaterial soul in a material body. More important for our purposes, he proposed criteria for determining just when a developing fetal body gains a human soul. His work was based on observation as well as theory. He was familiar with various writings by the Hippocratic physicians, which contained descriptions of spontaneously aborted fetuses, and he may well have studied some fetuses himself. His explanation of human reproduction and fetal development, as well as the criteria he developed for determining when one of us begins, were to dominate both secular and religious thought for two thousand years. The main features of his account are as follows.

When semen mixes successfully with blood in the uterus, the mixture congeals, preventing further menstruation. The semen or seed retained in the uterine blood begins to develop, much like a seed develops once it is planted in the ground. The seed first develops in a vegetative way, growing and becoming differentiated into distinct parts, much as a plant develops its stem, branches, and leaves. At this first stage, the fetus has a vegetative soul.

Later, this vegetative fetus acquires the ability to feel. The feeling of touch develops first, and then seeing, hearing, smelling, and tasting follow as the bodily parts supporting these sensations appear. With the beginning of feeling, the fetus passes from the vegetative stage to the second stage of its development—the animal stage. It now has an animal soul.

A third stage—the specifically human stage—appears when the fetus acquires what Aristotle called the "rational soul," the source of rationality. Unlike sensation, which resides in a part of the body such as the eye or the skin, rationality is not identified with any part of the body but with the immaterial soul. The immaterial rational soul not only thinks but animates the human body. It makes the fetus one of us, and each of us continues to exist as one of us until the rational soul ceases to animate the body. At this point, we still have a human body, but it is dead. The rational soul is so closely entwined with the body that it ceases to exist when the body dies or, conversely, we could say that the body is so closely associated with the soul that it dies when the soul ceases to animate it.

Aristotle's answer to the question "When did I begin?" is therefore as follows: A fetus becomes one of us when the rational soul permeates the developing fetal seed sometime after the appearance of sensation or feeling, which marks the animal stage. Just how long after the animal stage the rational soul appeared, Aristotle did not, and could not, say. But he was sure that the rational soul could not appear before the animal soul. And just how long after the seed began to grow did the animal soul or sensation develop? Aristotle's answer strikes us as bizarre today: sensation developed after 40 days of growth if the fetus is male, after 90 days if it is female.

What led him to this conclusion? We do not know for sure, but it seems to have been prompted by his observations of sexual development in fetuses. Apparently he assumed that the fetus had to be sexually differentiated before sensation could appear. Since he thought—erroneously—that the penis appeared about the fortieth day (he was probably observing the little tail that was still intact on some early aborted fetuses, and thought it was the penis) and the vaginal opening about the ninetieth day, he concluded a male fetus could acquire a rational soul any time after the fortieth day, but the female fetus could not acquire the rational soul until at least the ninetieth day. The delayed appearance of the rational soul in the female fetus was accepted practically without question in our culture for almost two thousand years.

Aristotle's concept of a new one of us, and the criteria he used to verify the presence of one of us, are now clear. Each of us began as a seed planted in the uterus. The seed first grew as a vegetable, and then, some time after the biological development of sexual differentiation, sensation appeared. At some point after sensation, the rational soul appeared. The emergence of the rational soul in the male fetus about the sixth week, and in the female fetus about the thirteenth week, is what makes the fetus one of us.

It should be no surprise that Aristotle's explanation of the beginning of human life was an important factor in his moral evaluation of abortion. Simply put, he thought abortions became a serious moral problem once sensation occurred since the invisible rational soul, and therefore one of us, could be present any time after that. In practice, since he could not determine whether a fetus was male or female, this meant he considered most abortions after the fortieth day unethical. His research had convinced him that some fetuses could feel by that time, and thus might possess a rational soul.

Hebrew Bible

The first book of the Hebrew Bible, the book of *Genesis*, records two versions of the myth of creation, including the creation of Adam and Eve. In both versions, however, the first humans appear as adults, so the biblical accounts of the beginning of the human race do not address our concern, the fetal beginning of each of us.

The most relevant biblical text for our purposes occurs in the book of *Exodus*. *Exodus* 21:22 reports a legal question about a man who attacked a pregnant woman. She lived, but miscarried. The biblical question centered on what should be the penalty for the criminal who caused the destruction of her fetus. If he killed one of us, he is a murderer, and the penalty is death; if the fetus is not one of us, a lesser penalty is sufficient. *Exodus* advocates the lesser penalty, suggesting that the Hebrews did not consider the unborn fetus one of us.

Beginning around 250 B.C.E., at Alexandria in Egypt, the ancient books of the Hebrew Bible were translated into Greek. The translators, however, changed the text of *Exodus* 21:22 in a significant way. While the original Hebrew text simply stated that the penalty for a criminal action resulting in the destruction of a fetus is a fine and not the death penalty, the Greek translation of this passage says that destroying a developed fetus, one with a human form, is punishable by the death penalty. Making the penalty for destroying a formed fetus the same as the penalty for murder is important because it implies the formed fetus is one of us.

Since the Hebrew text makes no distinction between early and formed fetuses, the statement in the Greek translation advocating the death penalty for the destruction of a formed fetus does not belong in the Bible. It reflects, rather, the position of the Greek translators at Alexandria, a position that could have been shaped by Aristotle's well-known doctrine of fetal development originating in the previous century.

In any event, the Greek version of the Hebrew Bible agrees in large measure with Aristotle's idea that an early fetus is not one of us, but that a more developed fetus, one that is formed, is one of us. And it was the Greek translation of the Hebrew Bible, along with Aristotle's similar account, that influenced so many later Jews and Christians living in the classical Greek-speaking world. When the Latin language began to replace Greek in the vast Roman Empire, the early Latin versions of the Hebrew Bible were actually translations of the Greek translation, and not of the original Hebrew. Only in the late fourth century, more than 600 years after the Greek translation, did St. Jerome make the first major Latin translation of the Hebrew bible directly from the original text.

By this time, however, it was too late for the biblical position (destruction of a fetus is not killing one of us) to dislodge the Greek distinction between unformed and formed fetuses, and its implication that destroying a formed fetus is killing one of us. Thus the prevailing idea of our culture became the more conservative philosophical position of the Greeks: destruction of a formed fetus is killing one of us.

Early and Medieval Christianity

Early Christian theologians such as Jerome (340?–420) and Augustine (354–430) accepted, along with almost everyone else, the Greek conception wherein a fetus becomes one of us at some point in its development. They thought the destruction of a fetus at any stage of development was immoral, but that it was not the destruction of one of us unless it occurred after the point in its development when God created a human soul and infused it in the developing fetal body. No one knew when this happened, but the tendency was to think it did not happen before there was sufficient development of the fetus to support feeling or sensation. The most widely held idea in Christianity seems to have come not from the Bible, but from Aristotle: the rational soul was formed in the male fetus during the sixth week, and in the female fetus during the thirteenth week, and only the destruction of these formed fetuses counts as killing one of us.

The classical Greek doctrine of the delay before a fetus became one of us received the official support of the Roman Catholic Church in the great collection of church law completed by Gratian around 1140. This collection, and the decrees subsequently added to it, had a long-lasting influence—it remained the foundation of Church law until a new Code of Canon Law was published in 1917. Gratian's *Decretum*, as the collection was called, accepted the standard explanation: a fetus did not become one of us until the human soul entered the fetal body some weeks after conception.

Gratian's position was subsequently confirmed in one of the official papal decrees, or "decretals" as they were called, approved by Pope Gregory IX during his reign from 1227 to 1241. A previous pope, Innocent III, had ruled that a monk causing a miscarriage of his mistress' early fetus was not subject to the ecclesiastical penalties for murder unless the fetus had been "vivified." In Gregory's collection of laws, a fetus was considered "vivified" from the point in its development when the soul was infused into it.

The idea of the rational soul's delayed arrival in a fetus received further confirmation in the twelfth and thirteenth centuries when Aristotle's works, long largely unknown in the Europe of the Dark Ages, were rediscovered and quickly became central texts in the curricula of the new universities. Thomas Aquinas (1224–1274), the scholar many recognize as the most influential thinker of this time, did not hesitate to embrace a position consistent with Aristotle as well as with Jerome and Augustine: The early fetus is not one of us. "In the generation of man first there is a living thing, then an animal, finally a man . . ." (*Summa Theologiae* II II, q. 64, a. 1) The fetus becomes one of us when the rational soul is infused, an event he thought happened after at least 6 weeks of fetal development in the male, and 13 weeks in the female.

Thus, consistent with the Christian tradition up to this point, Aquinas thought the deliberate destruction of a fetus before it is animated with the rational soul was morally wrong, but not murder. Commenting on the famous passage in *Exodus*, Aquinas wrote: "A person who strikes a pregnant woman does something wrong, and therefore if the death of the woman or of the *animated* fetus follows, he cannot escape the crime of murder." (*Summa Theologiae* II II, q. 64, a. 8 ad 2, emphasis added.)

To sum up, in the classical conceptual framework, each of us is considered a combination of body and soul. The body is material and organic, and the soul is immaterial and inorganic. The body arises from a seed mixing with bloody fluid in the uterus. This mixture congeals, and the seed grows and begins to take on a life of its own. Its life is first vegetative, then it becomes sentient as it achieves the ability to feel, and finally it becomes one of us when the rational soul arrives. In this conceptual framework, each of us is a composite of a human body and an immaterial rational soul, a composite that first appeared no sooner than forty days into the pregnancy.

Of course, the fundamental metaphor is all wrong. The metaphor for the beginning of one of us is not a planted seed, but a fertilized egg. Vegetables and flowers begin from planted seeds, but animals do not, and each of us definitely does not so begin. The father of a child is not analogous to a farmer sowing seed in the ground, but to a cock fertilizing eggs. The mother of a child is not analogous to the ground where the seed grew, but to a hen producing eggs.

Breakdown of the Classical "Seed" Explanation

In the seventeenth century, two major factors began to undermine the two-thousand-year-old explanation of when one of us begins. The first was the effort of some to move the time of the soul's infusion into the body earlier and earlier, almost to the very beginning of fetal development. The second was the series of discoveries in the biology of human reproduction that forced us to revise radically the classical conceptions of human reproduction.

Since no one working with the classical explanation could say just when the human or rational soul arrived in the zoological fetus, the exact time when a fetus became one of us was always open to debate. In the early part of the 17th century, some physicians began to argue for a very early infusion of the rational soul. A Flemish physician, Thomas Feyens, thought the soul was infused the third day after the semen mixes with the blood in the woman's body, and a Roman physician, Paolo Zacchias, thought the soul was infused almost immediately after the semen came in contact with the blood. Zacchias's opinion gained credibility for many European Catholics when he was honored by the Pope as the outstanding physician of the Roman Catholic Church in 1644.

Moving the arrival of the human soul to the first few days or hours after the semen mixes with the blood makes the beginning of each of us practically coincide with what we now call fertilization. At that time, of course, nobody yet knew that a spermatozoon fertilizes a human egg. In fact, no one knew the human female had eggs! But this discovery and others were about to come.

By the end of the seventeenth century scientists were becoming aware of the flaws in the classical biological understanding of human (and animal) reproduction. A major technological breakthrough, the microscope, helped them tremendously. As we know, grinding lenses a certain way can magnify objects and let us see things we never saw before. Galileo, using these lenses in a telescope, explored the night sky and produced the evidence showing that the fundamental classical assumption of cosmology—that the sun and other stars circle the earth—was simply false, even though it looks true and has biblical support.

Others used ground lenses in microscopes to explore bodily fluids. They soon discovered that the classical assumption of reproduction—that we begin as a seed—was simply false. From the study of reproduction in birds, where rather large eggs obviously play a pivotal role, they began to suspect that a human female might have eggs, and that a new fetus began when sperm fertilized one of these eggs, not when semen mixed with blood in the uterus. At this point, however, no one had seen the tiny human egg, so the process was still poorly understood. If the human female had eggs as large as those of a small bird, undoubtedly the riddle of human reproduction would have been solved much earlier.

It was not until 1827 that scientists achieved good observations of the microscopic human egg, or ovum, and produced the first rough scientific model of our modern understanding of human reproduction. They now realized that the sperm was not a seed that would grow in the moist environment of the uterus, but one of two biological pieces, the other being the ovum.

Later it was discovered that the spermatozoon and ovum each have only half the chromosomes of the other human cells, and that the merger of the male and female sex cells is what produces a normal human being with somatic cells of forty-six chromosomes. Then, less than half a century ago, the DNA molecule was discovered. We learned that the fertilized ovum contains a unique genetic structure of more than one hundred thousand genes, and that every cell of the human body that develops from that fertilized ovum will manifest that same genetic identity.

The discovery that new human life originated from the fertilization of an egg, and not from a seed planted in the woman's body, was provocative. The transition from two germ cells (ovum and spermatozoon) to one zygote in fertilization is undeniably a momentous development, and it suggested to some that it must be the moment when the rational soul arrives. If this explanation is accepted, then it is logical to say that the destruction of a fertilized ovum is the destruction of one of us. And if each of us has a right to life, then it is logical to say this right to life is being violated if the embryo or fetus is arbitrarily destroyed.

None of those embracing the body–soul model of describing who we are can ever know for sure, of course, when a soul would be infused in a fetus because both the philosophical and Christian traditions have always insisted that the soul was immaterial and hence beyond empirical observation.

Since no one can ever produce any empirical or scientific evidence that a soul has arrived, the moment of the soul's infusion will always remain a somewhat arbitrary interpretation. The radical change happening at fertilization, and the resulting zygote with its complete set of human genes, could well be the moment, but could just as well not be. In any event, since they can never know for sure, some argue that, to be on the safe side in our respect for human life, we should treat every fertilized ovum as a new one of us.

Others, of course, disagree. They agree with the biological facts, but they argue that we cannot call the early embryo—something invisible to the naked eye and lacking a brain—one of us. They suggest we should not consider the embryo or fetus truly a member of our species until a later stage of development appears, perhaps brain life, or viability, or birth, or even the end of infancy. This disagreement is bound to continue for some time because what is at issue is no longer the biological facts—we understand them pretty well—but people's interpretations of them.

Modern Concepts of Who We Are

Unhappy with the classical philosophical and Christian concepts of the imma-terial soul–material body composite, some modern philosophers and psychol-ogists have suggested the concept of person or personhood as the best way to think of each of us. But we run into all sorts of problems about defining what a person is. Some conceive person so broadly that it includes everything from a fertilized ovum to a human body that has been irreversibly vegetative for decades. Others define person so narrowly that it includes only those with self-consciousness, or with rationality, or with moral agency, or with rights that must be respected, or with some combination of these features.

If we cannot agree on a conception of what constitutes a person, then we cannot agree on the criteria to verify when a fertilized egg becomes a person, and when a permanently unconscious patient ceases to be a person. The debates about personhood are so interminable it seems best to avoid the concept altogether.

Another modern concept is that of the "self," a concept closely associated with person and exposed to its difficulties as well. For the influential philoso-pher John Locke, our personal identity is not secured by a "thinking thing" or mental substance that endures while we experience the many and various thoughts in our lives, but by the consciousness that accompanies our thinking. I not only think of a house, but I am conscious of my thinking of the house. My thoughts and actions come and go, and are of all different kinds, but my consciousness of the different thoughts and actions, past and present, remains ever the same, and this is what secures my personal identity. This conscious-ness is my "self." All this points to a position claiming a human being is not simply a body, nor simply a body with a substance called mind, but a body with something more, a self.

The concept of self, however, no less than the concept of person, is also the subject of great controversy, so it seems best to avoid using it. What we want to retain, however, is the notion of the "something more" that is captured in the ideas of soul, mind, person, and consciousness. Our concept of what we are will have to account for this, for otherwise it will collapse into the counterintuitive extreme we have identified as reductionist—the tendency to say that we are nothing more than biological organisms.

Critique of the Classical Conceptions

The most widely employed classical concept of ourselves is the material body–immaterial soul model originating with Socrates and Plato and modified by subsequent philosophies and Christian theologies. The classical concept remains firmly entrenched in the thoughts and language of many. It is supported by various Christian teachings insisting that, although the body dies, the soul lives on for eternity. It also underlies the modern philosophical concerns about what is called the "mind–body" problem.

The classical body–soul conceptual framework has merit but, unfortunately, there are no criteria to verify when something human gains or loses the immaterial soul or mind. While those accepting the conceptual framework will agree that you or I are undoubtedly composites of a material body and an immaterial soul, and that the soul has departed from the body taken to the morgue, there is no such agreement about the early stages of human development, nor about later stages of deterioration where some signs of life are still present.

We can all perceive an embryo under a microscope and we can verify that it has forty-six human chromosomes, but does it have an immaterial soul? Some proponents of the body–soul concept believe it does, others believe it does not. Again, we can all see the permanently unconscious patient in the hospital, but does that body have an immaterial rational soul? Some will say yes but others, knowing all feeling has been irreversibly lost, will see no reason for saying her body retains its immaterial rational soul.

The concept of the material body–immaterial soul composite fails us when we need it most; that is, at the edges of life when we ask when one of us begins, and when one of us dies. And it fails us because there are no criteria to show that a rational soul is present in any human body, especially a human body not manifesting any signs of sensation or thought.

At the root of the difficulty is the nature of the soul. It is thought to be immaterial, and the immaterial by definition cannot be perceived. There is simply no way we can empirically confirm the presence of an immaterial soul in a human body, which, of course, is why some people simply deny the existence of souls and advocate a materialism whereby we are nothing but our bodies. For those accepting the concept that each of us is a composite of body and soul, there is no way to settle the arguments about whether the soul arrives at fertilization, or at implantation, or at the development of the primitive streak, or at the beginning of brain life, etc. And there is no way to settle the arguments about whether or not a permanently unconscious human body still retains its immaterial soul.

And the modern concepts of mind, person, and self do not fare any better than the classical concept of soul. There is no way of knowing whether a fetus or neonate has become a person or a self, or whether a PVS patient is still a person with rights or a self that is one of us.

The problems generated by the classical and modern concepts suggest that we need a new concept describing and defining what we are. We need to begin again the effort to develop a concept of ourselves and to define, at least to some extent, what each of us is. Once the concept is developed, we can ask about the criteria to verify when something is one of us and when it ceases to be one of us.

A NEW CONCEPTUAL FRAMEWORK

We will avoid two extreme positions in developing a concept of ourselves. In the first, each of us is conceived as primarily immaterial. Socrates and Plato came close to one extreme position by locating the meaning and value of our humanity in the soul. In their view, the body is reduced to a receptacle for the rational soul, a receptacle that actually hinders the soul's life of rationality by clouding its clarity and disturbing its serenity. Descartes also veered in this direction by according primacy to the mind, which he described as a thinking thing (*res cogitans*). In his view, the body is reduced to an extended thing (*res extensa*) that operates like a machine.

The second extreme goes in the opposite direction. It conceives of us as material, as nothing but a body with its complex interactions. It dismisses the existence of any immaterial soul or mind. Some forms of cognitive science, behaviorism, Marxism, and scientific psychology embrace this general position.

Neither of these positions does justice to what most people feel about themselves. Most of us do not experience our bodies as receptacles for our souls, nor as machines housing a mind; we experience our bodies as truly ourselves, yet we experience ourselves as something more than our bodies.

The development of a new concept of ourselves will begin with the most obvious reality of our experience: we are living human bodies in the world. Now there are two ways of thinking of the living human body. In the first way, the human body is conceived as exclusively biological; it is any living body with the human genetic code. In this sense, a brain-dead patient with ventilator support is a living human body. The biological sense of human body requires only (a) a living body and (b) a full human genetic code.

There is a great temptation to think of the living human body as exclusively biological. It is not only convenient, but most of our philosophical and Christian traditions conditioned us to think of the body this way by proposing doctrines slighting the body and emphasizing the soul, or mind, or personhood, or the self as the primary sources of human value, dignity, and identity. If one devalues the body, as many philosophical and theological traditions do, then it is easy to think of it as merely biological.

The second way of thinking of the living human body is much richer, and it acknowledges the "something more" we mentioned earlier. It conceives the body as psychological as well as biological. In this view, the body is not a receptacle with a soul placed in it, nor is it an extended thing with a mind somehow linked to it (Descartes had suggested the pineal gland was the link between mind and body), nor is it a biological entity distinct from the consciousness accompanying our thinking, but the human body is a *perceiving body*. If we adopt this second way of conceiving the human body, then a living body with a human genetic code is not properly one of us unless the body also perceives. To be one of us, the body must be biologically human *and* psychic. The second sense of the living human body conceives the body as both biological and psychological. The psychic is not *in* the body; the body *is* psychic.

The conception of myself as a psychic body arises from my personal experience. If I reflect on my experience, I become aware that I experience myself as a psychic body. I do not experience myself simply as body, nor do I experience myself simply as soul or mind or self or person living in my body. Rather, I experience myself as a psychic body, a body that perceives and is aware that it perceives. My body is not mine, my body is me.

The basic and everyday word best suited for conveying the idea of the psychic body is awareness. The psychic body is a body that perceives, or has the capacity for perceiving, its environment. The phrase "capacity for perceiving" is added to cover those exceptional instances when a psychic body may temporarily lose its awareness—perhaps through trauma or anesthesia—but still retains the capacity to regain it. (When we speak of awareness in this text, we will always understand the word as designating both actual awareness and the capacity to regain awareness temporarily lost.)

We now have a working concept of what we are. Each of us is a human individual psychic body. A body is human if it has human DNA. A body is individual if it is an identifiable whole, and not a part of a whole (as is a kidney, which is not a whole, but a part of a human body). And a body is psychic if it perceives or, if it has lost awareness, still retains the ability to perceive.

This working concept of who we are allows us to identify three criteria for determining when a body is one of us. One criterion is human DNA, the second criterion is existence as an individual whole, and the third criterion is awareness, or the capacity for it if awareness has been temporarily lost.

Unlike concepts involving notions of soul, mind, self, and person, the concept of the psychic body lends itself to criteria that can verify whether or not a body is one of us. We can test for human DNA (although most of the time it is not necessary because we recognize a human body). We can recognize a human individual (we do it every day). And we can ascertain perception in most cases by our experience, and in difficult cases at the beginning and the end of life, by our knowledge of what neurological structures and functions are needed for it, and by neurological examinations.

The working concept of the psychic body, and the criteria whereby we can know whether a particular body is one of us, can help answer our two questions: When does one of us begin, and when does one of us die?

WHEN DOES ONE OF US BEGIN?

When I conceive of myself as a psychic body, the question "When did I begin" asks when my individual psychic body began. To answer the question, we need science to tell us about the development of a fertilized ovum into an individual psychic body. The individual that is me did not begin until the fertilized egg became an individual psychic body. Thus we want to know when the fertilized egg becomes an individual body, and when that individual body becomes psychic.

The Fertilized Egg Becomes an Individual Body

A few recent discoveries help us to understand when it is appropriate to say an individual human body has developed from a fertilized ovum. First, fertilization is a complicated interaction lasting about twenty-four hours. The sperm and ovum fuse into a genetic entity of forty-six chromosomes called a zygote in a process spanning about a day. This means any position claiming that a new one of us begins at "the moment of conception" or "the moment of fertilization" is misleading; there is no moment of conception or fertilization.

Second, the fertilized ovum or zygote is not yet something that will inevitably develop into an individual human body and become one of us. We now know that a high number of zygotes, more than a third, are lost in the first two weeks of life. Fertilization normally occurs in a fallopian tube, and implantation of the fertilized ovum in the uterus begins several days later. Evidence now indicates that many zygotes do not implant successfully. The fertilized egg passes through the uterus and is sloughed off with the endometrial lining two weeks after ovulation during what appears to be simple menstruation.

If the fertilized egg or zygote is understood as one of us, then these women carried a baby but never knew it. If the zygote is understood as one of us, then tragic deaths occur with astonishing frequency—almost as many zygotes die this way as there are pregnancies. If a baby is present in the uterus once fertilization is completed, then millions of babies die each year in the United States as they are spontaneously discarded in the first few days of life. Although this terrible waste of early human life is not a definitive argument that a zygote is not one of us, there is something suspect about claiming a zygote is one of us when so many are naturally lost.

Third, we know the zygote is not necessarily the beginning of a new individual body, despite its unique genetic structure. The zygote will sometimes, albeit rarely, split in two, and each side of the split can become one of us. Sometimes the splitting of the human embryo is spontaneous and sometimes, as we learned in late 1993, the splitting is the result of deliberate intervention. And two zygotes will sometimes, albeit rarely, fuse to become one entity that develops into one of us.

If we say a zygote is one of us, then we are also saying that one of us can become two of us, and that two of us can become one of us. This makes no sense. The possibility of zygotes splitting or fusing suggests the zygote is not yet what we mean by one of us. The zygote is obviously human life, but not so obviously a human individual because it has not yet reached the stage where it cannot become two instead of one, or become one after it was two. In the first week or so after fertilization, the embryo has not yet reached a stage of development where it has established itself as an individual body.

The biological facts about wastage, splitting, and fusion suggest that one of us has not yet begun before implantation and a stage of development where the embryo will be but one of us. This analysis shows how implausible it is to say one of us begins in the first two weeks after fertilization when so many embryos are lost and the individual identity of the embryo is not yet definitively established.

The Individual Body Becomes Psychic

More important, we want to know when the individual body becomes psychic because that is when a fetus becomes one of us. It may not be possible, at least for awhile, to pin down just when perception or awareness begins in a fetus, but growing evidence indicates many weeks of development are needed.

The neural pathways for perception or awareness run from sensory receptors in the skin to sensory areas in the cerebral cortex. The first sensory receptors in the skin appear about the seventh week of fetal development around what will be the mouth, and then spread to the rest of the body. The fetal neocortex appears in the eighth week and achieves its full complement of neurons by the twentieth week. Most important, the pathways connecting the sensory receptors to the sensory areas in the cerebral cortex are also completed about the twentieth week. Only when these pathways are operative does a fetus begin to perceive.

Perception or awareness occurs at the cortical level, and it requires both a considerable degree of cortical maturity and the establishment of neural pathways from the sensory receptors in the body to the sensory areas in the cerebral cortex. This suggests that perception certainly does not begin before the eighth week of fetal development, and probably not until some time later. If each of us is a psychic body, then a new one of us does not begin until the psychic body develops; that is, until the fetus perceives, something that cannot happen until some months into the pregnancy.

This may seem like a revival of the older body–soul or body–mind developmental theories embraced by many philosophical and theological traditions. Indeed, there are similarities, but there are also important differences. First, in the traditional theories a fetus with awareness is not yet one of us; in our theory the perceiving fetus, a fetus with awareness, is one of us.

Second, in the traditional theories the fetal body becomes one of us when the immaterial soul arrives by divine creation or some other mysterious process. In our theory the fetal body becomes one of us when its sensory receptors are linked with its cortical sensory areas and it begins to perceive. The arrival of one of us is not a mysterious, unexplained event, as it was for Aristotle, or a direct creative intervention by God, as it was in Christian theology, but a natural development of the fetal body itself. The fetus simply becomes a perceiving body at the appropriate stage of its development, and a perceiving human body is what we mean by one of us.

The body *is* psychic. We are not saying that our body contains a psychic entity called a soul or a mind, nor that our body is a composite of body and soul, nor that our body is matter informed by a rational soul, as suggested in the philosophical doctrine of hylomorphism, the matter–form model Aquinas ingeniously suggested to account for the individuality of the body–soul composite each of us is. Rather, we are saying that our body is at once biological and psychological. The psychological does not inform the biological, and the biological does not contain the psychological; both aspects are entwined in a mutual and complementary way.

The biological and the psychological are two sides of the human body. Human existence is not exclusively or even primarily biological, nor is it exclusively or even primarily psychological. Philosophies of materialism and of idealism both slight the full concept of a human being. Each one of us began when the fetus became a psychic body, a body that is at once biological and psychological; that is, when the genetically human fetus became an individual perceiving body.

The claim that each one of us begins many weeks into fetal development is derived from how I conceive myself. Once we conceive of ourselves as psychic bodies, we can provide a plausible and verifiable response to the question of when one of us begins. Each of us began when the individual body with our genetic code became sentient; that is, when it began to feel, to be aware, to perceive.

This view of what each one of us is and when each one of us begins to be will be, as are all other interpretations, highly controversial. Some will insist the fertilized ovum is a new one of us; they run the risk of devaluing the psychic dimensions of human existence. Others will insist human existence cannot begin until much later, perhaps at viability (which is achieved around the beginning of the third trimester), or perhaps as late as infancy; they run the risk of devaluing prenatal and neonatal human existence. The end of the controversies is nowhere in sight.

The suggestion that we should conceive of ourselves as psychic bodies, and that a new one of us begins when the fetal body becomes psychic, is simply one of many answers to the question "When did I begin?" It is an answer based on the idea that each of us is an individual human body sufficiently developed so that it is not capable of dividing or fusing, and is capable of perception. This approach will not please everyone, but neither will any other approach. No one expects that everyone will agree on when one of us begins. All we can hope is that the question will be approached in an orderly and thoughtful way, first by developing a concept of ourselves and then by looking for criteria that will show when a fetus becomes one of us and when one of us dies. The classical conceptions of body and soul, and the modern conceptions of body and mind, no longer serve us well. Perhaps some such concept as psychic body will help.

WHEN DOES ONE OF US DIE?

The end of life is also an important determination in health care ethics. We do not want to treat dead human bodies as if they were patients, nor do we want to make the horrible mistake of considering a living patient dead.

Determining death has become even more pressing in recent decades because of two advances in medicine—life-support systems and organ transplantation. Life-supporting technology can sometimes sustain cadavers for weeks, and organ transplantation encourages us to determine the exact moment of death so organs can be removed as quickly as possible.

In discussing the determination of death, the distinction between concept and criteria is once again important. The concept of death is what we mean by "death" and "dead." We all have a good idea of the concept of death. We know what it means when a friend or relative has died. We think of death as meaning someone has "left this world," "passed away," "departed," "passed on," or "is gone."

The criteria of death refer to the evidence that indicates someone is dead. Criteria enable us to verify that death has occurred. Sometimes the criteria are obvious. Anybody looking at a human body that has been dead for a few hours observes a whole series of changes that lead to one conclusion—the person died some time ago. A significant drop in body temperature, loss of normal color, rigor mortis, and biological disintegration are all clear criteria for indicating death.

These indications, however, are not sufficiently refined for medicine because they appear only several hours after death and, if life-support equipment is being used, they may not appear for weeks or even months after death. Medicine therefore uses two more refined criteria for determining when someone is dead. The first has a long history; the second was developed in the past few decades. The first criterion centers on circulation and respiration; the second on brain function.

The Cardiopulmonary Criterion of Death

According to the cardiopulmonary criterion of death, a person is dead if the functions of the cardiopulmonary system have irreversibly ceased. The pulmonary system provides oxygen and the cardiac system distributes the oxygenated blood. The contributions of these systems are crucial for life. If air is not taken in by the lungs and if blood is not pumped by the heart, organs begin to die. It matters little which function—cardiac or pulmonary—ceases first because the cessation of either will soon cause the cessation of the other.

Note that we did not say that the destruction of the heart or lungs is a criterion of death, because it is not. We know today that we can remove a person's heart and lungs, and she can remain alive as long as something else, perhaps a heart–lung machine or a transplant, provides the functions of the heart and lungs. Note also that we said *irreversible* cessation of cardiopulmonary functions is the criterion for death. Temporary cessation of the cardiopulmonary functions does not mean the person is dead. Some cessations of pulse and breathing are reversible, although seldom after twenty minutes or so. In rare cases such as drug overdoses or hypothermia (low body temperature, usually caused by submersion in cold water), people can be revived after several hours without air or detectable pulse. Often, unfortunately, their neurological recovery will not be complete because irreversible brain damage is likely after prolonged oxygen deprivation.

The lack of pulse and breathing is something physicians and other trained medical personnel can observe with great accuracy and, except for cases of drug overdose or low body temperature, it does not take long for the cessation of cardiopulmonary functions to become irreversible. In most situations, then, the cardiopulmonary criterion of death provides adequate evidence of death within a few minutes after it occurs. It serves us well in most cases.

Several decades ago, however, a problem emerged. The development of life-support systems enabling unconscious people to live for extended periods of time meant respiration could be prolonged long after it would have naturally stopped. Techniques for long-term feeding were also developed. Patients were fed through a tube entering the nose and running down into the stomach or through a tube surgically inserted into the gastrointestinal system. With good care and antibiotics to fight infection, irreversible cessation of the cardiopulmonary functions could now be prevented for long periods of time.

Some patients on advanced life-support systems had experienced the loss of all brain function. Were it not for life-support systems, they would have irreversibly lost cardiopulmonary functions and been declared dead. With the life-support equipment, they lived for weeks and even months. This led many to wonder whether the life-support systems were preserving life or preventing natural death. The cardiopulmonary criterion of death did not seem appropriate for cases where life-support systems kept hearts and lungs working for people without any brain function. This suggested that another criterion of death was needed. The obvious candidate was the irreversible loss of all brain functions.

The Brain-Death Criterion of Death

In 1959 French neurophysiologists published results showing that some unconscious patients sustained by respirators lacked all awareness and all electrophysiologic activity in their brains. Moreover, when these patients finally died of irreversible cardiopulmonary arrest despite the life support, autopsies revealed extensive areas of necrotic brain tissue. This showed that their brains had been dead for some time, just as any organ of the body can die if it is not properly nourished by oxygenated blood. In fact, sometimes the tissue had been dead so long that it had begun to digest itself in a process called autolysis, a phenomenon that normally occurs in a dead body some time after death.

The French physicians concluded that these patients had not really been in a coma while they had been on the life-support systems, but in a state "beyond coma," a state they called "coma depassé." Their brains were dead, but the technology was sustaining cardiopulmonary function so their bodies were alive. Thanks to a respirator, the bodies absorbed oxygen and were able to maintain the body temperature, pulse, and color of the living. The big question was: Are patients with dead brains and living bodies alive or dead?

At about the same time as life-support systems were creating a class of patients in "coma depassé," another development was beginning—organ transplantation. In the early kidney transplantations, organs were retrieved from living donors with close tissue matches to the recipient, but it was immediately recognized that most organs would come from cadavers once drugs could be developed to fight rejection by the recipient's body. Using organs from cadavers presents a problem because the organs have to be fresh, that is, as fully nourished by a healthy blood supply as possible. Without this nourishment, the organs rapidly degenerate and become unusable.

In other words, transplant teams want living organs, but they can only take them from dead patients. They need a way to determine death as soon as possible after it occurs, and they also need a way to determine when a patient dies while life-support systems are nourishing the body and making it look quite alive.

In 1968 an ad hoc committee of the Harvard Medical School published an important report outlining criteria for determining what it called "irreversible coma," the "coma depassé" first described by the French physicians. It outlined several clinical tests and also called for the use of an electroencephalogram (EEG) to show the absence of electrical activity in the brain. It recommended that these tests be repeated in twenty-four hours. These criteria became known as the "Harvard criteria." Their accuracy was demonstrated repeatedly in the ensuing years, for no patient diagnosed to be in "irreversible coma" according to these criteria ever recovered. These criteria, of course, were not really verifying the presence of an irreversible coma, but of something else, something that would soon be called brain death.

A consensus began to emerge that patients whose brains had permanently ceased to function should not be described as in an irreversible coma, but as dead. Their cardiopulmonary functions supported by respirators made it look like they were alive, but they were not. They were not living in a state "beyond coma" or in an "irreversible coma"—they were simply dead. In other words, a new criterion of death was emerging. If vital signs such as pulse, respiration, normal body temperature, etc., were being maintained by life-support systems, but the brain had irreversibly ceased to function, then it was thought that we should consider this as evidence the person was dead. Along with the original criterion of death—irreversible cessation of the cardiopulmonary function—there was now a second criterion—irreversible cessation of all brain functions.

When life-support equipment is not being used, brain and cardiopulmonary functions will cease almost simultaneously, so the brain-death criterion is of little practical value in most deaths. But when life-support equipment is being used, the mutual dependency of the cardiopulmonary and brain functions can be broken. The life-support equipment can sometimes maintain the cardiopulmonary functions for days and even months after all brain functions have ceased. The new criterion of death, irreversible cessation of all brain functions, is designed for just such a situation. It allows us to say that people with adequate circulation and respiration (thanks to life support), but with irreversible loss of all brain function, are truly dead.

For a time there was extensive debate about the brain-death criterion, but a consensus soon emerged. In 1970 Kansas became the first state to recognize brain death as a legal criterion of death. Today almost all states recognize the brain-death criterion, either by legislation or by case law derived from court decisions. Unfortunately, the laws are not identical in every state, and revisions are still being made. Some state laws, for example, speak of the cardiopulmonary and brain-death criteria as two separate but equal criteria, while some other states make the cardiopulmonary criterion primary and accept the brain-death criterion only when the cardiopulmonary criterion cannot be used because life-support systems are in use.

In the early 1980s, a Uniform Determination of Death Act (UDDA) was approved by the Uniform Law Commissioners, the American Bar Association, the American Medical Association, the American Academy of Neurology, and others, and adopted verbatim by a number of states. It reads as follows:

> An individual who has sustained either (1) irreversible cessation of circulatory and respiratory functions, or (2) irreversible cessation of all functions of the entire brain, including the brain stem, is dead.

Although this statement is actually quite clear, confusion over the brain-death criterion of death persists. People use the words "brain-dead" and "brain death" in misleading ways. It would be well if we could abandon these phrases and speak, instead, of the neurological criterion for death, but it is undoubtedly too late for that. Since people will likely continue to use the expression "brain death," we should attempt to be clear about what it means.

First, when we speak of brain death we are speaking of the whole brain. We are saying that the entire brain, including the brain stem, has irreversibly ceased to function. The brain stem is about three inches long and joins the spinal column to the brain itself. It is considered a part of the brain and is the primary center for the control of respiration and blood pressure. If it has ceased to function, there will be no spontaneous breathing and cardiopulmonary functions will cease almost immediately unless a ventilator is used. The bodies of brain-dead people always need this equipment—no truly brain-dead person is being kept alive simply by a feeding tube. Irreversibly unconscious patients breathing without a ventilator are not brain-dead. (Conversely, not every irreversibly unconscious patient on a ventilator is brain-dead.) The brain-death criterion of death, therefore, never refers to what some misleadingly call cerebral or neocortical death, the death of the cerebral hemispheres or the neocortex. It refers always to complete brain death, the irreversible cessation of all functions of the entire brain, including its stem.

Second, brain death is a definitive criterion of death; that is, it is an observable fact that allows us to say someone is dead. If someone has suffered brain death, then he is not alive. If he is on life-support systems, he will look very much alive because cardiac and pulmonary functions, as well as normal body temperature and skin color, continue. But if physicians have correctly diagnosed brain death, then the person is truly dead. This means he does not die when the life-support technology is disconnected and his breathing suddenly stops; he was already dead when the life-support system was removed. In effect, the life-support system was removed from a corpse.

Unfortunately, many people continue to think life-support systems keep brain-dead patients alive. Newspapers, for example, sometimes print stories about brain-dead pregnant women being kept alive in an effort to save the fetus and brain-dead babies being kept alive while suitable organ recipients are sought. If these women and babies are truly brain-dead, then they are simply dead, and it is incoherent to say that they are being kept alive. It looks like the life-support equipment is keeping them alive, but this is not so because dead people cannot be kept alive. What is really happening is this: the life-support equipment is supporting the biological life of a corpse in an effort to save the fetus or to salvage fresh organs. People become confused because they see the classic signs of life—pulse, temperature, color, and breathing—but once we know all brain functions have irreversibly ceased, we know the individual is really dead.

Third, the role of the electroencephalogram (EEG) in determining brain death is often misunderstood. It is not true to say a "flat" EEG, one that shows no electrical activity in the brain, indicates people are brain-dead. Nor is it correct to say an EEG showing electrical activity indicates people are alive. The EEG was a requirement in the tests set forth by the Harvard criteria of 1968, but since then most published criteria for determining brain death rely on a clinical diagnosis, usually by a neurologist, and use the EEG only in a secondary role for confirmation. One reason for this is that the EEG is not always a good indicator of brain death. Sometimes people with a flat EEG are actually not brain-dead, and sometimes the EEG indicates activity when in fact brain death has occurred.

Fourth, brain death is difficult to diagnose in children, especially in the first year of life when neurological development is incomplete. In the mid-1980s a special task force on brain death in children produced helpful criteria tailored to three age groups: over one year; between two months and one year; and between seven days and two months. The task force recognized the difficulty in applying brain-death criteria to children and declined to recommend criteria for infants less than a week old.

Fifth, despite widespread public acceptance of the brain-death criterion, some problems still linger. Among them are the following.

1. Some states have not yet passed laws defining neurological indications of death, and this leaves some physicians living in those states uncomfortable about using the brain-death criterion.
2. Some religious groups, including Orthodox Jews, object to the brain-death criterion. This has led some to suggest that people should be able to refuse the use of the brain-death criterion for determining their death, or the death of family members, if they so desire. Such a proposal, however, while considerate for individuals, would cause social problems. Societies need to know clearly whether someone is dead or not, and third-party payers for treatment understandably do not want to pay for treatment on legally dead patients.
3. Some people associated with right-to-life or pro-life groups still feel uncomfortable with the brain-death criterion, although their opposition to it is not as widespread as it was a decade or so ago. The underlying fear was, and to some extent still is, that acceptance of the brain-death criterion encourages a tendency to accept euthanasia and abortion.
4. Some neurologists and ethicists are concerned that the brain-death criterion is not as solid as it once seemed. Specifically, if brain death means the "irreversible cessation of all functions of the entire brain, including the brain stem," then some patients diagnosed as dead by

this criterion are not really dead since small nests of brain cells may continue to survive. The functions of these cells are meaningless as far as survival goes, but they are still functions of the brain, and hence "irreversible cessation of all functions of the entire brain, including the brain stem," has not yet taken place.

Neocortical or Cerebral Death

Brain death (that is, the irreversible cessation of all brain functions, including those of the stem) is the only acceptable neurological criterion of death at this time. There are proposals, however, that we should accept another neurological criterion for death—neocortical or cerebral death. As the Multi-Society Task Force on PVS noted in its 1994 consensus statement, the term neocortical death is limited in its usefulness because it does not denote a distinct clinical entity. For those advocating acceptance of a neocortical criterion of death, however, the notion of neocortical death centers on the permanent loss of functioning sensory areas in the cortex. The neocortical functions supporting awareness irreversibly cease when certain parts of the brain, usually the neocortex or the thalamus (a small area inside the brain beneath, and somewhat surrounded by, the neocortex), are permanently damaged, perhaps by lack of blood for more than a few minutes due to a cardiac arrest or a cerebral accident, perhaps by a severe head trauma.

The major neocortical function that interests us here is awareness. The ability to be aware depends on cortical areas in our brains. If this part of the brain has permanently ceased to function, the person will never again become aware of anything. People suffering what is called neocortical death are permanently unconscious. They are in either an irreversible coma or an irreversible vegetative state. They are not brain-dead because at least some of the brain stem continues to function. Sometimes enough of the stem functions so they can live without life-support equipment.

Although coma and vegetative state are sometimes confused, they are really two distinct phenomena. Coma patients look as if they are in a deep sleep. Their eyes remained closed and they cannot be aroused. Patients in vegetative state usually go through alternating periods of sleep and arousal. When aroused, their eyes are open and their facial expressions can vary from something akin to smiling to something akin to crying. Sometimes they can make sounds as if they were trying to talk. Although aroused, they are unaware. Patients in either a coma or a vegetative state are totally unconscious. It is very important not to confuse the arousal observed in PVS patients with awareness.

Some patients in a coma will recover some awareness; others will suffer cardiopulmonary arrest in a relatively short time without recovering any awareness. Sometimes, however, the coma will become a vegetative state, and vegetative states can last for years or even decades. Once a vegetative state is established, it is known as a persistent vegetative state or PVS. Most persistent vegetative states are actually permanent vegetative states. The loss of all neocortical functions is irreversible.

Since most vegetative states follow a period of coma, the family often interpret the appearance of arousal associated with a vegetative state as an indication that the patient is recovering from the coma. Unfortunately, the arousal associated with vegetative state is not a sign of recovery; the patient remains totally unconscious, and the longer a patient is unconscious, the less likely is recovery.

Some people suggest that patients suffering the irreversible loss of all neocortical functions, which means the loss of all awareness, should also be considered dead by a criterion they call neocortical death. These patients are "gone," since all that remains is a human body living irreversibly on a vegetative level. At the present time, however, neocortical death, unlike brain death, is not recognized as a criterion of death.

On the theoretical level, there is no reason why the permanent loss of all capability for awareness could not be an accurate indication that one of us is no longer here; that is, that one of us has died. If we accept the idea that each of us is a psychic body, then the end of the psychic body is the end of one of us. True, the human body may live on in a vegetative state, sometimes for years or even decades, thanks to the use of feeding tubes for medical nutrition and hydration. But a permanently vegetative body is not a psychic body; it is not one of us. Each of us is more than a vegetative body—each of us is a perceiving body. Once all capability for perception is irretrievably lost, the body, although still a living human body, is no longer one of us. A permanently vegetative human body is but the remains of what was one of us.

Even if one does not accept the concept of a psychic body, there are good reasons for believing the neocortical criterion for death is actually consistent with what most people think of life and death. As we have seen, many people think each of us is more than a human body. They speak of a human being as some kind of compound involving body and soul, or body and mind, or body and something called "personhood." The neocortically dead are not such compounds—they are simply vegetative bodies. There is no evidence of a human soul, or mind, or personhood. In fact, there is not even any potential for feeling on the sense level, let alone on the rational, mental, or personal level. All that remains is a vegetative body, a living organism that will survive, if nourished, but without the ability to feel anything.

Nonetheless, there are good reasons for arguing against supporting any effort to make what some call neocortical death a legal criterion of death, at least at this time. First, we have learned from the experience of using brain death as a criterion for death that any neurological criterion of death can be easily misunderstood. Although brain death has been widely accepted as a legal and moral criterion of human death for more than two decades, a great deal of confusion still lingers in the minds of health care providers and of the general public.

It is not easy for some to accept the fact that an individual on life-support systems with normal pulse, color, and temperature is dead. Many still think that brain-dead patients on respirators die when the life support is removed and the breathing stops. This is why some physicians still make the time of life-support removal the time of death, despite the fact it may have been determined days earlier that the patient had suffered brain death. The continuing confusion over brain death, years after public policy has accepted it as a criterion of death, is a powerful argument for not making any effort at this time to have neocortical death accepted as a criterion for death, at least not in the near future.

Second, any move to make neocortical death a criterion of death at this time will be needlessly divisive in our society. Many opposed to euthanasia can be expected to argue against a neocortical-death criterion either because they believe it is a form of euthanasia or because they see it as a slippery slope that will lead to euthanasia. Many opposed to abortion can also be expected to resist the neocortical criterion. Their fear is that the support of a position whereby bodies suffering neocortical death are considered dead would make fetuses without neocortical development vulnerable to abortion.

Given the problems that would arise if we tried to have something like a neocortical criterion of death accepted as social policy, it seems better to leave things as they are. And there is no compelling reason to change the social policy. People can leave advance directives stating they do not want their vegetative bodies sustained after they have suffered the permanent loss of all awareness and, in the absence of such directives, good ethical reasoning supports a proxy making the same decision for a patient.

Instead of presuming these patients would want their bodies maintained indefinitely in a vegetative state, we should assume the opposite is true unless there is clear and convincing evidence to the contrary. And if people do want their permanently vegetative bodies maintained indefinitely, it would not be unreasonable to require them to arrange funding for what might last for years and cost from $350 to $500 a day ($126,000 to $180,000 a year). Keeping neocortically dead bodies alive in a persistent vegetative state for years or even decades is simply unreasonable. It provides no benefit for the patient and is a burden for many others.

ETHICAL REFLECTIONS

Determining just when an individual human life begins and ends is difficult. The beginning of a new genetic human entity is now relatively easy to fix at the end of the fertilization process but, as we saw, this entity is not yet a definitive individual entity because it might fuse or split. After about fourteen days it does become a definitive individual but, except for those who view human beings solely in physical or biological terms, this is not enough to provide a definite answer for when one of us begins. Sometime after several months into the pregnancy the fetus becomes capable of sensation. Although we do not know exactly when the fetus begins to perceive, the development of perception may well be the transition in the process that began with fertilization best suited to indicate the presence of a new one of us. Before this time, the fetus is a human being but does not possess human existence. It has not yet developed beyond a vegetative body, and a vegetative human body is not yet one of us.

We have to admit, however, that designating transitions in embryonic and fetal development remains a somewhat arbitrary exercise. We do know that a spermatozoon just beginning to penetrate an ovum is not yet a new genetic human being, and most of us readily admit a viable fetus is very much one of us. But the intervening weeks between the beginning of fertilization and the beginning of viability are a gray area. Since science cannot say when one of us begins, it remains a matter of interpretation. And, as we know, people have their own reasons (and agendas) for choosing various points in the process as the precise moment when the developing entity becomes one of us.

To some extent, then, there is a time in the process of fetal development when we cannot say for certain whether or not we are faced with an individual human life that is one of us. This gray area raises an ethical concern. Some would say human life is so important that, even if we are not sure a developing embryo or fetus is one of us, we must treat it as if it were. Others feel that morality does not require us to treat what might be one of us the same as what is certainly one of us. Here, again, our response rests with what is reasonable. The more probable it is that we are dealing with one of us, the more careful we have to be. We undermine our own good when we cause harm without adequate reason to what is, or could be, one of us.

Two further remarks about the beginning of life are in order. First, our moral well-being depends to some extent on treating all human life, even before it becomes individuated and sentient, with respect. A recently fertilized embryo in a laboratory is not just another cluster of cells. It is a new human life, and it will be good for us to treat it with respect. The morally virtuous person treats all life, especially all human life, with a high degree of dignity and care.

Second, our suggestion that we consider the appearance of the sentient fetus as the appearance of a new one of us suggests an analogy with brain death. The analogy says that just as we consider brain death an indication that human existence is over, so we should consider the absence of brain life in a fetus an indication that human existence has not yet developed. Thus some say we should consider human life as beginning with brain life and ending with brain death. This implies we should consider a fetus without brain life as if it were a body without brain life; that is, as if it were dead.

The symmetry is neat and provocative, but the analogy has serious drawbacks. There is a significant difference between a fetus without brain life and a human being that has lost brain life and is brain-dead. The fetus is alive and the brain-dead patient is dead. The brain-dead patient is dead because he has suffered the irreversible loss of all brain functions. The fetus has not suffered any such loss, and therefore is not dead. The patient is brain-dead because he once had a living brain and it died; the fetus is not brain-dead because it never had a living brain, and therefore its brain did not die. A brain cannot be considered dead if it never lived—death always follows life. True, neither the six week fetus nor the brain-dead individual has brain life, but the former is alive (although not one of us) and the latter is dead. The fundamental difference between life and death undermines the analogy between an early fetus and a brain-dead patient.

For these reasons, comparing an early fetus with a brain-dead patient does not seem like a good idea. The early fetus is not dead but alive; it simply has not yet developed awareness. The lack of any awareness may mean, as we suggested, that the fetus is not yet one of us, but it does not mean the fetus is dead. The fetus is very much alive, very much human life with a potential for awareness, and we achieve our good by treating it with the respect we have for human life, which is something more than the respect we have for the dead. Good moral reasoning presupposes that we can separate the dead from the living. A brain-dead patient is dead; a developing fetus is living.

SUGGESTED READINGS

A very helpful book for material covered in the first part of this chapter is Norman Ford. 1988. *When Did I Begin: Conception of the Human Individual in History, Philosophy and Science.* Cambridge: Cambridge University Press. Ford believes a new human individual begins with the appearance of the "primitive streak" in the embryo at about the 15th day of its development. The primitive streak is a thickening of cells at the caudal or tail end of the embryonic disk, and it marks the future longitudinal axis of the developing embryo. Ford argues, convincingly, that the development of the primitive streak marks the beginning of the human individual. We have argued that a human individual is not yet one of us until it becomes a psychic body, an event that occurs several months after the primitive streak appears.

Also helpful are: Bonnie Steinbock. 1992. *Life Before Birth: The Moral and Legal Status of Embryos and Fetuses.* New York: Oxford University Press; chapters 1 and 3; Clifford Grobstein. "The Early Development of Human Embryos." *Journal of Medicine and Philosophy* **1985**, *10*, 179–82; Hans-Martin Sass. "Brain Life and Brain Death." *Journal of Medicine and Philosophy* **1989**, *14*, 45–59; Richard McCormick. "Who or What is the Preembryo?" *Kennedy Institute of Ethics Journal* **1991**, *1*, 1–15; Thomas Shannon and Allan Wolter, "Reflections on the Moral Status of the Pre-Embryo." *Theological Studies* **1990**, *51*, 603–26; Lisa Cahill. "The Embryo and the Fetus: New Moral Contexts." *Theological Studies* **1993**, *54*, 124–42; Carlos Bedate and Robert Cefalo. "The Zygote: To Be or Not To Be A Person." *Journal of Medicine and Philosophy* **1989**, *14*, 641–45; Thomas Bole. "Metaphysical Accounts of the Zygote as a Person and the Veto Power of Facts." *Journal of Medicine and Philosophy* **1989**, *14*, 647–53 and "Zygotes, Souls, Substances, and Persons." *Journal of Medicine and Philosophy* **1990**, *15*, 627–35; Joseph Donceel. "Immediate and Delayed Hominization." *Theological Studies* **1970**, *31*, 76–105; Mario Moussa and Thomas Shannon. "The Search for the New Pineal Gland: Brain Life and Personhood." *Hastings Center Report* **1992**, *22* (May–June), 30–37; Lorette Fleming. "The Moral Status of the Foetus: A Reappraisal." *Bioethics* **1987**, *1*, 15–34; and M. C. Shea. "Embryonic Life and Human Life." *Journal of Medical Ethics* **1985**, *11*, 205–09.

The concept of the "psychic body" is suggested by a number of contemporary philosophies, among them the process philosophy of Alfred North Whitehead and the existential phenomenology of Maurice Merleau-Ponty. Whitehead's process philosophy, sometimes called the philosophy of organism, is strongly opposed to any bifurcation of reality into physical and mental substances such as body and soul. Rather, all reality is described as comprising both physical and mental processes entwined in various degrees. The processes fall into six major categories: the microscopic events of atomic physics, macroscopic inorganic things (e.g., stones), living cells, vegetative life, animal life, and human existence. Both animal life and human existence have sufficient mental feelings so that they have what Whitehead called, in his technical language, "hybrid prehensions;"

that is, a physical–mental consciousness or awareness. Before it develops these hybrid prehensions, the embryo is not a process we recognize as human existence; after it loses them irreversibly, it is no longer a process we recognize as animal or human existence. See Whitehead. 1968. *Modes of Thought*. New York: Free Press, pp. 156–57, and 1967. *Process and Reality*. New York: Macmillan, pp. 163–67.

Merleau-Ponty's philosophy also eschews the classical dualities of body and soul or body and mind; it makes the perceiving body primary. Our body is both object and subject, thing and consciousness, perceiving and perceived. A body that is not an object (a body unable to be perceived) does not enjoy human existence. And a body that is not a subject (a body unable to perceive) does not enjoy human existence. Hence, the embryonic bodies unable to perceive and the bodies locked in PVS do not enjoy human existence. "There is a human body when, between the seeing and the seen, between touching and the touched . . . a blending of some sort takes place—when the spark is lit between sensing and sensible, lighting the fire that will not stop burning until some accident of the body will undo what no accident would have sufficed to do . . ." "Eye and Mind," Carleton Dallery, trans. 1964. *The Primacy of Perception*, ed. James Edie. Evanston: Northwestern University Press, pp. 163–64. See also 1968. *The Visible and the Invisible*, Alphonso Lingis, trans. Evanston: Northwestern University Press, pp. 130–55. For the primacy of the psychic body in Whitehead and Merleau-Ponty, see Raymond Devettere. "The Human Body as Philosophical Paradigm in Whitehead and Merleau-Ponty." *Philosophy Today* **1976**, 10, 317–26.

The most important source for Aristotle's ideas on reproduction is his *Generation of Animals*. Although he was influenced by the recorded observations of the Hippocratic physicians, he rejected their views on reproduction. The Hippocratic texts on *The Seed* and *The Nature of the Child* hold that both the man and the woman contribute seed that forms the embryo. See G. Lloyd, ed. 1986. *Hippocratic Writings*, trans. J. Chadwick and W. Mann. New York: Penguin, pp. 315–46.

As we saw, Aristotle believed that only the man contributes seed. The woman contributes the material for the seed to act on. The famous second-century physician Galen thought both the man and the woman contributed seed, but it was the model of Aristotle that dominated the Western tradition. Unfortunately, it is a model that views the woman as passive in the generation of new life and makes her analogous to the dirt in which the valuable human seed is planted. The Islamic tradition, however, followed Hippocrates and Galen, and held that both the man and the woman contribute semen to the offspring. See B. F. Musallam. 1983. *Sex and Society in Islam: Birth Control before the Nineteenth Century*. Cambridge: Cambridge University Press, pp. 39–59.

Sometimes Aquinas' position that the fetus is not one of us before the infusion of the rational soul forty days into its development is slighted when his work is translated into English. The passage cited in the text about an attacker being guilty of homicide if he kills either a pregnant woman or her *animated* fetus reads in Latin ". . . si sequatur mors vel mulieris vel puerperii *animati*, non effugiet homicidii crimen . . ." A well-known English translation, however, leaves out the word "animati" and makes the passage say: ". . . if either the woman or the foetus dies as a result, he will be guilty of the crime of homicide . . ." 1974. *Summa Theologiae*, Marcus Lefebure, trans. New York: McGraw Hill, vol. 38, p. 47. This inaccurate translation leaves the reader with the impression that Aquinas is saying the destruction of a fetus at any stage of development is homicide, and this simply is not true. According to the Latin text, only the destruction of a fetus after it is animated by the rational soul is homicide.

Two good starting points for understanding the issues associated with determining when one of us dies are the President's Commission report entitled *Defining Death*. Washington: U.S. Government Printing Office, 1981, and the report of the New York State Task Force on Life and the Law entitled *The Determination of Death*. Albany: Health Education Services, 1986. See also Robert Veatch. 1989. *Death, Dying, and the Biological Revolution*, revised edition. New Haven: Yale University Press, chapters 1 and 2; David Lamb. 1985. *Death, Brain Death and Ethics*. Albany: State University of New York Press; Karen Gervais. 1986. *Redefining Death*. New Haven: Yale University Press; and Richard Zaner, ed. 1988. *Death: Beyond Whole-Brain Criteria*. Norwell: Kluwer. For brain death in children, see "Report of a Special Task Force: Guidelines for the Determination of Brain Death in Children." *Pediatrics* **1987**, *80*, 298–300.

The following articles are also helpful: Christopher Pallis. "Whole-Brain Death Reconsidered—Physiological Facts and Philosophy." *Journal of Medical Ethics* **1983**, *9*, 32–37; Daniel Wikler. "Conceptual Issues in the Definition of Death." *Theoretical Medicine* **1984**, *5*, 167–80; Raymond Devettere. "Neocortical Death and Human Death." *Law, Medicine and Health Care* **1990**, *18*, 96–104; Michael Green and Daniel Wikler. "Brain Death and Personal Identity." in Marshall Cohen et al., eds. 1981. *Medicine and Moral Philosophy*. Princeton: Princeton University Press, pp. 49–77; James Bernat. "How Much of the Brain Must Die in Brain Death?" *Journal of Clinical Ethics* **1992**, *3*, 21–26; and Robert Veatch. "The Impending Collapse of the Whole-Brain Definition of Death." *Hastings Center Report* **1993**, *23* (July–August), 18–24.

For an interesting article on death and the permanently unconscious, see Alan Shermon. "The Metaphysics of Brain Death, Persistent Vegetative State, and Dementia." *The Thomist* **1985**, *49*, 24–80. This article is noteworthy because Shermon, employing the classical medieval Christian concept of body and soul, suggests that it is more appropriate to say a patient in irreversible coma or persistent vegetative state is dead than to say he is still living. This is so because there is no reason to think a rational soul still permeates the irreversibly unconscious body, and the departure of the rational soul is what marked death in medieval Christian thought.

The consensus statement of the Multi-Society Task Force on PVS (with membership drawn from the American Academy of Neurology, Child Neurology Society, American Neurological Association, American Association of Neurological Surgeons, and American Academy of Pediatrics) is a valuable review of the latest thinking about persistent vegetative state and related conditions such as coma, brain death, locked-in syndrome, and dementia. It appears as a two-part report entitled "Medical Aspects of the Persistent Vegetative State." *NEJM* **1994**, *330*, 1499–1508 and 1572–1579.

7

Life-Sustaining Treatments

A life-sustaining or life-prolonging treatment is a medical intervention designed to prolong the patient's life rather than to cure the problem threatening his health. Of course, the distinction between life-sustaining treatments and other medical and surgical treatments is not a sharp one. Treatments promoting the restoration of health often prolong life; and treatments prolonging life often promote the restoration of health.

Nonetheless, the distinction is a helpful one in situations where the major impact of a treatment is more the prolongation of life than the restoration of health. A ventilator, for example, supports respiration but does not always contribute to the restoration of health—sometimes it merely enables the patient to live longer with his disease. The same may be said for dialysis when the patient is not a candidate for a transplant—the dialysis merely enables him to live longer with renal disease. On the other hand, some treatments—a kidney transplant, for example, or chemotherapy—are treatments designed to restore health.

The life-sustaining aspect of some interventions is most easily noticed when the restoration of health is no longer possible. Consider, for example, a patient suffering from multiple life-threatening problems associated with advanced AIDS and approaching the end of her life, which is expected at any time. If she begins to suffer respiratory distress, a ventilator will keep her alive a little longer, but will not restore her health. Consider, again, an infant born with anencephaly and having difficulty breathing. Ventilation can sustain his life, perhaps for months, but will not contribute anything to the amelioration of the anencephaly. In situations such as these, the ethical question centers on when it is reasonable to employ life-sustaining treatments and when it is not.

Our main concern in this chapter will be respirators and ventilators. Every life-threatening disease, even those not directly affecting the respiratory system, will eventually threaten respiration. Now that we have the technology designed to support respiration when spontaneous respiration is no longer possible, a major moral problem has emerged over when it is good to use it.

We will also consider briefly two other examples of life-sustaining therapy—dialysis and surgery. Dialysis is designed to support kidney function by purifying blood when the renal system can no longer perform this function adequately, and some surgeries are directed more to prolonging life (and delaying death) than to curing the disease threatening to shorten life.

166

VENTILATORS

Early in this century, an American engineer named Philip Drinker designed the first respirator. The patient was placed inside an enclosed tank, and cycles of positive and negative pressure were used to push air into the lungs and then evacuate it. The popular name for the cumbersome and now obsolete Drinker respirator was "iron lung."

Smaller machines providing air under positive pressure, through tubes in the patient's throat, were soon developed. They were called respirators, although today they are more often called ventilators. In this chapter, we will use the words "respirator" and "ventilator" interchangeably to designate the electrically powered devices providing air through a tube inserted either down the throat (intubation) or into an opening cut into the side of the neck (tracheotomy). These respirators and ventilators are marvelous life-saving inventions, but they have created a host of moral dilemmas.

Sometimes ventilators are clearly necessary for survival—if they are withdrawn the patient will die almost immediately. At other times they play a subsidiary role, either assisting the patient's breathing or providing a backup should the breathing falter. If a patient cannot live without the ventilator, it is truly a life-sustaining treatment.

Those still using the distinction between ordinary and extraordinary treatments in medical ethics invariably consider the respirator an extraordinary means of preserving life. As we noted in chapter three, however, this distinction is ambiguous, and thus not always helpful in ethics. The ventilator is a good example of this ambiguity. When the respirator was introduced, ethicists, moral theologians, and judges (impressed by the advanced technology) tended to consider it an extraordinary treatment. This made it more comfortable for them to say withdrawing a ventilator could be morally justified in some situations.

In one important sense, however, a respirator or ventilator is not extraordinary treatment; in fact, it is quite ordinary. A respirator does not provide medicine but air, an ordinary basic need of human life. It is most often used not to correct a medical problem, but to enable a person with a medical problem to breathe. Mechanical ventilation thus resembles medical nutrition and hydration supplied by feeding tubes. The ventilator tube supplying air to the lungs through an incision in the throat is analogous to a gastrostomy tube supplying nutrition and hydration through an incision in the stomach. And the ventilator tube inserted through the mouth is analogous to a nasogastric feeding tube inserted through the nose. If we remove a feeding tube, the person dies from lack of nutrition and hydration; if we remove a needed ventilator, the person dies from lack of air.

Ventilation is frequently initiated in emergency situations when there is little or no time for careful decision making. If the need is temporary, ventilation seldom presents a moral dilemma. Sometimes, however, the need is long-term or even permanent, and the patient will remain on a ventilator indefinitely, perhaps for life. It is the long-term uses of ventilators that create most of the ethical issues. Many patients kept alive by ventilators are suffering from life-threatening medical problems. Some of them do not want their lives prolonged by the machine, yet declining mechanical ventilation means an earlier death for those who cannot breathe without it. It can be distressing for a physician to withdraw a respirator when she knows her patient will thereby suffer respiratory arrest, often soon after the withdrawal.

Many ventilator-dependent patients are so sick they can no longer make decisions for themselves, and this complicates the moral issue. If they have not given advance directives, their proxies must determine what is in their best interest. If the proxy believes mechanical ventilation is not in the patient's best interest, she has little choice but to request withdrawal. Many proxies are reluctant to do this, especially if the patient will be conscious when the ventilator is removed. It is difficult for a proxy to request something that will result in the death.

Withdrawing a ventilator from a ventilator-dependent patient is, and should be, an extremely serious affair. The people doing it, as we saw in chapter three, are not simply "allowing the disease to cause death." They are playing a causal role, along with the disease, in the patient's death at this time, although their actions are not necessarily unethical or immoral.

So unnerving is the connection between withdrawing the needed ventilator from a patient and the patient's death that many still insist their actions of withdrawing the life-support equipment do not play any causal role in the subsequent death. They insist that the withdrawal of a ventilator merely "lets the patient die," and that the disease is the sole significant cause of death. We have already suggested the questionable nature of this description in chapter three. It is more accurate to acknowledge that both the respirator withdrawal and the disease play causal roles in the death. Thinking this way enables us to see more clearly our responsibility for the death resulting from the withdrawal.

We will now consider some moral issues associated with several important legal cases involving ventilators. Our consideration of cases in this and subsequent chapters will follow the outline of prudential reasoning presented in chapter two. The format is not a rigorous method. It is, rather, an illustration of how prudential deliberation and moral judgment might unfold in situations suggested by the cases.

THE CASE OF KAREN QUINLAN

The Story

This is one of the most famous cases in health care ethics. It marks the beginning of the widespread public debate about stopping life-sustaining therapies, and of court interventions in health care decision making.

In April 1975 Karen Quinlan, then twenty-one, felt faint after drinking at a local bar. Her friends took her home and helped her into bed. When they checked on her a short time later they found she had suffered a cardiopulmonary arrest, probably caused by the combination of alcohol and the prescription drugs she was taking. An ambulance responded, and the emergency personnel administered cardiopulmonary resuscitation, restoring her pulse. She was transported to a local hospital and placed on a ventilator. After some complications developed, a tracheotomy was performed the next day.

Nine days later she was transferred to St. Clare's Hospital, a larger facility. Here she was kept alive in the intensive care unit by the respirator and by a feeding tube that ran through her nose and into her stomach. She remained unconscious, although she displayed alternating periods of sleep and arousal. When her eyes were open, they moved randomly.

The months dragged on with no improvement. Parts of her body became rigid and she lost weight, dropping from one hundred fifteen to about seventy pounds by September. As nearly as could be determined, she would never regain any awareness of anything.

Karen's family asked that the respiratory support be withdrawn. A local priest helped them to see the technology as an extraordinary means of preserving life, and therefore not morally required according to the opinions of Catholic moral theologians and of Pope Pius XII himself in a 1957 address to anesthesiologists. The hospital insisted it could not honor the family's request unless the person making it, Karen's father, was legally appointed Karen's guardian.

The Quinlans went to court and Karen's father, Joseph Quinlan, asked to be appointed her guardian with the power to authorize "discontinuance of all extraordinary procedures" for sustaining life. Hearing this, the court appointed him guardian of her property, but not of her person. This meant Joseph could make decisions about her property but could not authorize the withdrawal of the respirator. The court then appointed another guardian, a guardian *ad litem*, to represent Karen in the case. Karen's guardian *ad litem* saw his role as preserving her life and, therefore, argued against withdrawal of the respirator. The legal process had now become, as so often happens, a battle. The patient's family wanted the respirator removed, the guardian *ad litem* wanted it continued.

During the legal hearings, the lawyer for the attending physician joined with the guardian *ad litem* in opposing removal of the respirator. He argued that removing respirators from living patients was not standard medical practice. Now there was another battle, a battle between the family and the physician.

In his decision of November 1975 the judge sided with the guardian *ad litem* and the attorney for the physician; he declined to give Karen's father the authority to have the respirator stopped. The Quinlans then appealed, and the case went to the New Jersey Supreme Court. Before looking at this court's landmark decision and how Karen was subsequently treated, we will pause to examine the ethical issues. We will try to determine what behavior is "according to right reason," where right reason is the prudence of the moral agents involved in the dilemma. We want to know how the moral agents involved in this tragic situation can find a way to live well, or at least to avoid the worse.

Ethical Analysis

Situational awareness

We are aware of the following facts in the Quinlan story.

1. After several months Karen was irreversibly unconscious in a persistent vegetative state. She could not, and would never again, feel anything. She was beyond experiencing the burden of pain or the benefit of

any treatment or nourishment. She was, according to testimony, not lying peacefully in bed as if asleep but was ". . . emaciated, curled up in what is known as flexion contracture. Every bone was bent in a flexion position and making one tight sort of fetal position. It's too grotesque, really, to describe in human terms like fetal." She was expected to die if the respirator was removed.

2. Karen had not prepared any written directives or communicated any specific instructions to her family about withdrawing respirator support for her if she ever became irreversibly unconscious. This is not surprising; few people were making advance directives at the time and, even today, it is not something most young people think of doing.

3. Since Karen had lost decision-making capacity, proxies (in this case her parents), had to make decisions for her. Since Karen's wishes had not been clearly communicated, her parents could not really use the substituted judgment standard for proxy decision making. They could say, based on their experience of living with their daughter, what they thought she would have wanted. They may have been convinced of this, but they could not report her explicit instructions about respirators because she never left any. Nor could they use the other usual standard for proxy decision making, the best interests standard, because permanently unconscious persons have no inter-ests—they cannot experience anything. A proxy making a decision for the permanently unconscious Karen can only ask what is the reasonable treatment for the vegetative body. He has to rely on what we have called the reasonable treatment standard.

4. The physician was reluctant to withdraw the respirator, and this is understandable. Respirator withdrawal from living patients was not a widely accepted medical practice in 1975. Moreover, the New Jersey attorney general was opposed to the withdrawal, and the threat of possible criminal charges would make anyone nervous about withdrawal. And the physician's lawyer later argued in court that he believed withdrawing a respirator from someone who needs it imposes a death sentence on the person.

We are also aware of the following good and bad features in the story.

1. We would expect Karen's death if the respirator was removed. Dying and death are bad, although in this case the person dying would not experience the process in any way, and the bad associated with the death was reduced by the massive damage already suffered by the brain. Nonetheless, every human death is bad; that is why we regret and mourn death.

2. Karen's life, as all life, was good, although it was not a good for her since she was not aware of it. Nonetheless, human life, even very damaged and very old human life, is an important good.

3. The suffering of the family was bad. Their suffering was caused by Karen's tragic condition, but also by the opposition of the physicians to their wishes for their daughter and by the stressful ordeal of the legal proceedings.

4. The distress the physicians would experience if they withdrew the respirator is another unfortunate aspect of the case. They had to deal with fear of prosecution, with ominous advice from attorneys, with a situation for which there was not yet a recognized medical tradition, with their own recognition that stopping life support does play a causal role in bringing about a patient's death, etc.

These are just some of the good and bad features in the story thus far. Most are directly linked to the central question—is it ethical to withdraw life support from a permanently unconscious patient? To answer this question we will ask what behaviors of the major moral agents in the case (here the parents and the physicians) would be reasonable; that is, what response in the situation would enhance their living well. And if any of their deliberate behaviors would bring about what is bad, we will ask what overriding reasons would justify this.

Prudential reasoning in the Quinlan story

We begin reasoning in an ethics of prudential judgment by asking two fundamental questions: What is truly good for the moral agents, and how can they achieve it? We distinguished two ways a moral agent achieves the good and lives well. First, he enhances the good whenever he can reasonably do so. Second, he eliminates the bad features in the situation whenever possible. And if his deliberate behavior gives rise to anything bad (that is, anything causing suffering, damage, or death) it is always for overriding reasons that are strong enough to compensate for the bad features resulting from his behavior.

We will now look at this dilemma about withdrawing a respirator from the perspectives of the patient, the proxy, and the physician.

Patient's perspective.   Karen was unable to function as a moral agent. She was forever beyond being a moral agent because she was beyond making decisions for her own good. In fact, she was beyond experiencing any good or bad. There is no patient perspective in this kind of situation when the patient left no advance directives.

Proxy's perspective.   Joseph Quinlan was a primary moral agent in this story. If his decision were carried out, the expected result would be the death of his daughter. He knew this, and still wanted the respirator withdrawn. The death of a person is bad. His decision to stop life support for his daughter would be immoral unless he had an adequate reason to justify the bad outcome, death. Did he have a reason capable of justifying the death his decision would cause?

A proxy in this situation could begin by realizing how the bad features accompanying Karen's death are much less than they would be in the death of a normal person her age. The usual harms we associate with death will not occur when Karen dies. First, much of her brain is already destroyed, and there is no reasonable hope that she will ever regain consciousness. People dying in a state of permanent unconsciousness really do not lose that much, and they do not suffer. Death will not take that much more from Karen—she has already lost everything but vegetative life. And if Karen ever did regain consciousness, it would be terrible for her—her rigid, contorted body would cause her significant discomfort and pain.

Second, Karen's actual death will cause only minimal harm to her loved ones, since so much of Karen has already been destroyed by the brain damage that reduced her life to a vegetative state.

Third, Karen's death will cause no real social harm; society has already lost any possible contributions she could have made. Moreover, society's interest in preserving life, an important interest we must not forget, is not undermined when the life has become irreversibly unconscious and is sustained by a mechanical respirator and feeding tubes.

The proxy might also ask how much good the life-support treatment is achieving. It does no good for Karen—she is beyond experiencing any good or bad. Nor is it doing good in the eyes of the family because the use of ventilation to sustain a vegetative body without any capacity for awareness makes no sense. Nor is it accomplishing any good for society or the common good; in fact, it can be argued that this kind of a situation actually undermines the common good by its unreasonable use of financial resources contributed by others in the society.

In the ethics of Aristotle and Aquinas, each moral agent follows the guideline: "act (and feel) according to right reason" where the right reason is prudence, and the reasonable is what achieves the agent's good in the circumstances. Joseph Quinlan's basic options were two: continue the ventilation sustaining a permanently unconscious body or discontinue ventilation, an action that would result in the death of a permanently unconscious body. He was convinced that withdrawal of the respirator was the more reasonable response—the less worse option. It is hard to fault the moral reasoning.

Providers' perspective.   The attending physician, Dr. Robert Morse, and other members of the health care team at St. Clare's Hospital were not convinced that withdrawing the respirator could be morally justified. Their position is not unreasonable, especially if we situate the story in its proper moment in history. At the time this story unfolded in the mid-1970s, many physicians and nurses were understandably upset about removing life-sustaining treatments from living people, and for good reasons. It was not yet a widely accepted move in medical practice, a thorough ethical analysis justifying respirator withdrawal in appropriate situations had not yet been developed, and the threat of legal action was real. Many physicians would have found withdrawal of life-sustaining treatment morally disturbing at the time. It would be less so today, however, because so much ethical dialogue and progress on the matter has taken place, along with some supportive court decisions.

Based on these considerations, there are sound reasons for the physicians' reluctance to withdraw the respirator. The reasonableness of their position is, on the other hand, weakened by the fact that they were forcing treatment on a helpless patient over the proxy's strong objections.

The clash between proxies and providers creates another twist in the story. It is one that occurs frequently. What is the most reasonable way for physicians to respond when a proxy asks them to do something they think is seriously immoral? The answer is relatively straightforward: since they cannot compromise their moral integrity and do what they think is morally wrong because somebody asks them to, they will arrange for alternative provisions for care, and then withdraw from the case. This response was already well worked out by the time the Quinlan story happened. A few years before, in 1973, the United States Supreme Court had declared most restrictions on abortion by state legislatures unconstitutional. What then, should physicians and nurses opposed to abortion do when their patients are seeking abortion? It was generally agreed that they could, and morally should, step aside.

If the physicians had a moral problem with the withdrawal of Karen's respirator, one reasonable response would have been to turn her care over to others and then step aside. The physicians chose not to do this, however, and thus another chapter in the Quinlan story began. Before we consider the moral issues embedded in this chapter of the story, however, we will return to the supreme court's decision in the case.

The Supreme Court Decision

The New Jersey Supreme Court reversed the decision of the lower court in March 1976. It allowed the appointment of Joseph Quinlan as Karen's guardian with the authority to have the respirator discontinued. The court found that the state certainly had an interest in preserving human life, but that the constitutional right to privacy extends to decisions about medical treatment. It found that the state's interest in preserving life weakens, and the person's right to privacy grows, as medical interventions become more invasive and the prognosis for recovery diminishes. It further found that a person's right to privacy can be asserted by a guardian when the patient is incompetent.

Mr. Quinlan then requested removal of the respirator. Apparently the physicians were still unhappy with this decision. Instead of simply removing the machine, they began a process of weaning Karen from it. They withdrew the respirator support, for brief periods at first, and then gradually extended the time until, a month later, she was able to live without it. By June she was off the respirator and was then transferred to a nursing home where, twisted into an unnatural position and totally unconscious, she lived for another ten years. Eventually she developed pneumonia, and her parents requested that antibiotics be withheld. She died in June 1986 from overwhelming infection.

We will never know for sure whether Karen would have died in 1976 if the respirator had been simply removed. But it was not. The physicians at St. Clare's apparently decided that every effort should be made to preserve her vegetative life despite her father's request, which was supported by the New Jersey Supreme Court and by a long Catholic moral tradition allowing people to forego means of preserving life that are considered extraordinary.

Ethical Reflection

Here we take the perspective of an ethicist. We try to make moral judgments about some of the ethical dilemmas faced by moral agents in the story.

The proxy's decision to withdraw the respirator in these circumstances seems reasonable. So does the decision of the New Jersey Supreme Court to allow the proxy to make such a decision. The initial decision of the physicians to continue the respirator can also be justified as reasonable if we remember that the situation happened in the 1970s, when the issue of respirator withdrawal had not yet been extensively deliberated and debated. However, once the court decision was given, the decision of the physicians to stay on the case and try so hard to wean Karen from the respirator does not seem reasonable. Their efforts were successful—Karen survived without a respirator for another ten years—but it was of no benefit to her.

The physicians' decision to wean rather than simply withdraw the respirator was morally problematic in that it brought no good to the patient, was not consistent with the desires of the proxy, and imposed a decade of expensive and useless care on a vegetative body. It is difficult to defend the physicians' actions after the supreme court decision. If they could not in good conscience withdraw the respirator in accord with the proxy's directions, the reasonable ethical response at that point would have been withdrawal from the case.

As you might well imagine, this case generated enormous publicity, and all sorts of opinions were voiced. Some people thought it would be tantamount to murder if the life-sustaining treatment were stopped. Others thought it was cruel for patients and their families to be trapped by a medical establishment so fixated on treatment that it would impose life-prolonging interventions regardless of their benefit for the patient or the wishes of the family. The public uproar was to be expected because new ground was being broken in legal and medical morality, and it takes time for new situations to be absorbed by the medical, legal, and ethical professionals as well as by the rest of society. Today, the removal of a respirator from a permanently unconscious patient at the request of an appropriate proxy would not create a legal or moral problem for most people. But it was not so easy for those involved in the Quinlan case; they were breaking new ground.

THE CASE OF BROTHER FOX

The Story

Brother Fox, a member of a Catholic religious order, arrested during surgery for a hernia repair in October 1979. It left him unconscious, and shortly thereafter he was diagnosed as being in a vegetative state with no chance of recovery. He was eighty-three years old at the time. His religious superior, Father Philip Eichner, asked that the respirator be withdrawn. When the hospital and the physicians caring for Brother Fox refused, he turned to the courts. He argued that Brother Fox had explicitly said more than once in discussions about the Quinlan case that he did not want to be kept alive on a respirator if he was in a similar condition.

The trial court judge approved the respirator withdrawal, but the district attorney appealed the ruling. On appeal, the case went to the Appellate Division of the New York Supreme Court. This court affirmed the lower court ruling, but its decision was also appealed. During this appeal process, Brother Fox died while still on the respirator. In order to establish a legal precedent, New York's highest court, the Court of Appeals, agreed to hear the case even though Brother Fox was now dead. Before looking at the decision of the highest New York court, we will consider the story from an ethical point of view.

Ethical Analysis

Situational awareness

We are aware of the following facts in the Fox story.

1. Brother Fox was permanently unconscious with no hope of recovery.

2. He had made it clear that he did not want a respirator used to keep him alive if this ever happened to him.

3. His proxy was thus able to use the substituted judgment criterion of proxy decision-making and report that Brother Fox had previously indicated he did not want a respirator in these circumstances.

4. The hospital and physicians refused to abide by the patient's request as reported by the proxy, and this brought the case to court.

We are also aware of the following good and bad features in the Fox story.

1. Brother Fox was expected to die when the respirator was removed, and death is always bad. Death was not, however, a bad thing for Brother Fox because his permanent loss of consciousness had removed him from experiencing any bad or, for that matter, any good. Nor was it bad for others at this point, because he was already permanently unconscious.

2. The expense of treatment that provided no good the patient could experience and that the proxy wanted stopped is a bad feature of the case. Somebody was spending money for health care services that would never provide any benefit the patient could experience.

3. The hospital and the physicians were distressed about withdrawing the respirator, and this distress was not surprising at this point in history. The Quinlan case had happened in New Jersey, not New York, and there was no guarantee that New York would not try to prosecute them if they removed life support from a living patient and the patient died. And the Fox story happened soon enough after the Quinlan story that we really cannot say at this point that removing respirators from permanently unconscious patients was a recognized medical practice.

Prudential reasoning in the Fox story
What is good for the people involved in this situation, and how can they achieve it? What is bad, and how can they avoid it?

Patient's perspective.   Brother Fox was unable to communicate anything, but he did leave instructions about what he thought was reasonable. He had decided that withdrawing his life-support equipment after the permanent loss of consciousness was a reasonable thing to do. He was correct—there are no reasons for using medical technology to sustain permanently unconscious patients.

Proxy's perspective.   Father Eichner was also acting reasonably by reporting Brother Fox's instructions to the providers. This is exactly what a proxy is supposed to do. Anything else would have been unethical.

Providers' perspective.   The hospital and physicians were against the withdrawal. Their position is not totally unreasonable, given the moment in history when the case happened. But it is not very strong either, given the legal precedent (the Quinlan case) in the neighboring state and a growing body of commentary at the time indicating there are strong moral reasons supporting respirator withdrawal when the treatment provides no benefit the patient will experience and it is clear that the patient would not want the treatment.

The Court of Appeal's Decision

The highest court in New York, the Court of Appeals, approved the proxy's decision to withdraw the respirator. It confined its ruling to cases where the incapacitated patient is fatally ill with no reasonable chance of recovery, and where we have "clear and convincing evidence" that the patient had given instructions to withdraw the respirator in this kind of situation.

This story differs somewhat from the Quinlan story because, thanks to the extensive publicity surrounding the Quinlan case, Brother Fox had left clear instructions about what he wanted. Once this was evident, the courts had no trouble granting Father Eichner's request. Other courts had long recognized a person's right to refuse medical treatment, and the New York courts sensibly argued that such a right should not be lost just because the person becomes incapable of exercising it.

We should note, however, the court's insistence that there be "clear and convincing evidence" of the incapacitated person's previous wishes. "Clear and convincing evidence" is a legal phrase denoting the highest level of evidence in civil cases. It is very difficult to obtain unless the patient left explicit instructions about treatment. Most states do not require such a high standard of evidence for proxy decision making. Only two states, New York and Missouri, have been consistently demanding it. Years after the Fox case, the United States Supreme Court was asked whether Missouri's insistence on "clear and convincing evidence" was so strict that it was unconstitutional; that is, so strict that it deprived citizens of their constitutional right to refuse medical treatment. The U.S. Supreme Court found, in the Cruzan case that we will consider in the chapter on medical nutrition and hydration, that it was not unconstitutional for states to insist on the strict "clear and convincing" standard in these cases. Fortunately, most states do not insist on such a high standard of evidence for establishing what we think the now incompetent patient would want.

Ethical Reflection

The court's argument based on the patient's right to reject medical treatment does not, of course, settle the moral question. The moral question is whether or not Brother Fox's prior decision to reject life-sustaining treatment in the event of permanent unconsciousness was morally reasonable. As was mentioned earlier, it seems clear that it was, as was the behavior of his proxy, Father Eichner. The reluctance of the hospital and physicians to abide by the information given them by the proxy was also a reasonable position in 1979 when many were not yet morally comfortable with respirator withdrawal. Today, however, it would not be easy to defend morally a refusal to withdraw a respirator in a case such as this.

The actions of the district attorney, however, were more problematic. He chose to appeal the trial court judge's decision, thus dragging out the ordeal. On the other hand, the patient was not suffering, and the appeal did move the case to the appellate level and eventually to the highest state court. This provided an opportunity to set a legal precedent for this kind of case. The decision thus added burdens to the proxy and caregivers, but also contributed to a legal clarification for people living in New York.

THE CASE OF WILLIAM BARTLING

The Story

William Bartling was a sick man in 1984. The California resident was seventy years old and had been hospitalized six times in the previous twelve months. His problems included severe emphysema, hardening of the arteries, an abdominal aneurysm, and inoperable cancer of one lung. His lung had collapsed during the biopsy that found the lung cancer, and a ventilator was necessary to support his breathing. In view of his condition, doctors had no reasonable hope that he would ever again live without the ventilator. Since patients on ventilators in 1984 were usually kept in intensive care units, this prognosis meant that he would probably be confined to the ICU of the hospital for the rest of his life. Although he was suffering from depression, there was general agreement that he had not lost his capacity to make his health care decisions.

William's ability to communicate was hindered by the ventilator tube surgically inserted into his throat, but he was able to indicate repeatedly that he wanted the ventilator removed. After he pulled the tube out several times, his hands were tied to the sides of the bed. He also wrote a statement saying he did not want the life support continued, appointed his wife proxy with durable power of attorney so she could order the respirator removed, and signed documents releasing the physicians and hospital from liability if they withdrew the treatment.

His physician seemed ready to respect his decision to refuse treatment until legal counsel advised the hospital administration to continue the ventilator. Bartling's lawyer then went to court in an effort to have his client's decision to refuse treatment respected by the hospital. He also filed a complaint against the physicians and the hospital for treating Bartling without his consent, and for violation of his constitutional rights.

The day before the court hearing in June 1984, attorneys visited William Bartling in the ICU to take his testimony in a legal deposition. His attorney asked him three questions:

1. "Do you want to live?" Bartling indicated that he did.
2. "Do you want to continue to live on the ventilator?" Bartling indicated that he did not.
3. "Do you understand that if the ventilator is discontinued or taken away you might die?" Bartling indicated that he did.

The court found that Mr. Bartling was seriously ill but competent. Before considering its decision, however, we will reflect on the ethics of the case.

Ethical Analysis

Situational awareness

We are aware of the following facts in the Bartling story.

1. Despite some depression, William was capable of making important decisions.

2. He was seventy years old and had several serious medical problems, including inoperable lung cancer. It was unlikely that he could ever live without the ventilator or leave the ICU.

3. His decision to withdraw the respirator remained constant over many months. It was also supported by his effort to use every means possible to have his wishes carried out by himself or by others.

4. The physicians and the hospital refused to honor Bartling's decision to withdraw the respirator.

We are also aware of the following good and bad features in the Bartling story.

1. If the ventilator was removed, everybody expected Bartling's death. Unlike Karen Quinlan and Brother Fox, he would experience his dying because he was conscious. His suffering and death are clearly bad.

2. If the ventilator was not removed, Bartling's distress would continue. To prevent him from withdrawing the ventilator himself, his hands had been tied. Continuing the respirator and tying his hands were frustrating to William Bartling; they conflicted with his wishes and he knew what was happening.

3. If the ventilator was not removed, his family would be distressed; they wanted his wishes carried out. The whole frustrating process was an additional bad situation for Bartling's family, who were already distressed over his life-threatening illness.

4. The physicians and the hospital were worried about adverse legal consequences if the ventilator was removed, thanks to the legal advice they had received. Such worries are understandably upsetting but, as we will see, were not well grounded in this case.

Prudential reasoning in the story of William Bartling

What is good in this situation and how can the persons involved achieve it?

Patient's perspective.   William was in the best position to judge whether, all things considered, this treatment was really reasonable for him. He did not want to die, but neither did he want to continue the uncomfortable life-sustaining respirator. The respirator would not cure any of his diseases, and one of them (the inoperable lung cancer) was ominous, especially given his problem with emphysema. He had sought hospital treatment six times in the past twelve months, but had now decided it was better to stop the life support than to live with the two new factors: the ventilator and the cancer. It is difficult to think his position was unreasonable, that is, unethical. The life support was providing some good—it was preserving his life for the moment—but it was also causing him a great deal of physical and emotional suffering. He did not want to kill himself; he simply wanted the treatment bringing him more burden than benefit stopped.

Proxy's perspective.   Since William was still capable of making his decisions, there was no role for a proxy at that time. Ironically, if he had lapsed into irreversible unconsciousness, a judge may well have accepted his wife's testimony that there was clear evidence that he did not want the ventilator, and then allow its withdrawal under the precedent set in the Fox case. Thus, Bartling's decision might very well have been accepted if he were unconscious, but it was not being accepted while he was still conscious and able to indicate exactly what he wanted. It is difficult to see the reasonableness of this.

Provider's perspective.   From a legal point of view, one could claim the physicians had some reason to fear litigation if they removed the ventilator and this conscious man died. However, it is hard to think they were worried about criminal prosecution—only a year earlier a California court had found that charges of murder could not be brought against two physicians who had ordered first a respirator and then tubes providing nutrition and hydration to be removed from an unconscious patient at the request of the family.

Moreover, the highest courts in New Jersey and New York (the Quinlan and Fox cases) had already established the right of people to refuse ventilators, and a decision in Florida for a case very similar to Bartling's (the Perlmutter case, which we will mention shortly) had also favored this right. In addition, the California living will law (the California Natural Death Act) was in place at the time of Bartling's request. It would have allowed William to refuse the respirator if he were considered terminally ill, something his physicians declined to say since they thought he might live for more than a year. All things considered, the worries of the physicians and of the hospital about legal liability were more imaginary than real. Nonetheless, the questionable legal advice they received did make the fear of litigation real to them, and exposure to prosecution is certainly something people want to avoid.

From a moral point of view, however, the decision of the attorneys to recommend against withdrawing the ventilator was problematic. The patient did not want it, and his physicians did not want to force it on him, but that is precisely what the legal advice encouraged them to do. Moreover, the decision of the hospital to fight Bartling's request in court is highly unreasonable behavior. It set up an unfortunate relationship of conflict between the institution and a patient, and the conflict could easily have been avoided. The attorneys for the hospital and the physicians did not have to fight for continuation of the ventilator in court; in fact, they could have supported the right of patients to refuse burdensome life-sustaining treatment and simply sought a declaration of immunity to protect themselves if the respirator were withdrawn.

The Court Decisions

The trial court refused to support William's decision to remove the ventilator. It said the right to remove life-sustaining treatment extends only to the comatose or to the terminally ill. The court also refused to grant a subsequent request of Bartling's lawyer—he sought to have the hospital untie Bartling's hands so he could withdraw the ventilator himself.

The case received widespread publicity in September 1984, when Mike Wallace showed dramatic documentary footage of Bartling, in his ICU bed, giving his deposition on the television program *60 Minutes*, and also reported how the judge refused to let his wishes be followed.

Bartling's lawyer appealed the decision of the trial court judge. During the appeal William Bartling died, still tied up and on the respirator. Later the California Court of Appeals reversed the lower court. It ruled that the right to refuse treatment is not confined to the comatose or to the terminally ill, but is based on the constitutional right of privacy enjoyed by all citizens. This decision would have allowed withdrawal of the respirator if William had still been alive.

Ethical Reflection

There seems to be no reason for saying William Bartling was behaving immorally by deciding to stop the uncomfortable treatment that was providing so little benefit for him at this point in his life. Another person in his position might decide differently, however, and that could also be a morally justified position. Prudential judgments often vary among individuals. In this kind of case, an ethicist could very well acknowledge two reasonable decisions: one patient may want the respirator continued, another may want it withdrawn. The primary moral agent, the patient, is thus not making a decision between two options, one ethical and the other unethical, but between two ethically reasonable options.

This does not mean there is no right answer in this kind of case, because there is. The right answer in this kind of case is the answer given by the patient, the person in the best position to figure out how to achieve his good or, in this tragic situation, how to avoid the worse. For Bartling, as for so many others, the respirator could not cure his life-threatening problems; it could only sustain his breathing in the face of severe emphysema and lung cancer. He decided the burdens of the life-sustaining treatment in the ICU as his life ebbed away simply were not worth the benefit it provided.

Let us look at those opposing Bartling on legal grounds, which were later shown to be invalid. There are serious questions about whether the great harm the legal delay and court actions caused the patient and his family can be morally justified. It is difficult to think of any adequate reasons for putting the patient and his family through this ordeal when other options were legally available. Instead of using the courts to fight the patient's wishes, the physicians and hospital could have presented themselves to the court as parties seeking legal protection for respecting a patient's decision to refuse treatment. This legal approach would have been more kind to the patient and his family. And it may have affected the trial judge's decision because, once the hospital stopped opposing withdrawal of the respirator, the central legal issue would emerge more clearly—the patient's legal right to refuse unwanted treatment.

There was no need for the hospital to use the legal system to force unwanted treatment on the patient. This is especially so since an earlier case in Florida had already resolved the issue in favor of the patient with decision-making capacity. In the 1980 landmark case known as *Satz v. Perlmutter*, the Florida Supreme Court affirmed the decisions of lower courts to honor the request of a conscious patient (suffering from amyotrophic lateral sclerosis—

Lou Gehrig's disease) to have his respirator removed. The earlier Florida case had another similarity to the Bartling case—Mr. Perlmutter had also tried to remove the respirator himself but hospital personnel had tied his hands so he could not.

Although the first ethical dilemmas about the use of ventilators centered on patients or proxies trying to remove them, lately ethical issues have emerged when proxies have insisted on prolonging ventilation long after it benefits the patient. Two such cases have received wide publicity. We will consider the first, involving an elderly woman named Helga Wanglie, next; and we will consider the second, involving a baby known as Baby K, in the chapter on neonatal life.

THE CASE OF HELGA WANGLIE

The Story

In December 1989, eighty-six-year-old Helga Wanglie broke her hip. She was successfully treated at the Hennepin County Medical Center in Minnesota, and then discharged to a nursing home. In January 1990 she was back in the hospital with respiratory distress, and a respirator was necessary. In early May, still on the respirator, she was transferred to a chronic care facility where, two weeks later, she suffered a cardiopulmonary arrest. She was resuscitated and readmitted on May 31 to the medical center, where she was diagnosed as being permanently unconscious with chronic lung disease that would require a respirator for the rest of her life. It soon became clear that she was in a persistent vegetative state.

By the end of 1990, almost a year after Helga had become respirator-dependent and months after the diagnosis of persistent vegetative state, her attending physicians felt strongly that the ventilator and other life-support systems were medically inappropriate treatments since they could not serve any of the patient's interests. Helga's husband Oliver, however, wanted the life-sustaining treatment to continue. He felt that only God should take life, and said that Helga would not have wanted anything done to shorten her life.

In December 1990 the medical center advised Mr. Wanglie in writing that it did not believe treatment considered inappropriate by physicians should continue, but that it would continue the life-sustaining treatment if he obtained a court order mandating it. During this time, both the hospital and the family tried to find another facility willing to accept Helga as a patient. None would accept her.

When the Wanglie family made no move to seek a court order for treatment, the medical center filed a legal petition on February 8, 1991, seeking appointment of a conservator for the patient. Ordinarily, a guardian *ad litem* would be appointed to perform this function, but Minnesota did not have a guardian *ad litem* process, so the hospital sought appointment of the conservator to protect the interests of the patient.

The medical center had serious doubts that Helga's proxy, her husband, was making the right decision, so it was seeking to have the court appoint a conservator to represent her. The center hoped the court-appointed conservator would say that the ventilator was not beneficial to Helga, paving the way for its removal. The hospital's legal move was undermined when Helga's husband filed a petition asking that he be appointed the conservator.

On July 1, 1991, the court did appoint a conservator for Helga—her husband. He continued to insist on the ventilator, and the medical center continued to provide it. Three days later, Helga died. During the last fourteen months of her life, Helga, a permanently unconscious woman in her late eighties with no hope of recovery, had her vegetative body sustained by a respirator at the medical center. It was reported that Medicare paid about $200,000 for her first hospitalization at the center, and that a private HMO paid over $500,000 for the second admission that ran from May 1990 to July 1991.

Ethical Analysis

Situational awareness

We are aware of the following facts in the Wanglie story.

1. Helga was in persistent vegetative state. She could experience neither benefit nor burden from life-sustaining treatment.

2. She had not made it clear that she would want a ventilator keeping her alive if she ever lapsed into persistent vegetative state, but there are several reasons to think that she may well have wanted it. Although her husband first said he did not know what she would have wanted, he later indicated, in a letter to the medical center dated December 3, 1990, that she had always said she did not want anything done "to shorten or prematurely take her life." Moreover, it was known that her religious views included the idea that only God gives and takes life, and that her moral views were strongly pro-life.

Unfortunately, a precious opportunity to learn Helga's wishes was lost. She was a conscious patient in the hospital on a respirator from January until May 1990, yet published reports do not indicate that anyone attempted to determine her wishes while she was still capable of stating them.

3. Her husband was her proxy and, thanks to the court, also her conservator. He wanted the ventilator continued. His decision was apparently based on his familiarity with her wishes, although this did not become clear until physicians asked him to consider withdrawing the ventilator.

4. Her physicians came to the conclusion that ventilation was not appropriate medical treatment for her. Although Dr. Stephen Miles, an ethicist serving as consultant to the physicians caring for Helga, declined to characterize the ventilator as futile treatment because it was sustaining vegetative life, a newspaper story in the *Chicago Tribune* of January 10, 1991, reported that other physicians involved in the case sought relief in the court because they did think the ventilator was futile treatment after the diagnosis of PVS. And an attending physician, who joined the case later, spoke of the respirator as "nonbeneficial" in that it could neither heal Helga's lungs nor restore her awareness.

We are also aware of the following good and bad features in the Wanglie case.

1. Without the respirator Helga would die, and death is always bad.

2. Withdrawal of the respirator would cause distress to Oliver and to his two adult children, who also opposed the withdrawal.

3. Continuation of the respirator would cause distress to the providers, who felt it was inappropriate. The respirator, however, caused no distress or burden to Helga, nor any benefit, because she was totally and irreversibly oblivious to it.

4. Continuation of the respirator required considerable financial support, and this was eventually a burden on insurance plans and the people paying into them.

Prudential reasoning in the story of Helga Wanglie

What is good in this situation and how can the persons involved best achieve it, or at least avoid the worse?

Patient's perspective.   It is hard to comment on this because we do not know for sure whether Helga would have insisted on the ventilator to sustain her life once it had deteriorated into a persistent vegetative state. The fact that her husband of 53 years at first took the position he did not know what she would want, and then after some months said that she had stated she would not want anything done to shorten her life, is cause for concern.

If a patient did want a ventilator continued after months of irreversible vegetative existence, it is difficult to see how moral reasons could justify that desire. Patients in persistent vegetative state experience no benefit from treatment, and both the costs and the responsibilities of care it imposes on others are significant burdens. Burdening others with what offers no benefit to oneself is difficult to justify as a morally admirable position. This leaves only a religious argument to justify a patient's insistence that life support be continued for her vegetative body; namely, the belief that God, and not anyone else, is the one to decide when death should come.

Religious beliefs are notoriously hard to critique. While some very important religious thinkers—the thirteenth century theologian Thomas Aquinas is perhaps the most notable example—insisted that no moral position derived from religious faith could ever contradict reason, not every religious person embraces such a position. Many claim what is unreasonable to the human mind is not unreasonable in the eyes of God, and further claim that they can know how God sees certain apparently unreasonable situations. In the hands of these people, the religious argument becomes a trump card. It trumps reason. Once it is played, no other reason can undermine it. The religious belief, no matter how unreasonable, becomes, in the mind of the believer, the reason for the decision. No reasoning from moral philosophy or prudence will ever appear cogent to a person basing her apparently unreasonable position on a religious belief.

Proxies' perspective.   If Oliver and his two adult children really thought Helga wanted the ventilator continued after months in persistent vegetative state, then this is a reason in favor of their requesting continuation of the treatment. However, it is not of itself a sufficient reason. Simply because someone wants something does not mean what is wanted is morally good.

If she had wanted a treatment that was clearly absurd, they could not in good conscience be a party to providing it for her. When a proxy acts on the basis of substituted judgment (that is, when a proxy makes the decision based on what he or she knows the patient wanted) there is a presumption that the proxy is presenting a decision that is morally acceptable or at least morally plausible.

While many would argue that respirators for PVS patients in their eighties is an immoral use of personnel and resources because the treatment provides no benefit the patient can experience, some people do see the preservation of human beings in persistent vegetative life as morally good, or at least not morally evil. Helga's family apparently did believe the treatment was morally correct, so it was proper for them to request it. Their moral beliefs, judging from published reports, were based more on a religious conviction than moral reasoning, but religion is an important source of moral judgment for many people.

To carry out their religious conviction, however, they had to ask a hospital, physicians, and nurses to provide treatments these people did not think were appropriate. In effect, they were forcing their morality on others, yet they had little choice but to do so because Helga needed professional care and hospitalization. Helga's vegetative life was a value to them, a good they saw through the eyes of their religious conviction, and a good they wanted to pursue.

Providers' perspective.   The providers did not see any good in the treatment at this point, except for the possible comfort it gave to the family. Did they think continuing the treatment was therefore immoral? That is a separate issue. It is one thing to say the treatment is not doing the patient any good; it is another to say the treatment is immoral.

What did the providers think? Perhaps they thought using the ventilator on a PVS patient was immoral and that they had to stop it, but if this is so, one of their moves was curious. In December 1990, after Helga was in PVS for about six months, the hospital's medical director wrote Mr. Wanglie and said medical consultants, the attending physician, and he (the medical director) did not believe the hospital was obliged to provide inappropriate medical treatment, but would do so if a court ordered it. If the medical director and consultants thought the inappropriate treatment was also unethical, they could not in good conscience make such a statement—legal immunity does not make something immoral moral. Thus their position, assuming they are people of moral integrity, was that the treatment was medically inappropriate, but not morally so.

Their position is coherent if we distinguish, as we should, between good clinical practice and clinical ethics. In this case, a strong argument can be made that good clinical practice indicates that the ventilator supporting the irreversibly vegetative life of an elderly PVS patient for many months is not an appropriate clinical treatment and should be discontinued. This is not the same as saying, however, that continuation of the ventilator is unethical. Claiming continued mechanical ventilation on this unconscious patient is not clinically good does not automatically mean it is not ethically good. What is clinically good is not always ethically good, and what is clinically bad is not always unethical.

Is the continuation of the ventilator not only medically inappropriate but unethical as well? Perhaps, but there are reasons for saying it is not. First, a ventilator does not cause PVS patients any burden or discomfort because they are not aware of anything done to them. This removes a major source of ethical concern—the harm we may be causing a patient. Second, her family claims, or came to claim after several months, that she did not want life-sustaining treatments withdrawn before she died. Since we cannot ask her to verify this, the better course is to give them the benefit of the doubt and assume she, unlike most people, would want to be kept alive indefinitely in a persistent vegetative state. Apparently she considered vegetative life a value, and so does her family.

The view of some that vegetative life is valuable is not completely absurd. The value of vegetative human life is recognized in law. If, for example, a stranger walked into a hospital with a gun and shot a PVS patient dead, we know exactly what the charge would be—murder. Current law supports the idea that a PVS patient is still a living human being, and thus the idea that the ventilator is supporting something of value—human life—is not patently absurd.

In a pluralistic society, respect has to be given (within reason) to the religious and moral considerations patients may have, but which their physicians may not share, as long as such consideration does not force the providers to compromise their moral integrity. In this case, the physicians consider the ventilator medically inappropriate but, judging from their willingness to continue it if a court ordered them to do so, not morally evil. Thus the providers would not be violating their moral convictions by continuing what they thought was unreasonable medical treatment.

This may have been an extraordinary situation where the hospital and the physicians should have continued the medically inappropriate treatment. There are several reasons for saying this. First, the providers did not think the treatment was morally evil, only medically inappropriate; second, the proxy's refusal to accept withdrawal was for sincerely held religious reasons; third, the treatment was not causing the patient any suffering; and fourth, the treatment was not damaging the financial condition of the institution.

Ethical Reflection

The clash in the Wanglie case was ultimately a clash between the religious convictions of the family and the clinical convictions of the physicians. It could also have developed into a clash involving the insurance company, but that did not happen in this case because the HMO did not object to paying for life-sustaining treatment long after consciousness was irreversibly lost.

The Helga Wanglie story is almost the exact opposite of the Karen Quinlan story. Both women were in persistent vegetative state, and neither had left clear advance directives. In Karen's case, however, the family wanted the respirator stopped and her physicians did not, while in Helga's case the family wanted the respirator continued and her physicians did not. Karen's case helped us clarify a proxy's ability to refuse treatment for a permanently unconscious patient; Helga's case raises questions about a proxy's ability to insist on treatment considered, with good reason, medically inappropriate by physicians. This is a new kind of situation and, unlike the right to refuse treatment, we have not yet developed a consensus about the right of a patient or proxy to demand treatment physicians do not consider appropriate.

From the ethical perspective we have been developing, it can be argued that treating Helga is reasonable, given her religious beliefs and the instructions of her family, and the fact that treatment caused no harm to her. However, the actions of the hospital—asking the family to get a court order for treatment and then, when they refused, trying to have the court appoint a conservator who would authorize the treatment withdrawal—are strategies difficult to understand as morally reasonable. The efforts of the hospital to find another institution to care for her, however, were reasonable. And it was morally appropriate for the hospital to continue her care—which was reported as excellent—when no one else would accept her as a patient.

Certainly, it is troubling for physicians to give expensive life-sustaining treatment when they feel it is inappropriate, but when the treatment causes the patient no harm, the bad features of providing the treatment are significantly reduced. Of course, other bad features remain. Among them are the high costs of treatment providing no benefit to the patient and the distress health care professionals experience when they are asked to provide treatments they consider, with good reason, unreasonable. But as long as the physicians and nurses cannot establish that these disturbing factors provide reasons sufficiently strong to override the family's reasons for treatment, they are not compromising their ethics by providing a treatment that causes the patient no harm. Here, what is at least arguably bad clinical practice—using respirators on PVS patients for months—is not necessarily immoral because of the respect one tries to have for sincerely held religious beliefs.

Of course, if the hospital were being forced to provide for the care without compensation, then the drain on hospital funds would be a significant factor for consideration. But that is not the case here—the third party payers made no move to question the treatment. In some ways, the payers of the treatment have stronger reasons for being morally disturbed over the treatment than the physicians. It is certainly harmful for insurance programs to pay out significant sums of money for inappropriate medical treatments of no benefit to the patient.

The day may come when third party payers and HMOs will limit payments for the life-sustaining treatments they will agree to provide. Perhaps, for example, they will explain to their membership that payments for life-sustaining treatment will cease a certain number of months after a confirmed diagnosis of persistent vegetative state. The family of a PVS patient would then have the option of withdrawing the treatment or seeking other sources of funding.

Finally, it must be said that an ethics of right reason finds nothing to justify the position taken by Helga's husband and family, and perhaps by Helga herself. It simply does not seem reasonable for a patient or family to want ventilation continued indefinitely once persistent vegetative state has been definitively diagnosed. Nonetheless, given the religious issue, continuing the harmless treatment—despite its expense and the upset it caused physicians and nurses—may have been the less unreasonable response in this case.

DIALYSIS

Although research on rabbits suggested as early as 1913 that a machine could perform some kidney functions and thus reduce the chemical imbalances associated with kidney failure, it was not until the 1940s that efforts were made to use such a device for patients with chronic renal disease. Less than 20 years later, hemodialysis became a reality. The dialysis machine does the work of a kidney, purifying the blood by removing waste products from it. Normally, the procedure takes about five hours and is repeated three times a week.

When dialysis was perfected in the late 1960s there were more patients than machines, and difficult decisions had to be made about who would be given the treatment. Selection committees were soon formed. In some areas, these committees were called "God squads" since their decisions were, indeed, decisions of life or death for those with serious kidney disease who were unable to obtain a kidney transplant.

In 1972 Congress responded to the shortage of dialysis machines by amending the Social Security Act to guarantee dialysis treatment for all those needing it, regardless of age or other disability. Within a short time, a sufficient number of dialysis centers were established and the number of patients grew. In November 1993 the *New York Times* reported that almost 200 thousand patients with kidney failure were being dialyzed in the United States, that the annual cost was approaching $7000 million ($7 billion) dollars, and that by the year 2000 the annual cost would be more than $10 billion for about 300 thousand patients.

Dialysis is not a perfect answer to the problem of serious kidney disease. It does not cure the disease, and the patient experiences frequent discomfort during the treatment. Moreover, it cannot quite match the work of healthy kidneys, and as time goes on, the disease gains ever so slowly. For example, statistics show that the life expectancy of a forty-nine-year-old dialysis patient is about seven years, compared with about thirty years for the general population.

After years of dialysis, some patients experience mounting health problems. In a few cases they decide to decline the treatment, judging that the mounting burdens outweigh the benefits. Sometimes, as the following story shows, family members must decide when the burdens of dialysis outweigh the benefits.

THE CASE OF EARLE SPRING

The Story

Earle Spring was a vigorous man in his seventies when he developed serious kidney disease. He consented to dialysis and underwent the treatments despite the dizziness, leg cramps, and headaches they caused. As time went on, he became senile and lost his decision-making capacity. He began to resist transportation to the dialysis center and to pull the tubes out of his arm. Heavy sedation was necessary to control his disruptive behavior. His physicians thought he could live for months with dialysis. Survival for five years was conceivable, but not probable. He was not a candidate for a kidney transplant. There was no hope his senility could be reversed, so he would remain in a state of mental confusion the rest of his life.

Since his wife was also advanced in years, the court appointed his son temporary guardian in January 1979. Earle's son, with the consent of his mother (Earle's wife), immediately asked the probate court to issue an order stopping the dialysis. The judge appointed a guardian *ad litem* to investigate the facts in the case. Within a few weeks, the guardian *ad litem* finished his investigation and filed a report recommending continuation of the dialysis.

The judge deliberated until May 1979 and then issued an order for the cessation of dialysis. The guardian *ad litem* objected and filed an appeal.

While the appeal process was under way, the probate court judge had second thoughts about his order directing cessation of dialysis. In July 1979, realizing that he should not be making the treatment decision for Earle, he vacated his original order for ending the dialysis. He then issued a new order directing Earle's wife and son, with the attending physician, to decide whether or not to continue the dialysis. The guardian *ad litem* also appealed this ruling.

In December 1979 the appeals court affirmed the probate judge's July ruling directing the family and physician to make the decision about withholding dialysis. The guardian *ad litem* again objected and filed another appeal, this time to the Massachusetts Supreme Court. Meanwhile, of course, three times a week, the incompetent and protesting Earle was heavily sedated and given his dialysis treatment. It was now eleven months since his son, his legally appointed guardian, had first requested stopping his dialysis.

Unlike the two lower courts, the Massachusetts Supreme Court acted swiftly. In January 1980 it ruled that the probate judge's original order issued in May, the order for the cessation of dialysis, was correct, and that his subsequent ruling in July (directing the family and physician to make the decision) later affirmed by the appeals court, was not correct.

The supreme court said dialysis should be stopped, but not because the family and physician believe it is more of a burden than a benefit. Rather, it should be stopped because Earle "would, if competent, choose not to receive the life-prolonging treatment." The basis for withdrawing the dialysis from a patient who willingly accepted it when he had decision-making capacity cannot be, in the eyes of the court, the family and physicians determining what is now in his best interests. Instead, a judge must determine, thanks to substituted judgment, that the patient changed his mind about dialysis after he lost his decision-making capacity and now would, if competent, choose to stop his dialysis.

At this point, after more than a year, the legal system was at last allowing the family's wishes about Earle's treatment to be followed, and the dialysis should have been stopped. But nurses at the nursing home where Earle was now a patient raised questions about his incompetence. They claimed he was competent, and that he was indicating he wanted to live. They took their concerns to the press and it became a headline story. A right-to-life group asked the court to let them enter the case to fight for Earle's life.

The guardian *ad litem* brought this to the attention of the court. It immediately ordered the dialysis continued while it arranged for a panel of five physicians to determine whether or not Earle was truly incompetent. These physicians examined Earle and reported that he was indeed entirely and irreversibly incompetent. Before the court acted on this report, Earle died on April 6, 1980, still receiving dialysis. The cause of death was listed as cardiopulmonary failure. The Spring family sued the nursing home and was awarded a financial settlement to compensate for the actions of the staff who made their loved one's case a public spectacle and thereby delayed the cessation of treatment they believed was not in Earle's best interests.

Ethical Analysis

Situational awareness

We are aware of the following facts in the Spring story.

1. Earle was seventy-eight and suffering from irreversible renal failure. Dialysis could extend his life for months, perhaps years. While he had decision-making capacity, he had agreed to undergo dialysis, but a court later determined he was incompetent. There is no evidence about whether or not he would want dialysis continued in the circumstances he faced—increasing age, bothersome side effects, and organic brain syndrome, the source of his confusion. We simply cannot say, on the evidence presented, whether he would have wanted the dialysis continued until the day he died, or whether he would have wanted it stopped at some point in his mental and physical deterioration. His vigorous protests against the dialysis cannot be taken at face value because they are the protests of a man without decision-making capacity or legal competence. He was so confused he no longer recognized his wife or son. Nonetheless, his struggles did indicate that the treatments were causing him significant emotional stress.

2. His primary proxy was his son. Although Earle's wife believed, based on her knowledge of him gained in their marriage of fifty-five years, that he would not want to continue to live in his condition of senility and dependence on dialysis, the son did not have any explicit evidence of what Earle would have wanted for himself in these circumstances. The basis of the son's decision to forego further dialysis, then, was largely what he thought was in his father's best interests at that point in his life. He believed that dialysis was no longer appropriate for him and that he probably would not have wanted it. His mother agreed, as did the nephrologist.

3. None of the three courts thought the dialysis had to be continued. Only the guardian *ad litem* continued to argue for it. It was his legal actions—the appeals he made from the decisions of the lower courts, and then his reopening the question of Earle's competency after the supreme court decision—that kept Earle on dialysis for 15 months after his family, with the approval of the courts, decided it should be stopped.

We are also aware of the following good and bad features in the story.

1. We would expect Earle's death relatively soon if dialysis were stopped. The loss of a human life is always bad.

2. Earle was suffering side effects from the dialysis and protested vigorously when efforts were made to place him on the dialysis machine. The treatment was thus a significant burden to him and offered no cure for his disease. In his state of confusion, it was impossible to explain to him how the treatments could help him, so the discomfort had no meaning to him.

3. The family was suffering distress because they could not have their senile husband and father treated the way they thought he should be treated and the way the courts agreed he could be treated.

4. Newspaper reports indicated that some providers in the nursing home were upset that the dialysis would be stopped, and their discomfort was a bad feature, albeit not a significant one if the withdrawal was morally reasonable. The guardian *ad litem* may also have been personally upset by the possibility of stopping the dialysis and thought he had to exhaust every legal option to keep Earle on the life-sustaining treatment.

Prudential reasoning in the story of Earle Spring

Patient's perspective.   Earle had lost decision-making capacity. He had earlier decided dialysis was worth the burden, but we have no evidence indicating what he would have decided about the dialysis in the situation he eventually confronted, and we will never know. There is no patient perspective in moral reasoning when a patient has lost decision-making capacity and had left no indications about how he wanted to be treated in the future.

Proxy's perspective.   Earle's son was the legal guardian of his father; he was the primary moral agent. He had the difficult task of figuring out what was in the best interests of his father, a man suffering from incurable but controllable renal failure and organic brain syndrome or senility. Dialysis was causing him distress, but it could keep him alive a little while longer. The son believed it was reasonable to stop dialysis at this point. His father had already experienced renal failure and could not receive a new kidney. His rational faculties had collapsed as well, so the burdens and benefits of the treatment could not be understood by him. His body and mind were irreversibly disintegrating. Given his strong reactions against the dialysis treatment and the uncomfortable burdens it imposed on him without any meaningful benefit to him, the son concluded it was reasonable to stop the treatments. It is hard to argue that his position is unreasonable.

Providers' perspectives.   There is no indication in the supreme court findings that any physician involved in Earle's care had any problem with discontinuing the dialysis. Some of the staff in the nursing home where he spent the last months of his life, however, did disagree with the decision. They claimed that he might be competent, and that he told them that he did not want to die. Every indication, however, indicated that he was truly incapable of making health care decisions and legally incompetent, so it is difficult to understand the reasonableness of their claim.

The courts' position.   All three courts allowed the dialysis to be discontinued. This seems a reasonable position. Heavily sedating a senile seventy-eight-year-old patient with no hope of either mental or renal recovery in order to provide the life-prolonging treatment is not a reasonable course of action when the treatments are so upsetting to the patient.

The guardian *ad litem*'s position.   Perhaps his first appeal was reasonable, but his subsequent efforts, even after the supreme court decision, are not easy to judge reasonable. A guardian *ad litem* in a treatment case has no legal obligation to use every legal ploy possible to keep a patient alive. His primary responsibility is to investigate the facts in the case, to report them to the judge, and to recommend to the judge what treatments he thinks are best for the patient. In its decision, the supreme court noted that a guardian *ad litem* is expected to present only reasonable arguments for treatment and has no duty to present arguments for treatment that are not meritorious or to seek endless appeals in cases.

Ethical Reflections

The decision to discontinue dialysis on an elderly patient with irreversible kidney disease when the treatment obviously causes him great distress is a reasonable one. The treatment is burdening him significantly but doing little more than prolonging life in a nursing home for a patient who has lost, due to senility, meaningful contact with reality and his loved ones. If he had quietly acquiesced to the treatment and was living in peace, the decision to stop dialysis at this time would not be so readily defensible, but it might still be reasonable at some point. It is not reasonable to attempt reversal of every renal failure, any more than it is reasonable to attempt reversal of every respiratory or cardiac failure. In some cases, it is in a patient's best interests to forego life-sustaining treatments, especially if they are causing him significant burdens with little gain beyond the continuation of a severely compromised life.

A word needs to be said about the reasoning of the courts. The first probate decision and the final supreme court decision insist that judges should be the ones to order treatment stopped or continued once the case comes to court. On the other hand, the second probate decision, confirmed by the appeals court, said the family and the physicians should decide on the appropriate medical treatment. The second approach is more reasonable. While the courts must protect the lives of vulnerable people who have not left advance directives, they are not in a good position to determine proper medical treatment for a person whom they do not know. When appropriate proxies are available, and when there is evidence they are acting in good faith and with good reasons, the courts should allow the normal process of treatment decisions to unfold.

Since the Spring case, efforts have been made to acknowledge this approach in legislation by granting civil and criminal immunity to proxies making health care decisions in good faith on the basis of best interests for patients without advance directives. Such a law did not exist in the Spring case, but the supreme court could have followed the appeals court and allowed the family to make the decision, a decision the court agreed was acceptable. This would avoid the situation whereby courts are saying to families: "Your decision is correct but we are the ones to make it."

We should also remember that the basis of the supreme court's reasoning is suspect. It acknowledged that "there was no evidence that while competent he had expressed any wish or desire as to the continuation or withdrawal of treatment in such circumstances." Yet it claimed to know what Earle would have wanted in such circumstances if he were competent. If the court found no evidence as to what Earle would have decided in such a situation, it is difficult to see how the court can say he would have decided on withdrawing dialysis. As we noted, the Massachusetts court takes this approach because, while it recognizes the right of a patient to decline treatment, it will not allow anyone but the patient to make the decision. If the patient is incompetent, then it falls to a judge to decide what he would have decided if he were competent, a rather difficult challenge whenever the court acknowledges there is no evidence about the patient's desires before he became incompetent.

Underlying this position is a fear about introducing judgments about the quality of life in such cases. In a previous Massachusetts case, known as *Superintendent of Belchertown State Hospital v. Saikewicz* (1977), the first major treatment decision case in the state, the supreme court had rejected the idea that the value of life can be equated with the quality of life. It said that a poor quality of life can never be a deciding factor in a proxy's decision to withdraw treatment from the patient. This means that the court will not allow a proxy to use the best interests standard for the withdrawal of life-sustaining treatment. All cases pertaining to the withdrawal of life-sustaining treatment, then, must be construed as instances of substituted judgment, and it makes no difference whether the wishes of the incompetent patient are known, or whether the patient is a child who was never able to express any wishes about treatment.

In an ethics of right reason, however, judgments about the quality of life are absolutely necessary. They are the only way we can say what is reasonable or unreasonable in the circumstances. As the quality of life irreversibly deteriorates, the reasons for burdensome life-sustaining treatments become less cogent. It is hardly reasonable, for example, to subject very elderly and frail patients without advance directives or decision-making capacity to respirators or dialysis to keep them alive a little longer.

In the final analysis, then, the decision to stop dialysis in this situation belongs with the family and is morally justified. Given the best interests of the patient, the decision to withhold the life-sustaining treatment was more reasonable than the decision to continue it in the circumstances.

SURGERY

Sometimes surgical interventions are associated more with life-sustaining efforts than with correcting medical problems. The surgeries to insert gastrostomy or tracheostomy tubes are cases in point. And the amputations necessary to prolong the life of diabetic patients are another example of life-sustaining surgery. We really cannot say the amputation of a limb cures the gangrene affecting it, nor can we say the amputation contributes to a cure of the disease causing the death of the tissue.

Sometimes patients do not think the life-sustaining surgery is a reasonable intervention in the circumstances, and they decline it. The following case illustrates how this can happen and shows how difficult it can be for families.

THE CASE OF ROSARIA CANDURA

The Story

Seventy-seven year old Rosaria came to this country from Italy in 1918. She married, had a family, and was living in her own home when the case began in late 1977. She had been depressed and unhappy since her husband's death in 1976, and suffered from diabetes. Her relationship with her children (a daughter and three sons) was marked by a degree of conflict, and she really did not want to live with any of them.

Struggling against gangrene in her extremities, she had consented to the amputation of a toe in 1974 and to a part of her foot in November 1977. In April 1978 gangrene was found in the remainder of her foot, and she consented to the amputation of her leg.

On the morning of the surgery she changed her mind and the operation was cancelled. She was discharged to her daughter's home. Around May 9, after encouragement from a physician she had known for years, she again consented to the amputation, but then reversed her decision a second time.

It was clear from her testimony, and from the testimony of others, that she was confused on some matters. Her train of thought sometimes wandered and her conception of time was distorted. She was sometimes hostile with certain physicians and combative when questioned about the possibility of surgery. She expressed a desire to get well but, discouraged by the failure of the earlier amputations to stem the gangrene, was afraid the amputation of her leg would not be successful in controlling the problem. Her opposition to the surgery soon became definitive. She was quite clear on this point and gave every indication that she understood the consequences of declining the amputation.

Her daughter, Grace Lane, was understandably upset over her mother's refusal of the life-sustaining surgery. Grace asked the probate court to appoint her the guardian for her mother with the authority to give consent for the surgery. The court approved her request, but the guardian *ad litem* appealed the ruling. He felt it had not been proven that Rosaria was incompetent, and therefore that no guardian should make any decision about her surgery.

Before looking at the outcome of his appeal to a higher court, we will consider the case from an ethical perspective.

Ethical Analysis

Situational awareness

We are aware of the following facts in the Candura story.

1. Rosaria suffered from diabetes and life-threatening gangrene. Only the amputation of her leg could save her life. Two previous amputations had failed to stem the spread of gangrene in her leg.

2. She was confused about some things, and was somewhat unhappy and depressed. She had vacillated about the amputation, twice agreeing to

it and twice changing her mind. In the final analysis, however, she seemed clearly opposed to it.

3. Grace believed her mother should have the life-prolonging surgery, and sought guardianship so she could give consent to what she, the physicians, and most everyone else believed was appropriate medical treatment.

4. The judge in probate court agreed with Grace, and appointed her guardian of her mother so she could give consent for the surgery.

We are also aware of the following good and bad features in the case.

1. Rosaria's death, which could probably be delayed by the surgery, would be unfortunate.

2. The amputation of her leg would cause pain, suffering, and a difficult sense of loss. It would also undermine the ability of this strong-willed seventy-seven-year-old year old woman to live in her own home.

3. Her daughter was naturally distressed and upset that her mother was declining life-prolonging treatment. At least one physician was also upset and had tried to have Rosaria change her mind.

Prudential reasoning in the Candura case

Patient's perspective.   Rosaria was in the best position to determine whether, all things considered, the amputation of her leg was reasonable. She would be experiencing the pain resulting from the surgery, and she would have to live with the loss of her leg. There was no indication she wanted to die; in fact, she told the judge she would like to get better. But she did not want the life-prolonging surgery. In her mind, the burdens of another amputation, and its consequences in her life, outweighed the benefits of life without her leg. For the past few years she had felt great loss over the death of her husband and the amputation of her foot. Well aware that the two earlier amputations were not enough to prevent the life-threatening problems associated with gangrene, she simply did not see the sense of undergoing another great loss, her leg.

It would be hard to argue that her decision was unreasonable. Of course, another person in her position may think the surgery would be reasonable, and it would also be hard to argue with his decision. Often in ethics, especially when we are coping with difficult choices when both courses of action are burdensome, one can defend the reasonableness of both. In other words, Rosaria's decision to decline the surgery is morally justified because the burdens she would experience outweighed the benefits, but another person's decision to have the surgery could also be morally justified if he would experience more benefit than burden from the amputation.

The only remaining moral question, then, is whether or not she has the capacity to make such a decision. Evidence indicated she was sometimes confused about some things, but there was no indication that she had lost the capacity to make the decision about amputation. In fact, the evidence indicated the contrary. When her physician sought informed consent for the surgery, he did not hesitate to obtain it from her, something he never would have done if he thought she had lost decision-making capacity or was incompetent.

Daughter's perspective.   Rosaria's daughter was naturally upset that her mother was declining the surgery. She thought Rosaria should have the amputation that was expected to prolong her life. So she decided to ask the probate court to appoint her the guardian for her mother so she could authorize the surgery. If she was convinced that her mother had lost the capacity to make decisions, her efforts to be appointed guardian and make the decision for her were appropriate since children are usually the proper proxies for their parents.

The physician apparently refused to accept the daughter's consent for the surgery, so she took the matter to probate court. Here the judge agreed with her by concluding that Rosaria was "incapable of making a rational and competent choice to undergo or reject the proposed surgery to her right leg." The judge's finding reminds us that the daughter's belief that her mother had lost her capacity to decide about the surgery had some merit. Thus her move to be appointed guardian was a reasonable one from a moral point of view.

The Court Decision

The appeals court did not agree that Rosaria was incompetent. It noted that a person is presumed competent unless and until it is established by evidence that he or she is not competent. And the burden is on the person petitioning for guardianship to prove the person is incompetent. The court acknowledged that Rosaria was confused on some matters, but not on the issue of the surgery, where she "exhibited a high degree of awareness and acuity." The court also acknowledged that her decision may well have been irrational from a medical perspective, but the irrationality of a decision does not prove a person is legally incompetent. As we all know, competent people make irrational decisions every day.

The court also pointedly remarked that nobody had questioned Rosaria's competence the two times she had consented to the surgery. And it noted that surgeons were still prepared to amputate if she gave consent, an indication that they still considered her capable of giving informed consent for the surgery, despite the ruling of the probate judge.

Since the court did not find Rosaria incompetent, it dismissed her daughter's petition that she be appointed guardian. It acknowledged that Rosaria's decision may be regarded as unfortunate, but insisted that she could not be forced to have the surgery. The law protected Rosaria's right to accept or reject treatment, whether or not the decision was a wise one.

Ethical Reflection

If Grace really thought her mother had lost decision-making capacity, and we have no reason to believe she did not, then her efforts to be named proxy were reasonable. If a parent cannot make decisions for herself, then it is laudable for the children to try to make the right decisions for her.

We must remember, however, that a proxy first tries to make a decision based on what she thinks the patient wants—the substituted judgment standard. If Grace thought her mother had lost decision-making capacity and that she had to function as her proxy, her first efforts would have been to report what her mother's wishes were. Only if she had no way of knowing what this might have been could she have proceeded to make decisions for her mother based on what she thought was in Rosaria's best interests.

As we might expect, the appeals court based its decision on the constitutional right to privacy that allows a person to decline life-sustaining treatment in most cases. The law allows people to accept or reject treatment regardless of whether the decision is wise or unwise. This is not enough for good ethics, however, because the ethicist will not consider a decision acceptable unless it is reasonable. But in this case, as we noted above, there are good grounds for thinking Rosaria's decision was a reasonable one for a person in her circumstances.

OTHER LIFE-SUSTAINING TREATMENTS

The ethical reasoning about accepting or rejecting other life-sustaining treatments is the same as we employ for ventilators, dialysis, and surgery. The moral agents involved, primarily the patient or proxy, and the physicians, will try to figure out what will achieve the balance of good over bad, or at least what option is less worse.

This is true even if the life-sustaining treatment is simple and routine. Consider respiratory therapy, for example. In a situation where a person receiving respiratory therapy is found to have rapidly developing terminal cancer, a decision to withhold further respiratory therapy may be reasonable. Many patients would see no sense in prolonging life with this therapy when all it does is set up a situation where they will suffer a few more days or weeks as they die from the incurable cancer. In the last analysis, the ethics of all life-sustaining treatments revolves around what is reasonable or unreasonable, given the circumstances and the consequences of the treatment. The good and bad features—the benefits and burdens of what we deliberately do—have to be considered so we can determine as best we can what is reasonable under the circumstances.

Unfortunately, most situations where life-prolonging treatments are an issue are tragic situations—no behavior really leads to a significant degree of well-being or happiness. People suffering from serious medical problems and permanently dependent on life-sustaining treatments have no attractive options. Prolonging a declining or sick life with these treatments or surgeries does not really result in a good life, and foregoing the life-prolonging treatment soon leads to no life at all. The only moral challenge of people trapped in these tragic situations is to determine whether accepting life-prolonging treatments is less worse than declining them. This is a highly subjective prudential determination, and should be respected by others involved in their care.

SUGGESTED READINGS

For a succinct introduction to what ventilation entails, see Martin Tobin, "Mechanical Ventilation." *NEJM* **1994,** *330,* 1056–61. The New Jersey Supreme Court decision in the Quinlan case is *In re Quinlan,* 355 A2d 647 (1976). Lengthy excerpts from the decision appear in many places, among them Tom Beauchamp and LeRoy Walters. 1982. *Contemporary Issues in Bioethics,* second edition. Belmont, CA:

Wadsworth Publishing Company, pp. 365–72; and Munson, *Intervention and Reflection*, pp. 172–74. Eight years after Karen died, her family authorized publication of the neurological findings contained in the postmortem report. Perhaps the most interesting fact was that the most severe damage was not, as expected, in the cerebral cortex but in the thalamus, suggesting the critical role this area of the brain plays in awareness. See Hannah Kinney et al., "Neuropathological Findings in the Brain of Karen Quinlan." *NEJM* **1994,** *330,* 1469–75.

There are many commentaries on the Quinlan case. See Joseph Quinlan and Julia Quinlan, with Phyllis Battelle. 1977. *Karen Ann: The Quinlans Tell Their Story.* New York: Doubleday Anchor; Gregory E. Pence. 1990. *Classic Cases in Medical Ethics.* New York: McGraw-Hill, chapter 1; Richard McCormick. 1981. *How Brave a New World: Dilemmas in Bioethics.* Washington: Georgetown University Press, chapter 19; and Veatch, *Death, Dying and the Biological Revolution,* pp. 118–23.

See *In re Eichner* (*In re Storar*), 52 N.Y.2d. 363 (1981) for the New York Court of Appeals decision in the Brother Fox case. Since Brother Fox was unconscious, the case was brought to court by his religious superior, Father Eichner. The name Storar refers to a second case involving treatment which the court resolved in the same decision. See also George J. Annas. "Help from the Dead: The Cases of Brother Fox and John Storar." *Hastings Center Report* **1981,** *11* (June), 19–20; Richard McCormick and Robert Veatch. "The Preservation of Life and Self-Determination." *Theological Studies* **1980,** *41,* 390–96; Paul Ramsey. "The Two Step Fantastic: The Continuing Case of Brother Fox." *Theological Studies* **1981,** *42,* 122–34; and John Paris. "Court Interventions and the Diminution of Patients' Rights: The Case of Brother Joseph Fox." *NEJM* **1980,** *303,* 876–78.

See *Bartling v. Superior Court,* 163 Cal. App. 3d 186 (1984), and *Bartling v. Glendale Adventist Medical Center,* 184 Cal. App. 3d 97 (1986) and 184 Cal App. 3rd 961 (1987) for the decisions in the Bartling case. For background to the early court battle, see George Annas. "Prisoner in the ICU: The Tragedy of William Bartling." *Hastings Center Report* **1984,** *14* (December), 28–29. The citation for the Perlmutter case is *Satz v. Perlmutter,* 379 So. 2d 359 (1980).

The court proceeding relevant to Helga Wanglie is *In Re: The Conservatorship of Helga M. Wanglie,* No. PX–91–283 (Probate Court Division, 4th Judicial District, Hennepin County, Minnesota). A physician-ethicist who was involved in the case has written several articles on the family's demand for continued respirator support; see Steven Miles. "The Informed Demand for 'Non-Beneficial' Medical Treatment." *NEJM* **1991,** *325,* 512–15; and "Legal Procedures in Wanglie: A Two-Step, Not a Sidestep." *Journal of Clinical Ethics* **1991,** *2,* 285–86. See also two articles by Marcia Angell. "The Case of Helga Wanglie." *NEJM* **1991,** *325,* 511–12; and "After Quinlan: The Dilemma of the Persistent Vegetative State." *NEJM* **1994,** *330,* 1524–25.

For the Massachusetts Supreme Court decision involving dialysis for Earle Spring, see *In the Matter of Earle Spring,* 405 N.E.2d 115 (1980). The citation for the Saikewicz case is *Superintendent of Belchertown v. Saikewicz,* 370 N.E.2d 417 (1977). A helpful commentary is George Annas. "Quality of Life in the Courts: Earle Spring in Fantasyland." *Hastings Center Report* **1980,** *10* (August), 9–10, For a study of withdrawing dialysis, see Steven Neu and Carl Kjellstrand. "Stopping Long-Term Dialysis: An Empirical Study of Withdrawal of Life-Supporting Treatment." *NEJM* **1986,** *314,* 14–20. The Massachusetts Appeals Court decision involving Rosaria Candura's refusal of surgery is *Lane v. Candura,* 376 N.E.2d 1232 (1978).

The literature about providing, withholding, and withdrawing life-sustaining treatment is, as can be imagined, very extensive. Among the helpful basic resources are: *Deciding to Forego Life-Sustaining Treatment,* President's Commission for the

Study of Ethical Problems in Medicine and Biomedical and Behavioral Research, originally published by the U.S. Government Printing Office (1981) but now available from Indiana University Press. The *Guidelines on the Termination of Life-Sustaining Treatment and the Care of the Dying*, a 1987 report of the Hastings Center is also helpful.

An early article of historical interest is Charles Fried. "Terminating Life Support: Out of the Closet." *NEJM* **1976**, *295*, 390–91. See also the historical development in two important articles by a group of physicians: Sidney Wanzer et al. "The Physician's Responsibility Toward Hopelessly Ill Patients." *NEJM* **1984**, *310*, 955–59 and Sidney Wanzer et al. "The Physician's Responsibility Toward Hopelessly Ill Patients: A Second Look." *NEJM* **1989**, *320*, 844–49. For an excellent study of shared decision making in the withdrawal of life-sustaining treatment (ventilation, dialysis, and vasopressors) from twenty-eight patients in an intensive care unit, see David Lee et al, "Withdrawing Care: Experience in a Medical Intensive Care Unit," *JAMA* **1994**, *271*, 1358–61.

The role of the courts in cases involving life-sustaining treatments has been both extensive and important. Although it is now somewhat dated, an article by a judge of the Massachusetts Appeals Court provides a good analysis of the trend in court decisions through 1986: Christopher Armstrong. "Judicial Involvement in Treatment Decisions: The Emerging Consensus." In Joseph Civetta, Robert Taylor and Robert Kirby, eds. 1987. *Critical Care*. Philadelphia: J. B. Lippincott Company, pp. 1649–55. More current is Alan Meisel. "Legal Myths about Terminating Life Support." *Archives of Internal Medicine* **1991**, *151*, 1497–02, and "The Legal Consensus About Forgoing Life-Sustaining Treatment: Its Status and Prospects." *Kennedy Institute of Ethics Journal* **1992**, *2*, 309–345; and Robert Veatch. "Forgoing Life-Sustaining Treatment: Limits to the Consensus. *Kennedy Institute of Ethics Journal* **1993**, *3*, 1–19.

In 1992 the National Center for State Courts in Williamsburg, Virginia, produced its "Guidelines of State Court Decision Making in Authorizing or Withholding Life Sustaining Medical Treatment." These guidelines will undoubtedly be widely consulted by judges and attorneys involved in future cases. The New York State Task Force on Life and the Law has published *Life-Sustaining Treatment: Making Decisions and Appointing a Health Care Agent*. Albany: Health Education Services, 1987.

8

Cardiopulmonary Resuscitation

In this chapter we will consider the ethical aspects of attempting cardiopulmonary resuscitation in hospitals and nursing homes. We know that over three-quarters of the roughly 2 million people who die in the United States every year die in hospitals or chronic care facilities. Every person who dies suffers cardiopulmonary arrest, so we know that about 1.5 million potential cardiopulmonary resuscitations can be attempted every year in our health care facilities.

Attempted resuscitation in a health care facility is an emergency procedure involving a high level of activity by a team of physicians, nurses, and technicians. One or two nurses insert IV lines and administer strong drugs, sometimes directly into the heart. Another nurse does chest compressions that may result in injuries, especially in the elderly. A respiratory therapist or anesthesiologist intubates the patient, and a physician applies electric shocks to stop the fibrillation, the useless fluttering of the heart, that often occurs. Despite the latest equipment and a high level of expertise, the effort often fails to revive the patient or, if it does revive the patient, leaves him with extensive brain damage caused by lack of adequate blood circulation in the brain.

Clearly there are reasons why some cardiopulmonary arrests in hospitals and other facilities should not trigger these resuscitation efforts. The dying person may be a hospice patient, for example, and not want resuscitation. Or the patient may be so sick and frail that the shock treatments and chest compressions of cardiopulmonary resuscitation would be unreasonable—the harm they inflict outweighs the slim chance of limited benefit they offer.

After a brief consideration of terminology relevant to cardiopulmonary resuscitation, this chapter will consider the history of resuscitation efforts, the effectiveness of these efforts, the move to withhold these efforts in some cases, the development of institutional policies for not attempting resuscitation, a typical hospital policy for withholding resuscitation efforts, and a look at some lingering ethical questions about attempting resuscitation. The chapter will conclude with an analysis of several key cases involving cardiopulmonary resuscitation.

TERMINOLOGY

Strictly speaking, there is a difference between cardiac arrest and respiratory arrest. For our purposes, however, we can ignore the difference. The cardiac and pulmonary functions are closely linked. Loss of blood flow soon causes damage to the respiratory centers of the spinal cord and brain, so the person stops breathing. Conversely, lack of oxygen causes damage to the cardiovascular centers of the spinal cord and brain, so the heart stops beating. In other words, a cardiac arrest leads very quickly to respiratory arrest, and respiratory arrest leads very quickly to cardiac arrest. Since cardiac and pulmonary arrests are so closely related, we will consider them as one and the same event, and speak of cardiopulmonary arrest. We will also refer to the attempts aimed at reversing these arrests as a single action—cardiopulmonary resuscitation, often known simply as CPR.

Unfortunately, the terms "cardiopulmonary resuscitation" and "CPR" are misleading. Resuscitation means revival, yet the cardiopulmonary resuscitation often fails to revive the patient. Despite the efforts at CPR, the heart and lungs do not restart, and the person dies. We should really understand the treatments designed to reverse a cardiopulmonary arrest not as "cardiopulmonary resuscitation" but as "attempting cardiopulmonary resuscitation." And the physicians and nurses working at the scene of an arrest are not "doing CPR"; they are "attempting CPR."

This distinction may seem insignificant, but it is important in ethical considerations. Suppose, for example, you are making decisions for an elderly and sick parent, and a physician asks whether you want your mother to be resuscitated if her heart stops. The natural response to this question will almost always be affirmative; of course you want your mother to be revived. But if the physician asks whether you want nurses and physicians to *attempt* resuscitation if her heart stops, and if he explains what these attempts involve, and how often they fail to prevent death or, if they do prevent death, leave the patient with a damaged brain and body, you might not be so quick to give an affirmative answer.

It is well, then, to remember that CPR does not really mean cardiopulmonary resuscitation, but the attempt at cardiopulmonary resuscitation. And we should think of physician's orders not to intervene in the event of a cardiopulmonary arrest not as "Do Not Resuscitate" orders but as "Do Not Attempt Resuscitation" orders, and the abbreviation "DNR" (do not resuscitate) should really be "DNAR" (do not attempt resuscitation).

A BRIEF HISTORY OF RESUSCITATION ATTEMPTS

Attempts to resuscitate people have a long history in medicine. That history reached a turning point in the middle of the last century with advances in anesthesia and surgery. Chloroform, administered to mask the pain of surgery, sometimes caused cardiopulmonary arrests. Physicians naturally sought ways to reverse these arrests, but it was not until the middle of this century that effective treatments were developed. By the 1940s, it was learned that a combination of drugs, electric stimuli, and heart massage could sometimes restart stopped hearts. At first the heart massage was internal—as a last-ditch effort surgeons opened up the chest so they could actually get their hands on the heart—but it soon became clear that the heart could be massaged effectively by external chest compressions.

Attempts at resuscitation became more frequent, first in hospital operating and recovery rooms, then in emergency rooms and intensive care units, especially cardiac care units, and finally throughout the institution. Hospitals trained special teams and positioned the equipment they would

need in the event of an arrest. Since there is no chance to reverse a cardiopulmonary arrest after the first few minutes—recent figures indicate the chance
of success drops significantly after six minutes—the resuscitation team must
respond immediately.

Before the widespread use of electronic beepers, the fastest way to assem-
ble the members of the resuscitation team was by announcement throughout
the hospital over the loudspeaker system. Since it would be inappropriate to
announce something like "Heart attack in room 329," the notification was
usually given in a coded form. Some hospitals, for example, used the coded
expression "Code Blue—room 329" to alert the code team without upsetting
other patients and visitors. In time, attempting resuscitation became known
as "coding" someone or "calling a code," and physicians' instructions not to
attempt resuscitation were often called "No Code" orders.

Gradually, attempts at resuscitation spread to other areas of health care.
Emergency medical technicians and paramedics were trained and provided
with equipment that could be brought to the scene of an arrest. Nursing
homes also trained their staffs in the procedure and provided the equipment
needed to attempt resuscitation. Police officers and firefighters were also
trained, and a vast public education campaign was mounted so anybody could
begin emergency CPR by blowing in a person's mouth and by rhythmically
pushing down on the chest to massage the heart. What began as an intervention by physicians in an operating room soon became a widespread emergency
treatment.

THE EFFECTIVENESS OF ATTEMPTING CPR

Just how successful are the attempts at CPR in hospitals? The answer varies,
of course, and depends on many factors. But a brief glance at several studies
will give a general idea.

A 1983 report from the Beth Israel Hospital in Boston, a teaching hospital,
traced 294 attempts at resuscitation and found the following:

294	attempts at CPR
−166	deaths during the attempted CPR
− 31	deaths within 24 hours
− 56	subsequent deaths in hospital without discharge
41	discharged (14% of those coded)

A 1988 study at the Houston Veterans Administration Medical Center
traced 399 attempts at resuscitation and found the following:

399	attempts at CPR
−238	deaths during the attempted CPR
− 15	deaths within 24 hours
−124	subsequent deaths in hospital without discharge
22	discharged (6% of those coded)

A 1991 study conducted at Rhode Island Hospital, a teaching hospital in Providence, found that, of 185 patients brought to the Emergency Department in cardiac arrest with emergency personnel performing CPR, only sixteen survived long enough for admission to the hospital. None of these patients improved sufficiently for discharge; they all died in the hospital. Fifteen of them never regained consciousness. The average time before death in the hospital for these sixteen patients was about twelve days, although one patient remained alive for 132 days. Authors of the study questioned whether it was good medicine for emergency department personnel to attempt CPR when the arrest happened outside the hospital.

A 1988 study of forty-nine very-low-birth-weight babies suffering cardiopulmonary arrest revealed only four survived, and three of these suffered from neurologic deficits.

On average, attempts at CPR are successful about one-third of the time in hospitals, and fewer than a third of the resuscitated patients live to be discharged. It must be remembered, of course, that many of these patients were in the hospital because they were very ill, and some of them would never have recovered sufficiently for discharge even if they had not suffered the arrest that led to the successful CPR.

The figures help us place resuscitation efforts in perspective. Since the emergency treatment often brings a burden to the patient and frequently fails, we have to ask when it is reasonable to initiate CPR in a clinical setting. And patients have to consider whether it makes sense for them to be subjected to it. For a patient to figure this out, of course, he needs some idea about how often attempted CPR brings little or no benefit.

An interesting study conducted at the Presbyterian–St. Luke's Medical Center in Denver in the early 1990s revealed the following. When patients over sixty were asked whether they wanted CPR attempted if they arrested, forty-one percent said they did. But when they were informed of the probability of survival until discharge (somewhere between ten and seventeen percent), the number dropped to twenty-two percent. When the same patients were asked whether they wanted CPR attempted if they had a life expectancy of less than one year, eleven percent said they did. But when they were informed of the probability of survival until discharge (somewhere between zero and five percent), the number dropped to five percent, fewer than one out of twenty.

This reminds us how unreasonable it is to attempt reversal of every cardiopulmonary arrest. In other words, in many cases the ethical reaction to a cardiopulmonary arrest is to do nothing, to make no effort to save the patient's life. Emotionally, this is not easy. When physicians and nurses see an arrest, and have the training and equipment designed to reverse it, it is not easy to do nothing when they know the outcome is death. On the other hand, attempting CPR in some cases strikes almost everyone as ridiculous. It makes no sense, for example, to work at reviving a dying cancer patient every time she arrests. Several decades ago, it became clear that we would have to learn how to withhold efforts to revive some people experiencing a cardiopulmonary arrest.

LEARNING TO WITHHOLD CPR

As could be expected, once people learned how to attempt cardiopulmonary resuscitation, they tended to do it whenever a patient suffered an arrest. They soon realized, however, that this presumption of intervention was frequently a mistake because the treatment failed, left the patient alive but with neurological damage, or succeeded only in prolonging the life of a dying patient for a limited time. This left physicians and nurses in a difficult dilemma. If they attempted to revive every patient, they would often be providing inappropriate medical treatment; if they did not attempt to revive a patient, they might be letting someone die who could have benefited from being saved, and they could be subject to accusations from the family about medical negligence.

In 1974, a National Conference on Standards for Cardiopulmonary Resuscitation and Emergency Cardiac Care acknowledged both the value of attempting CPR in some cases and of withholding it in others, especially when it was a case "of terminal, irreversible illness where death is not unexpected." In such cases, the conference recommended writing the DNR order in the patient's progress notes so all providers would be aware that CPR should not be attempted if an arrest occurred.

Despite these recommendations, some providers felt morally obliged to continue making every effort to save life whenever a patient arrested. Others did acknowledge that attempting CPR was inappropriate in some situations, but found it difficult to acknowledge that treatment was being withheld from patients suffering respiratory or cardiac failure. It became clear that some guidelines were needed.

In 1976, two Boston hospitals instituted written policies—known as DNR (Do Not Resuscitate) policies—guiding the withholding of efforts to revive patients suffering an arrest. The policy of Massachusetts General Hospital centered on the physician—it allowed physicians to decide when attempting CPR was not medically appropriate, and then to write the DNR order in the medical record. The policy of Beth Israel Hospital, on the other hand, centered on the patient—it allowed patients to refuse CPR efforts, in advance, regardless of their medical condition, and it required physicians to have the consent of the patient or proxy before writing a DNR order.

The need for sound moral thinking and dialogue about attempting CPR, as well as the need for good hospital policies, became more apparent after a well-publicized New York grand jury investigation in 1984. The grand jury investigating the death of an elderly patient in the intensive care unit at La Guardia Hospital found that hospital administrators and representatives of the medical staff had decided, in an effort to minimize legal exposure, that patients and families would not be consulted about DNR orders, and that the orders would not be written in the patients' medical records. Instead, the DNR orders would be signified by small purple dots affixed to file cards kept by the nurses. As a result, no DNR order could be traced to any physician. The only record of it, the file card with the purple dot, was discarded when the patient was discharged or died.

The case investigated by the grand jury is summarized later in the chapter as "The Story of Maria M." It illustrates how the failure to face ethical dilemmas openly can create serious clinical and ethical abuses in patient care, and in the relationships between physicians and nurses.

On 8 February 1984, the New York grand jury made a number of important recommendations regarding the withholding of attempted CPR. They included: (1) the decision not to resuscitate should be made jointly by the physician and the patient, or by the physician and the patient's proxy; (2) the order should be a permanent part of the medical record; and (3) the physician, or the patient, or the proxy can revoke the order at any time.

The need for policies embodying these recommendations was underscored within weeks of the grand jury report. On 25 March 1984, eighty-seven year old Rose Dreyer died at New York Hospital after suffering an arrest. She had been admitted ten days earlier for pneumonia and, without consulting her or her family, the staff had determined that CPR would not be appropriate. The staff followed its custom of deciding unilaterally which patients would not be resuscitated. Their names were then circled in red on cards that were discarded after discharge or death. When Mrs. Dreyer arrested, no one attempted CPR.

The New York State Health Department brought administrative charges against the hospital, which admitted it had violated the woman's rights by withholding CPR without her or her proxy's consent. The charges were dropped when the hospital accepted a fine and agreed to develop written guidelines for withholding CPR, guidelines that included informed consent by patients or their proxies, and the entry of all DNR orders by the physicians in the permanent medical records of patients.

Today, most hospitals and long-term care facilities have helpful written DNR or No Code policies in place. These policies are, for the most part, morally sound and very helpful. By considering the elements in a good DNR policy and an example of what a DNR policy looks like, we can learn much about the ethics of attempting and withholding efforts to revive people in cardiopulmonary arrest.

IMPORTANT ETHICAL ELEMENTS FOR A DNR POLICY

A morally sound DNR policy will include the following provisions.

1. Physicians have the responsibility of initiating discussion about CPR with the patient or proxy if there is some reason to think a cardiopulmonary arrest may occur. Examples of reasons for thinking an arrest might occur are: a previous arrest, known respiratory or heart problems, terminal illness, irreversible loss of consciousness, etc.

Attempting CPR is a medical treatment, and patients or proxies should be involved in choices about medical treatment. Many patients and proxies will not know that they can decline resuscitation efforts unless their physicians tell them. And they have to be told in advance because there is no time for discussion when an arrest occurs. If an arrest occurs when there is no DNR order, the providers will usually consider it an emergency and treat to save life. Physicians should therefore initiate discussions about treatment in the event of an arrest in order to avoid having CPR attempted when it is not wanted or when it is not medically appropriate. The importance of stressing that physicians should take the initiative in discussing DNR orders with their patients is underlined by several studies showing that only twenty percent of hospitalized patients with DNR orders discussed their wishes about resuscitation efforts with their physicians.

2. Patients (or their proxies) have the final word on accepting or rejecting CPR efforts. Attending physicians, however, will assist the patient or proxy in thinking through the risks and benefits of attempted CPR, and in reaching an informed decision.

There is a strong legal and moral tradition against forcing unwanted treatment on people, and this gives the patient or proxy the last word on accepting or rejecting CPR attempts. The ideal, however, is to have the decision-making process shared by both patient or proxy and the physician. The participation of nurses in the decision-making process is often helpful as well.

3. If resuscitation efforts will be withheld, the physician will write the DNR order in the medical record.

Recording the DNR order in the medical record provides a permanent record of the order, the process leading to the decision, the reasons for it, and the person responsible for it. This eliminates the chances for the kinds of confusion and abuse that surrounded some DNR decisions in the past.

4. The patient or proxy may cancel the DNR order at any time. The cancellation becomes effective as soon as the patient or proxy tells the physician or nurse of his decision to cancel the DNR order.

This provision allows the patient the opportunity to reconsider his or her refusal of treatment, and to have any change of mind respected. It is important to note that the patient (or proxy) can cancel the order by simply telling a nurse of his desire to cancel it. The DNR order does not remain in effect while the nurse notifies the physician; it is cancelled as soon as the patient or proxy cancels it. The immediate cancellation of a DNR order at the request of the patient or proxy is morally necessary lest a code team be placed in the unethical position of forcing unwanted treatment on a patient. Or course, the patient's physician should be notified of the cancellation as soon as practicable.

5. The physician will automatically review the DNR order at frequent intervals, perhaps as often as every twenty-four hours.

Regular review of the DNR order is necessary to prevent the continuation of the order after the circumstances prompting it have ceased to exist. A patient on DNR status may improve to the point that attempting CPR would be a reasonable intervention in the event of an arrest. If the order has not been reviewed and, where appropriate, cancelled, the improving patient will not be given CPR and could be deprived of beneficial treatment.

6. If CPR is initiated, the attempted resuscitation will be genuine; that is, providers will do everything they can to revive the patient. In exceptional cases, fully informed patients may have indicated a desire for limitations on the efforts to revive them. Perhaps they want some efforts at CPR, but also want to exclude certain aspects normally associated with the procedure—intubation or defibrillation, for example. Their desires should be respected.

In most cases, however, these prior limitations will not exist, and the resuscitation team will do everything it can to resuscitate the patient.

When patients without a DNR order suffer a cardiopulmonary arrest, providers almost inevitably attempt to save their lives. Sometimes, however, the resuscitation efforts are obviously inappropriate, and the providers feel terrible about performing CPR. In the past, this dilemma was sometimes solved by what were called "show codes" (much activity but little that was effective) or "slow codes" (making the right moves so slowly that death would occur before any great harm from resuscitation efforts was done to the patient). These are not good solutions. Both "slow codes" and "show codes" are deceptive, and they compromise the ethical integrity of health care providers. Good ethics requires us to establish the DNR status of a patient likely to suffer an arrest as soon as possible. If this has not been done, and a patient whose condition is such that resuscitation efforts are not an appropriate response suffers an arrest, the morally sound response is to withhold the treatment if it is inappropriate, not to fake it.

7. A DNR order applies only to withholding CPR in the event of an arrest; it does not indicate in any way that other life-sustaining treatment should be withheld, diminished, or withdrawn.

Sometimes providers presume an order not to resuscitate implies that other interventions to sustain life need not be provided. This is not so. For example, a DNR order does not mean a ventilator should be withheld from a patient suffering respiratory distress, or that efforts should not be made to stabilize an erratic heartbeat. There may be good reasons for abating other treatments, but those decisions are separate issues, and a DNR order has no direct bearing on them.

8. A DNR order for a patient under anesthesia requires special consideration. If a patient has a DNR order, the surgeon should discuss, during preoperative conversations, the question of attempting CPR during the anesthesia and the immediate postoperative period. Often, but not always, it is reasonable to suspend the DNR order while anesthesia is in effect.

During anesthesia and surgery, an arrest can be much more effectively countered by CPR efforts. Some of the equipment is already in place, and the physicians can take immediate action. Moreover, the arrest may well be the result of anesthesia, and the anesthesiologist is trained to reverse this. Yet there are cases where CPR would not be appropriate in the operating room. A hospice patient, for example, undergoing surgery for pain relief may wish to maintain her DNR order during the surgery. Such a request is morally reasonable and should be respected by surgeons and anesthesiologists. If they cannot agree to it, they should seek others to provide the surgery or anesthesia, and then withdraw from the case.

9. Ordinarily, a DNR order does not require court approval. In some cases, however, recourse to legal counsel and perhaps to a court is appropriate.

Seeking court decisions about medical treatment is very much the exception, not the rule. Judges are not really in the best position to make decisions about medical treatment. Nonetheless, there are exceptions. Sometimes family members may be hopelessly divided over whether a DNR order should be written for a patient incapable of indicating what is desired; sometimes a proxy may want CPR, but the physician is convinced that attempting it is a medical error. These kinds of cases sometimes end up in court.

A good policy will include most, if not all, of these provisions. Institutional DNR policies are usually developed by hospital ethics committees, and then approved by the medical staff and the administration. What follows is a rather generic example, taken from a number of actual DNR policies, of what a hospital DNR policy looks like.

———*XYZ Hospital Policy for "Do Not Resuscitate" Orders*———

Introduction

Cardiopulmonary arrest occurs at some point in every person's life. When it occurs at XYZ Hospital, the commitment of the staff to the health and well-being of the individual establishes an ethical and legal presumption in favor of attempting resuscitation (CPR) to preserve the person's life.

In some circumstances, however, this presumption gives way to other considerations, and it is sometimes appropriate to omit CPR attempts. This policy provides direction for attempting or not attempting CPR. The goal is to protect the moral and legal integrity of both patients and staff by preventing CPR attempts that are unwanted or unreasonable.

Informed Consent

1. Discussion of CPR and DNR orders provides the patient with the opportunity to give or to refuse consent for this medical treatment should the need for it arise. The discussion will be sufficiently informative to allow *informed* consent; that is, the patient must be informed of the benefits and burdens, as well as the risks and approximate statistical chances of a successful outcome. Discussion about CPR does not imply in any way that a DNR order is appropriate.

2. In order to prevent attempting resuscitation on a patient who would not want it, the attending physician will discuss CPR and DNR orders with a patient or, if the patient does not have decision-making capacity, with the proxy whenever:

- The patient requests it.
- The patient is not expected to live more than a year.
- The patient has a serious and irreversible illness or disabling condition.
- The patient has suffered irreversible loss of consciousness.
- The patient had, or is likely to have, a cardiopulmonary arrest.
- The physician has reason to believe the patient would not want CPR.

3. The attending physician will not simply provide facts and information, but will assist the patient or proxy in reaching an informed decision about CPR. Discussion with the patient's nurses is also important because they will often be the only ones present when an arrest occurs, and their participation in the discussion better enables them to withhold efforts designed to save the patient's life.

4. The physician will obtain the informed consent of the patient or proxy before issuing a DNR order. If the physician is convinced that a patient with decision-making capacity will suffer serious harm from a discussion of CPR and that withholding resuscitation is the only appropriate medical treatment, he or she may issue the DNR order without the informed consent only after (a) making every effort to ascertain the patient's wishes without subjecting him or her to immediate and serious harm; and (b) writing the reasons for not obtaining the informed consent in the patient's record.

5. Patients who have not yet reached their eighteenth birthday are minors and not considered capable of deciding to forego CPR unless they are emancipated minors. However, minors should be involved in the decision-making process to the extent their age and maturity allow.

6. If the patient has lost decision-making capacity, the proxy should first try to report the patient's wishes about CPR. If these are not known, the proxy should make an informed decision based on the patient's best interests. If there are no family members or significant others to serve as proxies, the attending physician will consult the hospital administration. A court may have to appoint a guardian.

7. If the attending physician is convinced that attempting CPR would be medically inappropriate for the patient, but the patient or proxy insists on CPR in the event of an arrest, he will make every effort to reach a consensus on appropriate treatment. If the patient or proxy persists in demanding treatment that the physician considers medically inappropriate, it may be necessary for the physician to provide alternative arrangements for the patient's care and then to withdraw from the case. A physician cannot in good conscience allow inappropriate treatment for his or her patient.

Documentation

1. When a patient or proxy has decided to forego CPR, the attending physician will write "Do Not Resuscitate" or "DNR" on the patient's chart.

2. Within twenty-four hours of writing the DNR order, the physician will document the discussion that led to the DNR order.

3. Unless discontinued on review, the DNR order remains in effect for the duration of the hospital admission.

4. A patient with decision-making capacity, or the proxy, may cancel the DNR order at any time.

5. The DNR order automatically expires upon discharge. If the patient or proxy wishes to continue the DNR order at another facility, the physician will so notify the facility.

6. In extraordinary situations, the attending physician may issue the DNR order by telephone. In such cases, the physician will write the order in the record within twenty-four hours.

Review

1. The attending physician will evaluate the DNR order on a daily basis.

2. If the physician feels the DNR order has become inappropriate, he or she will reopen discussion with the patient or proxy.

Implementation

1. A fully informed patient may desire limitations on CPR (such as no defibrillation). If the attending physician believes these limitations are appropriate, he or she will note them in the patient's orders, and those providing CPR will abide by the patient's wishes.

2. All other attempts to resuscitate will be maximum efforts. "Slow codes" and "show codes" compromise the ethical integrity of health care providers because they are deceptive.

3. A DNR order applies only to CPR. It does not indicate in any way that other life-sustaining treatment will be withheld or withdrawn, including intubation, medication for cardiac problems, etc.

Emergency Department

1. CPR will be attempted for any person needing it in the Emergency Department unless it is clear that the patient or proxy does not want it. In that case, the physician will issue a DNR order.

2. If, after CPR has begun in the Emergency Department, it is discovered that the patient or proxy does not want it, it may stopped unless the person in charge of the team believes stopping at this point will result in damage to the patient that continued CPR efforts can prevent.

Reassessment Before Anesthesia and Surgery

1. Cardiopulmonary arrest during anesthesia and surgery differs from arrests in other situations in two important ways: it is likely that the interventions triggered the arrest and it is more likely that CPR will be successful. In addition, some procedures that are part of emergency CPR are routine in the operating room. Hence, there are good reasons for suspending DNR orders during anesthesia and surgery.

2. However, suspending the DNR order is not in the best interests of every surgical patient, and some patients do not want resuscitation attempted under any circumstances. Therefore, before surgery, the anesthesiologist and surgeon, in consultation with the attending physician, will discuss with every DNR patient or the proxy the status of the order during the surgery and the immediate postoperative period.

3. The surgeon will document in the medical record the patient's desire regarding the continuation or suspension of the DNR order during anesthesia and surgery and, if it is suspended, when it will resume.

4. If the patient or proxy wants the DNR order to remain in effect and the anesthesiologist or surgeon does not believe the decision is medically appropriate, he may decline to participate in the case. If either does decline, he will assist the attending physician to find an anesthesiologist or surgeon willing to provide treatment in accord with the patient's wishes regarding resuscitation attempts.

****

Most current DNR policies reflect several decades of ethical reflection and are morally sound. They do not, however, solve all the problems associated with cardiopulmonary resuscitation. Some questions surrounding CPR efforts still linger, as the following examples show.

LINGERING QUESTIONS ABOUT DNR ORDERS

The Question of Unreasonable CPR Efforts

Sometimes proxies or patients refuse to give consent for a DNR order when resuscitation is clearly an inappropriate medical response to an arrest. By refusing a DNR order, the patients or proxies in these cases are really ordering, by default, other people to provide inappropriate medical treatment. This sets up a difficult situation.

In an effort to resolve the difficulty, some suggest that providers could say that the inappropriate CPR would be futile for a patient, and therefore it should not be attempted even if there is no DNR order. But, as we saw in chapter three, we have to be careful about the word "futile." The 1988 New York Public Health Law on DNR orders defined futile CPR as either the failure of CPR to reverse the arrest or the expectation that the patient will suffer repeated arrests in a short time period before death (NY Public Health Law. Article 29-B, section 2961). Certainly CPR without the possibility of reversing the arrest is futile, but it is not so certain successful CPR with the expectation of future arrests would be perceived as futile by everyone. Some people think human life is so valuable that even a short gain is worthwhile.

The 1991 *Guidelines for the Appropriate Use of Do-Not-Resuscitate Orders* issued by the Council on Ethical and Judicial Affairs of the American Medical Association noted that futility is likely to be interpreted in different ways by different physicians, and thus is not a judgment the physician or proxy can make. Rather, "judgments of futility are appropriate only if the patient is the one to determine what is or is not of benefit, in keeping with his or her personal values and priorities." This is an excellent point, and reminds us that the notion of futility is not really something a physician should rely on when refusing possible life-saving interventions.

In the ethic we are using, the important point is not whether the physician or proxy can make a distinction between treatment that is futile and treatment that is not futile, and then describe CPR in some cases as futile, but whether a treatment is a reasonable intervention in the circumstances. Normally, providers are not acting morally when they are providing unreasonable treatment.

What does a provider do when a patient or proxy refuses consent for a DNR order, and the provider is convinced the resuscitation efforts would be medically and morally wrong? Physicians and nurses cannot justify behaving wrongly even when a patient requests it. The solution, however, is not to refuse the treatment because it is "futile"—the distinction between futile and not futile treatment is too ambiguous—but because it is bad medicine and contrary to ethical clinical practice. Physicians and nurses should simply refuse to provide treatment that is not reasonable. The basis of their refusal rests on their conviction that the requested treatment is bad medicine and immoral, not on the questionable distinction between "futile" and "not futile" treatment.

Refusal of inappropriate resuscitation efforts is not always easy in practice. The unique nature of CPR—patients automatically receive it unless a physician has written an order against it—enables patients and proxies to demand it, in effect, by simply refusing to give consent for a DNR order. Nonetheless, providers cannot abdicate their responsibility to provide only appropriate treatment, and may have to refuse CPR efforts, or try to withdraw from the case. This can be very difficult in practice, and thus moral problems linger when patients and proxies expect CPR efforts in inappropriate situations.

No completely satisfactory answer can be given to this problem of unreasonable CPR, but physicians and nurses must find a way to avoid giving their patients unreasonable medical treatment. As we shall see, some court decisions are beginning to recognize this. Physicians and nurses cannot always go along with patients and proxies who want "everything done" for the patient. The circumstances in which providers are morally justified in declining treatment against the wishes of the patient or proxy, however, are not yet worked out in the ethical conversation of our culture.

The Question of Conditions for DNR Orders

Early DNR policies and court decisions tended to restrict the DNR order to terminally ill patients or to those whose death was thought imminent. Newer policies acknowledge the prerogative of patients with decision-making capacity to decline CPR just as they would decline surgery or chemotherapy. In other words, they need not be faced with terminal illness or imminent death before declining CPR.

If the patient does not have decision-making capacity, however, the situation is still not clear. The 1988 New York law governing DNR orders, for example, does not allow a DNR order at a proxy's request unless the patient is terminally ill or permanently unconscious, or unless the resuscitation will be medically futile or impose an extraordinary burden on the patient (NY Public Health Law. Article 29-B, section 2965). Unfortunately, the law does not define "extraordinary burden" (perhaps because, as pointed out in chapter 3, it is impossible to define "extraordinary"), and so the extent of the restriction on the proxy's decision to request a DNR order is not clear. Clearly, though, the New York legislation intended to make the proxy's authority to request a DNR order more narrow than that of the patient.

On the other hand, the 1990 Massachusetts Health Care Proxy Act empowers the patient's health care agent (the proxy) to make any decision the patient could have made. Since a patient has the unconditional authority to refuse any treatment, there are no conditions that must be met before a properly designated Massachusetts proxy can refuse CPR on behalf of the patient, provided, of course, the proxy's decision adheres to the criteria of proxy decision making. In Massachusetts, then, a designated health care agent can decide on a DNR order even though the patient is not terminally ill or permanently unconscious.

Attempting CPR on Neonates

Attempting CPR on newborns poses special problems. As we mentioned earlier, CPR does not seem a reasonable intervention for very-low-birth-weight babies, and hence probably should not be attempted. There is something morally worrisome about attempting to resuscitate, sometimes repeatedly, an infant who weighs about 750 grams (one pound, ten ounces) or less. The whole issue of CPR for premature or seriously defective infants is a delicate one that needs much more extensive analysis than it has received in the ethical literature. Parents and neonatologists have to balance providing helpful treatment with protecting the infants from traumatic treatment interventions of little real benefit.

Attempting CPR During Transfers

Patients are often sent in ambulances to other facilities for treatment. If a patient with a DNR order arrests during a transfer, the ambulance crew will almost always start CPR despite the DNR order. They will claim that it is an emergency, so treatment must be given. Moreover, many ambulance companies order their people to do everything they can to save a life.

It is very difficult to justify this practice from a moral point of view. If the DNR order was appropriate in the hospital, there is no reason to believe it should be ignored while the patient is temporarily outside the hospital. Some legislatures are beginning to address this issue and to formulate a public policy that will allow ambulance and other emergency personnel to abide by legitimate DNR orders without fear of liability.

DNR Orders After Discharge

Some patients are discharged from hospitals to other facilities such as rehabilitation hospitals or nursing homes. Such a move puts the status of the DNR order in question. In one sense, the hospital's medical order ceases on discharge; in another sense, it is still appropriate for many of these patients to remain on DNR status. If the new facility accepts the DNR order, there is no problem; if it does not, then the process that led to the original DNR order has to begin again at the new facility. In other words, the physician and the patient or proxy must go through the informed consent process all over again, even though the patient's condition may not have changed. This is a rather cumbersome exercise, and there is always the danger the patient may have an arrest before it is completed. This could mean resuscitation will be attempted despite the wishes of the patient or proxy not to have it.

More work needs to be done in this area so patients will not receive treatment they do not want, or which is not appropriate. One solution is to have the new facility accept the hospital's DNR order on a temporary basis, and then reformulate the order in accord with its own institutional policy.

Overriding DNR Orders

Overriding a DNR order and attempting CPR on a "No Code" patient is hard to justify because, in effect, the providers are forcing treatment on a patient against his, or his proxy's, wishes. One situation where some do acknowledge the possibility of ignoring the DNR order and of attempting CPR occurs when the arrest was caused by the providers. For example, a physician may have mistakenly ordered, or a nurse may have mistakenly given, the wrong medication, thereby causing respiratory arrest.

There are good reasons for trying to reverse this arrest regardless of the DNR order. First, we can assume that the patient or proxy did not have this kind of arrest in mind when he consented to the DNR order. Second, it would be very difficult for the physician or nurse, now aware of the potentially fatal mistake, to live with the fact he did nothing to correct it. If a mistake caused the cardiopulmonary arrest, there are good reasons for making attempts to save that life by overriding, if necessary, a DNR order.

DNR Orders in Public Places

In 1993, the press reported a controversial situation in Maine. A thirteen year old girl named Corey Brown was suffering from mental retardation, spastic cerebral palsy, and severe scoliosis. Her mother had decided, in consultation with the pediatrician, that a DNR order was appropriate, and it was written. The mother and the pediatrician believed that attempting CPR on Corey Brown would be unreasonable because, even if it succeeded, it would almost certainly leave her more damaged than she already was.

A problem arose when the mother asked personnel at the school where Corey was a special needs student to respect the DNR order. The idea that a student might suffer cardiopulmonary arrest in class, and that no one could attempt to revive her, upset some teachers. The school committee, however, agreed to respect the DNR order.

The civil rights office of the U.S. Department of Education in Boston then filed a complaint against the school committee, claiming that withholding CPR from Corey was discriminating against her on the basis of her disabilities. In other words, since students without Corey's medical problems would receive CPR if they arrested at the school, withholding CPR from Corey would amount to withholding medical treatment on the basis of her disabilities, and thus be discriminating against her on the basis of handicap. Such discrimination, of course, is illegal.

The school committee then reversed itself, and refused to honor the DNR order. This decision undermined Corey's medical care, and the prerogative of her mother and pediatrician to decide what is in her best interests. It also set up an incoherent situation: if she arrested at school, people would try to revive her; if she arrested in other places, including her pediatrician's office, the DNR order would be honored, and people would not try to revive her.

Finally, a compromise plan was developed whereby the school made it a policy not to honor DNR orders for students, but school officials agreed to work out an individual medical plan for Corey to prevent her from receiving medical treatment against her mother's wishes. The problem of children with DNR orders attending schools, churches, synagogues, camps, youth organizations, etc., is bound to arise again. It is one more example of the lingering questions still surrounding DNR orders.

The lingering questions surrounding cardiopulmonary resuscitation are not easy to resolve, but one of the first steps we can take to sort out these remaining moral issues is to distinguish between two kinds of cardiopulmonary arrest. The first kind of arrest is expected. If we know a person is seriously ill, or dying, or very elderly, we also know that a cardiopulmonary arrest will occur at some point soon. These arrests are not really emergencies. They are not surprises, and resuscitation efforts are seldom a reasonable response.

The second kind of arrest is unexpected. It occurs suddenly and without warning. Sometimes we do not know the cause—a person might just collapse. At other times we do know the cause—it might be an accident, a fire, a near drowning, or a shooting. When an arrest is unexpected, attempting CPR is often a reasonable response.

The fundamental approach to CPR is, therefore, one of prudence. Patients deliberate to decide what is good for them, given the circumstances. Proxies try first to acknowledge what the patient wanted. If this substituted judgment is impossible, they try to figure out what is in the best interests of the patient. And if the patient has no interests because of irreversible unconsciousness, then a DNR order is the only reasonable treatment decision. Physicians will share in this decision-making process by providing adequate information about what attempted CPR involves, its physical and neurological risks, and the rather slim chances of a truly beneficial outcome. They will also help the patient or proxy decide whether or not attempting CPR would be a reasonable response in the circumstances if a cardiopulmonary arrest occurred.

We will now consider several cases that illustrate the history and complexity of decisions not to attempt resuscitation. These cases will help make us familiar with the early problems associated with CPR efforts, problems that led to the policies we have today, and they will also provide us with opportunities for engaging in the process of making moral judgments about withholding or providing treatments to reverse cardiopulmonary arrest.

THE CASE OF MARIA M

The Story

On 11 January 1981, Maria M was brought to the emergency room at La Guardia Hospital and eventually admitted. She developed respiratory problems and on 11 February, with her daughter's consent for the tracheotomy, was placed on a respirator. Her condition worsened. In March, a feeding tube was surgically inserted because a fistula in her throat was allowing food to enter her lungs. The cause of her problems was not known and hence no one was saying that she was terminally ill, and no one mentioned that CPR might be withheld if she arrested. Through all this, Maria was coherent and able to communicate somewhat with her daughter and providers. Sometimes she indicated that she wanted to return home, with a respirator if necessary. At other times she disconnected the tubing of the ventilator, leading some to think she did not want the equipment used.

At one o'clock in the morning of 27 March the monitor at the nurses' station showed the heart of this seventy-eight-year-old woman was failing. A nurse and a medical student went to the room (no physician or resident was in the ICU at the time) and found the respirator disconnected. The student started chest compressions as the nurse connected the tubing. Then, according to the testimony of two nurses, the student said: "What am I doing? She's a no-code." The student stopped the CPR and no "code" (in this hospital the resuscitation team was summoned by announcing "Code 33" over the public address system) was called. The student later disputed the nurses' testimony, but a resident arriving a few minutes after the arrest testified that the student had ceased CPR and had called him not to help resuscitate Maria, but to pronounce her dead.

When the resident examined Maria, he found her heart still beating faintly. He resumed chest compressions but in vain, and Maria died. Later, one of the nurses asked the student why he stopped CPR and why he had indicated Maria was not to be coded. He claimed a cardiologist had given him a DNR order orally; the cardiologist denied he ever gave such an order.

When physicians informed Maria's daughter of her mother's unexpected death, they told her everything possible had been done to save her life. They also requested permission for an autopsy, but the daughter refused. A few nights later, the daughter received a phone call from someone claiming to be a nurse at the hospital. The caller told her that her mother died unnecessarily because she was considered a DNR patient. The daughter notified authorities, and an investigation, including an autopsy, followed. It showed that Maria had died of cardiac arrest after disconnection from the ventilator. How the ventilator was disconnected is a mystery the grand jury could not solve. Somehow the alarm switch was turned off and the tubing neatly tucked behind and under her pillow, yet she was thought incapable of performing either action.

In the course of its investigation, the grand jury became aware of the deliberate effort by the physicians at the hospital to avoid any tangible evidence that some patients would not be given CPR if they arrested. The subterfuges included the practice of sticking the adhesive purple dots on the nurses' cards that we discussed earlier.

Many of the nurses were deeply concerned over withholding resuscitation efforts from patients without informed consent and without any notation about the treatment decision in the patient's permanent medical record. Some also felt that the adhesive dot system was unreliable, and indeed it was. One nurse, for example, had a card for a patient named Daisy S who had died at the hospital on 5 January 1982. There were two purple dots on it, yet all the physicians treating Daisy denied any knowledge of these dots, which were, in effect, orders not to attempt resuscitation if she arrested. And some nurses also felt it was unfair for physicians to expect them to document the DNR decisions with the purple dots on the cards in their file, when the physicians were unwilling to document the decision in the medical records.

Clearly, as the grand jury indicated, this was an intolerable situation. One of the reasons for telling the story of Maria is to show how careless things had become in some hospitals before people took seriously the ethics of DNR orders and the need for hospital policies to secure an ethically credible response to cardiopulmonary arrests.

A second reason for telling the story of Maria is to provide us with the opportunity to consider a case where we can ask whether a DNR order would, or would not, be the reasonable and moral thing to put in place. We want to bracket the conduct of the providers and hospital in 1981, and consider the ethical issues surrounding CPR for a patient such as Maria.

Ethical Analysis

Situational awareness

We are aware of the following facts in Maria's story:

1. Maria is seventy-eight, ventilator-dependent, and nourished by a feeding tube. She has serious respiratory problems but we really do not know why, and therefore we cannot say she is terminally ill or that her death is imminent. In recent weeks she had three surgeries: two were needed for the tracheotomy and one to insert the gastrostomy tube. Her prognosis is uncertain: she could improve, stabilize, or continue to decline.

2. Although she was coherent and able to communicate by writing notes and speaking during the brief periods the respirator was removed, no one attempted to discuss CPR with her. And, although the grand jury report indicates that she did discuss her general situation with her daughter and nurses, it makes no mention of discussions with her physicians.

3. Despite some coherence and ability to communicate, it is entirely possible this seventy-eight-year-old respirator-dependent woman would not be able to understand enough about CPR and the chances of a beneficial outcome to make an informed decision to accept or reject it. If this is so, and her physician has to make this judgment call, then her daughter would have a key role to play as proxy. If this is not so, then she needs a chance to consider her options.

We are also aware of these good and bad features.

1. Withholding CPR efforts means death is inevitable within moments if an arrest occurs. Maria's death, as any human death, would be unfortunate.

2. Attempting CPR causes trauma and often damages a patient. If it succeeds only partially, it leaves the person alive but in a condition worse than before. And in about five out of six cases, patients receiving CPR either die or never recover sufficiently to leave the hospital.

3. Not attempting CPR on Maria when neither she nor her family had agreed to decline it caused distress to her family, as the legal suit later brought by her family showed.

Prudential reasoning in Maria's story

Prudence asks two fundamental questions: What is my good and how do I achieve it? My good is what truly constitutes my fulfillment in life, what makes my life a good life, and this is living virtuously. The ethical task in any situation is for each person to figure out how he can live a good life in the circumstances.

Patient's perspective. The grand jury report indicates that, although Maria has some ability to understand and to communicate, her views on withholding or withdrawing life-sustaining treatment (the ventilator) and on withholding or attempting CPR cannot be conclusively determined.

Proxy's perspective.   Based on her knowledge of Maria, her daughter may have been able to make a good decision about attempting CPR and about other life-sustaining treatment, but she never had the chance. If she had the chance to make a decision about attempted resuscitation, she would make it on the basis of what her mother wanted or, if she did not know her mother's wishes, of what she thought was in her mother's best interests. And what would have been in her mother's best interests? Without knowing Maria, this is difficult to say. Since we do not know the nature of her problems, it is always possible she could recover from them. If so, attempting CPR if she arrested may have been reasonable. On the other hand, there are also reasons for thinking that resuscitation efforts would be unreasonable in these circumstances and that a DNR order to withhold CPR would have also been reasonable.

Providers' positions.   As we look back on this case today, we can see many areas where providers, chiefly the hospital administrators and physicians, suffered ethical lapses about the whole question of attempting CPR in the hospital. Good ethical reflection could have led them to realize that the system of subterfuge was not morally sound, and that any legal concerns about not attempting unreasonable resuscitations could be removed by taking appropriate legal steps. Physicians in Massachusetts had successfully sought judicial relief in a case involving the decision to withhold resuscitation efforts a few years earlier, and the physicians at La Guardia could have done the same.

The nurses on the floor when the arrest occurred were in a different situation. The circumstances surrounding Maria's arrest are murky. Somehow the respirator alarm had been shut off, and the tube had been withdrawn and tucked behind and up under her pillow, yet she was not deemed capable of making these moves herself. How should the providers have reacted when the heart monitor indicated trouble and they found the respirator tube withdrawn?

If a nurse does not know what a patient or proxy wants, and finds a respirator withdrawn without a proper decision-making process, then she has good reason to restore the respirator and attempt CPR if necessary. It is difficult to think inaction can be ethically justified in such circumstances. While it can be argued that attempting CPR on seventy-eight-year-old Maria whose respiratory problems require ventilation is unreasonable, the circumstances of this arrest—the disconnected respirator, the absence of any decision-making process involving the patient or proxy, and the unknown cause of her problems—all provide strong arguments for the nurses' attempts to resuscitate in this case.

Ethical Reflection

It is obvious that serious problems existed in this hospital relevant to withholding CPR efforts. There were real problems in many hospitals about CPR in the early 1980s, and it is good to remind ourselves of them so we can better appreciate the need for open dialogue and policy, not secrecy and purple dots, in these matters of moral concern. It should be noted that, as a result of Maria's case, the hospital took immediate steps to correct its CPR protocols.

For a patient in Maria's condition today, what would be the ethical decision about attempting CPR? The answer is not clear; this may be a case where there are two right answers. It is not difficult to see how some patients in her position might prefer to decline CPR efforts. Others, of course, might prefer CPR in the event of an arrest. If the patient in an ambiguous situation has decision-making capacity, the decision is hers to make, and neither option is morally unreasonable.

However, when a proxy has to decide, and does not know whether or not a patient wants resuscitation efforts in the event of an arrest, the decision in this kind of case is a difficult one. It is hard to know what is in Maria's best interests. If a patient is receiving respiratory support, as Maria was, a DNR order is often a reasonable response. If a patient has a cardiopulmonary arrest while on life-support systems, it often indicates that the arrest is associated with the end of life, rather than with an unknown or readily reversible condition.

On the other hand, it may be reasonable to delay writing a DNR order for a patient in Maria's condition. The cause of her respiratory problems was not yet known, and there was no evidence that she was suffering from a terminal illness. However, if a DNR order is not written in this kind of case, and the weeks on the respirator stretch into months, or if the patient suffers an arrest but is revived, the reasons supporting a DNR order grow stronger. At some point, it does become unreasonable for a proxy not to consent to a DNR order for an older patient who has lost decision-making capacity and is supported indefinitely, perhaps permanently, by a respirator.

What was clearly unreasonable in this case, of course, was the whole DNR situation at that hospital. As we noted, these situations are now largely a thing of the past in American health care, thanks to the widespread adoption of thoughtful institutional DNR policies.

Based on the grand jury account, then, we have reasons for saying both a decision for CPR (declining a DNR order) and a decision against it (consenting to a DNR order) would be morally justifiable decisions for a proxy to make. Actual situations, however, are much richer than the reports we read of them, so it is entirely possible that a proxy actually involved in this kind of situation would be able to discern better the more appropriate moral response.

THE CASE OF SHIRLEY DINNERSTEIN

The Story

The first major court case directly involving CPR happened in 1978, a few years before the case of Maria. Shirley Dinnerstein was a sixty-seven year old woman suffering from Alzheimer's disease. In 1975 her complete disorientation, frequent psychotic outbursts, and deteriorating ability to control her bodily functions required intensive nursing care in a nursing home. In February 1978, she suffered a massive stroke that left her paralyzed on one side. She was admitted to Newton–Wellesley Hospital, a teaching hospital located in a suburb of Boston, in a near vegetative state, unable to speak. She was fed by a nasogastric tube and, in addition to her Alzheimer's disease and stroke, suffered from uncontrollable high blood pressure and life-threatening coronary artery disease. Her life expectancy was no more than a year, and the most likely immediate cause of her death was expected to be, if not another stroke, a cardiopulmonary arrest.

In view of the circumstances, her attending physician recommended that CPR not be attempted in the event of an arrest. Her son, also a physician, and her daughter, with whom she had lived, agreed. But the physicians and family had a problem. They were in Massachusetts, and a recent (1977) decision of the Massachusetts Supreme Court concerning chemotherapy for an incompetent patient named Joseph Saikewicz required "judicial resolution of this most difficult and awesome question—whether potentially life-prolonging treatment should be withheld from a person incapable of making his own decision." "Judicial resolution" means, of course, going to court so a judge can decide whether the treatments can be withheld.

At the time of the Dinnerstein case, many lawyers were telling physicians that the Massachusetts Supreme Court decision about Saikewicz required physicians to obtain judicial approval before withholding any potential life-prolonging treatment. Based on this perception, the hospital, the physician, and Shirley's two children sought in probate court a determination that a DNR order for Shirley could be written without judicial approval or, if that were not possible, that judicial approval be given for such an order. The court appointed a guardian *ad litem* for Shirley. He apparently thought a patient in this situation should be resuscitated if possible, and opposed the DNR order. This set the stage for a court battle.

The probate court sent the case to the appeals court without a decision. Before looking at its decision, we will consider the case from an ethical perspective.

Ethical Analysis

Situational awareness

We are aware of the following facts in the story of Shirley Dinnerstein:

1. Shirley is without decision-making capacity and is a terminally ill patient whose wishes about CPR are not known.

2. Her children and physician think the DNR order is in her best interests. That is to say, they do not think attempting resuscitation would be in her interests if she arrests. Shirley is dying, and they expect an arrest may well be the immediate cause of her death.

We are also aware of these bad features:

1. The DNR order will result in Shirley's certain death if an arrest occurs, and any human death is bad.

2. Attempting CPR in the event of an arrest will probably result in discomfort and further damage to her.

3. Attempting CPR would also, presumably, cause distress for the physicians and her family because they do not think that it is appropriate.

4. The Massachusetts Supreme Court in the *Saikewicz* decision apparently required judicial intervention in cases involving the withholding of life-pro-

longing treatment from patients without decision-making capacity, and this is a factor the hospital and physicians must consider.

Prudential reasoning in the Shirley Dinnerstein story

Patient's perspective.   We do not know from the case what Shirley would have wanted.

Proxies' position.   Her children have made what appears to be the more reasonable decision, given the circumstances. In fact, it is somewhat difficult to see how we could say the decision to attempt CPR is a reasonable one in this kind of case.

Providers' perspective.   Their position is also reasonable. In view of Shirley's terminal condition, and the decision of her children, they are comfortable ordering resuscitation attempts withheld in the event of an arrest which, if it occurs, will not surprise anyone. In the legal climate of the time, however, they understandably perceive a legal risk if they order CPR efforts withheld. The hospital deserves credit for not sweeping the matter under the rug or using "purple dots," but seeking declaratory relief from the courts on this matter. This helped clear the air for the hospital and physicians, and also set a legal precedent acknowledging that the proper place for decisions about CPR is in the clinic, not the courtroom.

The Court Decision

The appeals court realized that, since everybody has a cardiopulmonary arrest when they die, it made no sense to require court approval for withholding CPR efforts every time a patient is dying. It therefore agreed with the physicians and family, and declared the DNR order in this situation would not violate the law. It further said that the question of DNR is "not one for judicial decision, but one for the attending physician, in keeping with the highest traditions of his profession, and subject to court review only to the extent that it may be contended that he has failed to exercise 'the degree of care and skill of the average qualified practitioner, taking into account the advances in the profession'."

The court distinguished the Dinnerstein case from the Saikewicz case. In *Saikewicz*, the issue was chemotherapy for an incompetent patient, and the court saw this as a treatment designed to bring remission from a disease—leukemia. In *Dinnerstein*, the issue was CPR for an incompetent patient, and the court did not see this as a treatment that could bring any cure or relief from Shirley's medical problems, and thus concluded the requirement of judicial resolution in *Saikewicz* did not apply in *Dinnerstein*.

Other courts have seen it within their purview to decide whether or not the guardian for a patient can request a DNR order. This happened, for example, in a Delaware case known as *Severns v. Wilmington Medical Center* in 1980. At the present time, however, the placing of a patient on DNR status in accord with current hospital DNR policies seldom requires judicial overview if patient or proxy consent is given and the physician agrees that the DNR order is appropriate. And some state legislatures have developed helpful laws. New York, for example, has a Public Health Law providing for DNR orders affecting people with and without decision-making capacity.

Ethical Reflection

An ethicist looking at a situation such as the one faced by Shirley Dinnerstein's family will conclude rather easily that, in the absence of knowing the patient's wishes, the most reasonable course of action is a DNR order. Attempting CPR is seldom reasonable for terminally ill patients at the end of life when an arrest is expected. There are no good reasons to justify the real and possible harms it will cause the patient. If the resuscitation efforts fail, they needlessly burden a dying patient; if they succeed, the seriously ill patient remains alive, but little has been gained. The terminal illness has not been reversed, and the likelihood of another cardiopulmonary arrest has increased. Attempting to restart the heart of a dying patient each time it stops is not an easy intervention to justify morally.

THE CASE OF BETH

The Story

Beth was born in September 1986, and several months later was in an automobile accident. The straps of her car seat were wrapped around her neck. She suffered extensive brain damage that caused permanent loss of consciousness. Her breathing was supported by a ventilator with its tube surgically inserted through an incision in her trachea, and her nourishment was provided by a gastrostomy tube surgically inserted into her stomach.

The Massachusetts Department of Social Services (DSS) had been given legal custody of Beth several weeks after she was born, but her mother retained physical custody. Thus it was that DSS and the mother moved jointly in July 1987 to have the district court judge issue a ruling about her future treatment. They thought a DNR order was appropriate, and the judge agreed. He found that Beth would, if competent, choose not to have CPR if she arrested. He also ordered a surgical intervention to lessen the chance of aspiration, which could result in food getting into her lungs.

The court-appointed guardian *ad litem* appealed the judge's decision requiring the DNR order. He argued that nothing in the judge's findings entitled him to say that Beth would choose to decline CPR if she were competent. He also argued that the state's interest in protecting human life should prevail in this case because CPR would impose neither a personal burden on the patient (she is permanently unconscious) nor a financial burden on the parents (Beth is a ward of the state). The case went to the Massachusetts Supreme Court.

The Supreme Court did not issue its decision until years later—in March 1992. By this time Beth was five and a half years old and, as expected, still in a persistent vegetative state. Before looking at the court decision, we will consider the ethical aspects of the DNR order.

Ethical Analysis

Situational awareness

We are aware of the following facts in the story of Beth:

1. Beth is a young ventilator-dependent child in a persistent vegetative state. She will never regain consciousness.

2. Her mother (unmarried at the time she was born) and father, as well as DSS, which has legal custody of her, and her physician, all think it is unreasonable to attempt cardiopulmonary resuscitation if she arrests. Hence they desire a DNR order to prevent anyone from attempting CPR.

3. The judge also thinks CPR should not be attempted, but for a different reason. He bases his conclusion on the substituted judgment standard; that is, he claims somehow to know what Beth, an infant, would decide if she were capable of deciding what treatments she would want while in her persistent vegetative state.

4. The court-appointed guardian thinks CPR should be attempted if she arrests. He argues that trying to preserve her life at no burden to her or cost to her parents outweighs letting her die.

We are also aware of these good and bad features:

1. If Beth arrests and no CPR is attempted, she will die. Every human death, even that of a vegetative body, is bad because human life, even in a persistent vegetative state, has some value, albeit minimal, and its loss is a disvalue.

2. Although Beth's treatment does not cause her any discomfort it is difficult, according to testimony, for her mother to see her life prolonged by medical interventions that she does not think are reasonable.

3. Considerable public funds are being spent for treatment providing no benefit the child can ever experience.

Prudential reasoning in the story of Beth

Patient's perspective.   Clearly the patient, a child in a persistent vegetative state, has no way to deliberate morally about whether or not attempted CPR is good for her if she suffers a cardiopulmonary arrest. It is incoherent to say the patient in this case—an infant—has any wishes about what kind of treatment she might prefer.

Proxies' perspective.   After the onset of irreversible unconsciousness, the parents and DSS, which had retained legal custody of Beth, think attempting CPR on this ventilator-dependent child in a persistent vegetative state is not appropriate because it will not do any good the child can experience. Their reasoning is morally sound; it is difficult to justify trying to resuscitate irreversibly vegetative bodies whenever they suffer cardiopulmonary arrest.

Providers' perspective.   The physician testified a DNR order was consistent with good medical ethics and, again, it is hard to disagree with this position.

Guardian *ad litem*'s perspective.   It is difficult to find any cogent moral reason supporting his position that Beth should be given emergency CPR if she arrested. A guardian *ad litem* acts to protect the interests of patient, but a permanently unconscious person has no interests. It is inconsistent to say a permanently unconscious person can have an interest in anything. Nothing is important to these patients because they cannot experience anything. The guardian *ad litem* had no moral basis to oppose the parents by insisting that efforts be made to resuscitate Beth. As the Massachusetts Supreme Court noted in the *Spring* case, the guardian *ad litem* has no duty to present arguments that are not meritorious. Arguments advocating resuscitation efforts on people in persistent vegetative state have no merit because they provide no benefit the patient can experience.

The Court Decision

In a 4–1 decision, the Massachusetts Supreme Court upheld the district court judge's decision that Beth would, if competent, choose to have CPR withheld. The court also stated that "the emotional disturbance which the ward herself, if competent, would experience as a result of her condition cannot be underestimated." The court thus imagined how an infant without any capacity for experience would actually experience her persistent vegetative state if she were not in a vegetative state. Most commentaries, both ethical and legal, agree with the court that CPR should not be attempted, but find the court's claim to know what a permanently unconscious baby would want or feel a baffling position. Such a claim is certainly not based on any evidence.

The dissenting justice in the case criticized his colleagues on this very point. He argued that it is impossible to say we know what a child would decide about CPR if she were competent to decide. The court's decision, he said, rests on imagination—imagining that a young child is competent, and then imagining what she will decide about CPR if she is in a persistent vegetative state and arrests. As he so correctly put it, the "route by which the court arrives at its conclusion is a *cruel charade* which is being perpetuated whenever we are faced with a life and death decision of an incompetent person" (emphasis added).

Ethical Reflection

Attempting CPR on any patient in persistent vegetative state is something very difficult to justify from a moral point of view. These patients are not terminally ill—some live for decades—but no treatment provides any benefit they can experience. Successful CPR can do no more than return them to the minimal existence of vegetative state. It is not easy to give moral reasons for attempting to reverse a cardiopulmonary arrest suffered by one of these patients.

The dissenting justice's criticism about how the court reached its decision is noteworthy. Making a decision for others on the basis of substituted judgment is impossible if there is no evidence for saying what the patient would want. When we do not know what an incapacitated patient would want, the correct standard to use is best interests. And if the patient is permanently unconscious, she does not really have any interests, so all we can do is ask what is the reasonable way to behave toward a permanently unconscious patient. Unless there are exceptional circumstances (perhaps the patient is an organ donor, and extending his life can be done without causing suffering and will facilitate the transplantation), it is difficult to see any reason for attempting emergency CPR on a permanently unconscious child already ventilator-dependent because of serious respiratory problems.

SUGGESTED READINGS

Chapter 7 of the President's Commission report entitled *Deciding to Forego Life-Sustaining Treatment*, 1981, pp. 231–55, is a good introduction to decisions involving resuscitation. The report includes a long appendix (pp. 493–545) presenting the DNR or No Code policies of selected institutions. Although these policies are somewhat dated (they make no provision for retaining a DNR order in the operating room, for example), they do give the reader an idea of what a DNR policy is. The Joint Commission on Accreditation of Healthcare Organizations expects hospitals to have an appropriate DNR policy; see the *Accreditation Manual for Hospitals* (1991), pp. 77–78.

The report of the New York State Task Force on Life and the Law entitled *Do Not Resuscitate Orders*. 1986. Albany: Health Education Services, is also a valuable document. The second edition (1988) includes the 1987 New York law on orders not to resuscitate which became effective on 1 April 1988, making New York the first state to enact legislation governing the withholding of cardiopulmonary resuscitation. For comments on the New York law, see Tracy Miller. "Do-Not-Resuscitate Orders: Public Policy and Patient Autonomy." *Law, Medicine & Health Care* **1989,** *17*, 245–54; and John McClung and Russell Kamer. "Legislating Ethics: Implications of New York's Do-Not-Resuscitate Law." *NEJM* **1990,** *323*, 270–72.

See also the section on "Guidelines on Emergency Interventions" in *Guidelines on the Termination of Life-Sustaining Treatment and the Care of the Dying*. Hastings Center, pp. 43–52; "Standards and Guidelines for Cardiopulmonary Resuscitation (CPR) and Emergency Cardiac Care (ECC)." *JAMA* **1986,** *255*, 2945–46; and the "Guidelines for the Appropriate Use of Do-Not-Resuscitate Orders." *JAMA* **1991,** *265*, 1869–71.

For the study of attempted CPR at Boston's Beth Israel Hospital, see Susanna Bedell et al. "Survival After Cardiopulmonary Resuscitation in the Hospital." *NEJM* **1983,** *309*, 569–76. For the study of attempted CPR at Rhode Island Hospital, see William Gray et al. "Unsuccessful Emergency Medical Resuscitation—Are Continued Efforts in the Emergency Department Justified?" *NEJM* **1991,** *325*, 1393–98; see also the editorial on pp. 1437–39. For the study of attempted CPR on babies of very low birth weight, see John Lantos et al. "Survival After Cardiopulmonary Resuscitation in Babies of Very Low Birth Weight: Is CPR Futile?" *NEJM* **1988,** *318*, 91–95. Also valuable is G. Taffet et al. "In-Hospital Cardiopulmonary Resuscitation." *JAMA* **1988,** *260*, 2069–72, and Robert Wachter et al. "Life-Sustaining Treatment: A Prospective Study of Patients with DNR Orders in a Teaching Hospital." *Archives of Internal Medicine* **1988,** *148*, 2193–98. The study of patients changing their minds about receiving CPR if they arrest is Donald Murphy et al. "The Influence of the Probability of Survival on Patients' Preferences Regarding Cardiopulmonary Resuscitation." *NEJM* **1994,** *330*, 545–49.

Many fine commentaries on the ethical issues involved in CPR have been published in the past ten years. We can mention several: Andrew Evans and Baruch Brody. "The Do-Not-Resuscitate Order in Teaching Hospitals." *JAMA* **1985,** *253*, 2236–

39; Leslie Blackhall. "Must We Always Use CPR?" *NEJM* **1987,** *317,* 1281–85; Donald Murphy. "Do-Not-Resuscitate Orders: Time for Reappraisal in Long-term-Care Institutions." *JAMA* **1988,** *260,* 2098–101; J. Chris Hackler and F. Charles Hiller. "Family Consent to Orders Not to Resuscitate: Reconsidering Hospital Policy." *JAMA* **1990,** *264,* 1281–84; Tom Tomlinson and Howard Brody. "Futility and the Ethics of Resuscitation." *JAMA* **1990,** *264,* 1276–80; Stuart Young-ner. "DNR Orders: No Longer Secret, But Still a Problem." *Hastings Center Report* **1987,** *17* (February), 24–33; Kathleen Nolan. "In Death's Shadow: The Meaning of Withholding Resuscitation." *Hastings Center Report* **1987,** *17* (October–Novem-ber), 9–14; Giles Scofield. "Is Consent Useful When Resuscitation Isn't?" *Hastings Center Report* **1991,** *21* (November–December), 21–36; and K. Faber-Langendoen. "Resuscitation of Patients with Metastatic Cancer: Is Transient Benefit Still Fu-tile?" *Archives of Internal Medicine* **1991,** *151,* 235–39.

For the recent debate over retaining DNR orders during anesthesia and surgery, see Robert Truog. "'Do-Not-Resuscitate' Orders during Anesthesia and Surgery." *Anesthesiology* **1991,** *74,* 606–08; Cynthia Cohen and Peter Cohen. "Do-Not-Resus-citate Orders in the Operating Room." *NEJM* **1991,** *325,* 1879–82; and Robert Walker. "DNR in the OR: Resuscitation as an Operative Risk." *JAMA* **1991,** *266,* 2407–11. A sidebar in this article includes "Suggested Policy Guidelines for Intraoperative Do-Not-Resuscitate (DNR) Orders" (p. 2410).

For different perspectives in the case involving a DNR order for the sixteen-year-old student in a school, see the six brief articles in the *Kennedy Institute of Ethics Journal* **1992,** *2,* 1–23. The story of Maria M was constructed from the "Report of the Special January Third Additional 1983 Grand Jury Concerning 'Do Not Resuscitate' Procedures at a Certain Hospital in Queens County," dated 8 Febru-ary 1984. The Grand Jury was impaneled in January 1983 at the request of the Deputy Attorney General and Special Prosecutor for Nursing Homes, Health and Social Services. The story of Shirley Dinnerstein is based on *In the Matter of Shirley Dinnerstein,* 380 N.E.2d. 134 (1978). The story of Beth is taken from the *Care and Protection of Beth,* 587 N.E.2d. 1377 (1992).

9

Medical Nutrition and Hydration

Medical techniques for providing nutrition and hydration have introduced another major area of ethical concern. While providing nutrition and hydration for the sick is normally considered a part of good patient care, there are times when it can be questioned. For example, a dying patient experiencing considerable suffering may well question the reasonableness of prolonging life a little while longer by using feeding tubes. And the proxy for an irreversibly unconscious patient may well question the reasonableness of maintaining the unconscious body with feeding tubes for months, years, or even decades.

Providing nutrition by tubes or lines is not always morally reasonable. In fact, it could be immoral if the burdens it places on the patient outweigh its benefits, or if it wastes resources while providing no benefit to the patient, or if the patient with decision-making capacity does not want it. Moral deliberation endeavors to discern those situations where medical nutrition and hydration is reasonable and contributes to the human good, and those situations where it does not.

Before considering some typical cases where supplying nutrition and hydration by medical interventions was morally problematic, two preliminary considerations are in order. First, we need some idea of the techniques and technologies used for supplying nutrition and hydration. Second, we need to examine the conceptual and linguistic presumptions underlying, and frequently distorting, much of the discussion about feeding tubes and IV lines.

THE TECHNIQUES AND TECHNOLOGIES

There are three major medical procedures for supplying nutrition and hydration.

Peripheral IV (Intravenous) Lines

About a hundred years ago, physicians began administering saline solutions directly into the veins of the arm. This was the beginning of the familiar IV lines running into arms that we see so often today. Since adequate long-term nutrition is not practicable with these IV lines because of infections and other problems, they are best viewed as temporary and not really adequate means for supporting human life indefinitely. They rarely present major ethical concerns, although occasionally ethical questions do arise about starting or withdrawing them.

Feeding Tubes

Surgical insertion of a feeding tube into the stomach was first attempted in the nineteenth century, but the practice did not become widespread until several decades ago. Since a feeding tube introduces nutrients into the gastro-intestinal system, it is sometimes called enteral nutrition. (Other ways of placing nutrients in the body, most notably those using veins, are called parenteral.)

There are two general types of feeding tubes, the gastrostomy tube and the nasogastric tube. The gastrostomy tube (often called a G-tube) is normally inserted under local anesthesia through the abdominal wall into the stomach or into the small intestine. A new technique inserts the tube through the throat into the stomach, captures the end with a thread inserted through the abdominal wall, and then pulls the end out through the small abdominal incision. In both cases, the patient is left with a small tube sticking out of the stomach area. Once in place, the tube is relatively comfortable.

The nasogastric tube (often called an NG tube) runs through a nostril and into the stomach by way of the esophagus. Once inserted, it stays in place and, unfortunately, can irritate the nasal passages and cause vomiting. Pneumonia sometimes follows as the aspirated contents of the stomach get into the lungs. Many semiconscious or sleeping patients manifest an instinc-tive reaction to pull the nasogastric tube out; it is often necessary to tie their hands so they cannot dislodge it.

Gastrostomy and nasogastric tubes are connected to a line from a bag of liquid nutrition, and the nourishment flows slowly under gravity at a controlled rate into the stomach. Both G-tubes and NG tubes can provide total nutritional needs for indefinite periods of time, decades if necessary.

Total Parenteral Nutrition (TPN)

In the 1960s, physicians were inserting a line into a large chest vein to measure pressure in the heart. It was soon discovered that specially prepared nutritional fluids could be inserted into this central vein, enough to supply complete nutrition for indefinite periods of time, and total parenteral nutrition became a reality. Early problems with infections at the site were reduced by new types of catheters that separated the entry through the skin from the entry into the vein. The procedure provides a way to nourish patients whose gastrointestinal system cannot tolerate the nutrition introduced through feeding tubes. Total parenteral nutrition is often called TPN.

The solutions used in TPN are less like food than the fluids used in tubal feeding. They are not really the kind of fluids we would ingest, and they must be prepared and delivered under sterile conditions. They contain the electrolytes, amino acids, sugars, fats, minerals, vitamins, etc., that the body normally produces after digestion. Despite the additional complexity of TPN, however, patients receiving it are no longer confined to hospitals. Some now receive TPN in nursing homes and, with nursing care, even at home.

More recently, another medical technique for parenteral nutrition has been introduced. A catheter is inserted into a vein in the arm, and then threaded through this vein into the central vein in the chest. The fluid nourishment thus runs into what looks like a peripheral IV line, but the internal catheter is actually carrying it to the central vein in the chest. This new procedure can provide more nutritional support than a peripheral IV, and for a longer time, but is not yet used for indefinite total nutrition. It is sometimes called PPN, partial parenteral nutrition.

In this chapter, when we speak of feeding *tubes*, we mean the G-tubes and the NG tubes inserted into the gastrointestinal system;, and when we speak of *lines*, we mean the peripheral and central feeding lines inserted into the venous system. For reasons that will become clear, we will use the phrase "medical nutrition" for both the feeding tubes and the venous lines.

Before considering some of the moral issues surrounding these ways of nourishing people, we need to consider the language we use to talk about the medical techniques for providing nutrition.

CONCEPTUALIZING MEDICAL NUTRITION AND HYDRATION

Whenever we are confronted with new realities in medical practice, we tend to think of them in terms of the classifications and descriptive categories already familiar to us. When nutrition by tubes or lines became a reality, two familiar classifications were available; we could think of it as feeding someone or we could think of it as a medical treatment. The interventions are a kind of feeding because they provide nutrition and hydration rather than medicine or medication, and nutrition and hydration are things everyone needs to live whether ill or healthy. The interventions are also a kind of medical treatment because medical research and practice developed the procedures, and because health care professionals first insert, and then monitor, the tubes and lines. Nourishing people this way is not something the untrained person can accomplish.

Yet the interventions are, in important ways, unlike both other forms of feeding and other forms of treatment. In assisted feedings with bottles, cups, spoons, or straws, the recipients are able to swallow what goes into their mouths. With feeding tubes and lines, the person is not swallowing— the nourishment flows directly into the stomach or veins.

On the other hand, the tubes or lines are also unlike other forms of treatment. The procedures do not provide medicine or medication, but what we all need to live—nourishment and hydration. If we withhold or withdraw the tubes or lines, the person will not die of the disease, but from malnutrition and dehydration, or from diseases such as pneumonia that would not be fatal were it not for the weakened state caused by the malnutrition and dehydration. Moreover, there is a symbolism attached to providing nourishment that is not found in providing treatment. Humans have always fed their children, and sharing nourishment with the needy or with guests has great personal and cultural significance. It makes us feel guilty to have nutritional substances, and then not give them to those unable to nourish themselves.

Nourishment by tubes or lines, then, does not fit neatly into either traditional classification—it is neither a typical kind of feeding nor a merely medical treatment. If we try to use either classification, we have to force or "shoehorn" the procedures into it. Medical nourishment resists being classified with feeding the hungry, but it also resists being classified with other forms of treatment or medication.

It may seem that concern over how we classify nourishment by tubes or lines is a linguistic quibble without importance. But this is not so. The moral judgment of many people is significantly influenced, and sometimes determined, by how they classify the procedures they are evaluating. Thus, those classifying intravenous or tubal nourishment as medical treatment inevitably defend the morality of withdrawal whenever it seems unreasonable, and those classifying the procedures as feeding inevitably claim withdrawal is immoral as long as the body accepts the nourishment.

An example of how classifications play an important role in the moral evaluation of feeding tubes can be seen in the two different positions taken by Roman Catholic bishops on the nourishment of patients in persistent vegetative state. Normally the bishops speak as one on moral matters, but they have taken different positions on medical nutrition, and each position owes much to the way they classify the procedures. The bishops of New Jersey, in a brief filed with the state Supreme Court, described the nutritional support of PVS patient Nancy Jobes as clearly distinct from medical treatment, and concluded withdrawal of the feeding tube would be immoral. In contrast, the bishop of Rhode Island described the nutritional support of PVS patient Marsha Gray as "artificially invasive medical treatment" and concluded withdrawal of the feeding tube would be moral. The bishops of Texas later aligned themselves with the bishop of Providence, while the bishops of Pennsylvania later sided with their colleagues in New Jersey.

What is happening here is clear. If people describe the tubes and lines as feeding, then they will consider withdrawing them as starving people to death, and they will argue that the tubes and lines must always be used as long as the body will accept the fluids. If, on the other hand, people describe the tubes and lines as medical treatment, then they will consider withdrawing them as withdrawing a medical treatment, and they will argue that the tubes and lines may be withdrawn whenever life-prolonging medical treatments could be withdrawn. In many debates about nourishment by tubes and lines, the descriptive classification chosen before the debate even begins determines the moral judgment. Serious moral reasoning about the issue never has a chance to begin.

If nourishment by tubes and lines is not well described as feeding nor as medical treatment, how can we classify it? It is best understood as a new kind of human action, one that combines the notions both of feeding and of treating, but is reducible to neither. We should not shoehorn these procedures into either of the more traditional descriptive categories (feeding or treatment), but develop a new classification, something like "medical nutrition and hydration." By not describing the procedures simply as feeding, withdrawal of the procedures will not be considered as "starving the patient to death." And by not describing the procedures as medical treatment, withdrawal will not be considered as if it were simply another case of stopping a medical treatment. In our analysis of cases involving feeding tubes and lines, we will not classify the interventions in either of the traditional categories (feeding or treatment), but in terms of a new hybrid classification we will call "medical nutrition and hydration" or, more simply, "medical nutrition."

In the past ten years, numerous cases about medical nutrition have emerged from the courts, and we will now review several of them.

THE CASE OF CLARENCE HERBERT

The Story

In May 1981, fifty-five-year-old Clarence Herbert presented at the emergency room of the Kaiser Foundation Hospital in Harbor City, California, with intestinal problems. Two operations were required. He was recuperating at home in July when he developed kidney problems, and he spent another brief time in the hospital. By the end of August his progress looked good, and he was back in the hospital for surgery to close the ileostomy that had been necessary to allow his bowel to recover from its original problems. The surgery was, as expected, routine, but he suffered cardiopulmonary arrest in the recovery room. CPR saved his life, but his brain was so badly damaged he lapsed into a coma. He was placed on a respirator and transferred to the ICU.

The next day, August 27, his physician, Dr. Barber, indicated in the medical record that Mrs. Herbert, who had been told her husband would not recover, wanted "no heroics." The following day he wrote that she wanted the respirator removed, and that she had consented to an autopsy. He left an order for the nurses to remove respiratory support, but the ICU nurses refused to withdraw the respirator. When a consulting neurologist requested more tests on the comatose patient, Dr. Barber cancelled the order to remove the respirator.

The additional tests confirmed extensive brain damage, and the family renewed their request to withdraw the respirator. The next day, Dr. Barber privately stopped the respirator for a few moments and observed that Clarence was unable to breathe on his own. He told the family that their husband and father would probably die very quickly when the respirator was removed. They understood and gathered around the bed for his final moments. Dr. Barber then disconnected the respirator tube from the endotracheal tube in Clarence's throat. Much to everyone's surprise, he started breathing on his own.

Other than breathing spontaneously, his condition remained the same and the family continued to feel that his comatose state should not be sustained by treatment. According to court testimony, they even objected to certain routine procedures used by hospital personnel in caring for comatose patients. On August 31, after continual consultation with the family, Dr. Barber removed the peripheral IV lines. Six days later Clarence Herbert died. His autopsy report listed dehydration, brain damage, and pneumonia as the causes of death.

Immediately after Clarence's lapse into a coma, disagreements about his care had arisen between his doctors (Dr. Barber and his surgeon, Dr. Nedjl) and the nurse in charge of the ICU, Sandra Bardenilla. In particular, she was upset about the failure of the physicians to order a misting device to prevent choking after the respirator was removed, and about the withdrawal of IV support so soon after the patient became comatose. Frustrated about her attempts to resolve the problems within the hospital structure, she filed a complaint with the Los Angeles Department of Health Services. After an investigation, the Department gave the information to the Los Angeles District Attorney.

A year later, in August 1982, both doctors were charged with murder and conspiracy to commit murder. The murder charge made the case national news.

A magistrate reviewed the case and ordered the complaint dismissed, but the Superior Court of Los Angeles County ordered it reinstated. Attorneys for the physicians appealed. Before considering the decision of the court of appeal, we will examine the case from an ethical point of view. We want to use the case as an example so we can deliberate about the morality of withdrawing nourishment from an unconscious patient.

Ethical Analysis
Situational awareness
We are aware of the following facts in the Herbert story.

1. Clarence is unconscious but breathing without respirator support. Although the court described him as being in a vegetative state that was likely to be permanent, we know today that such a diagnosis was a little premature. Normally, the diagnosis of a vegetative state that is likely to be permanent takes more than a few days. Moreover, comas and vegetative states are not really the same. It does seem a fact, however, that Clarence was unconscious and unlikely to recover.

2. It is not entirely clear what Clarence would have wanted. The court did find that he had said to his family that he did not want to "become another Karen Quinlan." At this time (1981), Karen had been living in a vegetative state without respirator support for several years, so it is quite possible Clarence did mean to say he did not want to be fed by tubes or lines if he became permanently unconsciousness and lapsed into a state similar to Karen's.

3. The proxy decision maker, Clarence's wife, and the children signed a document, along with two nurses as witnesses, before the respirator was removed. It said: "We the immediate family of Clarence LeRoy Herbert would like all machines taken off that are sustaining life. We release all liability to Hosp. Dr. & Staff."

4. The physicians' actions do not indicate they had any problem with withdrawing the respirator and, when Clarence did not die, the IV lines.

5. The hospital's legal counsel had circulated a memo dated 21 August 1981, advising physicians to obtain legal consultation before withdrawing life-sustaining treatment. Clarence's physicians knew of this memo—the neurologist had attached a copy to the front of Herbert's chart—but they chose to ignore it, apparently because they believed treatment decisions were something between physicians and the family.

We are also aware of these good and bad features in the case.

1. If Clarence is truly irreversibly unaware, then no benefits or burdens, no good or bad, will affect him; he is beyond experiencing anything. His death, of course, as any human death, even the death of someone in a permanent coma or persistent vegetative state, is bad, but not for him. And if he continues to live in a state of permanent unconsciousness, the preservation of his life is a good, but not for him, and it could well be a burden for others.

2. His family, acting on his previous remarks and on their understanding of what is the best thing to do, think the treatment should be stopped. They will suffer distress if it is continued against their wishes.

3. At least some of the nurses were upset at the way the case was handled. Sandra Bardenilla later told an interviewer that she was disturbed that there were no guidelines for this kind of case, that the family had consented to an autopsy before Clarence was dead, that the respirator was to be disconnected before the neurologist had run a confirmatory EEG, that a misting device had not been ordered to keep his airway clear after the respirator was removed and he continued to breathe, and, finally, that hydration was stopped after only a few days of coma. "God, you mean if you don't wake up in three days, this is what can happen to you?" she was reported to have said.

Prudential reasoning in the Clarence Herbert story

Patient's perspective.   Clarence is no longer able to make decisions, but he may have concluded earlier that he would not want feeding tubes to keep him alive indefinitely if he were like Karen Quinlan, that is, in a permanently unconscious state. Most would agree that this is a reasonable position for a person to take. In fact, wanting to be kept alive indefinitely in a state of permanent unawareness strikes most people as unreasonable.

Proxy's perspective.   If Clarence had previously indicated he would not want his life sustained if he became permanently unconscious, then his wife's request to withdraw medical nutrition and hydration is easily justified. In fact, it would be difficult to justify her failure to request withdrawal in these circumstances. If Clarence had not made his wishes known but was truly irreversibly unconscious, then the request to decline medical nutrition and hydration is also easily justified. The problem, of course, is that it is difficult to diagnose permanent unconsciousness in the first few days after it begins.

Providers' perspective.   It is morally reasonable for physicians to honor a request from a patient or proxy to withdraw medical nutrition and hydration in appropriate circumstances, and permanent unconsciousness is certainly an appropriate circumstance for withdrawal. If a patient left advance directives for withdrawal, they should be followed. If he did not, then the appropriate proxy is morally responsible for making the decision. Some would say that the best interests standard would justify a proxy's decision to withdraw medical nutrition and hydration. Since a permanently unconscious patient has no interests in anything, however, it is better to base the decision on simple moral reasonableness—it is not reasonable to sustain a human body once all awareness has been permanently lost.

The Court of Appeal's Action

The California Court of Appeal ordered the superior court to drop the murder charges. That ended the legal action. A murder trial never took place, but the close call made an indelible impression on many physicians.

Several aspects of the court of appeal's findings are relevant to the ethics of health care. They are:

1. The court conceived administering nourishment and fluid by IV lines as treatment akin to respirators and other forms of life support, and not as feeding or providing food and water. As we pointed out, once nourishment by lines or tubes is described as treatment, the tendency is to acknowledge that this medical treatment is not always appropriate. And, in matters of medical treatment, the courts tend to defer to the competence of physicians in determining whether to begin, withhold, or withdraw it.

2. The court conceived the removals of the respirator and the IV lines not as withdrawing treatments, but as withholding them. Apparently the court thought withholding treatment was legally less sensitive than withdrawing it, and wanted to construe the physicians' behavior in a favorable light. After all, if the doctors merely withheld treatments that they thought were inappropriate, then it is difficult to think of them as murdering the patient.

But how could the judges say disconnecting a respirator or ordering IV lines removed is "withholding" treatment? They explained it this way: each pulsation of a respirator and each drop of IV fluid is a discrete or separate self-contained application of a treatment. Thus the court conceived disconnecting the respirator not as withdrawing life-sustaining treatment, but as withholding the next pulsation, and it conceived pulling out IV lines supplying nutrition and hydration not as withdrawing nourishment, but as withholding the next drop that would have entered the line.

The court thereby held that the doctors did not perform any action that would have killed Clarence since their behavior consisted only of omissions. "(W)e conclude that the petitioners' *omission* to continue treatment under the circumstances, though intentional and with knowledge that the patient would die, was not an unlawful *failure* to perform a legal duty . . ." (emphasis added).

Needless to say, conceiving the actions of respirator withdrawal and IV disconnection as omissions is very peculiar. It is also unnecessary. We have already pointed out, in our discussion of the distinction between withholding and withdrawing treatments, how the decision to withdraw is easier to justify than the decision to withhold from a moral point of view. Once we are using the life-sustaining treatment, we know what it can do and what it cannot do, and this places us in a better position to determine whether or not it is a reasonable treatment for the patient.

3. The court rejected the distinction between ordinary and extraordinary treatment, claiming it begs the question. Thus it avoided the argument, advanced by some, that nourishment by tubes or lines must always be provided

because it is ordinary treatment. It suggested that the crucial distinction is between proportionate and disproportionate treatment. This is determined by weighing the benefits gained by the patient with the burdens the intervention imposes. This position is very close to the ethical approach we have been advocating, where the norm is what is reasonable in the circumstances.

4. The court acknowledged that a proxy decision maker should first base her decision on the patient's desires to the extent they are known, and only then on what she thinks is best for the patient. Thus the court embraced the widely accepted criteria for proxy decision making: the proxy first tries to use substituted judgment; if that fails, she resorts to best interests. Of course, if Clarence is truly irreversibly unconscious, he has no interests and the best interests standard will not apply. In this case, however, the court did find that Clarence had indicated he would not want to be kept alive by machines or "become another Karen Quinlan," and this allowed it to say his wife was relying on the substituted judgment standard.

5. The court remarked that seeking judicial intervention in treatment decisions is "unnecessary and may be unwise." In other words, the California court agreed with the Quinlan court in New Jersey (and disagreed with the Saikewicz court in Massachusetts) that the legal setting is not the proper place to make decisions about medical treatment.

This case is the first and only time to date that physicians have been charged with murder for withdrawing medical nutrition and hydration from a patient at the request of the family. And the court of appeal protected the physicians by refusing to let the murder trial proceed. To this day, some physicians and nurses, and some attorneys, believe that there is a real threat of criminal prosecution for withdrawing medical nutrition. This case, in which the murder indictment was thrown out before the trial even began, and the absence of any other cases where physicians have been charged with murder for removing feeding tubes show that the threat of criminal prosecution is more imagined than real. Prosecutors simply have not been charging physicians with murder when feeding tubes or lines are withdrawn at the request of the patient or proxy.

Ethical Reflection

Withdrawal of medical nutrition and hydration from a patient known to be permanently unconscious is not difficult to justify morally, especially if we have indications that the person would not want to be kept alive this way.

Many of the circumstances in this case, however, were less than morally acceptable. Specifically, the decision to withdraw nutrition was made too soon after the coma began. It is not always easy to diagnose permanent unconsciousness, and prudence would indicate that at least a few weeks are needed to verify that a patient breathing without respirator support was truly irreversibly unconscious. Hence, the nurse's position—that things went a little too fast and without sufficient attention to supportive care—is more reasonable than the physicians' willingness to withdraw the IV lines so soon after the cardiopulmonary arrest.

Moreover, the communication between the physicians and nurses was inadequate, and the communication between the physicians and the family also seems to have been poor, judging from the subsequent claims of the family that they did not understand Clarence's condition when they agreed to withdraw the treatments. The failures of communication between the physicians and family may have been the fault of the physicians, or of the family, or of both. The main thing to note is that good ethics demands good communication. Physicians and nurses must make sure that patients and proxies really grasp what they are saying.

THE CASE OF CLAIRE CONROY

The Story

In 1979 Thomas Whittemore became the legal guardian for his aunt, Claire Conroy. She had lived a very simple life; in fact, she had lived all her life in the house of her childhood. She had never married, had worked for the same company all her life, and had few friends. She had been close to her three sisters, but they had all died. Thomas was her only surviving blood relative, and he had been visiting her weekly for a number of years. As far as he knew, she had feared and avoided doctors all her life. When his wife once took her to an emergency room, she had objected vigorously. By the time she was about 80, she was suffering from an organic brain syndrome that caused periodic confusion. Thomas then placed her in a nursing home, where she became increasingly confused, disoriented, and physically dependent.

In 1982 she was hospitalized for four months. One of her problems was a gangrenous left foot thought by her physicians to be life-threatening. Two surgeons recommended amputation, but Thomas refused to give informed consent because he was sure that she would not have wanted the surgery. Despite the dim prognosis, she lived. During the same hospitalization, an NG tube was inserted to supplement her nutritional intake. After three months it was removed, but attempts to feed her by hand were not sufficient, and so it was reinserted. She was discharged to the nursing home, where another attempt was made to nourish her without the tube in January 1983. This effort also failed.

Later that year, when it became apparent that the feeding tube would be permanently needed, Thomas sought to have it removed on the grounds that she would never have consented to its insertion in the first place. By this time she was suffering from arteriosclerotic heart disease, hypertension, and diabetes. Her left leg was gangrenous to the knee. She could not speak, and physicians were not sure just how much pain she felt. Perhaps she was uncomfortable because she did pull and tug at her bandages, feeding tube, and catheter.

Her attending physician, Dr. Kazemi, and the nursing home administrator, a nurse named Catherine Rittel, did not think the feeding tube should be removed. Thomas Whittemore then went to court. The case is important because no court had ever before authorized the removal of feeding tubes.

He filed his petition on January 24, 1984, and the case was argued a week later. A consulting physician, testifying on behalf of the nephew, said he thought that it was appropriate to remove the feeding tube with the nephew's consent. He felt that Claire did not have long to live, could never experience significant recovery, and was possibly suffering. During the hearing, a seminary professor of Christian ethics (Ms. Conroy was a Roman Catholic) testified that removal of the tube would not, in his view, be a violation of Catholic teaching because the medical nutrition should be considered extraordinary treatment, and therefore optional, in these circumstances.

The trial court judge decided the case on February 2, 1984. He allowed removal of the feeding tube, stating that prolonging her life with its burdens by medical nutrition was pointless, and might even be cruel. The guardian *ad litem* appealed to the superior court, appellate division. During the appeal process, Ms. Conroy, still on the NG tube, died on February 15, 1984. Nonetheless, aware of the public need for judicial review on this kind of situation, the superior court agreed to hear the case.

The appellate court reversed the decision of the lower court, arguing that withdrawal of the NG tube would not simply be letting Claire Conroy die, but would be tantamount to active euthanasia or killing her. This decision was appealed, and the case went to the New Jersey Supreme Court. Before examining its decision, we will look at the story from an ethical point of view.

Ethical Analysis
Situational awareness
We are aware of these facts in the Conroy story.

1. Claire, in her eighties, was suffering from several serious problems. She was failing and would not live long. She was conscious, but mostly passive and incapable of making treatment decisions for herself. Her nephew was the appropriate guardian, and the court found he had no conflict of interest in requesting withdrawal of the NG tube.

2. Her proxy was requesting withdrawal of the feeding tube based on what he believed she would have wanted. She had never said explicitly that she would not want feeding tubes, but her lifelong aversion to medical care supported his position. Her physician was against the withdrawal.

We are also aware of these good and bad features in the case.

1. Without the NG tube, Claire would die, and a human death is always bad. Moreover, she may have suffered somewhat as she died from malnutrition and dehydration.

2. Using medical nutrition to keep her alive in her dying months prolonged her suffering and discomfort, yet achieved little benefit beyond an added period of life that had already lost so much.

3. The NG tube could have been causing her distress. All her life she had declined medical treatment, and we have no reason to think she had changed her mind and would want it now. Confused though she may have been, she may well have been upset with the NG tube, but so weak and incapacitated that she could not refuse the interventions.

4. Keeping her alive was undoubtedly upsetting to her nephew because he believed it was against her desires. It is difficult for caring proxies to see their patient's wishes disregarded.

Prudential reasoning in the Claire Conroy story

Patient's perspective.   Given the limited life expectancy and health problems (which include diabetes, a gangrenous leg, heart disease, high blood pressure, and no control over bodily functions), a patient not expecting to live long might well think declining medical nutrition and hydration is the appropriate moral response. Of course, Claire was too sick to decide this at the time but, judging from what we know of her, she did feel this way before she deteriorated, and it is not an unreasonable view.

Proxy's position.   A proxy acts morally when he tries to present what the patient would have wanted, provided what the patient would have wanted is not clearly immoral. In this case, there are good reasons for believing Claire would not want her life prolonged with medical nutrition and hydration and, if this was her position, the proxy's request to stop the medical nutrition is easily justified; in fact, it would be rather difficult to justify any other proxy decision in this kind of case. If a proxy has good reason for thinking that the patient would not want the NG tube continued in the circumstances, his failure to request withdrawal would be morally questionable. Thomas was on solid moral ground when he requested the feeding tube withdrawn from his aunt.

Providers' position.   There are also good moral reasons for doing what the providers did in this case. In the earlier stages of the patient's illness, they provided needed nutrition with the NG tube, but they saw it as something temporary and twice tried to wean her from it. Temporary use of a tube for nourishment is morally justified in most cases. Of course, if Claire had clearly refused tubal feeding while she had decision-making capacity, either personally or through advance directives to her proxy, it would have been unethical for providers to force the tubal nourishment on her.

As it became apparent that Claire's medical nutrition and hydration would be permanent and that she would die within a short time even if it were continued, the reasonableness of the tubal nutrition declined to the point where its withdrawal can be morally justified. Moreover, if her proxy could show that she would not have wanted indefinite medical nutrition at the end of her life, it is arguably unethical for physicians to continue it.

It was also appropriate for the providers to seek a judicial opinion before withdrawing the feeding tube. In 1983 it was not well-established that the withdrawal of a feeding tube would not be considered equivalent to illegal euthanasia and, in fact, the superior court did so consider the proposed withdrawal. Even today, withdrawing medical nutrition from conscious patients without evidence that this is what they would want is a very sensitive issue from a legal point of view. Prudent legal advice and judicial intervention were important protections for providers before any legislation or case law had established support for withdrawing medical nutrition from conscious patients without decision-making capacity.

The Supreme Court Decision

In a long decision dated January 17, 1985, the New Jersey Supreme Court reversed the ruling of the superior court and concluded that a proxy may direct withdrawal of tubal nourishment in some cases, provided certain procedures are followed. It argued that the right to self-determination can outweigh the state's interest in preserving life and that, as the Quinlan decision by the same court a few years earlier had shown, this right is not lost when a person becomes incapable of exercising it personally. The court ruled that a proxy can direct withdrawal of medical nutrition if any one of three tests or standards can be met. The court described these standards as follows.

1. *Subjective:* Here the proxy knows what the patient would have chosen to do. This knowledge can be the result of written or oral advance directives, or come from knowing the reactions of the person to similar cases. The knowledge might also be deduced from a person's religious beliefs, or from a consistent pattern discernible in prior decisions about medical treatment.

2. *Limited-objective:* Here the patient's wishes are not so clear as they would be with the subjective standard, but there is some trustworthy evidence that she would have refused the treatment and, in addition, the patient is suffering unavoidable pain that outweighs the benefits of continued life.

3. *Pure-objective:* Here we have no trustworthy evidence that the patient would have refused the treatment, but the burdens of pain and suffering are so great that the proxy can reasonably conclude they outweigh the benefits of continued life.

According to the New Jersey court, any one of these standards would legally justify, in principle, a proxy's decision to withdraw medical nutrition from a conscious patient. The question now is: Did the request of Claire's proxy meet any of these standards? According to the state supreme court, it did not.

The court felt that the evidence at trial was inadequate to satisfy any of the three standards. If Claire Conroy were still alive at the time of the decision, then, her nephew would have had to present additional evidence before it would have been legal to withdraw the nasogastric tube. If he wanted to use the subjective test, he would have to show more clearly that she would not have wanted the tubal nourishment. If he wanted to use either objective test, he would have to show better that she was suffering so much it overrode the benefits of continued life. Perhaps he could have presented additional evidence that would satisfy the court's requirements but, since she had died almost a year earlier, there was no need for him to pursue the issue, and the court declined to remand the matter for further proceedings. Thus the case of Claire Conroy ended at this point.

The court also commented on several distinctions that are now familiar to us. It rejected the distinction between actively hastening death by terminating treatment and passively allowing a person to die of a disease, claiming that the description of conduct as active or passive is a notion so elusive it is of little value in decision-making situations.

The court also rejected the use of the distinctions between withholding and withdrawing treatment, and between ordinary and extraordinary treatments. The court recognized the emotional significance of feeding, but saw a distinction between feeding by bottle or spoon and feeding by tube and lines, which is a medical procedure. It also pointed out that receiving nourishment by means of a tube can be seen as equivalent to breathing by means of a respirator; both interventions enable a body to perform a vital function it can no longer manage on its own. Since withdrawing respirators is morally justified in many cases, so must be withdrawing feeding tubes.

We should note that the Conroy decision was rather limited in its application—it applies only to patients in nursing homes. It also required the physician to follow certain detailed procedures. These included notifying the New Jersey Ombudsman Office of the intended withdrawal and obtaining confirmation of the patient's diagnosis and prognosis by two physicians not affiliated with the nursing home. In addition, if either objective standard is being used, the patient's family members or, in their absence, the next of kin must concur with the decision to withdraw the medical nutrition.

The Conroy case was important because it was the first time a state supreme court ruled that, in some circumstances, medical nutrition and hydration could be withdrawn from a conscious patient without decision-making capacity. The court also recognized that a competent person has the right, based on common law and on the Constitution, to reject medical treatment regardless of the person's medical condition or prognosis, and that this right remains intact even when the person becomes incapacitated.

Ethical Reflection

An ethicist could rather easily conclude, along with the moral theologian who testified in the trial court, that it is morally reasonable for a proxy to request withdrawal of medical nutrition and hydration for a person in Claire's condition and with her history of refusing most medical interventions throughout her life. Keeping people in their eighties with limited life expectancy alive by using tubes and lines for nourishment at the end of their lives does not make a lot of sense when we have good reason to believe they would not want the interventions.

Some will consider the case of Claire Conroy as an argument for active euthanasia. If it is morally justified to withdraw medical nutrition and hydration from a conscious patient, they argue, then it seems reasonable and compassionate to give the person a lethal injection rather than to allow the slow death caused by malnutrition and dehydration. Unlike the cases where the patient is unconscious, a person in Claire's position might suffer when her feeding tube is withdrawn and, since the fatal outcome is inevitable without nourishment, waiting days for death seems senseless.

This argument has a certain appeal but is not a convincing argument for active euthanasia. The key is to prevent suffering when the NG tube is removed, and if we can prevent suffering without taking the drastic step of having a physician kill the patient, then good ethics suggests we do so. Once we sedate a person suffering is not a question, and no compelling reason for euthanasia remains. True, the sedation of a patient just waiting for death after nutrition is withdrawn creates a situation no one really likes, but euthanasia creates an even less desirable scene—physicians killing patients.

THE CASE OF ELIZABETH BOUVIA

The Story

In February 1986, twenty-eight-year-old Elizabeth was a patient at the High Desert Hospital in Lancaster, California. She had been afflicted since birth with cerebral palsy, and quadriplegia had left her immobile except for some movement in her fingers, head, and face. She also suffered from degenerate and crippling arthritis causing so much pain that a permanent catheter had been placed in her chest for regular doses of morphine. It gave her some, but not total, relief. Her mind was clear, and she had earned a college degree. Her weight hovered around 65 to 70 pounds. She had stopped eating solid food when the food was causing her nausea and vomiting. The hospital's physicians, fearing her liquid diet would be inadequate, had inserted a nasogastric tube.

She had dictated advance directives to her lawyers and signed them with a pen in her mouth that marked an "X" on the paper. These directives indicated she did not want nourishment by tubes, but her physicians ignored them.

Undoubtedly, part of the reason why they inserted the NG tube was their knowledge of the circumstances surrounding her previous hospitalization in 1983. At that time—shortly after she had checked into the Riverside General Hospital—there was some indication that she had decided to starve herself to death and wanted medical support as she died. Physicians at Riverside prevented her suicide by inserting an NG tube, and a court had supported the hospital's position. Elizabeth did not appeal that ruling, and she eventually began eating again, so the NG tube was removed. Thus the physicians at High Desert Hospital in 1986 may well have thought she was making another attempt to commit suicide, and they were trying to prevent it by using a nasogastric tube, something the physicians at Riverside had done with court approval three years earlier.

Her lawyer asked the court to issue an injunction ordering physicians at High Desert Hospital to remove the NG tube. The court refused, arguing that disconnecting life-support equipment could only be done if the patient was unconscious and terminally ill. Elizabeth was neither unconscious nor terminally ill; testimony indicated that she might live another 15–20 years, if adequately nourished.

In April 1986, the California Court of Appeal reversed the trial court's decision and directed the lower court to order the NG tube removed. Medical nutrition was withdrawn, and the providers at High Desert Hospital began feeding Elizabeth as much as she could tolerate. This turned out to be sufficient. She left the hospital and remains alive as this is being written.

The court of appeal argued that competent adults have the right to refuse life-sustaining medical treatment even if they are not terminally ill and unconscious. It also reminded providers that "no civil or criminal liability attaches to honoring the refusal by a competent and informed patient of medical treatment."

Ethical Analysis

We now want to consider this case from an ethical point of view. It can serve as a paradigm case for people with decision-making capacity who are experiencing a high level of pain and suffering with little hope of any significant improvement. If spoon feeding causes them additional distress, is it morally reasonable for them to decline it? And if they do decline the uncomfortable spoon feeding, is it morally reasonable for them to decline medical nutrition as well?

Situational awareness

We are aware of the following facts in the Bouvia story.

1. Elizabeth was severely ill, and her pain was only partially controlled by morphine. Her prognosis for improvement was slight, although her life could continue for decades. She was accepting some liquid nourishment, but not enough to sustain her life indefinitely because the food caused her physical distress. She did not want medical nutrition by tubes or lines, but a nasogastric tube was nonetheless inserted. Due to her illness, she was powerless to resist the nasogastric tube inserted against her will. A gastric tube may have been more comfortable for her, but she had not given informed consent for the surgery to insert it. She wanted the nasogastric tube removed.

2. Her providers and the first judge to review the case believed the tube should remain. They viewed the situation as an attempted suicide rather than as a refusal of medical interventions providing nutrition and hydration.

We are also aware of these good and bad features in the case.

1. Elizabeth was not able at this time to receive adequate nourishment orally. The feeding tube was preserving her life, and human life is a good.

2. Removal of the NG tube would be a causal factor in her death, and human death is always bad.

3. Oral nourishment caused Elizabeth distress and discomfort, but so did the NG tube, which she did not want.

4. If providers believed she was once again trying to commit suicide, then withholding or withdrawing the tube could cause them distress. Many physicians and nurses would not want to help patients, especially those not terminally ill, to commit suicide.

Prudential reasoning in the Bouvia story

Patient's perspective.   Elizabeth had been thrown into a terrible and tragic situation. As one judge wrote: "Fate has dealt this young woman a terrible hand. Can anyone blame her if she wants to fold her cards and say 'I am out?'" And in 1983 her intentions at Riverside apparently were to commit suicide.

In 1986, however, she was no longer trying to commit suicide; she was simply refusing the oral nourishment that was causing her distress and the medical nutrition supplied by an NG tube. Is the refusal to eat reasonable for someone in her position? It would be difficult to say it is not. Food caused her so much distress that her refusal to eat does not seem unreasonable, especially in view of her tragic situation. And if she declined to eat, must she accept a feeding tube? Again, it seems not. She knew, better than any of us, what a burden it is to live like this, and her desire not to use feeding tubes to prolong this painful life was not an unreasonable response. If a person can no longer eat naturally, then it may well be reasonable for her to decline feeding tubes in some situations, and this seems like one of them.

So incomprehensible to us is the position of a patient locked into such a terrible condition that it almost seems arrogant to second guess her preferences. It would be difficult for anyone to say, given her unfortunate situation, that her decisions to refuse food her body does not tolerate well and to decline tubes for nourishment are morally unjustified.

Proxy's perspective.   There is no proxy here—Elizabeth is competent and capable of making her own decisions.

Providers' position.   What is the right thing for providers to do when patients cannot eat adequately, and then refuse to accept feeding tubes? When the patients are as damaged as Elizabeth was, and experiencing significant pain and suffering, there seems little doubt that they should acknowledge the patient's desires. This conclusion becomes clear when the alternative is considered. If a patient with decision-making capacity refuses a feeding tube and her wishes are ignored, it creates a situation where physicians are forcing medical interventions on her. In this case, they could physically do this because Elizabeth was too helpless to resist. But the thought of taking advantage of her paralysis to force an unwanted feeding tube through her nose is not a comfortable one, especially since her anguish at being treated this way was evident.

The motivation of people working in health care to save lives is a wonderful thing, but it cannot override the wishes of patients with decision-making capacity, who are in a better position to know what is best for them. Forcing treatment or tubes for nutrition on competent adults against their wishes is difficult to justify. It violates respect for them and pushes medicine back into its paternalistic mode. Certainly, it was difficult for providers to remove the NG tube, which they thought she needed to live, but it should be more difficult for them to force tubes into helpless people against their will and to refuse to withdraw them when the patient with decision-making capacity clearly wants them out.

Ethical Reflection

If we look on this case from the vantage point of our ethical approach, the patient's decision to forego nourishment by tubes is reasonable, as would be the decision to accept medical nutrition. There is a point where a suffering person may reasonably decide that the burdens of treatment and medical nutrition fall so far short of the benefits that it is more reasonable to decline the interventions, even if it means death, than to accept them. Nothing Elizabeth could choose would help her live well or have a good life in any meaningful sense of these terms. She was trapped in a tragic situation and could only choose the less worse.

It is difficult to find cogent reasons for requiring a person suffering from an incurable painful situation to accept tubes and lines for nourishment. The idea that each person should live reasonably and take reasonable care of her life is not undermined when a person, whose body is almost totally immobile and generating so much pain that continual morphine is required, opts to decline treatment or nutrition. Nor is it unreasonable if a person in this situation opts for treatment and medical nourishment. In tragic situations such as these, providers can allow some leeway for the suffering patient to decide what interventions are acceptable. In some cases, and this may well be one of them, the patient has plausible reasons for both accepting and rejecting medical nutrition.

Not to be overlooked, however, is Elizabeth's earlier request for assistance in committing suicide. During her 1983 hospitalization, she did want help in starving herself to death. In today's debate about physician-assisted suicide, some might argue that her providers should have helped her end her life. Although not terminally ill, she was suffering significantly and had little hope of meaningful improvement. Since she had decision-making capacity and was freely requesting assistance in suicide, compassion suggests to some that she should have been given that assistance.

But her physicians did not help her commit suicide when she was at Riverside General Hospital, and the fact that years later she continues to eat suggests that we should be careful when suffering patients ask for help in killing themselves. Their requests cannot always be taken at face value; sometimes the determination of these patients to kill themselves is only temporary.

Elizabeth had reasons other than her medical problems for being depressed in 1983. She had developed a pen pal relationship with a man in prison, and they became a couple when he was released. A glimmer of good fortune came into her life, but he abandoned her when she became pregnant. Then she suffered a miscarriage. It is not surprising that significant depression would follow these experiences, especially for someone in her circumstances.

However, her survival to this day indicates a will to live that reasserted itself after that temporary desire to commit what some would call a "rational suicide." This reminds everyone in the debate about physician-assisted suicide just how difficult it is to know when the desire of a suffering patient with decision-making capacity for help in committing suicide is truly a definitive stance. Few people want to help a patient commit suicide when the patient would have changed her mind if she had the chance.

THE CASE OF MARY O'CONNOR

The Story

Mary had worked in a hospital for years before her retirement in 1983. Two years later she began suffering a series of strokes. At first her two daughters, both practical nurses, cared for her at home, but her deteriorating condition necessitated transfer to a nursing home in February 1988. The strokes left her bedridden, partially paralyzed, severely demented, and unresponsive despite the daily visits of her daughters. She was, however, thought to be still somewhat conscious. She was nourished by spoon feedings but had difficulty swallowing. There was no doubt that she was incapable of making health care decisions. Her daughters served as her proxies.

Before her strokes, she had repeatedly stated for years that she did not want her life prolonged by artificial means. From her experience working in a hospital, she was aware of how some patients lingered thanks to life-sustaining treatments. She thought it was "monstrous" that they were kept alive when they were not going to get better. After a hospitalization for a heart attack in 1984, she again repeated her feelings that she would not want life-support systems maintaining or prolonging her life if they could not restore a reasonable degree of health.

By June 1988 her condition had so deteriorated that the nursing home transferred her to the Westchester County Medical Center. The hospital wanted to insert a nasogastric tube for nourishment. The attending physician thought the tubal nourishment might extend her life for several months or "perhaps a year or two." Her daughters refused permission for the tube, saying she never wanted this kind of life support. The physicians asked the hospital ethics committee for its opinion; it advised the physicians that it would be inappropriate to withhold nutrition and hydration. The daughters still refused permission for the NG tube. The hospital then sought authorization from the court to insert the tube.

The Westchester County court found that Mrs. O'Connor's wish to decline life support was clear enough, even though she had not specifically discussed NG tubes or possible disability due to strokes. In deference to her wishes, the court refused to order the feeding tube.

The medical center appealed, and in August 1988 the appellate division upheld the lower court's decision by a narrow 3–2 margin. The medical center again appealed, this time to the court of appeals (the highest court in New York). Its decision came in October 1988. During these legal proceedings Mrs. O'Connor was nourished by peripheral IV lines.

Before looking at the final court decision, we will consider the case from an ethical point of view.

Ethical Analysis

Situational awareness

We are aware of the following facts in the O'Connor story.

1. Mary was seventy-seven, still somewhat conscious, but generally unresponsive and unable to eat as the result of strokes. Although not really terminally ill in the sense that she was suffering from a fatal disease, her life expectancy was not long and her neurological damage was irreversible.

2. She had a long history of repeatedly expressing her desire not to be kept alive by life-support systems if they would not help her get better. She had frequently stated that she wanted nature to take its course and that she did not want to become a burden to anyone.

3. Her proxies, her two daughters, declined the nasogastric tube because they were convinced that she never would have wanted it in these circumstances. Their convictions were based on her remarks over the years before the strokes left her incapacitated.

We are also aware of the following good and bad features in the case.

1. If she was not nourished she would die, and death is always unfortunate. The feeding tube was preserving her life, and all life has value.

2. If she was nourished by tubes she could well be upset, given her previous desires. Medical nourishment was also upsetting to her daughters because they knew that she did not want medical interventions in these circumstances.

3. Providers would presumably have felt uncomfortable about withholding nourishment, especially when the ethics committee advised them that medical nourishment should be provided. It is unclear from the court testimony, however, whether the daughters had the opportunity to present their side to the committee. The discomfort of the physicians and of the hospital was so strong that the medical center twice appealed the rulings of the lower courts. The distress of the center and its personnel over withdrawing her feeding tube is an additional bad feature in the case.

Prudential reasoning in the O'Connor story

Patient's perspective.   Is it morally reasonable for a person in Mary's position to decline tubal nourishment in advance? Much of her life had already been lost and not much time remained for this bedridden seventy-seven-year-old unresponsive victim of multiple strokes and a heart attack. She felt strongly that death was a part of nature, and that nature should just take its course. Unlike Claire Conroy, she did accept medical care and hospitalization but, like her, she dreaded being kept alive by life-sustaining treatments if she could not recover in a meaningful way.

Mary's long-standing moral position about how to live and die well appears most reasonable. No good except the prolongation of unresponsive life for a year or so at most could be achieved by medical nutrition, and the intervention would bring a number of bad consequences. These include the discomfort and possible complications of the NG tube and the distress of her daughters over her being kept alive this way.

Proxies' perspective.   Given the wishes of their mother, the only morally reasonable course of action for the daughters was what they did. If they had consented to what they knew she did not want, their actions would have been morally indefensible. Mary had been around a hospital for years and she knew how life support was being used to keep people alive when it could offer little benefit except prolongation of a life already extremely diminished by illness.

Providers' perspective.   This was a little more complex, and the court testimony did not elaborate on the reasons for their position. To their credit, they did consult with the ethics committee, which supported their position in favor of nutrition. On the other hand, the practitioners (and the ethics committee) should have been aware by this time (1988) of the trend in law and ethics to respect the wishes of incapacitated patients that were voiced before they lost the ability to make treatment decisions. The physicians and the medical center decided to ignore these wishes and the wishes of her proxies, and to force medical nourishment into Claire.

It is difficult to think of a strictly ethical reason that would justify the harm they thereby caused her and her daughters. It is not, however, difficult to find a legal reason for their position. They had reason to believe that withdrawing the tube might expose them to legal liability, so it was prudent for them to seek court authorization before carrying out the daughters' request to withdraw the feeding tube.

However, once the trial court had granted that authorization, one is at a loss to find a reason justifying their appeal to the appellate division and then, when they lost at this level, their additional appeal to the supreme court in the state. Once they had a court authorization to withdraw the feeding tube, the reasonable ethical response would have been to withdraw it or, if that violated their conscience, to arrange for transferring Mary to other providers. There was no need for the medical center to take an adversarial role against Mary and her daughters in this case, especially after a court approved of the daughters' request to withdraw medical nutrition.

The Court of Appeals Decision

In a 5–2 opinion dated October 14, 1988, the court of appeals found that Mrs. O'Connor's prior statements did not constitute "clear and convincing evidence" that she would not want feeding tubes if she became incapacitated. The court held that everyone has a right to life, and no patient should be denied any medical care unless "clear and convincing" evidence shows that the patient wanted to decline a particular type of treatment. The court dismissed Mary's earlier statements about not wanting to be kept alive on life support as not being clear indications of what she wanted. In the words of Chief Justice Sol Wachtler, her statements were nothing more "than immediate reactions to the unsettling experience of seeing or hearing of another's unnecessarily prolonged death."

Two of the justices wrote a strong dissent to the decision. They claimed that the justices supporting the decision had "trivialized" Mary's remarks of many years by not taking them seriously. The decision of the court is unworkable, they argued, because it means people cannot have their wishes to decline medical procedures respected unless they anticipate exactly what procedures might be an option in various circumstances that might develop. The dissenting justices argued that "Mary O'Connor expressed her wishes in the only terms familiar to her, and she expressed them as clearly as a lay person should be asked to express them. To require more is unrealistic, and for all practical purposes it precludes the right of patients to forego life-sustaining treatment."

The reasoning of the dissenting justices in this case is far more reasonable from a moral point of view than the reasoning in the decision written by the

Chief Justice himself. Mary's wishes were clear enough, and most reasonable given her circumstances.

The legal problem could have been avoided, of course, if Mary had written advance directives about tubal feeding. And, ironically, it could have been avoided if Mary had appointed a durable power of attorney, as the decision acknowledged in a footnote. At that time, New York law allowed people to appoint a durable power of attorney with the authority to make health care decisions, including the withdrawal of medical nutrition, without explicit advance directives about specific treatments.

It is important to notice how the supreme courts of New York and New Jersey differ in the matter of withdrawing medical nutrition. In the Conroy case, the New Jersey court allowed a proxy to use the best interests standard in certain situations, but the New York court did not allow this standard in the O'Connor case. In New York, the court requires the proxy to use the substituted judgment standard, and the evidence that the patient would not want the medical nutrition must be of the strictest kind—it must be "clear and convincing."

However, the strict requirement of "clear and convincing evidence" used by the New York court in its 1988 decision about Mrs. O'Connor has now been partially negated by the 1990 New York Health Care Proxy Law. This law allows a proxy designated on a signed proxy form to make treatment decisions without producing clear and convincing evidence that the decisions are what the person wanted, even though the person has not been appointed a durable power of attorney. Hence if Mary's case had happened a few years later and if she had designated one of her daughters as her health care agent under the new law, the medical nutrition could have been withdrawn.

Ethical Reflection

The decision to decline medical nutrition in these circumstances is morally justifiable. Mary is not trying to commit suicide; she merely wants to be left alone and let nature take its course. She does not want additional medical interventions if they cannot offer her any more than some additional bedridden months in a hospital in a conscious but unresponsive state. Many people imagining themselves in a similar state would undoubtedly find her position reasonable. She sees no benefit in living that outweighs the burdens of her irreversible situation. She believes it is good for her to let nature take its course. The intentions of her providers to use tubal feeding may well have been nobly motivated, but there are no compelling moral reasons why Mrs. O'Connor should have been subjected to medical interventions she did not want at the end of her natural life.

THE CASE OF NANCY CRUZAN

In recent years there have been a number of legal cases involving the nourishment of patients in a persistent vegetative state. Many of these patients survive for years, even decades, thanks to feeding tubes and basic nursing care, yet they will never regain any consciousness. A trend has developed wherein courts allow proxies to stop the medical nutrition and hydration if there is evidence that these patients would not have wanted it continued in a persistent vegetative state.

Among the most celebrated cases where courts have allowed the withdrawal of medical nutrition and hydration of PVS patients are:

1. Paul Brophy, Massachusetts Supreme Court, 1986.
2. Nancy Jobes, New Jersey Supreme Court, 1987.
3. Marsha Gray, Federal District Court (Rhode Island), 1988.
4. Carol McConnell, Connecticut Supreme Court, 1989.

The most noteworthy recent case, however, is that of Nancy Cruzan. It is the only case involving the withdrawal of medical nutrition that went to the United States Supreme Court. The decision came in June 1990.

The Story

In January 1983 Nancy's car went off the road into a ditch. She was found lying face down and not breathing. Emergency personnel began CPR; it restored her breathing, but she never regained consciousness. A year later, it was clear that she was in a persistent vegetative state. She could conceivably live for decades without any prospect of regaining the slightest level of awareness. After several years her parents, acting as her guardians, asked that the gastrostomy tube be removed; they claimed she had made remarks indicating she would not want any life support keeping her alive unless she could live at least halfway normally. Her physicians and the hospital refused to stop the medical nutrition. Her parents went to court in 1988.

The evidence indicating that Nancy would want the medical nutrition withdrawn consisted primarily of statements she had made to a roommate about a year before the accident. This person reported that she had said she would not want to live if she ever faced life as a vegetable. After hearing the evidence, Judge Charles Teel of the Jasper County Circuit Court authorized the withdrawal of the medical nutrition. His order was not carried out because a guardian *ad litem*, supported by several state officials, appealed to the Missouri Supreme Court.

The Missouri Supreme Court reversed Judge Teal's decision. It said that medical nutrition cannot be withdrawn from a PVS patient unless there is "clear and convincing" evidence that this was the patient's wish. The court also noted (correctly) that Nancy was not terminally ill and was not suffering. Thus it saw no reason to act contrary to the state's interest in preserving life, no matter how minimal the life had become. ". . . (T)he state's interest is in life; that interest is unqualified." In other words, the quality of a life has no bearing on the state's interest in preserving that life.

The Missouri court acknowledged that the doctrine of informed consent gives people a right to refuse treatment, and that this right persists even when they are incapacitated, but the court insisted that a proxy cannot exercise this right except (1) under the requirements of the state Living Will statute or (2) in situations where the evidence of the patient's wish to decline medical nourishment is "clear and convincing."

Missouri and New York are the only states insisting on "clear and convincing" evidence that an incapacitated patient had previously indicated she does not want medical nutrition and hydration before a proxy's request to withdraw medical nutrition can be honored. (Two other states, Maine and Illinois, have applied this standard of evidence to refusals of other life-sustaining treatments, but not specifically to the withdrawal of feeding tubes and lines.)

The phrase "clear and convincing evidence" is important, although there is no precise definition for it. "Clear and convincing evidence" falls somewhere between the evidential requirements in civil cases captured in the phrase "preponderance of the evidence" and the more strict requirement of evidence in criminal cases known as "evidence beyond a reasonable doubt." It is a very strict evidential requirement, as we saw in the O'Connor case.

After the Missouri Supreme Court ruled against them, the Cruzans appealed to the United States Supreme Court, and arguments were heard in December 1989. A major issue was whether Missouri's requirement of "clear and convincing evidence" was so demanding that it effectively violated a patient's constitutional right to refuse medical interventions. The due process clause of the Constitution gives one the liberty to refuse unwanted medical treatment, and most would argue that this liberty is not lost simply because a person has lapsed into unconsciousness. If unconscious people do not lose constitutional protection, then an environment must be maintained so their proxies can see to it that their wishes about treatment remain effective. The question is whether or not the demand that a proxy produce "clear and convincing evidence" is so strict that it, in effect, destroys the constitutional protection most people should enjoy when they become permanently unconscious.

Before looking at the decision of the U.S. Supreme Court in the Cruzan case, and its aftermath, we will examine the case from a moral point of view.

Ethical Analysis

Situational awareness

We are aware of the following facts in the Cruzan story.

1. About a year before the accident, Nancy had made some reference to the fact that she would never want to live as a vegetable. That had become precisely her status, and it would continue for the rest of her life.

2. Her proxies (her parents) believed the medical nutrition should be stopped because she would not want it in her condition.

3. Her physicians and the state of Missouri believed it should be continued because they had medical and legal interests in preserving life. Since the evidence of her previous wishes was not clear and convincing, as the state law governing living wills requires, and since she was not suffering, they saw no reason why their interest in preserving life should not prevail.

We are also aware of these good and bad features in the case.

1. Nancy's death, as any human death, would be unfortunate even though most of her brain had already ceased functioning.

2. Providing medical nutrition caused no burden or benefit to her because she could not experience anything. It did cause her parents distress, however,

because they were convinced she would not want it, and this is a bad feature of the case.

3. Withdrawing the nutrition would cause her physicians and state officials (the court records name the administrator of the Missouri Rehabilitation Center and the director of the Missouri Department of Health, acting in their official capacities, as opposing the Cruzans) some distress, judging from their strong stand against withdrawal.

4. The treatment and care of Nancy burdened the taxpayers of Missouri; they were paying most of the medical bills. Unfortunately, the public funds could not provide any benefit Nancy would experience.

Prudential reasoning in the Nancy Cruzan story

Patient's perspective.   Nancy had no perspective at this point, but did have some ideas before she lost consciousness about not wanting to live in a vegetative state. Were these ideas morally reasonable? Undoubtedly they were. The vast majority of people, most ethicists, and even the courts are in agreement that it is reasonable for people to want medical nutrition stopped if they fall into a persistent vegetative state. One is hard pressed to find any plausible reason why a person would want his irreversibly vegetative body kept alive for years.

Proxies' perspective.   The proxies acted in an admirable way. They knew what their daughter did not want, and they knew, after several years, that the continuation of medical nutrition and hydration was senseless. Since they had reason to believe their daughter would not have wanted the medical intervention continued indefinitely, they were on solid ethical ground when they requested its removal.

Providers' perspective.   The physicians disagreed with the parents about withdrawing the nutrition. This position can be justified if they felt withdrawal would be illegal under Missouri law because the evidence that Nancy would not want the tubal feeding was less than "clear and convincing." The physicians knew Nancy was not suffering, and if they thought the law required them to continue the feeding, this is a good reason for them to do so until a court resolved the legal issue.

Guardians *ad litem*'s perspective.   There were actually two guardians *ad litem* appointed in this case, and one of them took an interesting legal position. He thought that it was in Nancy's best interest to have the medical nutrition withdrawn, but he also thought it was important to have the case reviewed by the state supreme court. This was a new type of case in the state, what is called a case of the "first instance," and the state supreme court decision would therefore establish a legal precedent for Missouri. This guardian *ad litem*, therefore, took a rather contradictory position: he concluded Nancy's nutrition should be withdrawn, and then he appealed the judge's order allowing the withdrawal. And when the Missouri Supreme Court later ruled against withdrawal, the same guardian filed a brief urging the U.S. Supreme Court to reverse the decision of the Missouri court and to allow the withdrawal.

From a moral perspective, however, it seems that a guardian *ad litem*'s role is simply to determine what is right for the patient. Since the guardian in this case was satisfied with the lower court's decision to allow withdrawal of medical nutrition, his role in appealing its decision is difficult to justify from an ethical standpoint. Guardians *ad litem* are expected to determine what is best for the patient in the particular litigation; normally they would appeal a decision only if it goes against what they think is right for the patient.

Missouri's perspective.   The state decided to fight the parents after the first court ruled the medical nutrition could be withdrawn. Its position is difficult to justify morally. The state officials could have simply accepted the ruling of Judge Teel, but they did not. Why did the state of Missouri adopt an adversarial role against the family and appeal Judge Teel's decision to the state supreme court?

Perhaps the state officials felt obliged in conscience to do so. Perhaps they were also motivated by political considerations that extended beyond anything directly connected with the reasonable treatment of Nancy Cruzan. Published reports indicate that an intense political struggle between advocates of the right to life and advocates of the right to choose was unfolding in Missouri during the years when Nancy's family were trying to have the medical nutrition withdrawn, and Nancy's case happened to become a focal point of that political struggle.

In 1986 Missouri had amended its abortion act to read: "It is the intention of the . . . state of Missouri to grant the right to life to all humans, born and unborn . . ." If unborn humans have a "right to life," then so does an adult on life-support systems. Permitting the withdrawal of life support from an unconscious adult could undermine the claim that not yet conscious fetuses have an inviolable right to life. The intense state interest in fighting the wishes of Nancy and the request of her parents may have had more to do with the strong position of many state officials against abortion than with the question of withdrawing nutrition from a PVS patient.

But good ethical reasoning can see the difference between abortion and withdrawing medical nutrition from patients in PVS, just as people can see the difference between abortion and killing criminals for capital crimes, a practice that exists in Missouri and in many other states where many people are strongly opposed to abortion on the basis of the "right to life." To the extent the state officials' opposition to Nancy and her parents was motivated by their position on abortion, their actions were morally suspect, and the suffering they caused the family was a morally unjustified imposition. The Cruzan family may well have been a pawn in a burning political issue that has nothing to do with persistent vegetative state—the politics of abortion.

The U.S. Supreme Court Decision and Its Aftermath

The U.S. Supreme Court decided, in June 1990, that Missouri's insistence on clear and convincing evidence before a proxy could have a feeding tube removed was not so strict that it violated the Constitution, and it also noted that no such clear and convincing evidence is yet found in this case. In effect, then, the court ruled the medical nutrition could not be withdrawn. The court stated that a competent person has "a constitutionally protected liberty interest" in refusing unwanted medical treatment. It also said that, for purposes of this case, it can be "assumed" a competent person has "a constitutionally protected right" to refuse life-saving nutrition and hydration, but "this does not mean that an incompetent person should possess the same right . . ." Thus the court, by allowing states to adopt the "clear and convincing" standard, did little to protect the right of an incompetent patient to refuse medical nutrition and hydration, although much of the press seemed to read the decision as indicating otherwise.

On November 1, 1990, the Cruzans were back in Judge Teel's court in Carthage, Missouri. Three friends of Nancy's came forth to give "clear and convincing" evidence that she had told them she would never want to live like a vegetable, and her physician testified that it was no longer in her best interests to be medically nourished. The state of Missouri, which had originally opposed the withdrawal of medical nutrition, had by now withdrawn from the case.

On December 14, 1990, Judge Teel issued an new order, similar to his original order of 1988. He said again that the medical nutrition could be stopped. Only this time he was able to say, thanks to the new witnesses who had come forward, that the "court by clear and convincing evidence" finds Nancy's intent would be to terminate her nutrition and hydration, and thus her parents were authorized to have it stopped.

Despite strong protests at the hospital by groups supporting the right to life, the medical nutrition was stopped. On December 26 Nancy died while special state police details guarded her hospital room to keep the chanting and praying protestors at bay. It was almost eight years after she lapsed into the irreversible unconsciousness of a persistent vegetative state. A documentary of the case was subsequently shown on PBS television. It is well worth seeing.

Ethical Reflection

The decisions of Nancy and her parents are morally reasonable. The nutrition and hydration offered no benefit that Nancy could experience. Medical nutrition given to a permanently unconscious person is meaningless to that person, and the presumption should be that it is reasonable to discontinue it when permanent loss of consciousness is definitively diagnosed. In rare situations, there may be a reason for continuing it briefly. The person may be an organ donor, for example, and it may be reasonable to continue life support in order to enhance organ transplantation.

Most people intuitively sense that withdrawal of medical nutrition is appropriate when a person is in a persistent vegetative state. When asked, few people want their bodies kept alive indefinitely after all awareness has been irreversibly lost. There is no point in maintaining a permanently unconscious and meaningless coma or vegetative state. Once a person has lost all capacity for any awareness, he is no longer really one of us. Truly human existence is gone, only vegetative life continues. Intervention becomes meaningless, and if it imposes a burden on others, as it does, then it is arguably unreasonable and unethical to continue it.

Unfortunately, the state of Missouri apparently assumes, in effect, that most people would want to be kept alive in vegetative state. It requires a strong standard of evidence—the clear and convincing standard—before their families or other proxies can have the medical nutrition withdrawn. This makes the family's decision to withdraw medical nutrition look like the exception when, in fact, it is what most people consider a normal reaction to persistent vegetative state. The effort to keep an irreversibly vegetative body alive for years, and even decades, is what strikes most people as abnormal, not the request to stop meaningless treatment of no benefit to the patient.

Treating a PVS patient creates many burdens on the family, on the providers who feel it is unreasonable, and on those paying for it. These burdens can be justified if they are balanced by proportionate reasons, and there are seldom any such reasons when a person has lapsed into a persistent vegetative state.

Some people, however, do not feel this way. A small but vocal and well-organized minority takes a strong position against withdrawing medical nutrition from PVS patients. The *amicus curiae* or "friend of the court" briefs filed when the Cruzan case went to the U.S. Supreme Court provide an indication of just how divided people are on this subject. Among those supporting the position against Nancy and her parents were:

National Right to Life Committee, Inc.
United States Catholic Conference
National Association of Evangelicals
Baptists for Life and Southern Baptists for Life
Catholic Lawyers Guilds of Boston and New York
National Federation of Catholic Physicians' Guilds
Knights of Columbus
Roman Catholic Archdiocese of New Orleans
Missouri Doctors for Life

Among those supporting Nancy's parents were:

American Medical Association
American College of Surgeons
American Nurses Association and the American Association of
     Nurse Attorneys
National Hospice Organization
Catholic Health Association
Evangelical Lutheran Church in America
American Academy of Neurology
St. Joseph Health System
Center for Health Care Ethics, St. Louis University Medical Center

What ethical reasons do the opponents of withdrawing medical nourishment from irreversibly unconscious people give for their position? In general, several common threads run through their arguments. The first is a rights-based argument. They accept the political philosophy of Thomas Hobbes and

John Locke, and build an ethic on the right to life. It was this right, Hobbes argued, that secured everyone's self-preservation. If everyone has a right to life, then no one can kill anyone else. This right also gave the state its authority and power, because the state must preserve this right to life, especially when the person cannot defend it himself. The government in all its branches must therefore oppose any movement that undermines or might undermine anyone's right to life.

A second thread often found in the arguments of those opposing the withdrawal of medical nutrition and hydration from people in a persistent vegetative state is the fear of a slippery slope (that is, the fear that allowing the withdrawal of nutrition will inexorably lead to other actions they consider immoral). Most of those opposed to withdrawing nutrition from patients in PVS know the nutrition is of no interest or benefit to the patient. Their concern lies elsewhere. They fear these withdrawals will open the door to euthanasia, which they vehemently oppose. And they fear, as the Cruzan case suggests, that withdrawal of nutrition from a human being in vegetative state will open the door to abortion, especially the abortion of fetuses that have not yet achieved any awareness.

A third thread running through the arguments of those opposing withdrawal of nutrition from PVS patients is the conviction that any consideration of the quality of a patient's life is irrelevant to moral questions about preserving that life. In other words, it is not relevant that the life of a PVS patient has deteriorated to a purely vegetative state due to extensive neurological damage. Human life is human life; its value is intrinsic. Most people embracing the right to life approach in ethics allow no room for judgments about the quality of that life.

These arguments will not appear convincing in the ethical approach inspired by Aristotle and Aquinas that we have been employing. Making the political doctrine of rights the foundation of ethics is not without serious problems. It is not at all clear, for example, where these rights, never really noticed until several centuries ago, originated. Some say they come from nature (they are "natural" or "human" rights); others speak as if they come from God. And a moral philosophy based on rights frequently ends up in irresolvable conflict. One reason the abortion debate remains so persistent is that both sides rely on a rights-based position. One side bases its position on the right to life; the other side bases its position on the right to choose. The result is gridlock. The rapidly emerging euthanasia debate is now trapped in a similar stalemate: many opponents of euthanasia rely on the right to life; proponents rely on the right to choose and the right to die.

The slippery-slope argument is also weak. History simply cannot be predicted. The euthanasia practiced in Germany during the 1930s, for example, did not slide into an abortion movement. In fact, there was a strong antiabortion movement in the Germany of the 1940s, although it was not motivated by any respect for human life. There is simply no way to say withdrawing medical nourishment from PVS patients will be followed by more abortions or by euthanasia. In fact, the contrary can be argued: the willingness to withdraw unreasonable life-prolonging treatments weakens the fear of losing control that motivates some supporters of euthanasia. Certainly, there are slippery slopes in life, and some have a limited validity in moral reasonings, but sometimes we cannot avoid facing a slippery slope. When this happens, we can only proceed with caution and take the necessary steps to avoid sliding out of control into moral disaster.

Finally, the refusal of any quality of life assessment in moral judgments about human life is simply impossible. Certainly, making quality of life assessments is open to abuse, but we cannot do good ethics without considering the quality of life in some situations. The quality of life is an important aspect of the ethical question in many situations; it cannot be ignored in any ethics of prudence and prudential moral judgment. It is one of the important circumstances, and ethical judgments ignoring the quality of life are hobbled by their ignorance of this significant feature in the situation.

Although the withdrawal of feeding tubes and lines remains problematic for some, the fundamental moral norm of the ethical approach we have been employing indicates there are situations when it is morally justified. Using medical nutrition and hydration, as any behavior, is morally justified when it helps people achieve a good life, to the extent it can be achieved, or at least to embrace the less worse; and it is morally unjustified when it does not.

SUGGESTED READINGS

An excellent, albeit somewhat dated, introduction to the ethical dilemmas of medical nutrition is Joanne Lynn, ed. 1986. *By No Extraordinary Means: The Choice to Forgo Life-Sustaining Food and Water*. Bloomington: Indiana University Press. It includes essays on the medical procedures, the moral and legal issues, and the religious perspectives. Also helpful is Richard McCormick. "Nutrition–Hydration: The New Euthanasia?" which appears as chapter 21 in 1989. *The Critical Calling: Reflections on Moral Dilemmas Since Vatican II*. Washington: Georgetown University Press; Norman Cantor. "The Permanently Unconscious Patient, Non-Feeding and Euthanasia." *American Journal of Law & Medicine* **1989**, *15*, 381–437; William Curran. "Defining Appropriate Medical Care: Providing Nutrients and Hydration for the Dying." *NEJM* **1985**, *313*, 940–42; Rebecca Dresser and Eugene Boisaubin. "Ethics, Law, and Nutritional Support." *Archives of Internal Medicine* **1985**, *145*, 122–24; Robert Steinbrook and Bernard Lo. "Artificial Feeding—Solid Ground, Not a Slippery Slope." *NEJM* **1988**, *318*, 286–90.

Some health care facilities are attempting to develop institutional policies on nutrition and hydration similar to the policies for cardiopulmonary resuscitation. For an interesting example, see Monica Koschuta et al. "Development of an Institutional Policy on Artificial Nutrition and Hydration." *Kennedy Institute of Ethics Journal* **1991**, *1*, 133–38. The authors trace the development of the policy at Hospice of Washington. The actual policy is published, along with a brief commentary by John Robertson.

The court of appeal's decision in the Clarence Herbert case is *Barber v. The Superior Court of Los Angeles County*, 147 Cal. App. 3d 1006 (1983). Dr. Neil Barber was one of the two physicians whose murder charge was reinstated by the Superior Court of Los Angeles after a magistrate ordered it dismissed. The court of appeal's decision directed the superior court to vacate its order and prohibited it from taking any further action against the physicians. Good discussions of the case are found in David Meyers. "Legal Aspects of Withdrawing Nourishment from an Incurably Ill Patient." *Archives of Internal Medicine* **1985**, *145*, 125–28; and

Bernard Lo. "The Death of Clarence Herbert: Withdrawing Care is Not Murder." *Annals of Internal Medicine* **1984**, *101*, 248–51. The Meyers article also includes an analysis of the Conroy case.

The New Jersey Supreme Court decision in the Claire Conroy case is *In re Conroy* 486 A.2d. 1209 (1985). Among the many commentaries are: Bernard Lo and Laurie Dornbrand. "The Case of Claire Conroy: Will Administrative Review Safeguard Incompetent Patients?" *Annals of Internal Medicine* **1986**, *104*, 869–73 and the six articles that make up Part V of Lynn, *By No Extraordinary Means*.

The 1984 California Superior Court decision that refused to allow withdrawal of Elizabeth's feeding tube lest hospital staff become accomplices in her suicide is Bouvia v. County of Riverside, No. 159780 (Sup. Ct. Cal.), 1984. The later decision allowing her to forgo tubal feeding based on the right of a competent person to refuse medical treatment, including treatment furnishing nutrition and hydration, is *Bouvia v. Superior Court* (Glenchur), 179 Cal. App. 3d. 1127 (1986). For commentaries see George Annas. "Elizabeth Bouvia: Whose Space Is This Anyway?" *Hastings Center Report* **1986**, *16* (April), 24–25, and Robert Steinbrook and Bernard Lo. "The Case of Elizabeth Bouvia: Starvation, Suicide, or Problem Patient?" *Archives of Internal Medicine* **1986**, *146*, 161–64.

The decision of New York's highest court, the Court of Appeals, in the Mary O'Connor case is *In re O'Connor*, 531 N.E.2d 607 (1988). Bernard Lo et al. "Family Decision Making on Trial: Who Decides for Incompetent Patients?" *NEJM* **1990**, *322*, 1228–31 discusses this case and that of Nancy Cruzan. For other commentaries see Daniel Gindes. "Judicial Postponement of Death Recognition: The Tragic Case of Mary O'Connor." *American Journal of Law and Medicine* **1989**, *15*, 301–31; and George Annas. "Precatory Prediction and Mindless Mimicry: The Case of Mary O'Connor." *Hastings Center Report* **1988**, *18* (December), 31–33.

The U.S. Supreme Court decision in the Cruzan case is *Cruzan v. Director, Missouri Dept. of Health*, 110 S. Ct. 2841 (1990). The commentaries on the case and the Supreme Court decision are innumerable. Some examples: George Annas. "The Insane Root Takes Reason Prisoner." *Hastings Center Report* **1989**, *19*, (January–February), 29–31; and "Nancy Cruzan and the Right to Die." *NEJM* **1990**, *323*, 670–73; Marcia Angell. "Prisoners of Technology: The Case of Nancy Cruzan." *NEJM* **1990**, *322*, 1226–28; Lois Snyder. "Life, Death, and the American College of Physicians: The Cruzan Case." *Annals of Internal Medicine* **1990**, *112*, 802–04; David Brushwood. "Need for Clear and Convincing Evidence of a Patient's Wishes Before Artificial Nutrition and Hydration May Be Withdrawn." *American Journal of Hospital Pharmacy* **1990**, *47*, 2720–22; Alan Meisel. "Lessons from Cruzan." *Journal of Clinical Ethics* **1990**, *1*, 245–50; and Robert Weir and Larry Gostin. "Decisions to Abate Life-Sustaining Treatment for Nonautonomous Patients: Ethical Standards and Legal Liability for Physicians After *Cruzan*." *JAMA* **1990**, *264*, 1846–53. See also the four brief articles by William Colby, Pete Busalacchi, Charles Baron, and Joanne Lynn and Jacqueline Glover in *Hastings Center Report* **1990**, *20* (September–October), 5–11.

10

Reproductive Issues

There is some disagreement about just when a pregnancy begins. Some think a woman is pregnant as soon as an ovum in her body is fertilized. This view, however, gives rise to several difficulties. First, since more than a third of fertilized ova fail to implant, it forces us to conclude that the number of spontaneous abortions is quite high—several million every year in the United States alone. Second, it conflicts with how we think about the embryo transfer that occurs during in vitro fertilization (IVF). No one considers a woman undergoing IVF procedures pregnant when the embryos are transferred to her uterus—she is considered pregnant only if one of the embryos implants. And when they fail to implant, which is more often the case, the failures are not considered miscarriages or spontaneous abortions, but unsuccessful pregnancy attempts.

For purposes of discussion, we will say pregnancy begins when a fertilized ovum implants in a woman's body. Pregnancy is something that happens to a woman, not an ovum. It seems reasonable to say that a woman becomes pregnant when her body "con-ceives" or "takes hold" of the fertilized ovum. The Latin etymology of "conception" is *concipio*, and the roots of *concipio* are *com* and *capio*. These roots indicate conception connotes a grasping, a laying hold of, a taking in. This suggests a pregnancy begins when the woman "conceives," that is, when her body grasps the fertilized ovum.

The decision to consider implantation the beginning of pregnancy does not mean the embryo is less than human before implantation. A human embryo is certainly a new human life before it implants, but the emergence of new human life does not mean a woman is pregnant. The human life of children resulting from IVF, for example, began in the laboratory, but their mothers did not become pregnant until the embryos were transferred and became attached to the uterus. The question of when a new human life begins and the question of when a pregnancy begins are two different questions. There is nothing inconsistent about saying that a new human life begins at fertilization, and also saying that the pregnancy does not begin until implantation. And, as we noted in chapter six, there is nothing inconsistent about saying that a new one of us does not begin until some time after both fertilization and implantation.

The destruction of an embryo before implantation, whether the embryo is in the laboratory or in the woman's body, is a morally significant action. The deliberate destruction of human life is a serious matter, and always immoral unless justified by an adequate reason. Destruction of an embryo before implantation, however, is not what we mean by abortion. Since abortion presupposes that a pregnancy has begun, destroying an embryo before implantation, however unethical it might be, is not really an abortion.

We will consider abortion in the next chapter. In this chapter we will examine the techniques and technologies affecting reproduction. In the first part we will look at the medical interventions designed to prevent pregnancy (that is, contraception and sterilization), and in the second part we will look at the medical interventions designed to cause pregnancy.

CONTRACEPTION AND STERILIZATION

Contraception—a better word might have been "contra-conception"—describes any behavior where the intention is to prevent pregnancy. Thus a condom or a tubal ligation is contraceptive, but so is abstinence or noncoital sex when the intention is to avoid pregnancy. In ordinary discourse, however, we usually associate contraception with heterosexual intercourse, and we use the term contraception to describe the effort to prevent conception resulting from heterosexual intercourse.

Some do not consider contraception and sterilization moral issues. Indeed, most modern moral philosophers and health care ethicists scarcely mention contraception and sterilization. If they do mention sterilization, their concern is coerced sterilization—the sterilization of the retarded, or of criminals, or of irresponsible mothers.

Yet there are at least three reasons why we should consider contraception and sterilization the subject of moral reflection. First, from its very beginning until the midtwentieth century, Christianity, the most influential religious tradition of our culture, always condemned contraception as immoral, and a few Christian churches still do. Since there is nothing in the Bible about contraception, thoughtful people will ask why Christians were so opposed to contraception.

Second, until recently, many states in the United States had laws condemning the distribution and, in some cases, the use of contraceptives. Since laws are passed by elected representatives of the people, the laws against selling or using contraceptives suggested that many people thought something was wrong with contraception.

Third, many contraceptive interventions, and all sterilization procedures, are medical interventions posing some risk to the person, and whenever we do anything that risks damage to life, we are faced with an ethical issue. We now know that some contraceptive interventions have caused serious damage to women. Many women, for example, suffered great harm from using the Dalkon Shield, a type of intrauterine device (IUD). Behavior that risks causing damage to life is ethical only if we have adequate or proportionate moral reasons to balance the risks.

Contraception in History

Contraception has a long history. Ancient Egyptian, Greek, and Latin texts all reveal attempts to prevent conception, some of them quite crude. Contraception was also the subject of some early ethical concerns, especially when the survival of a people depended on reproduction. In a society needing a high birth rate to survive, preventing pregnancy was sometimes seen as immoral because it undermined the social good.

By the second century the Romans, despite their toleration of infanticide and the exposure of unwanted children, had laws against the ingestion of drugs thought to prevent conception or cause miscarriage. The reason for these laws is not entirely clear. Certainly, the Romans were concerned about the declining birth rate in the better families as the empire deteriorated, but they may also have been concerned about the serious side effects women experienced from these rather crude, and often ineffective, drugs.

The Hebrew Bible emphasized having children, but said nothing about the immorality of preventing them by contraception, probably because it was not widely practiced. The book of *Genesis* encourages people to increase and multiply, and most of the great biblical heroes reproduced with both wives and concubines. The twelve sons of Judah destined to become the patriarchs of the twelve tribes of Israel, for example, were born of four women, two of them wives and two of them mistresses. And the Bible shows no discomfort with Solomon's many wives and concubines—both were numbered in the hundreds. With notable exceptions such as Jeremiah, the central biblical figures set an example of reproduction, not contraception, yet contraception was never explicitly condemned.

Some religious critics of contraception once pointed to the biblical story of Onan, a son of Judah, as an indication of God's displeasure with people who frustrate the reproductive aspect of sex. Onan had been told by his father Judah to have children with Thamar, the widow of his wicked older brother whom God had slain. Onan did not want children by Thamar, so when he engaged in sexual intercourse with her, he withdrew before ejaculating. "Onan knew that the children would not be his own, so whenever he had relations with his brother's wife, he wasted his seed on the ground, in order not to raise up descendents for his brother" (*Genesis* 38:9). God then punished Onan the same way he punished his brother—he struck him dead.

Was Onan punished because his sexual behavior was contraceptive? Over the centuries many thought so, including Pope Pius XI, who used the biblical story in his 1930 encyclical letter on Christian marriage to support his condemnation of contraception. Today, however, most biblical scholars do not think Onan's death was a punishment for contraception. Nor do many of them think, as some have suggested, that it was a punishment for disobeying a law that required sons to beget offspring with a dead brother's widow—that particular law did not come until much later. God seems to have killed Onan not because he practiced contraception or broke a law, but because he disobeyed his father, a major offense in a patriarchal society.

The early Christians did not continue the Hebrew emphasis on reproduction. In fact, many of them claimed that virginity was superior to fruitful marriage. Having a family was simply not a central Christian concern. Jesus, a Jew who neither married nor fathered a family, often encouraged his followers to leave their families and follow him. As for contraception itself, not a word about it is mentioned in the Christian scriptures; it is neither condemned nor condoned.

If neither the Hebrew Bible nor the Christian scriptures contain any texts proscribing contraception, why did so many Christians condemn it throughout the centuries, and why does a major religious denomination, the Roman

Catholic Church, continue to condemn it to this very day? The roots of the contraception condemnation are not in the Bible but in Stoicism, the most powerful moral philosophy in the Greek and Roman traditions.

Stoicism dominated the ancient world from about 300 B.C.E. until Christianity began to emerge in 350 C.E. as the dominant religion of the vast Roman Empire. Two fundamental features of Stoic philosophy paved the way for a negative moral judgment about contraception. First, Stoics emphasized nature as the norm of morality. Living and behaving morally meant living and behaving according to nature. Second, they thought nature was imbued with reason, what the Greek Stoics called *logos*. Moral behavior is behavior according to reason, not behavior spawned by emotion or passion.

For the Stoic, then, sex will be moral when it is undertaken (1) according to its natural design and (2) in accord with reason, not passion. The morally good Stoic will not introduce into sexual intercourse any intervention contrary to nature and will not seek sex for passion or for pleasure, but for a reason, and the most obvious reason for sexual intercourse is reproduction. On two counts, then, the Stoic ethic was anticontraceptive: contraception is artificial, not natural, and contraception indicates that the sexual activity springs from passion rather than its purpose—reproduction.

The influence of Stoicism on Christianity was greater than is often realized. Much of it was subtle, but there are some explicit references. For example, a prominent early Christian writer, St. Jerome (340–420), quoted with approval the Stoic philosopher Seneca, as saying that a wise man ought not to love his wife with affection, but with judgment, and that nothing is more foul than for a man to love his wife like one loves an adulteress (that is, with passion but without the desire for children).

The person most responsible for shaping the traditional Christian theology that condemned contraception and permitted sexual activity only for reproductive purposes, however, was not Jerome but Augustine (354–431). Augustine converted to Christianity in his thirties. Before his conversion, he had lived with a woman for over a decade and fathered a child. He dismissed this woman, the mother of his son, when his mother selected another woman, a girl of about thirteen, for him to marry. While waiting for her to mature, however, he converted to Christianity and embraced a celibate life. He became a priest and later a bishop. He wrote numerous theological works, although he is probably best known for his rather personal *Confessions*, a moving story of his conversion that is widely read to this day.

In his book on marriage (*The Good of Marriage*) Augustine drew a parallel between eating and sex. The reason for eating is survival and, as long as we are eating to survive, we may enjoy whatever pleasure eating provides. Similarly, the reason for sex is pregnancy and, as long as married couples are engaging in sex for pregnancy, they may also enjoy whatever pleasure sexual intercourse provides. All sex initiated when pregnancy is not the goal, even sex between husband and wife, is morally defective because it lacks the reproductive purpose. In *The Good of Marriage* Augustine wrote that an unmarried woman having intercourse in order to have a child sins less than a married woman having marital intercourse with the hope of avoiding pregnancy.

Underlying Augustine's theology of sexuality, which was to dominate Christianity for a thousand years and which casts a shadow over some Christian theology to this day, is his rather idiosyncratic interpretation of *Genesis* 2:18. This biblical text depicts God creating the first woman, Eve, after noting it was not good for man to be alone. Augustine asked why it was not good for man to be alone, and what help a woman could possibly provide for for man. And he replied: "I do not see what other help woman would be to man if the purpose of generating were eliminated." In other words, the existence of women is helpful only for their role in reproduction. Augustine understood both sex and the creation of women in terms of the same purpose: pregnancy. In such a theology there is clearly no room for contraception. The only thing that justifies sex is reproduction; in fact, the only thing that justifies the existence of women is reproduction.

In his later book, *On Marriage and Concupiscence*, Augustine explained how sexual passion, what he called lust or concupiscence, is the effect of Adam's "original sin." He was convinced that God's original plan of human reproduction, even though it would have involved man and woman, did not require sexual arousal—that is, lust or concupiscence—on the part of either the woman or the man. Adam's original sin ruined all this, and so lust, Augustine thought, unfortunately now accompanies, at least in the male, sexual intercourse. Augustine also claimed, in *On Marriage and Concupiscence*, that the lust involved in intercourse is the specific disorder in the reproductive act that transmits Adam's sin to what will become a new human being. In his theology, every new human life begins in sin, an original sin that only the waters of Christian baptism can wash away.

Thus two bad features mark sexual intercourse—the concupiscence, a disorder caused by Adam's sin, and the transmission of Adam's sin to the embryo. Since every act of intercourse arouses concupiscence and multiplies sin in the world, it is something everyone should avoid unless there is an overwhelming reason for engaging in it. And there is one such reason, and only one: reproduction. Sexual intercourse is a terribly flawed action justified only for one reason, the intention to cause pregnancy, for without pregnancies the human species will die out.

There is no room for contraception or sterilization in such a theology. And, not surprisingly, we find an explicit condemnation of them in *On Marriage and Concupiscence*. Those trying to prevent pregnancy ". . . although they be called husband and wife, are not; nor do they retain any reality of marriage, but use the respectable name (of marriage) to cover a shame. . .Sometimes this lustful cruelty, or cruel lust, comes to this, that they even use sterilizing drugs . . ." The phrase "sterilizing drugs" (*sterilitatis venena*) was to become the central phrase used in almost all the theological and ecclesiastical texts condemning contraception and birth control for the next thousand years. Augustine reinforced his argument against contraception by recalling the story of Onan, whose efforts to avoid pregnancy were, according to Augustine's mistaken reading of the story, punished by God.

The condemnation of contraception continued in Christian moral theology throughout the Middle Ages. We find it in the penitential books that guided priests hearing confessions, in the legal decrees of the Roman Catholic Church, the church that dominated religious life in Europe from the fourth century until the sixteenth century, and in the writings of the philosophers and theologians teaching in the universities. The fundamental idea underlying the condemnation of contraception was always the Stoic argument from nature or natural law—contraceptive behavior is against nature, and morality is always "according to nature" or "according to the natural law." Furthermore, for the Christian, nature was designed and created by God, and thus contraception, a violation of nature, is also an act against God. Contraception is not only a crime against nature, but a rebellion against God's will; it is both unnatural and sinful.

By the sixteenth century, the original Stoic–Christian position against contraception came under increasing attack. A growing number of people, including some Christian theologians, began wondering whether contraception was always immoral. The Roman Catholic Church, however, stood firm. The great Council of Trent (1545–1563), called to reform abuses in this church and to clarify its position against the new Christian churches springing up in the Protestant reformation of Christianity, produced an official catechism. Unlike theological tomes read mostly by specialists, catechisms are used to educate the people at large about the central tenets of the Catholic faith. This catechism appeared in 1566 and, as might be expected, condemned contraception. But that is not all—the catechism considered contraception a form of homicide (that is, it equated it with murder). Lest this very strict position be overlooked, the editor-in-chief of the catechism, St. Charles Borremeo, issued a commentary on the catechism explaining how contraception is a sin against the biblical commandment "Thou shalt not kill." This placed contraception in the same moral category as murder.

The effort to consider contraception an act of homicide was renewed by Pope Sixtus V in 1588. He condemned both abortion and contraception, calling them murder, and advocated both excommunication from the church and the death penalty for those convicted of these crimes. Many theologians dissented from this extremely rigid papal teaching, and shortly after Sixtus's death a few years later, his successor repealed most of the penalties for contraception, while continuing to insist it was sinful.

Contraception and Christianity in This Century

Although some Christians continued to wonder whether contraception and sterilization were always immoral, most Christian churches maintained their absolute prohibition of contraception until the twentieth century, when a shift began to occur. The Church of England, the Anglican Catholic Church, had condemned artificial contraception in the Lambeth Conferences of 1908 and 1920. In the Lambeth Conference of 1930, however, the Anglicans reversed their position, holding that artificial birth control is ethical if practiced for morally sound reasons and if it is not motivated by selfishness.

Many other Christian denominations soon followed the Anglicans, and by 1959 the World Council of Churches took an official position, advising Christian couples that responsible parents should consider many factors, including the population problems of their region, in the decision to reproduce.

The World Council of Churches also took the position that once a responsible decision was made not to have a child, any appropriate method could be used. In other words, the World Council of Churches saw no moral difference between natural family planning, artificial barrier methods (condoms, etc.), sterilization, and anovulant drugs (birth control pills).

In 1930 the Roman Catholic Church also made a significant change in its centuries-old opposition to contraception. In the 1920s it was definitively established by medical science that a woman is fertile for only a few days each menstrual cycle, and that these days occur about two weeks after menses. This had been suspected for some time, but never established by scientific evidence. Now that the cycles of fertility were better understood a new question arose: is it moral for married couples to abstain from sex voluntarily during fertile days in order to avoid pregnancy? If they avoid fertile periods, there will be no pregnancy, yet no "unnatural" sexual behavior is involved. Is such behavior moral?

In 1930 somewhat surprisingly, Pope Pius XI officially stated that intercourse deliberately undertaken during the infertile periods before and after ovulation in order to avoid pregnancy was not contrary to the order of nature, and therefore could be practiced if there was a good reason for it. This represented a major change in traditional Roman Catholic teaching; the older theology had always insisted on the link between the purpose of sex (pregnancy) and the act itself. Now the Pope was saying that a couple, for a good reason, could deliberately choose to have sexual intercourse only during the infertile periods for the purpose of preventing pregnancy.

The deliberate effort to prevent pregnancy by having sexual intercourse during the infertile periods before and after ovulation was first called "periodic continence" or "the rhythm method;" today the practice is more commonly known as "natural family planning."

Although the acceptance of deliberate but natural family planning represented a significant change in the traditional Catholic linkage of sex and reproduction, there was no change in the Catholic teachings against other ways of planning families (artificial contraception). All the traditional prohibitions against artificial birth control remained in force.

In the 1950s the controversy over birth control in the Christian churches rekindled with the development of "the Pill." The birth control pill prevents pregnancy by preventing ovulation. Most Christian churches had no trouble accepting it, and a number of Roman Catholic theologians suggested the birth control pill could be accepted by the Roman Catholic Church as well. They argued that sexual intercourse was performed in a perfectly natural manner when a woman was "on the Pill." Using the birth control pill was therefore not that much different from the approved rhythm method or natural family planning.

In 1963 Pope John XXIII set up a commission to study questions of population in the world, something now recognized as a serious problem on the planet. The commission's investigations naturally led to questions of controlling births, and thus opened up the whole issue of contraception. Some church leaders urged that the question should be debated at the Second Vatican Council that was meeting at the time (1962–1965), but Pope Paul

VI ordered the question of contraception kept off the agenda. In 1966 the commission gave the Pope its findings: by a large majority it concluded that artificial contraception was contrary neither to Christian morality nor to the natural law. The commission acknowledged that contraception could be selfish and thus sinful, but that it need not be if there were good reasons for limiting births.

In 1968 Pope Paul VI published the official Roman Catholic teaching on artificial contraception and sterilization in an encyclical letter entitled *Humanae Vitae*. The Pope rejected the findings of the papal commission and repeated the centuries-old position: all forms of artificial contraception, including the Pill, are immoral.

He also rejected the commission's view that nothing in natural law shows that contraception is immoral. He argued this way: Jesus made Peter and the Apostles the authentic interpreters of all moral laws, both the law of the Gospel and the law of nature. The Pope and the bishops are the successors of Peter and the Apostles, so they are the authentic interpreters of the natural law today. According to their authentic interpretation, the natural law does forbid all forms of artificial contraception.

By saying the natural law, and not just church discipline, forbids contraception, the Pope was saying artificial contraception is immoral not only for Roman Catholics, but for all human beings. This is so because the heart of the natural law doctrine is that all human beings are subject to it.

The idea that religious authority is needed to provide authentic interpretations of the natural law was a rather startling departure from the centuries-old tradition of natural law in philosophy and in Roman Catholic theology itself. Although natural law can be understood a number of different ways, a key feature running through all the different versions is that it is knowable by *natural* reason; that is, it can be discerned by people using their own resources of understanding. Neither religious revelation nor religious authority is needed for us to know what natural law requires; it is natural precisely because it is discoverable by the natural reflection of intelligent people of good will. Biblical revelation and ecclesiastical authority were always understood as complementary to the natural law, but they were not needed to know what natural law allows and forbids. The whole point of "natural" law was that people could discern it by their natural powers of understanding and interpretation.

In the 1950s, however, some Catholic theologians had begun to back away from this traditional view of the natural law, largely due to the growing controversies over birth control. The more astute among them realized that no explicit natural law arguments against contraception exist. Thus some began to argue that human beings cannot always discern the natural law by natural reason alone, but need the Roman Catholic Church to explain it to them. In his influential *Medico–Moral Problems*, published in 1958, the prominent American theologian Gerald Kelley wrote: "Rather frequently, circumstances have made it necessary for the Holy See to explain the natural law as it applies to medical problems . . . the Church not only claims divine authorization to interpret the moral law; it also claims that its teachings are a practical necessity for a clear and adequate knowledge of this law."

Ten years later this idea—that in practice we cannot know some aspects of the natural law by unaided human reason but need guidance from the Pope—reappeared as the crucial rationale for the papal condemnation of artificial contraception. In the final analysis, then, the natural law is not so natural after all. In some cases, and contraception is one of them, it has to be interpreted by the Pope, and his interpretations are the authentic and authoritative interpretations binding for all human beings. Needless to say, many supporters of a natural law ethic, especially those not of the Catholic faith, have trouble accepting this view of the natural law. And of course many moralists, especially those of the past few centuries, do not take a natural law approach to ethics.

This detour into a consideration of artificial contraception, and the traditional Christian stance against it, may seem a little out of place in a text on health care ethics. After all, most people today do not consider birth control a moral issue. The failure to see contraception as a moral issue, however, is an unfortunate, if all too familiar, tendency in medicine to ignore the moral significance of reproductive questions. In recent years techniques were developed to prevent pregnancy, people wanted them, and so physicians provided them. And techniques were developed to enhance the chance of pregnancy, people wanted them, and so physicians provided them. But few people, until recently, saw the moral implications of these interventions.

Whether one agrees with the Roman Catholic Church or with the Church of England and the World Council of Churches on artificial contraception, at least their statements serve as a reminder that artificial contraception, and sterilization as well, raise moral issues. Interfering with the normal reproductive process is not a morally neutral activity.

And it is important, in a text on health care ethics, to ask what underlies the traditional Christian position against artificial birth control. The ideas prompting the traditional religious prohibitions of contraception are of historical interest even today.

First, in a time when sex was considered mostly from the male viewpoint, and chiefly as an outlet for passion, the effort of many people, among them the Stoics, was directed toward humanizing the sex drive. Philosophers and theologians were convinced men should not simply use women to satisfy their sexual hunger. Looking for a way to dignify human sexuality, they tried to link it with an environment of responsibility, the family.

Insisting on the link between sexual passion and family is a major factor in the humanization of sex. It elevates human sex above sexual activity in the forest and in the barnyard. The man having sexual intercourse with the intention of having a child is having intercourse with the woman he wants to be the mother of his child, and this generates a respect for her that would not be there if his actions were motivated by pure sexual need.

Second, the traditional Christian stance against contraception reminds us of the bad features associated with most contraceptive interventions. Many contraceptive interventions entail risks of unwanted side effects. Many of the early efforts to prevent conception caused health problems for women. Advances in medicine have reduced these problems significantly, but not completely. Surgeries that sterilize by tubal ligation or vasectomy, IUDs, anovulant pills, and Norplant are all medically controlled contraceptive techniques with some degree of risk, and the bad features have to be recognized in an ethics of right reason. In fact, almost anything done to prevent a pregnancy, even the use of a condom, introduces a disorder into sexual intercourse.

Morality urges us to avoid disorders in human behavior unless we have an appropriate reason to justify them. The traditional Christian prohibition against contraception reminds us that we cannot simply charge ahead and engage in contraceptive practices without thinking about the impact they will have on our lives. Specifically, we have to ask whether the interventions will truly contribute to individual and social human goods or undermine them; that is, whether contraceptive interventions are moral or immoral.

Contraception and the Law

The Christian churches were not the only major opposition to birth control in our culture; until recently, laws in many states restricted contraception. The ease with which people can obtain contraceptive devices and medical interventions in our country today is a relatively new phenomenon. Not so long ago the distribution and even the use of contraceptives were illegal in many places. The fact that these laws existed until recently is one more reminder that many of our predecessors thought something was wrong with contraception.

The laws banning contraceptives came under attack in the middle of this century, shortly after most of the Christian denominations accepted the morality of contraception. In 1961 a pharmacist in Connecticut challenged the state laws in a case before the U.S. Supreme Court known as *Poe v. Ullman*. Although the court dismissed the case on technical grounds, two justices dissented. They believed that the Connecticut law against contraception violated the constitutional right of privacy, and therefore should have been examined by the court. One dissenting justice, Justice Douglas, feared that the law banning contraceptives would lead to an intolerable situation: since it is the duty of police to enforce laws, we might ". . . reach the point where . . . officers appeared in bedrooms to find out what went on." Justice Harlan, the other dissenting justice, echoed the same concern for privacy.

It is important to note that Justice Harlan did not favor overturning the Connecticut law against contraceptives because he thought that contraception was morally acceptable. On the contrary, he was convinced that contraception was immoral and encouraged such "dissolute actions" as fornication and adultery. His only concern was that he thought it unwise to bring ". . . the whole machinery of the criminal law into the very heart of marital privacy, requiring husband and wife to render account before a criminal tribunal of their uses of that intimacy." The key word here is privacy; Harlan thought laws against contraceptives were bad because they make an intimate and private matter—what married couples do when they have sexual intercourse—a subject for criminal investigation and prosecution.

In 1965 Connecticut's law banning contraceptives was again challenged, this time in a famous case known as *Griswold v. Connecticut*. Under state law, Connecticut had imposed a criminal penalty on a physician for prescribing contraceptives for a married couple because he thought a pregnancy would be dangerous for the woman. The U.S. Supreme Court struck down the Connecticut law, explicitly recognizing a constitutional right of privacy, a right that was to play a major role eight years later in the even more famous *Roe v. Wade* abortion decision. Since *Griswold*, states can no longer prohibit married couples from using contraceptives because such a ban would "allow the police to search the sacred precincts of marital bedrooms for telltale signs of the use of contraceptives." In other words, using contraceptives is wrong, but invading the bedroom to enforce the law is a greater wrong because it would violate the couple's right to privacy during sexual intercourse.

This decision did not end the court battles about contraception. A few years later an outspoken advocate of birth control, Bill Baird, was arrested in Massachusetts for distributing contraceptives to anyone who wanted them. The Massachusetts law differed from the Connecticut law struck down in *Griswold* in two ways: it banned the distribution and sale of contraceptives, not their use, thus avoiding the repulsive idea of police checking whether people are using contraceptives when they have intercourse, and it banned the distribution of contraceptives only to unmarried people.

In the 1972 case known as *Eisenstadt v. Baird*, the U.S. Supreme Court struck down the Massachusetts law prohibiting the distribution of contraceptives to unmarried people. "If the right of privacy means anything, it is the right of the *individual*, married or single, to be free from unwarranted governmental intrusion into matters so fundamentally affecting a person as the decision whether to bear or beget a child." As the result of this decision, states cannot prevent the distribution of contraceptives to any adult, married or single.

In 1977 the U.S. Supreme Court struck down still another law restricting the distribution of contraceptives. New York had a law prohibiting the sale or distribution of contraceptives to minors under the age of sixteen. In its decision overturning this law, a decision known as *Carey v. Population Services International*, the court emphasized that ". . . the Constitution protects individual decisions in matters of childbearing from unjustified intrusion by the State." As the result of this decision, states cannot restrict the distribution of contraceptives to minors.

Several points emerge from this brief review of three U.S. Supreme Court decisions involving contraception. First, they remind us that many state legislatures had enacted laws against contraception, even for married people. The laws never could have existed unless a good number of elected representatives believed that there was something wrong with contraception.

Second, the court never disagreed with this view; it never said contraception was not immoral. It invalidated Connecticut's law because it was unenforceable without having police officers in the bedroom, and it invalidated the Massachusetts and New York laws because it thought the decision of individuals to have children is a private matter they should be able to pursue without government intrusion, regardless of whether they are unmarried or under sixteen years of age. The court never invalidated the laws prohibiting contraception because those laws incorrectly implied contraception was wrong; it invalidated the laws restricting contraception because these laws violated people's privacy.

The many laws against contraception remind us, as does the traditional Christian stance against it (and undoubtedly the two prohibitions are related), that in many people's minds contraception was immoral and should be illegal. The very fact so many people once considered contraception wrong helps to make us aware that moral issues might well be involved in contraceptive behavior.

Contraception and Ethics

Today a variety of contraceptive methods are available. They raise a special set of ethical issues in health care. Unlike standard medical treatments that are intended to correct what is dysfunctional, contraceptive medical interventions are intended to cause the dysfunction of what is functioning properly. Such interventions are morally acceptable only if they are justified by adequate reasons.

The most popular forms of contraception today are the following.

Sterilization by tubal ligation or by vasectomy.

Short-term barriers such as male and female condoms, diaphragms, cervical caps, contraceptive sponges, and spermicides.

Long-term barriers such as the intrauterine devices (IUDs). Some are effective up to six years; others for a year or more.

Anovulants, which include (1) birth control pills, providing protection against pregnancy a month at a time; (2) injections of Depo-Provera, providing protection for three to four months at a time; and (3) Norplant capsules implanted in the upper arm, providing protection for up to five years.

Antiprogestin drugs such as RU 486 that can be used as a contraceptive to prevent uterine implantation of embryos. Since the major use of RU 486 is to dislodge implanted embryos, we will consider this drug in the section on abortion. Depo-Provera also has an antiprogestin effect on the uterus.

The moral implications of these interventions are not all equal. Using an IUD or RU 486 to prevent the implantation of an embryo is more morally serious than using a barrier to prevent fertilization or using anovulant drugs to prevent ovulation. And permanent surgical sterilization is more morally serious than various reversible methods of contraception.

But the key ethical issue in these interventions is when, if ever, they contribute to the human good of the couple and of society despite the disorder they introduce into the reproductive physiology, and despite the risks and side effects that accompany most of them.

In deliberating about the morality of various contraceptive interventions, the following points may be helpful.

First, we now accord love in general, and sexual love in particular, a much more important role than did earlier peoples, who tended to see marriage in terms of children, social standing, political advantage, etc., and sex in terms of appetite and lust. Perhaps the greatest sign of this is the assumption we all make that we can simply choose our mates, and that we will mate with the one we love. In earlier times parents arranged marriages, and love was not a crucial factor. ·

The personal history Augustine records in his *Confessions* sums up the earlier practice: his mother picked a girl for him to marry, so he dismissed the woman he said he loved and with whom he had lived, with their son, for over a decade. And he saw nothing wrong with this. In those days, parents played a much larger role than love in their child's marriage, and the parents were more interested in the impact of the new in-law on the family than in the romantic love life of their child. To this day, many marriage ceremonies retain a trace of parental control in the ritual whereby the father of the bride "gives her away" to the man she is about to marry, implying she could not go to him, even if she loved him, without her father's permission.

And we consider sexual love a much more important part of human dignity than did our cultural ancestors. They tended to separate body and soul, and to see sex as an appetite of the body and a threat to the life of the soul. Today we do not think sexuality is a merely animal appetite or a disorder caused by the original sin of Adam; we understand it rather as an integral aspect of intimate human love when caring, commitment, and trust are present. And once the important role of sexuality in human love is appreciated, the traditional idea that every sexual act is morally acceptable only if it is open to pregnancy loses much of its cogency.

Second, we now live in a time when overpopulation is undermining human life in many areas of the world. What is now clear to us, and what was never dreamed of by our ancestors, is that without some form of birth control, the human population will one day overwhelm the planet. There is no serious disagreement about the need for birth control; the disagreement is whether natural family planning will be sufficiently effective or whether artificial methods of birth control will be needed to prevent the human misery and famine exacerbated by overpopulation. At this point in history, there is no evidence that abstinence or natural family planning will work, especially in those parts of the world where the population problems are most serious.

Third, contraception is not, considered in itself, something good. Contraceptive behavior, even natural family planning, is always a disorder, a bad feature, in sexual intimacy. Thus the argument is not between those who say contraception is always wrong and those who say contraception is good. It is, rather, between those who say contraception is always a moral evil and those who say it is always bad, but not a moral evil whenever there are sufficient reasons for introducing it into the interpersonal relationship.

Fourth, it is well to remember that contraception can be a moral evil, that is, unethical. This is so when it is motivated not by a seeking of the human good but by selfishness. It becomes a moral evil when it enables one to pursue more comfortably irresponsible and promiscuous sexual activity, or when it encourages people to make sex trivial, or reduces intercourse to lust without any caring.

Fifth, the morality of contraception can best be determined by considering the question as but one aspect of the entire interpersonal relationship.

Ethical reflection will therefore focus on the people in the relationship, on their history and circumstances, on their children, and on their present and future needs. It will also consider the good of society, a good that can change with the times. Today, for example, overpopulation threatens many parts of the world, whereas for most of human history underpopulation was the problem. Underpopulation suggests the reasonableness of prohibitions against artificial contraception; overpopulation suggests the opposite.

Sixth, any consideration of the ethics of contraception cannot ignore our present knowledge about human sexual biology, something our predecessors did not have. We are now aware of the high degree of randomness involved in the beginning of a new human life. We know hundreds of thousands of spermatozoa advance toward an egg that will normally accept only one, if any. At the moment each of us began as a fertilized egg, we know that if any other spermatozoon had fertilized that egg, the baby born nine months later would not have been the person each of us is. The immense statistical odds against any specific person being conceived and born means the interventions to regulate conception will not appear as unreasonable to us as they would to many of our ancestors, who thought contraception prevented a specific predestined child from being conceived. It was their ignorance of how human life begins that led some of them to draw an analogy between contraception and abortion, or between contraception and homicide.

Seventh, any moral deliberation about contraception cannot ignore how unexpected pregnancy can undermine the emancipation of women in society. As more and more women see their role in life expanding beyond that of wife and mother, the control of pregnancy becomes more important and more reasonable.

Finally, we are increasingly aware that longer life spans are making pregnancy and parenthood an ever-smaller chapter in a marriage. Reproduction is an important chapter in most marriages, but not the most important one. Most parents now live long after the children are gone, and this longevity reminds us that the primary players in marriage are not the children but the couple. The strength of the marriage bond is not primarily the children but the depth of the spouses' love and affection for each other, a love and affection embodied in sexual love. The intimacy of sexual love in the relationship is always for the partners, and only sometimes for pregnancy.

Although contraception is a moral issue and is sometimes contrary to the good of those practicing it and of society, no blanket condemnation of it is consistent with an ethics of right reason, where right reason denotes what will achieve the person's good. In our culture, the only remaining major condemnation of all directly intended sterilization and artificial birth control comes from a few religious leaders. For some believers, this is enough. For nonbelievers, and for many believers, it is not.

The intent in this section was to raise consciousness about the moral seriousness of contraception and sterilization and to enable us to situate the necessary moral deliberation in a historical context. This may help us reflect in a morally serious way on the paradigm case of contraception—the couple wishing to limit or avoid pregnancies in their relationship—as well as on numerous subsidiary issues. Some of these subsidiary issues are the following.

1. Some public schools are now dispensing contraceptives. The most common types are condoms and birth control pills, but some high schools have begun offering surgically implanted Norplant capsules for girls who want them. Distribution of contraceptives in high schools upsets many people and needs more reflection and dialogue.

2. A few courts are suggesting or ordering sterilization in criminal cases involving violent sex offenders. This demands serious ethical deliberation.

3. There is public pressure for sterilization. Some, for example, think women supported by public funds who continue to have children by unknown fathers, thus adding people to the welfare rolls, should be asked to accept sterilization as a condition of future welfare support.

4. Many hospitals sponsored by a religious organization opposed to contraception refuse to allow any sterilizations intended to prevent pregnancy, or any other contraceptive interventions. When the hospital is the only one available to people in the area, this refusal puts a serious burden on patients and physicians who are convinced these interventions are medically and morally justified in particular situations. In some cases, it results in needless surgical interventions. For example, when a woman in poor health with a large family requests in good faith a tubal ligation during a cesarean section, and the hospital rules will not allow it, she has to undergo another surgery for the ligation a few weeks later at another hospital.

5. Some suggest the sterilization of mentally challenged women who enjoy some degree of social freedom. The idea is to prevent them becoming pregnant by men taking advantage of them because they are not mentally and emotionally mature enough to avoid intercourse.

Issues such as these are the subject of intense debate in some quarters. In the ethical approach we have been suggesting in this text, the morality or immorality of contraception will be determined by whether or not the intervention, with its inherent disorder, risks, and side effects, is justified by moral reasons showing that the alternatives to contraception will do even more harm to the good life of the moral agents involved.

We turn next to the other side of the reproductive issue, and ask about the new techniques and technologies designed not to prevent, but to cause pregnancy.

MEDICALLY ASSISTED PREGNANCY

We will now discuss the most popular methods of artificial reproductive technologies and some of the ethical issues they raise.

Artificial Insemination

Artificial insemination (AI) was the first major success in assisted reproduction. A little over 200 years ago, the Italian priest Lazaro Spallanzani began artificially inseminating frogs and dogs. In 1790 a surgeon in Scotland successfully inseminated a woman with her husband's sperm, and the practice slowly began to spread.

It was not until the 1960s, however, that artificial insemination became popular in our country. It began as a treatment designed to correct infertility in married women when intercourse was impossible, or when the husband had a low sperm count. Before long, sperm from other men was also used. Sometimes it was added to the sperm of a husband with low sperm count, at other times it was the only sperm used.

Eventually, heterosexual women without a partner, and lesbian women with no desire for a male sexual partner, sought and received AI. This created a new kind of situation because the medical intervention in these cases cannot be considered a treatment for infertility—most of these woman are quite fertile. For this reason, as well as for concern for children deliberately conceived outside of marriage, some medical facilities decline to provide AI in these circumstances.

The man providing the sperm for AI is called a donor. If he is not the husband, however, the word is misleading. Sperm provided by third parties is not donated but sold to the physician or to a sperm bank. Usually the man remains anonymous so the mother and child do not know, and often can never know, the identity of the father. The father's genetic characteristics, however, are usually available to the woman using the commercial sperm.

AI is the most widely used reproductive assistance at the present time, playing a role in more than thirty thousand pregnancies a year in the United States alone. Some AI is done within marriage, but there are about seventy commercial sperm banks supplying more than three hundred AI clinics in the United States. The sperm banks advertise for sperm in various publications, including college newspapers. A recent advertisement in the Harvard Crimson, for example, promised $105 per week ($35 per sample) to qualified students providing sperm for artificial insemination.

AI is a relatively simple and inexpensive procedure. Sperm is obtained, usually by masturbation, and then inserted into the uterus during ovulation. To prevent transmission of disease, sperm from donors is tested for HIV and other problems. Some sperm banks now freeze the sperm for six months, and test the sellers' blood, semen, and urine monthly during this time for disease and drug use.

When the practice of AI using sperm bought from third parties or strangers became popular thirty years ago, little attention was paid to its ethical implications. People proceeded as if no moral issues were involved. Now there is increasing awareness that the procedure is not morally neutral, and the possibility that it can be the source of serious harms must be considered.

First, there is the matter of selling sperm by anonymous men who accept no legal or personal responsibility for their genetic offspring. While this does not seem to harm most men providing the sperm, there are indications that children born of AI can be distressed about their origins in the world. They come to know that half of their genetic material came from a father who provided it not in an act of sexual intimacy but as a commercial transaction, that the man has no interest in knowing or caring about them, and that he in all probability has so masked his identity that they will never know who he is.

Moreover, children of AI by an anonymous seller of sperm can face potential problems when they begin to mate. Since some men have donated sperm numerous times in the same geographical area, it is possible that people with the same father could unknowingly marry. This can create genetic as well as emotional difficulties because people conceived by AI are aware they might be marrying a half-sister or a half-brother. Other unhappy combinations are also possible. For example, a woman might someday marry the anonymous donor who provided the sperm used in the insemination of her mother, and thus find herself married to her father.

Some have suggested that the anonymity of the father in AI is akin to adoption, and most people accept adoption as a morally respectable procedure. But there is an important difference between AI with purchased sperm and adoption. In adoption, the child already exists and the adoption is an attempt to compensate for the breakdown of the family structure. The whole motivation behind the moral acceptance of adoption is that, in some difficult situations, it is good for the child who is already here. In AI, on the contrary, there is no child whose best interests are at stake. Rather, there is a deliberate effort to father a child by a man not related to the mother in any way, and most often that man will deliberately remain anonymous and uninterested in his genetic offspring. Adoption is an attempt to help a child born into a less than ideal situation; AI with purchased sperm is a deliberate attempt to produce a child with an unknown and disinterested genetic father.

Second, additional ethical issues arise with AI when the woman is not married. A woman without a partner may intensely desire pregnancy, but the long-term effects of children intentionally born to a single parent are not yet known. Most people do think, however, that children are better off and that the society is stronger if children have traditional family support, although many different versions of "family" have existed in history and continue to exist today. Children born of a lesbian woman may face additional problems in a society still uncomfortable with homosexuality when the sexual orientation of the mother becomes known by other children. Children are not always without cruelty when it comes to isolating their peers who may have an idiosyncratic feature in their lives.

For AI within marriage, using the husband's sperm, few ethical problems exist. Here the couple is simply trying to overcome a fertility problem and have a family. Even here, however, some see an ethical issue in the procedure used to obtain the husband's sperm. The Roman Catholic Church, for example, has a long-standing position that masturbation is a serious moral wrong, even for the purpose of producing a pregnancy. To avoid the sin of masturbation, some theologians suggest that the couple have intercourse using a condom with holes in it. By using a perforated condom during intercourse, the husband is not masturbating, nor is he practicing birth control because a sufficient quantity of sperm will escape from the condom into the vagina. After the sperm trapped in the condom is retrieved, the woman takes it to her physician, who then inseminates her as with any AI procedure. Other Catholic theologians do not agree with this position, and argue that Catholic husbands could masturbate to obtain sperm for reasons such as fertility treatments or medical diagnosis.

In Vitro Fertilization (IVF)

In 1978, after years of research, the first "test tube" baby, Louise Brown, was born in England. Since that time, more than 20,000 babies have begun life through fertilization in a petri dish, and more than 200 clinics now offer IVF in the United States. The first baby conceived by IVF in the United States was born in Norfolk, Virginia, late in 1981.

There are four major steps in the IVF process:

1. *Ovulation induction*. Before the procedure, hormonal products are injected into the woman to stimulate follicle growth and to prepare the eggs for retrieval at the proper time. This progress is monitored by ultrasound and blood tests to determine when ovulation is about to occur.

2. *Egg retrieval*. Two major options exist for the retrieval of the eggs: laparoscopy and vaginal ultrasound. In laparoscopy, several small incisions are made under a light general anesthesia in the abdominal wall so three instruments can be inserted. The first is a scope so the physician can see inside the abdominal cavity, the second is a device to grasp the ovary, and the third is a hollow needle to suck up the ripened eggs from the ovarian follicles. In vaginal ultrasound, either a local or spinal anesthesia is given, and an ultrasound probe with a sheathed hollow needle is inserted into the vagina. The physician, guided by the ultrasound picture on the monitor, then passes the needle through the vaginal wall to reach the ovary and suck out the ripened eggs. After the laparoscopy or the vaginal ultrasound, the retrieved eggs are immediately transferred to an adjoining laboratory, treated, and placed in a special fluid for several hours. The patient leaves the IVF center when the retrieval is completed.

3. *Fertilization*. The semen obtained from the husband (or from a commercial sperm supplier) is brought to the laboratory, washed, and prepared for fertilization. Then concentrated sperm is added to each petri dish and, if all goes well, a spermatozoon fertilizes the egg in the petri dish or "test tube." In 1993 physicians began capturing the tiny spermatozoon and then injecting it directly into an egg. This new procedure, called direct egg injection, promises to increase the chances of fertilization, especially when the spermatozoa have been unable or slow to penetrate ova. Once fertilized, the eggs are allowed to develop for about 48 hours. Then the woman returns to the hospital or clinic for the fourth step.

4. *Embryo transfer* (ET). A number of fertilized ova, usually four, are inserted through the cervix into the uterus that has been prepared by yet another injection to ripen it for implantation of the embryo. Most of the time none of the embryos will implant, but there is a chance of about one in five that one will. Occasionally several will implant, and then multiple births result. At the time of the transfer the embryo has about eight cells, considerably fewer than a normal embryo has when it arrives in the uterus.

Among the ethical concerns about IVF are the following.

1. Some people, most notably some religious leaders, have moral objections to obtaining sperm for IVF procedures by masturbation.

2. Some people have moral objections to a human fertilization process that occurs apart from sexual intercourse and outside the human body. They find the idea of a new human life beginning in a laboratory morally objectionable because they believe it degrades human dignity. Some of them argue that it violates a human right, the right of every child to be conceived naturally. The rights-based argument is problematic—it is difficult to claim that someone had a right before he becomes a someone; that is, to claim a child had a right before the fertilization that led to the child took place.

3. Many people think that IVF for married couples is ethical, but they have moral objections to using the fertility treatments for unmarried women. This is especially true if there is no fertility problem, and the IVF is used simply because the woman does not have (or does not want) a partner to father her child. They object for two reasons: (1) they see no cogent reason to use a fertility treatment when there is no infertility, and (2) they do not think it is good to cause a pregnancy deliberately outside the traditional family relationship of husband and wife. In IVF, it is possible to use purchased sperm and purchased eggs, and to transfer the embryo to a third party with no genetic or social relationship to the child. Thus, in a worst case scenario, adults may deliberately arrange for a future child to have many parents, perhaps as many as five: the man and woman raising the child, the man selling his sperm (the genetic father), the woman selling her egg (the genetic mother), and the woman receiving money for carrying the child in pregnancy (the gestational mother). The confusion of parenthood when IVF is extended beyond married couples using their own sperm and ova is a serious ethical concern.

Another twist to using ova from third parties surfaced in 1993 when it was reported that eggs could be retrieved from aborted fetuses, nourished so they would mature quickly, then fertilized by an IVF procedure to produce an embryo for transfer to a woman hoping to become pregnant. Using IVF in this way would produce a child whose mother was never born; in fact, it would produce a child whose mother was a dead fetus, and probably a dead fetus deliberately destroyed by her mother, the child's grandmother. There is no reason to believe that a child whose mother was a fetus destroyed by her grandmother would benefit from this arrangement, and many reasons to believe that she would suffer from it.

4. Another major moral concern relevant to IVF centers on the moral status of the embryo. In many IVF procedures, more eggs are fertilized than are needed at the time, so there is a question of what to do with the embryos that will not be transferred. Discarding a developing human embryo is obviously a moral issue since it is the deliberate destruction of a new human life.

Sometimes the embryos are frozen so they will be available for the woman in the future if she needs them, but this also raises moral issues. The freezing process destroys some embryos and, if those successfully frozen are not needed, they will have to be destroyed as well.

Several highly publicized cases have alerted the general public to the problems caused by freezing embryos. In 1983 Mario and Elsa Rios were killed in a plane crash, leaving frozen embryos in an Australian fertility clinic and an estate worth more than a million dollars. Questions about what to do with the embryos arose. If they were brought to term, they would inherit the estate; if not, others would receive it. A special panel suggested that the embryos should be destroyed, but the Parliament of the state of Victoria passed a special law protecting the embryos. At present, they remain frozen, and eventually will probably deteriorate beyond any chance for survival.

Another case arose in Tennessee when Mary Sue Davis and Junior Davis underwent IVF fertility treatments. Their excess embryos were frozen. After their marriage broke up, Mary Sue wanted to become pregnant with the frozen embryos, but Junior was now strongly opposed to her having his children. She considered the embryos her babies, and insisted she had a right to bring them to term. In September 1989 a judge gave custody of the embryos to Mary Sue because they are "children," and it is in the interests of children to be born. Mary Sue then married another man and changed her mind about wanting to use the frozen embryos. A year later the court of appeals overruled the circuit judge, and granted joint custody of the frozen embryos to Mary Sue and Junior. Then, in 1992, the Tennessee Supreme Court held that Junior could not be forced into fatherhood against his will. Finally, in June 1993, Junior announced that the embryos no longer existed.

The production of more embryos than will be immediately transferred into the woman is not the only problem in IVF; sometimes too few embryos are produced, thus reducing the opportunity for pregnancy. This has led some researchers to try splitting the human embryos produced by IVF in order to increase the number available for pregnancy. In 1993 several human embryos were actually split and, although no efforts were made to implant them, they did begin to develop normally after they were split. The procedures were widely reported in the media as "cloning" human beings, but it would be more accurate to say that the early embryos were simply split, much as they sometimes split spontaneously in the first few days of life, a phenomenon we explained in chapter six.

Among the possible abuses arising from splitting embryos in a laboratory is that one identical twin could be frozen and implanted years after her sister was born, perhaps because the parents wanted to see how the first one turned out. Yet, in the proper circumstances, the deliberate splitting of an early human embryo, if perfected, could be morally reasonable. This is especially true now that we know, as was pointed out in chapter six, that a few embryos spontaneously split in the first few days of development. If a married couple is seeking IVF as a last resort to have a genetic child, and cannot produce an adequate number of embryos during the IVF, it seems reasonable to see splitting these embryos as an appropriate way to produce more embryos and thus enhance the chances of pregnancy.

The American Fertility Society has determined that embryos in the first 14 days of development, while deserving of respect because they are human life, may be frozen for future use, discarded if not needed, or used for research with the parents' permission. Other national commissions and committees—

most notably in England, Australia, and Canada—have taken similar positions. But not all ethicists agree; some claim that respect for the human embryo requires fertilizing only the number of eggs to be transferred at the time of retrieval. This may cause additional inconvenience and expense for the couple, but these ethicists feel that the practice of fertilizing only what will be immediately implanted protects the origin of new human life and acknowledges the value of the human embryo in a way discarding or freezing them does not. Although their position is a minority view at the present time, there are good reasons for it.

The moral status of the embryo is the fundamental issue in IVF, and it is difficult to resolve. At one extreme are those who consider the embryo an unborn baby, and at the other extreme are those who think of it simply as human tissue. Both extremes are unreasonable. Most people fall somewhere in the middle and think that some special respect is appropriate for embryonic human life.

What might be a reasonable moral position at this time in regard to IVF? Perhaps a position that seeks a middle ground between outright condemnation and casual acceptance. That prudential position might find IVF reasonable for married couples of child-bearing age when all else has failed, and when the number of fertilized ova is restricted to the number that will be immediately returned to the woman's body. This is a starting point.

With more experience and ethical reflection on the process, a wider scope for IVF may be morally justified. It seems reasonable for couples who are carriers of serious genetic disease to resort to IVF in order to select only unaffected embryos for transfer. And it may be possible to give adequate reasons for splitting or freezing a couple's embryos, for example, despite the risks and damage to human life that these procedures promote. And it may be possible to give adequate reasons to justify using IVF with a couple's frozen embryos after menopause, despite our lack of knowledge about how postmenopausal pregnancies will affect the woman and child.

An ethics of prudence requires us to consider all the relevant circumstances and consequences of our behavior, and we simply do not yet know the consequences that will ensue from many of the different ways IVF can be used. Thus our moral judgments must be tentative and conservative lest we thoughtlessly harm ourselves and our chances for happiness.

We have been slow to recognize the ethical issues associated with the new reproductive technologies in the United States. Other countries have been more sensitive to the moral and social dimensions of the procedures, and are not so willing to allow IVF or other fertility treatments in every kind of situation. In late 1993, for example, Canada's Royal Commission on the new reproductive technologies issued its long-awaited report recommending, among other things, that IVF be limited to women with blocked fallopian tubes, and that men selling their sperm be limited to fathering no more than ten children. In many European countries, there are also growing movements to introduce restrictions on the use of the new reproductive technologies.

It is ironic, in a way, that the moral vacuum surrounding IVF in the United States was generated, at least in part, by moral concerns. During the Reagan–Bush years (1980–1992), the government, committed to an antiabortion position, withheld practically all federal support for IVF research. While this move did protect embryonic life, it also created, as we will see in chapter fourteen, an unfortunate situation. Without federal funding, IVF researchers sought private capital. Thus the IVF research in this country was supported by commercial interests, and commercial interests are driven largely by financial motives.

Fertility treatments are very profitable, and it matters little to some people involved in the new reproductive technologies whether the woman is married or not, whether the eggs are hers or purchased from another woman, whether the sperm comes from her husband or is bought from a sperm bank, whether the woman is heterosexual or homosexual, etc. What does matter is whether the client has access to funding and whether the chances of pregnancy are sufficiently high to make the procedures worthwhile.

As we will see in the chapter on research (chapter fourteen), if federal funding had been allowed for IVF research, the research would have been subjected to local review boards and could have been subjected to a national ethics committee as well. The reviews by local and national committees designed to protect the human subjects in research would have made the ethical issues associated with IVF far more prominent than they have been in the commercially funded research.

The morality of IVF cannot be determined by an ethics of rights. It is not enough for a woman or a couple to say "I have a right to have a baby" and conclude that IVF is morally justified. Nor is it enough for opponents to say "every child has a right to begin life in the body of the woman whose egg is fertilized." The morality of IVF is a morality of responsibility; we determine the morality of what we do by how it affects the human good. It is not difficult to recognize that infertility is a problem for couples desiring to reproduce their genetic children, and that some medical interventions to alleviate this problem are morally reasonable.

The ethics of IVF becomes much more shaky, however, when we go beyond what we have to do to overcome infertility in a couple and begin to buy and use eggs and sperm from third parties, or begin to cause pregnancies that will result in children whose fathers are anonymous and disinterested. Using IVF to help infertile couples have their own children is one thing many ethicists can readily accept; discarding and freezing human embryos is more difficult to justify; and the buying and selling of human sperm and eggs for purposes of reproduction is even more difficult to see as something good and noble.

Gamete Intrafallopian Transfer (GIFT)

In 1984 the reproductive technique known as GIFT was developed. The most important difference between IVF and GIFT is that the fertilization with IVF occurs outside the body, while the fertilization with GIFT takes place inside the body in a fallopian tube. GIFT is the procedure whereby gametes (sperm and eggs) are placed in the fallopian tubes before the egg is fertilized. The first two steps of the procedure are the same as they were for IVF, although the egg retrieval for GIFT is more frequently by laparoscopy. In the third step, some eggs are transferred by laparoscopy into the fallopian tubes along with the sperm. The entire procedure takes about an hour. Sometimes, of course, GIFT cannot help a couple because it requires at least one healthy tube, whereas the IVF procedure does not depend on healthy fallopian tubes.

GIFT avoids many of the moral issues found in IVF. First, the fertilization occurs in the body, not in a laboratory petri dish, and thus GIFT reduces the intrusion of medical manipulation into the beginning of human life. Second, GIFT avoids the sensitive questions about the moral status of the embryo in the laboratory or in the freezer. There are no extra embryos in GIFT to discard, freeze, or use for research; all the embryos are in the body, not the laboratory. There may be extra eggs, but discarding eggs does not present the same moral issues as does discarding embryos. Thus, many people uncomfortable with IVF from a moral point of view find it possible to consider GIFT a morally acceptable option.

Zygote Intrafallopian Transfer (ZIFT)

More recently, a process called ZIFT is gaining in popularity. ZIFT is similar to IVF. Ovaries are prepared; eggs are retrieved (usually by laparoscopy) and then fertilized in a petri dish. The zygotes (very early embryos) are then transferred, usually the day after they are retrieved, into the fallopian tubes rather than into the uterus as with IVF. The moral issues for ZIFT are, in general, the same as they are for IVF.

Ovum Transfer

In this procedure, one woman sells or donates her eggs for insertion into another woman whose ovaries are not producing healthy eggs either because of abnormalities or because she has passed menopause. Sperm is then inserted, either by AI or by intercourse. In late 1993 it was reported that a fifty-nine year old postmenopausal woman had become pregnant this way and delivered a child.

One moral issue with such a procedure is the use of eggs from a third party. This means the baby is not the genetic child of the woman. Moreover, the procedure can be used for questionable purposes not associated with infertility. It was also reported in 1993, for example, that a black woman married to a white man wanted a white child. She arranged for the insertion of an egg from a white woman; then her husband's spermatozoon fertilized this egg, producing a white baby. Among the several ethical issues in such a procedure is the issue of racism; good ethics requires that the intention of a racially mixed couple to avoid a child with any chromosomes from one race is not tainted with racism—the notion that one racial group is superior to others.

Surrogate Motherhood

Advances in the mastery of human reproduction have introduced still another phenomenon: surrogate motherhood. The general idea of surrogacy is that a woman unable or unwilling to become pregnant engages another woman to become pregnant in her place, with the understanding that this woman will give her the newborn child at birth. The conception of the child can happen in a number of ways. The most common is artificial insemination of the surrogate woman by the husband's sperm. This will make the husband and surrogate woman the genetic parents, and the wife an adoptive parent. If the wife is willing to undergo egg retrieval, it is also possible that her egg could be used in a process such as IVF, GIFT, or ZIFT to begin pregnancy in the surrogate. This will make wife and husband the genetic parents, and the pregnant woman is simply the gestational mother carrying a child genetically unrelated to her.

The idea that a couple experiencing infertility can enlist the aid of a fertile woman to bear a child for them is an ancient one. The Hebrew Bible (*Genesis* 16:17) records the story of childless Sarah telling Abraham to sleep with her maid Hagar so he could have a child. Abraham and Sarah were living in Egypt at the time. Abraham complied with Sarah's request, slept with her maid, and she became pregnant. The Bible gives no indication that using a maid, and an Egyptian one at that, for a surrogate mother by the childless couple was immoral. In fact, the customs of ancient Babylonia (modern Iraq), where Abraham and Sarah grew up, allowed the practice.

We should note that the notion of "surrogate" motherhood in these situations suffers from some linguistic confusion. Hagar, not Sarah, was the real mother of Abraham's first son, Ishmael. Hagar was both the genetic parent and the gestational mother. Today the "other" woman is called the "surrogate" mother. She does not become pregnant by intercourse with the husband, of course (that would now be considered adultery, although it was not so considered by the people of Abraham's time), but by artificial insemination. But if a woman becomes pregnant by intercourse or by artificial insemination and then delivers a child, she is not really the surrogate mother; she is, as was Hagar, the real mother.

If another reproductive technology such as IVF or GIFT is employed in the modern surrogacy arrangement, and the eggs of the wife are used, then it is true that the "surrogate" mother is not the genetic mother of the child. But there is still good reason to consider her the mother because she is the gestational mother—the one who conceives, carries, labors, delivers, and perhaps nurses the child. Merely contributing the egg to be fertilized does not make one a mother. We do not consider the women who sell their eggs the mothers of the children whom other women will conceive with these eggs. The woman with the strongest claim of motherhood is the woman who actually becomes pregnant and gives birth. Another woman may raise the child, and this makes her the mother in a real sense, but she does not thereby become the natural mother. And another woman may have donated the egg, making her the genetic mother of the child, but she is not the natural mother whose body supported the fetus for nine months and then delivered the baby.

We stress this because there is a value in beginning with our traditional ways of viewing motherhood, and then considering the new reproductive possibilities in light of them. Calling the artificially inseminated woman giving birth the "surrogate" mother implies that the woman who will pick up the baby after birth and raise the child is the "real" mother. But this is not so, and it demeans the woman who was pregnant and gave birth. It also sets the stage for a failure to appreciate the difficulty some women have in giving up a child after birth, despite their agreement to do so nine months earlier.

We should also recognize at the outset two very different settings for what is called surrogate motherhood. The more common kind of surrogacy is commercial. It involves a contract and the exchange of money. The woman is recruited by some kind of broker or agency, and then becomes pregnant, usually by artificial insemination. Her medical bills are paid, she signs a contract to give up the child, and she is paid a significant sum (around $10,000) when she does.

The second setting involves personal relationships and no money. By way of example, a woman may carry a child out of love for her sister who is unable to do so. The mother may have contributed her own egg, which is fertilized by the artificially inseminated sperm of her sister's husband, or accepted an IVF embryo resulting from the medically assisted fertilization of her sister's egg by the sister's husband. This kind of family surrogacy presents far fewer moral issues than the surrogacy involving strangers and money. In the case of the sisters, the child remains in the family, as it were, and the natural mother remains bonded in the role of aunt. Of course, the surrogate need not be a sister. In 1987 a forty-eight-year-old grandmother in South Africa gave birth to triplets who originated from an IVF procedure using her daughter's eggs and the sperm of her daughter's husband. She is thus the gestational mother of her grandchildren, and the grandmother of her own children, which will make her the great-grandmother of her grandchildren.

The effort to show that family surrogacy is reasonable and good has a better chance of succeeding than does any form of commercialized childbearing. After all, surrogacy for another member of the family is rooted in love, not money. But there is a subtle shadow of immorality lurking beneath the surface of this selfless love. The sister, or mother, or other female relative offers her body in a spirit of altruism that many find morally appealing, but others question. The pregnant woman becomes the altruistic woman giving and nurturing and providing for the needs of another who cannot become pregnant.

Extolling the maternal role of women for the sake of another, however, has a dark side—pregnancy and child rearing have often been used to turn women away from their own needs. As we become more sensitive to the ways women can be exploited and how victims of exploitation often willingly embrace the structures that exploit them, there will be doubts on the moral goodness of even family surrogacy where the woman undergoes pregnancy not for herself and her husband, but for the sake of a relative.

The moral analysis of surrogate motherhood must embrace all the relevant circumstances. It is not enough to say the family surrogate is acting out of love, not money, and therefore that the action is morally justified. We must also show how the action accords with the achievement of the human good. If family surrogacy places the women who do it in a position of exploitation, then the human good is undermined.

The fact that the woman chooses to be a surrogate is not enough to neutralize the moral questions. Migrant workers or illegal aliens may choose to work for below-minimum wage, but that does not mean they are not being exploited. While it is possible to volunteer to work for substandard wages, or even to work for nothing, more often than not the "volunteer" is in a psychological or social position where she just cannot say no. In other words, the choice is really the illusion of choice. And the same situation is an ever-present danger in family surrogacy, where the danger is that the choice to become pregnant for one's sister may not be much of a choice at all because the potential surrogate would feel so bad, perhaps even guilty, if she did not do it for her sister.

Despite this objection, some ethicists do not object to family surrogacy. What they widely criticize, however, is commercial surrogacy; that is, entering into a child-bearing contract involving money with a stranger who was provided by a broker for a fee. The moral arguments supporting this practice are shallow; they usually rely on a gratuitous claim to reproductive freedom and on the supposed right of people to have a child. Often they introduce the idea of how noble it is for a woman to help another woman have a child by becoming pregnant for her, and then experiencing the great joy of presenting her with the baby that will fulfill her life and needs.

We turn now to what is perhaps the most publicized case of commercial surrogate motherhood, the story of Baby M. It is a story where almost everything that could go wrong did go wrong. Thus it does not represent most contractual arrangements, but it is a good case to consider because we often learn more about things when they break down than when they function well.

THE CASE OF BABY M

The Story

In 1984 William and Elizabeth Stern decided to have a child. Later testimony revealed that William was very interested in having a genetic child, but there were no indications that Elizabeth felt strongly about becoming pregnant. There were also some indications that, despite lack of definitive medical diagnosis at the time, she had medical problems that discouraged her from wanting to become pregnant. There is no evidence that she was infertile. Both the Sterns were well-educated and well-employed—she is a physician.

They were soon to meet Mary Beth Whitehead. Mary Beth had dropped out of high school, was married with two children, and was in serious financial difficulty. After both mortgages on their home lapsed into default, she and her husband had filed for bankruptcy. In 1984 she applied to the Surrogate Mother Program in New York, but was rejected. Then she applied to a program with less rigorous screening, the Infertility Center of New York, and was accepted. The center brought the Sterns and Mary Beth together in January 1985.

They made a contract. It stipulated that Mary Beth would not smoke, drink, or use drugs during pregnancy; that she would seek prenatal care; that she would not abort the baby unless it endangered her health; that she would undergo amniocentesis or similar tests to detect defects; and that she would have an abortion at the request of William if the fetus was defective. If she had the abortion she would receive $1000; if the baby was defective and she refused an abortion at William's request, then he had no obligation to accept the child. When the child was born and handed over to the Sterns, Mary Beth was to receive $10,000; if the child was stillborn she was to receive $1000.

After nine attempts at artificial insemination, Mary Beth became pregnant. Her obstetrician advised against amniocentesis because she was in her twenties and at low risk for an abnormal fetus. William insisted, however, so she had the test, thus needlessly risking damage to the fetus. Everything was normal.

The baby was born on March 27, 1986. Those assisting at the birth were unaware of the surrogacy arrangement. Mary Beth's husband was listed as the father on the birth certificate, and Mary Beth began nursing the child. She named her Sara Elizabeth Whitehead. Several days later, the Whiteheads took Sara home and reluctantly surrendered her to the Sterns. Mary Beth became very upset and asked to have the baby back for a few days. The Sterns agreed. Once Mary Beth had her baby back, she left with the five-day-old infant for her mother's home in Florida.

She soon returned to New Jersey but kept the baby, so William Stern got a court order directing her to surrender the baby to him. She refused. With the order and five police officers, he then went to the Whiteheads' house, but Mary Beth passed the baby out a rear window before they could retrieve her. William and the police left empty-handed. The next day the Whiteheads fled to Florida, where they disappeared for almost three months. Florida police finally recovered the baby, and she was returned to the Sterns. They named her Melissa Stern. The Whiteheads returned to New Jersey and began legal action to recover Sara/Melissa.

In April 1987 a judge ruled that a contract is a contract, and thus "Baby M" belonged with the Sterns. Mary Beth appealed, asking the courts to declare any contracts signed by a surrogate mother void and unenforceable because no contract can force a mother to give up her child. In February 1988 the New Jersey Supreme Court, in a unanimous decision, agreed with her. It pointed out that laws forbid payments to induce women to give up their children; that a woman can give up her child for adoption only after birth; and that children cannot be taken from their mothers unless the mothers are shown to be unfit. The supreme court considered the child a baby conceived out of wedlock—the daughter of Mary Beth Whitehead fathered by a married man, William Stern. It then had to decide which parent—Mr. Stern or Mrs. Whitehead—should have custody of the child.

By the time of the state supreme court deliberations, Mary Beth had become pregnant by a person other than her husband (he had had a vasectomy). She then separated from her husband and married the father of her newest child in November 1987. Knowing this, the court gave custody of Sara/Melissa to William Stern in view of his more stable home life. And to Mary Beth, the child's mother, it gave visitation rights. It refused to allow Elizabeth Stern to adopt Sara/Melissa because Sara/Melissa's real mother, Mary Beth, did not want to give her up for adoption. For most of the year, Baby M is known as Melissa and lives in New Jersey with the Sterns, but every other weekend and during two weeks in the summer she is known as Sara and lives in New York with her mother—now Mrs. Mary Beth Gould—and her mother's four other children.

The court wisely noted that this kind of surrogate motherhood comes close to selling babies. In a stinging comment, it said that a surrogate contract ". . . guarantees separation of a child from its mother; it looks to adoption regardless of suitability; it totally ignores the child; it takes the child from the mother regardless of her wishes and her maternal fitness; and it does all this, it accomplishes all of its goals, through the use of money."

Ethical Reflection

In the minds of most ethicists commercial surrogacy is not an ethical dilemma because the bad features totally overwhelm any possible good features, and hence we will not do an ethical analysis of the story. Simply put, the bad features in this case are many and obvious, the good features are few or absent. Among the bad features are the following.

1. Deliberate and planned damage to the fullness of parenthood by separating maternal rearing from the maternal genetic and gestational aspects of motherhood.

2. Deliberate and planned distancing of a child from its genetic and gestational mother.

3. The undermining of human dignity by reducing human reproduction to a commercial contract, thus reducing the birth of a child to a legal arrangement akin to the sale of goods and services.

4. Payment of money for a child. Mary Beth was to receive $10,000 for the baby born live, but only $1000 if the baby were stillborn, thus showing that the major part of the payment was for a live baby, and not simply for the inconvenience of pregnancy, as some claimed. Children are not property, and buying and selling them treats them as property.

5. Potential future harms to a child who may one day discover her mother became pregnant with the idea of rejecting her at birth. There is, of course, no hard evidence that children born in these circumstances will be hurt by the discovery that their mothers planned to reject them as soon as they were born, but it is an ethical issue we cannot ignore until we are sure it would not happen. It is difficult to see how a person would not be hurt by such a discovery.

6. Potential future distress to a woman who may easily one day regret deliberately becoming pregnant with the intention of handing over her baby to strangers for money.

7. Potential custody battles over who gets a child deliberately conceived outside of marriage.

8. Potential degradation of the gestational mother, whose actions have some analogy with prostitution. In prostitution, a woman allows the use of her reproductive system to fulfill the needs of a stranger in return for money. If his needs are sexual gratification without reproduction, we call the agent who arranges it a pimp or procurer and the activity prostitution. If his needs are reproduction without sexual gratification, we call the agent who arranges it a broker and the arrangement "surrogate motherhood." Despite the more polite language of surrogacy, neither commercial arrangement is morally noble.

9. Payment for a live baby sets up exploitation of the gestational mother. It is not readily conceivable that a woman would become pregnant for a stranger unless she needed the money. Some say this is not exploitation if the woman freely chooses to do it. After all, they say, she has the right to use her body as she sees fit. But most would say the needy person choosing to become pregnant for a stranger is trapped into making a decision people would not make if they had enough money. Deciding to become pregnant by a stranger with a baby one intends to abandon at birth bespeaks a desperation that makes people vulnerable to exploitation. Desperate financial circumstances can undermine the ability to give truly voluntary consent. Surrogacy for money sets up a social phenomenon whereby the financially well-off can pay to use the reproductive systems of the less well-off, and this is a form of exploitation difficult to admire morally.

10. Potential harm to the surrogate's other children when they learn that their mother has babies and then gives them away for money, an unpleasant thought for children with their normal fears that their parents might abandon them.

Most ethicists can find no adequate reasons to justify commercial surrogacy, and thus there is widespread, albeit not total, consensus that it is immoral. Surrogacy within a family for altruistic reasons where no contract or money is involved fares better, yet many still have ethical objections to those arrangements. The reality of human existence is that some people of reproductive age want to have children but cannot. There are many techniques and technologies to help them, but it is naive to think all reproductive procedures and arrangements are morally noble. Surrogacy, especially commercial surrogacy, is most difficult to justify morally. Wanting a child very badly is not enough to make every means to have one morally reasonable.

We have considered reproductive issues at some length because most medical interventions to prevent pregnancy as well as to cause it involve bad features (that is, moral issues). While most texts on health care ethics now take reproductive interventions for pregnancy seriously, that was not always the case. Both AI and IVF became established medical practices before there was adequate moral reflection and dialogue. And few texts consider the moral issues involved in the medical interventions to prevent pregnancy.

What interventions designed to prevent or to cause pregnancy are moral, and under what circumstances, are frequently matters of moral dispute. We cannot settle these disputes, but the ethical approach we have been using suggests prudential reasoning will unfold within the following framework.

1. Sexuality is best lived in a stable and faithful relationship of love, caring, and trust.

2. Contraceptive interventions always introduce bad features in a sexual relationship; the interventions become moral evils whenever they are not reasonable and truly constitutive of the good of the couple and of society.

3. Reproductive interventions are also bad features in a sexual relationship; they become moral evils whenever they are not reasonable and truly constitutive of the good of the couple and society. The easiest reproductive interventions to justify are those involving infertile committed couples using

their own gametes and producing no surplus embryos. Introducing sperm and eggs produced by third parties for money, or trying to cause pregnancy outside socially acceptable family structures, seriously complicates the procedure and makes it all the more difficult to justify it morally. And surrogate motherhood for money has so many bad features that it is difficult to see how it could ever contribute to the human good of the adults involved, of a child reproduced in such a way, and of society itself.

SUGGESTED READINGS

The brief account of the history of contraception is drawn from John Noonan. 1986. *Contraception: A History of Its Treatment by the Catholic Theologians and Canonists*, enlarged edition. Cambridge: Harvard University Press. The quotations from Augustine are taken from here. Also helpful is James Brundage. 1987. *Law, Sex, and Christian Society in Medieval Europe*. Chicago: University of Chicago Press. For a brief summary of the good and bad features of various contraceptive interventions, see Daniel Mishell. "Contraception." *NEJM* **1989**, *320*, 777–86.

The idea that the leaders of the Catholic Church are needed to explain the natural law is found in Gerald Kelly. 1958. *Medico–Moral Problems*. St. Louis: Catholic Health Association, pp. 131–132. Kelly also wrote: "It follows, therefore, that the teaching of the Church is a practical necessity for an adequate knowledge of the natural law; and we should not be surprised when those who lack the benefit of this teaching are in error as to the existence or extent of some obligations . . . In our age, this guidance seems to be particularly necessary in the matter of artificial birth prevention . . ." (p. 153).

John Noonan has proposed a provocative, and seldom noted, strategy for reconciling artificial contraception with the current papal teaching that artificial contraception is against the natural law. Since nature restricts a woman's fertility to the few days surrounding ovulation, natural law proscribes using contraceptives only during these few days. In other words, Noonan claims that the official Roman Catholic position against all artificial birth control permits a couple with good reasons to use contraceptives (condoms and diaphragms, for example) any time except on the few days each month when fertility is thought to occur. See his "Natural Law, the Teaching of the Church, and the Rhythm of Natural Fecundity." *American Journal of Jurisprudence* **1980**, *25*, 16–37, reprinted as an appendix in *Contraception*, pp. 535–554. For one of the few reactions to this innovative proposal see Joseph Boyle. "Human Action, Natural Rhythms, and Contraception: A Response to Noonan." *American Journal of Jurisprudence* **1981**, *26*, 32–46. For Noonan's reply, see "A Prohibition Without a Purpose? Laws That Are Not Norms?" *American Journal of Jurisprudence* **1982**, *27*, 14–16. Noonan's ingenious effort to reconcile his church's position against artificial birth control with the practical need for contraception in some marriages is not necessary for Catholics who understand morality as primarily a matter of doing what achieves the human good in particular circumstances, and not primarily a matter of observing laws, principles, rules, or dictates.

The key cases in the legal history of contraception in the United States are *Poe v. Ullman*, 367 U.S. 498 (1961); *Griswold v. Connecticut*, 381 U.S. 479 (1965); *Eisenstadt v. Baird*, 405 U.S. 438 (1972); and *Carey v. Population Services International*, 431 U.S. 678 (1977).

Sterilization is widely recognized as an ethical issue when the person is a minor, retarded, or directed by a court or other agency to have the surgery. In 1927 the U.S. Supreme Court, remarking that "three generations of imbeciles are enough," ruled that state statues providing for compulsory sterilization of retarded people were constitutional (*Buck v. Bell*, 274 U.S. 200 [1927]). Punishing criminals by sterilization, however, was declared unconstitutional in *Skinner v. Oklahoma*, 316 U.S. 535 (1942).

Nonetheless, interesting legal and ethical cases continue to arise. In 1988, for example, Indianapolis newspapers reported that an unmarried pregnant woman was charged with murdering her four year old son. She was allowed to plead guilty to a lesser charge. Before sentencing, the judge indicated he would impose a reduced prison term if she agreed to sterilization after the child she was now carrying, conceived while awaiting the murder trial, was born. She had her baby, immediately surrendered him for adoption, and consented to the sterilization. This kind of case sets up a major ethical conflict. A psychiatrist had testified that she was sane and not a threat to anybody except her children, so the judge thought it was reasonable to shorten her prison term if she agreed to sterilization. But it is also reasonable to suggest that a person cannot give consent freely for a surgical procedure when the only alternative is spending time in prison, and therefore that the surgery was unethical.

For the personal and social ethics of artificial reproduction see: Kenneth Alpern, ed. 1992. *The Ethics of Reproductive Technology*. New York: Oxford University Press; Richard Hull, ed. 1990. *Ethical Issues in the New Reproductive Technologies*. Belmont: Wadsworth Publishing Company; Andrea Bonnicksen. 1989. *In Vitro Fertilization: Building Policy From Laboratories to Legislatures*. New York: Columbia University Press; Peter Singer and Deane Wells. 1985. *Making Babies: The New Science and Ethics of Conception*. New York: Charles Scribner & Sons; Steinbock, *Life Before Birth*, chapter 6; Machelle Seibel. "A New Era in Reproductive Technology: In Vitro Fertilization, Gamete Intrafallopian Transfer, and Donated Gametes and Embryos." *NEJM* **1988,** *318*, 828–34; Marcia Angell. "New Ways To Get Pregnant." *NEJM* **1990,** *323*, 1200–02; Arthur Caplan. "The Ethics of In Vitro Fertilization." *Primary Care* **1986,** *13*, 241–53; Edward Hill. "Your Morality or Mine? An Inquiry into the Ethics of Human Reproduction." *American Journal of Obstetrics and Gynecology* **1986,** *154*, 1173–80; Hans Tiefel. "Human In Vitro Fertilization: A Conservative View." *JAMA* **1982,** *247*, 3235–42; and Lori Andrews. "Legal and Ethical Aspects of New Reproductive Technologies." *Clinical Obstetrics and Gynecology* **1986,** *29*, 190–204.

Many organizations have issued position papers on the new techniques of assisting pregnancy. Some of the more important examples are the Ethics Committee of the American Fertility Society. "Ethical Considerations of the New Reproductive Technologies." *Fertility and Sterility* **1986,** *46*, supplement, 1–94; Committee on Ethics of the American College of Obstetricians and Gynecologists. 1986. *Ethical Issues in Human In Vitro Fertilization and Embryo Placement*. Washington: ACOG; the Department of Health and Social Security in Great Britain. 1985. *A Question of Life: The Warnock Report on Human Fertilization and Embryology*. New York: Basil Blackwell; the Roman Catholic Church. 1987. *Instruction on Respect for Human Life in its Origin and the Dignity of Procreation: Reply to Certain Questions of the Day*. San Francisco: Ignatius Press; and the U.S. Congress, Office of Technology Assessment. 1988. *Infertility: Medical and Social Choices*. Washington: U.S. Government Printing Office. For an excellent summary of the major committee statements, see LeRoy Walters. "Ethics and the New Reproductive Technologies: An

International Review of Committee Statements." *Hastings Center Report* **1987,** *17* (June), supplement, 3–9.

The New Jersey Supreme Court decision in the Baby M case is *In the Matter of Baby M*, 537 A.2d 1227 (1988). See also Phyllis Chesler. 1988. *Sacred Bond: The Legacy of Baby M*. New York: Times Books; Dianne Bartels, ed. 1990. *Beyond Baby M: Ethical Issues in New Reproductive Techniques.* Clifton, N.J.: Humana Press; George Annas. "Baby M: Babies (and Justice) for Sale." *Hastings Center Report* **1987,** *17* (June), 13–15; and "Death Without Dignity for Commercial Surrogacy: The Case of Baby M." *Hastings Center Report* **1988,** *18* (April–May), 21–24; Angela Holder. "Surrogate Motherhood and the Best Interests of Children." *Law, Medicine & Health Care* **1988,** *16,* 51–56; Ruth Macklin. "Is There Anything Wrong with Surrogate Motherhood? An Ethical Analysis." *Law, Medicine & Health Care* **1988,** *16,* 57–64; and Lisa Cahill. "The Ethics of Surrogate Motherhood: Biology, Freedom and Moral Obligation." *Law, Medicine & Health Care* **1988,** *16,* 65–71. Also helpful is the New York State Task Force on Life and the Law's report *Surrogate Parenting: Analysis and Recommendations for Public Policy.* 1988. Albany: Health Education Services.

On the hidden undesirable features of altruistic surrogacy (that is, the offer of a woman to bear another's child for love, not money), see Janice Raymond. "Reproductive Gifts and Gift Giving: The Altruistic Woman." *Hastings Center Report* **1990,** *29* (November–December), 7–11. Raymond notes: "altruism has been one of the most effective blocks to woman's self-awareness, and demand for self-determination. . . . The social relations set up by altruism and the giving of self have been among the most powerful forces that bind woman to cultural roles and expectations" (p. 9).

11

Prenatal Life

By prenatal life we mean the period of human life extending from implantation until the birth or extraction of the fetus. The developing human life is usually called an embryo through the eighth week of development, and then a fetus until birth. For the sake of simplicity, we will use the words "fetus" and "fetal" to describe prenatal human life from implantation until viability. Once a fetus is viable, it really should no longer be considered a fetus, but a baby within the mother. Viability—the expectation that the fetus can survive outside the uterus—normally occurs toward the end of the second trimester.

A heated controversy rages over just when a fetus becomes a "person." It is a controversy worth avoiding. The debate about the personhood of the fetus is endless and not resolvable. "Person" is one of those terms people define arbitrarily. Some say a newly fertilized egg is a person, while others insist we cannot speak of a person until a later stage of embryonic, fetal, or even neonatal development.

A more promising approach is to ask when the developing fetal body becomes "one of us." As was pointed out in chapter six, not every living human body is one of us. A brain-dead human being, for example, is no longer one of us, yet his human body may live for weeks or months, thanks to life-support equipment. And a fetus without the ability to perceive is not yet one of us because it is not yet a "psychic body." It makes little sense to say that a human body without the capacity for perception, because it has either irreversibly lost it or not yet developed it, is one of us. Human existence is never simply vegetative; it is always an existence with awareness, or at least the capacity for awareness, of its environment. Human existence does not mean something human "is"; it means something human "is-in-a-world." When the developing fetal body becomes psychic, it becomes one of us because its existence is now "in-the-world" by virtue of its awareness.

It is important to remember, however, that a fetus is human life before it becomes one of us. All human life is valuable, and thus an ethics of the good calls for special respect toward prenatal life from the beginning, not simply from the time it becomes a psychic body. No human life can be deliberately harmed or destroyed without adequate compensating reasons. What constitutes an adequate reason for damaging a fetus, however, varies with its stage of development. Once the fetus becomes a psychic body, only very serious reasons justify intentionally damaging it, and once the fetus is viable, the reasons justifying deliberate damage become even more serious, almost as serious as those justifying deliberate damage to a newborn. In this chapter we will consider but four of the many moral dilemmas associated with the way we treat prenatal life:

- the deliberate destruction of a fetus by invasive procedures (that is, surgical abortion);
- the deliberate destruction of a fetus by RU 486, a drug designed to dislodge a fetus from the uterus; some call this a medical abortion;
- the treatment of the fetus when the intervention conflicts with the well-being or wishes of the woman;
- the transplantation of fetal tissue.

Before taking up these issues, it will be helpful to acknowledge two major features of prenatal life.

1. Pregnancy makes a major impact on the life of the woman, and it may cause considerable discomfort. Pregnancy is sometimes accompanied by physical and psychological problems, and the physical risks are occasionally life-threatening. In view of a fetus' impact on her life, a woman obviously needs some control over whether and when she will become pregnant. It is, after all, her body that becomes pregnant, and each of us has an important interest in determining what happens to our bodies. Every discussion about pregnancy, therefore, is a discussion about a woman's life.

2. An embryo is a new human life. It is a living human being with a new genetic identity. While the fetus cleaves within another body for its existence until birth, it is genetically distinct from its human host. Every discussion about pregnancy, therefore, is also a discussion about a new human life.

Prenatal life, then, raises questions about two important human goods: (1) the woman's personal choices and responsibility for her life, and (2) the important reality of a distinctively new human life. It is precisely this dual nature of prenatal life, of course, that creates the major moral dilemmas.

ABORTION

The most conspicuous clash of these human goods occurs when abortion is the issue. In June 1994 the Allan Guttmacher Institute, a nonprofit organization that studies reproductive issues, reported that in 1992 there were about 1,529,000 legal abortions in the United States. More than one pregnant woman in four (27.5 percent) decided to terminate her pregnancy that year, a slight decrease over previous years. In round numbers, about 5.5 million women were pregnant in 1989, and 1.5 million of them chose to destroy the new human life.

This raises an obvious moral question: is the destruction of so much human life good or bad for people? Does it enhance or does it undermine our respect for living things? At a time when people are becoming more aware of a moral responsibility for animals, and for the environment itself, what is the appropriate ethical attitude toward this extensive destruction of prenatal human life?

Much of the debate about abortion in our country is couched in terms of rights—the right to life and the right to choose. And the public debate is also characterized by extreme positions—many people defending the right to life or the right of choice allow no exceptions to their positions. The result is a noisy and often ugly stalemate. Careless rhetoric has replaced careful thought, ill will has replaced good will, ideology has replaced reason, simplistic self-righteousness has replaced awareness of just how complex the whole question really is. The ideological right-to-life position tramples on a woman's prerogative to make choices about her body, and the ideological right-to-choose position fails to appreciate the human life of the fetus.

The intractable stalemate about the morality of abortion argued from uncompromising positions suggests we look elsewhere for moral insight. A moral reasoning that first acknowledges the complexity of the issue and then seeks a solution according to right reason may be helpful. The abortion issue is complex because it involves, among other things, two human lives, so many relevant circumstances, and such long-term effects.

Any adequate consideration of the ethics of abortion will include (1) something of the history of the dilemma, (2) acknowledgment of the bad features present in every abortion, and (3) recognition of the widespread agreement that some elective abortions are morally justified; that is, consistent with the human good, despite the destruction of human life they entail.

Abortion in History

Abortion is not a new moral concern. People have been having and doing abortions for a long time, and physicians and ethicists have been debating the ethics of the interventions for centuries. Some ancient commentators, as the Hippocratic Oath so vividly reminds us, thought abortion was always immoral. Others thought it could be justified in certain situations. The conditions most frequently proposed to justify abortion were: the pregnancy was endangering the health of the woman, population control was needed, or the pregnancy would cause extreme difficulty for the woman. An example of extreme difficulty would be the situation where society punished a woman's adultery by death, and abortion was the only way to conceal adulterous behavior.

Although neither the Hebrew Bible nor the Christian scriptures mention abortion, the influential translation of the book of *Exodus* from Hebrew into Greek (third century B.C.E.) revised the original biblical text to say that the destruction of a "formed" fetus was equivalent to homicide. (We pointed out this textual revision in chapter six.) Several centuries later the influential Jewish philosopher Philo of Alexandria associated abortion with infanticide, a practice he deplored. Considering abortion equivalent to homicide or infanticide is, of course, to consider it seriously immoral.

The Christian stand against abortion was strong from the beginning. An influential summary of Christian prohibitions composed in Syria around the year 100 explicitly listed the sin of abortion alongside sins of killing, stealing, adultery, and fornication. All the early Fathers of the Christian Church condemned abortion. After the Roman Empire, which covered much of Europe, adopted Christianity as its official religion in the fourth century, the Christian position against abortion became normative and was almost unquestioned for a thousand years in Europe.

The rise of medical education in the new universities springing up in the thirteenth and fourteenth centuries stimulated renewed interest in the ethics of abortion. At the beginning of the fourteenth century John of Naples, who taught at the universities of Paris and of Naples, argued that it is morally justified for a physician to perform an abortion of an early pregnancy to save the woman's life. Most moralists of the time declined to support his views.

By the end of the sixteenth century, however, the important Jesuit moralist Tomas Sanchez was arguing that abortion of an early fetus could be supported by plausible arguments in three cases: (1) serious danger to the woman's health, (2) fear of family reprisals for an extramarital pregnancy, and (3) avoidance of the injustice an adulterous pregnancy would cause a husband who would have to support a child he did not father. Sanchez thought the arguments for abortion in these circumstances were not simply "probable" but "more probable." "More probable" is a technical term in moral theology indicating arguments stronger than merely probable arguments, but weaker than arguments providing us with moral certitude.

The work of Sanchez prompted other Christian moralists to question the absolute prohibition against abortion more openly. They were aware that Christian morality had embraced the Biblical commandments against killing and stealing, yet had allowed exceptions to these laws of God in extenuating circumstances. They suggested the same approach could be used for abortion.

Although some Christian moralists began proposing exceptions to the traditional Christian prohibition against abortion at this time, papal authority and the leaders of the other Christian churches springing up in the sixteenth century were moving in the opposite direction. In 1588, for example, Pope Sixtus V issued an official document (called a papal bull) condemning all abortion at any stage of prenatal development without exception and, as we saw in the last chapter, all contraception as well. Lest there be any doubt about how serious the sin of abortion was in his mind, he ordered the heaviest penalties of church and civil law imposed on those performing any abortion, even an abortion necessary to save the woman's life. This meant the abortionist would be excommunicated and, if he or she lived in the territories where the church had civil jurisdiction, as it did in central Italy, would be executed. (History does not record anyone executed for abortion or for contraception; the penalties were never strictly enforced, and the successor of Pope Sixtus cancelled most of them.)

By the end of the nineteenth century, most Christian churches still considered all abortion immoral. Christianity, however, has not been the only historical factor shaping the American consciousness about abortion; there is also a legal history. During the nineteenth century, most of the opposition to abortion in the United States came from legal and medical sources, not from religious movements. Connecticut enacted the first state law against abortion in 1821. It was a limited law, forbidding only drugs used to induce abortions of "quickened" fetuses (that is, abortions after fetal movement is experienced).

By 1840, seven more states had placed restrictions on abortions after quickening. During this time, the abortion rate continued to climb in the United States. It reached, according to some estimates, 250 abortions for every 1000 live births. This represents about 20 percent of all pregnancies, a rate not too far below that of today (27.5 percent).

Abortions in the nineteenth century were often painful, unsafe, and botched. People performing them were not well-trained medically, and they operated on the fringes of the medical profession. Most people performing them were not physicians. It is not surprising, then, that reputable physicians became concerned, especially when women harmed by abortionists came to them for help. Many physicians, therefore, began to take a stand against the practice of abortion.

A turning point was reached when the newly established American Medical Association (the AMA) adopted an antiabortion stance at its annual convention in 1859. The physicians' position against abortion was influential, and it stimulated political action. As a result, by the end of the century, state laws against abortion were widespread in our country. They usually allowed one exception: an abortion necessary to preserve the life of a woman.

It is somewhat ironic how the struggle by physicians against abortion at this time was actually setting the stage for the current practice whereby physicians now have the exclusive authorization to perform abortions. By making all abortions illegal except those to save the woman's life, the only legal abortions were those performed by physicians trying to save a patient's life. For decades these abortions were few because abortion is seldom necessary to save the life of the woman. But when abortions for other reasons became legal in the twentieth century, society simply assumed physicians should continue to perform them, and thus elective abortion became a medical intervention only physicians could provide. This is what makes abortion a topic in medical ethics, and not merely a matter of choice or a legal question.

As time went on, some physicians used a very broad interpretation of abortions needed to "preserve the life of a woman." For a few, this phrase meant any abortion was justified if there was reason to believe that the woman would seek an illegal abortion if she could not obtain a legal one, and thereby would expose herself to life-threatening injuries and perhaps death.

By the 1950s a movement was well under way in the United States to reverse the laws against abortions, especially in one or more of these situations: (1) the pregnancy was dangerous for the woman, (2) the fetus was seriously defective, and (3) the pregnancy resulted from rape or incest. Soon the state laws began to change. By the early 1970s, nineteen states had relaxed their abortion laws to some extent, and four states (Hawaii, New York, Washington, and Alaska) allowed early abortions at the request of the woman without any justifying reason. Pressure for change was mounting, and the state legislatures were responding by liberalizing the abortion laws.

Then, in one stroke, the Supreme Court dramatically undermined the legislative process. In the famous decision known as *Roe v. Wade* (1973), it struck down almost all state laws restricting abortion. Seven of the justices found that most laws restricting abortion were unconstitutional because they violated a woman's "privacy," something not explicitly mentioned in the Constitution, but nonetheless guaranteed by it.

The name "Jane Roe" was used to designate the woman who challenged the abortion laws. This was her story. In the summer of 1969, she was walking home from work late in the evening when she was jumped and gang raped. She did not report the crime to the police. When she realized she was pregnant a few weeks later, she wanted an abortion, but abortion was illegal in Texas except to protect the life of the woman. Roe's lawyer, Sarah Weddington, challenged the Texas law, and a three judge panel, after listening to her story, ruled that she could have a legal abortion. Henry Wade, the district attorney of Dallas County, did not agree, and he appealed the ruling to the U.S. Supreme Court. The famous case is known as *Roe v. Wade*.

The U.S. Supreme Court ruled in 1973 that the Texas abortion law was unconstitutional. In *Roe v. Wade* it decided that:

- in the first trimester, states cannot make any laws regulating abortions;
- in the second trimester, states cannot make any laws regulating abortions unless they are related to the health of the woman;
- in the third trimester, states may make laws regulating abortions, and even forbid them, unless the abortion is necessary to preserve the life or health of the mother.

The real name of Jane Roe is Norma McCorvey. Her story was a lie— she was not raped. She had already given up custody of her first baby and released the second one for adoption at birth. Now she simply wanted to end her third pregnancy. Her subsequent admission that she lied about how she became pregnant and why she wanted the abortion does not, of course, affect the Supreme Court ruling. And she never had the abortion; she gave her baby up for adoption, and the little girl is now a young woman.

The history of abortion since Roe v. Wade has been marked by intense controversy. The tedious but valuable process that had begun to work its way through state legislatures was destroyed as seven men (the decision was 7–2) made, in effect, a new law for the land on a very important and controversial issue. They based their decision on a right, the right of personal privacy. They acknowledged that this right is not explicitly mentioned in the Constitution, but insisted its roots are found in the "penumbras" (or shadows) of the Bill of Rights and in the concept of liberty guaranteed by the fourteenth amendment to the Constitution. They also ruled that the right of privacy covering abortion is not unqualified; it "must be considered against important state interests in regulation."

The *Roe v. Wade* decision is extremely liberal. It does not allow states to restrict abortion at all in the first trimester, and allows restrictions in the second trimester only on how the abortions will be performed. In the second trimester, for example, states may insist on regulations governing abortionists and abortion clinics, as long as these standards do not unduly restrict a woman's access to an abortion. In effect, then, the Supreme Court decision allows abortion on demand during the first six months of pregnancy. No reason is needed to justify the decision.

We can see how extreme this decision is by comparing it to the positions other countries take on abortion. Abortion is now legal in every other Western country except Ireland, but the legal restrictions are more conservative. Most of the countries do not allow abortion on demand, but only for reasons judged adequate to justify it. Those few that do allow abortion on demand (examples are Norway, Sweden, Denmark, Austria, and Greece) generally restrict it to the first trimester. Sweden is the most liberal of the abortion-on-demand countries, allowing it through the eighteenth week, but this is still more conservative than what the law allows in the United States.

Roe v. Wade does not provide much protection for prenatal life. The fetus is not protected at all until the third trimester, and then it is not protected unless the individual states choose to restrict or forbid abortions. By 1989 only thirteen states had enacted laws protecting third trimester fetuses, which are really unborn babies.

The failure of the Supreme Court to offer any protection to prenatal life in the first two trimesters and its claim that abortion was somehow an almost unlimited "right" during these trimesters have caused intense political distress from the very beginning. The ruling sent the wrong message to many people. Many Americans could have accepted laws allowing early abortions in difficult situations as the lesser of two evils, but they almost instinctively react to a position that gives no indication that prenatal life is of any importance in the first two trimesters, and that views the choice to destroy a fetus as a constitutional right. In hindsight, we can see the great political mistake of *Roe v. Wade*: regardless of its merit in acknowledging and protecting a woman's choice about her pregnancy, it failed to acknowledge that prenatal human life in the first two trimesters is also something important and valuable.

The history of the abortion debate in the United States since *Roe v. Wade* has been largely the story of reactions to that Supreme Court decision. Many of the battles have gone to the Supreme Court as some people have tried to narrow the application of *Roe v. Wade* by passing state laws restricting abortion.

At first the Supreme Court took a dim view of the efforts of any state to restrict abortions and struck down most of the new laws as unconstitutional in light of the *Roe v. Wade* decision. As the years went on, however, new justices with more conservative ideas about abortion were appointed to the court, and its recent decisions tend to give states more room to make some regulations about elective abortions, as long as the laws do not impose an undue burden on the woman seeking an abortion. The following are some of the more notable positions on abortion taken by the Supreme Court after *Roe v. Wade*.

1. Some people claimed that *Roe v. Wade* implied people on welfare could have free abortions. This would mean that federal and state governments, using tax dollars, would be paying for abortions. In fact, in the first three years after *Roe v. Wade*, about a third of all abortions (almost 300,000 annually) were actually funded by Medicaid, a federal and state welfare program for poor people. Some states, however, refused to use tax dollars for abortions.

Connecticut was one such state, and its refusal to use Medicaid funds for elective abortions was challenged. Its refusal was upheld, however, by the U.S. Supreme Court in *Maher v. Roe* (1977). This decision means states may refuse to provide abortions for women on welfare, and most of them do refuse.

At about the same time, some members of Congress were trying to prevent the use of federal funds for abortions. In 1976 Congress passed an amendment first proposed by Representative Henry Hyde; the final version of this amendment prohibited the use of federal funding for abortion unless the woman's life was endangered. Since that time, the annual amendments restricting federal funding for abortion have been known as the Hyde Amendments. In 1993 Congress relaxed the Hyde Amendments' federal ban somewhat by requiring Medicaid (the state-run program partially supported by federal funds) to pay for abortions after rape or incest beginning April 1, 1994. Several states (among them Pennsylvania, Michigan, Arkansas, Louisiana, and Kentucky) have nonetheless refused to fund abortions in their Medicaid programs.

The day after the first Hyde Amendment was passed in 1976, it was challenged in federal court by Cora McRae. She lost her case when the Supreme Court upheld the constitutionality of the Hyde Amendments in *Harris v. McRae* (1980).

In view of *Maher v. Roe* and the Hyde Amendments, states need not, and the federal government cannot, fund abortions unless the pregnancy threatens the woman's life or is the result of rape or incest. In other words, the right of privacy that the Supreme Court invoked to allow a woman to choose abortion in the first two trimesters does not mean that welfare programs have to pay for it if she cannot afford to pay herself.

In this sense, *Roe v. Wade* does not give every woman the right to abortion on demand; it does not guarantee that she can have an abortion. Its position is more modest; it simply says that states cannot prevent a woman from having an abortion in the first two trimesters. It does not say that the state or the federal government has to provide the abortion for her—unless her life is endangered or, since 1994, the pregnancy was caused by incest or rape. A pregnant woman *cannot* argue: "*Roe v. Wade* gives women the right to an abortion; hence, if I cannot pay for my abortion, my medical care under a welfare program must provide it." A few states do pay for elective abortions, but they have gone beyond what *Roe v. Wade* requires.

2. A Missouri law allowed the husband or, if the pregnant woman was a single minor, her parents to veto a woman's abortion decision. When this law was challenged, the court ruled that these restrictions were unconstitutional in *Planned Parenthood v. Danforth* (1976).

3. A city ordinance in Akron, Ohio, required women under fifteen to obtain parental consent before an abortion. When this was challenged the court ruled, in a case known as the *City of Akron v. Akron Center for Reproductive Health* (1983), that minors of any age who have good reasons for not seeking parental consent may give consent for an abortion. States may, however, require that they appear before a judge in a confidential hearing to show that they are mature enough to make the abortion decision. The *Akron* decision upheld *Roe v. Wade*, but the majority on the Supreme Court dropped to 6–3.

The *City of Akron* decision also modified *Roe v. Wade* in an important way: *Roe* had said that states could not make laws regulating abortion in the first trimester; *Akron* said that states could make such laws as long as these laws do not unduly restrict the woman's right under the Constitution to have an abortion. And, in an important dissent, Justice O'Connor explicitly criticized the trimester framework employed in *Roe v. Wade*; she claimed it had no justification in law or in logic. Her criticism gained support in the years after *Akron*.

4. Pennsylvania's Abortion Control Act of 1982 stipulated that a woman considering abortion had to be given certain information that included the gestational age of the fetus, the physical and psychological risks of the abortion procedure, the assistance she could receive for having the baby and then giving it up for adoption, the financial liability of the father for the support of the child, and an offer to review literature that showed "the probable anatomical and physiological characteristics of the unborn child at two-week gestational increments from fertilization to full term, including any relevant information on the possibility of the unborn child's survival."

In *Thornburgh v. American College of Obstetricians and Gynecologists* (1986), the court found these restrictions were "overinclusive" and "not medical information that is always relevant to the woman's decision, and. . .may serve only to confuse and punish her anxiety, contrary to accepted medical practice." The court found that all this information went beyond what was needed for informed consent to abortion, and thus overruled the 1982 Abortion Control Act. *Thornburgh* also upheld *Roe v. Wade*, but the majority on the court dropped to 5–4.

The *Thornburgh* decision is not without a certain irony. On the one hand, the ruling protects the woman from being manipulated during the informed consent process by people trying to make her change her mind about the abortion allowed under *Roe v. Wade*. On the other hand, the ruling undermines the pregnant woman's ability to give truly informed consent by allowing abortionists to withhold information about the acceptable alternatives to abortion. As we saw in chapter four, truly informed consent means that the physician discusses all reasonable alternatives with the patient.

Withholding information about the side effects and alternatives to abortion might make it more probable that the woman will continue with her decision to have the procedure, but it also undermines her ability to make a truly informed choice. Our choices are not informed unless we have all the available relevant information. Thus—and this is the irony—the *Thornburgh* decision makes it easier for women to have abortions, but undermines an authentic "pro-choice" position. It strengthens the right to abortion on demand, but undermines the informed consent process necessary for sound choices about any invasive medical procedure. Justice Burgher made this very point in his dissenting opinion in *Thornburgh*. His remarks are all the more significant because he was one of the seven justices who originally voted for *Roe v. Wade*.

5. Missouri inaugurated a number of regulations aimed at restricting abortion. These included: physicians employed by the state may not perform abortions, state facilities may not provide abortions, and physicians performing abortions must try to determine whether the fetus is viable whenever there is question of an abortion at or beyond twenty weeks. These regulations were challenged and, in *William Webster v. Reproductive Health Services* (1989), the court ruled the state of Missouri could make these regulations. In effect, *Maher v. Roe* had already established that states could not be forced to fund

elective abortions, and this easily allowed the court to uphold state laws prohibiting nontherapeutic abortions in state hospitals and prohibiting physicians on the state payroll from performing abortions.

The Missouri regulation requiring physicians to determine viability of fetuses beyond twenty weeks of gestation, however, was not so easy for the court to resolve. *Roe v. Wade* had said the state cannot make regulations affecting fetal life before the third trimester, which begins about the twenty-fourth week. The Missouri twenty-week test thus contradicted the trimester framework of *Roe v. Wade* and would seem to be unconstitutional.

The court responded by saying the trimester framework of *Roe* is outmoded. Moreover, it saw no reason why a state's interest in protecting prenatal life "should come into existence only at the point of viability." In other words, in contrast to *Roe v. Wade*, the court now acknowledged that prenatal life is important before viability and that states might have an interest in protecting it. In *Webster*, the court does not see why ". . . there should therefore be a rigid line allowing state regulation after viability but prohibiting it before viability." Once the court accepted the view that the state has an interest in protecting prenatal life before the third trimester, it could easily conclude that the testing of fetuses at twenty weeks, which is in the second trimester, is constitutional.

6. After the 1986 *Thornburgh* decision, Pennsylvania enacted a new Abortion Control Act in 1989. It included the following restrictions: (1) the woman seeking an abortion must notify her husband in writing; (2) the physician must inform the woman of fetal age and the risks of abortion, pregnancy, and childbirth; and a counsellor must provide information about fetal development, alternatives to abortion, and possible state aid available if pregnancy continues; (3) a twenty-four-hour waiting period between consent and the abortion procedure; and (4) if the woman is a minor, at least one parent must also give consent, unless a judge waives this requirement.

This law was challenged and, in *Planned Parenthood Association of Southeastern Pennsylvania v. Casey* (1992), the court upheld all its provisions except the requirement of notifying the husband. This decision pleased neither the defenders nor the opponents of *Roe v. Wade*. Defenders thought that the court should have found the Pennsylvania law unconstitutional; opponents were disappointed that the court did not simply overturn *Roe v. Wade*.

The *Planned Parenthood* decision is important for what it said about the value of prenatal life. While it insisted that a woman has the right to choose abortion before viability without undue interference from the state, it also said that the state has legitimate interests in protecting both the woman's health and the "life of the fetus that may become a child" before viability. The decision allows states to regulate abortions before viability, provided the regulation is not an "undue burden" on the woman's right to have the abortion. The court concluded that the twenty-four-hour waiting period and the requirements for information about the risks, fetal development, and alternatives to abortion reflected Pennsylvania's legitimate interest in the life of the fetus. Thus, they were not unconstitutional or in violation of *Roe v. Wade* because they were not "undue burdens" on the woman.

These brief remarks give us some idea of the religious and legal history behind the abortion controversy. In the next section, we will consider the moral issues of abortion. Every abortion destroys human life, and that is bad. The bad features of abortion remind us that deliberate abortion will be immoral and unethical—unless there are adequate reasons justifying the destruction of human life.

Abortion Is Always Bad

As we have noted, most of the debate about abortion in the United States has been couched in the language of rights. Some argue that the rights of privacy and choice imply a right to destroy prenatal life regardless of the reason; others argue that the right to life implies few, if any, reasons are sufficient to justify destroying prenatal life. Some say the fetus's right to life trumps the woman's right to make decisions about what happens in her body; others say the woman's right to choose trumps the fetus's right to life. The debate reveals a fundamental weakness in arguments that use rights as trump cards—when more than one right is in play, no resolution is possible because each side considers its right the trump card.

An alternative approach is needed. Ethics is ultimately not about rights, but about what is good. Life, even prenatal life, is a very basic good. Ethics encourages us to cherish life, especially human life. Prenatal human life has a value, and this value is lost if we destroy it. Destroying any form of life— the environment, an animal, a fetus, a person—is bad, and ethics requires us to consider it immoral unless we have an adequate reason to justify the destruction.

We begin the ethical consideration of abortion, then, by considering it as something bad because it is a destruction of human life. Abortion is always a moral decision, and a serious one because it is the taking of human life. Our society has struggled hard to inculcate a presumption in favor of life, including the lives of the frail, the elderly, and the dying, and the lives of fetuses as well. Society has an interest in preserving that presumption, and so do we.

Since abortion is bad, we need serious reasons to justify it, or it will be immoral; that is, it will undermine our good. People will disagree, of course, over just what reasons are adequate to justify an abortion, but that is a separate issue. The important thing is to begin every discussion of abortion not with a claim based on rights—the right of a woman to choose it or the right of a fetus to live—but on the recognition that destroying human life—even prenatal human life—is a very serious action, and it should never be done without compelling reasons.

This ethical approach to abortion is nothing new. We have used it for centuries in questions about killing postnatal life. Our culture has always said "Do not kill . . . unless there are good reasons for killing." "Thou shall not kill" has always been understood to mean that killing is wrong, but some exceptions can be justified. What we say about killing postnatal life can also be said about destroying prenatal life. As we will argue in the next section, the presumption in favor of fetal life can sometimes be overridden by the woman's choice to have it destroyed, but that choice is an ethically sound choice only if the reasons supporting it are strong enough to justify the destruction of human life.

Areas of Agreement About Abortion

Once we recognize that abortion is always bad, we can ask whether any situation exists where it is nonetheless a reasonable course of action. The following examples are admittedly "easy" ones, at least for most people, but they do show how reasons justifying some abortions in difficult situations are plausible in an ethics of the good that cherishes human life.

Ectopic pregnancy

Some embryos implant outside the uterus, usually in a fallopian tube, although sometimes an embryo attaches to an ovary or to the cervix. If the pregnancy continues, the growing fetus will threaten the life of the woman before it becomes viable. The accepted medical response, once an ectopic pregnancy is diagnosed, is to abort it. The abortion will be a first trimester abortion, and few physicians or women, even those otherwise opposed to abortion, think it is immoral to perform these abortions.

These abortions are easy to accept in an ethics of right reason. The destruction of fetal human life is unfortunate, but it is the only reasonable action in the situation. Nothing can be done to save the fetus, which is not yet one of us, and if the pregnancy continues, it will cause the deaths of both the woman and the fetus. Once an ectopic pregnancy is diagnosed, the best we can do is to abort it as simply as possible.

In passing, however, we should note that one important religious denomination, the Roman Catholic Church, still opposes the abortion of an ectopic pregnancy. The Vatican condemned ectopic abortions in 1902. Some women with ectopic pregnancies adhered to the church teaching and, unfortunately, died as the result of their ectopic pregnancies.

By the 1930s, however, Catholic theologians found a way to save the lives of these women, and yet avoid the ban on aborting ectopic pregnancies. They applied the "principle of the double effect," a principle explained in chapter three, to the problem of ectopic pregnancies. If the site of the ectopic pregnancy is considered pathological (as the result of an embryo growing in or on it) and a threat to the woman's life, surgical removal of the site would have two effects, one good and one bad. The good effect is the removal of the pathological site threatening the woman's life; the bad effect is the destruction of the fetus. Since the intervention is directed toward the site, however, and not the fetus, it is not a direct abortion. The principle of double effect allows surgery to remove a life-threatening pathological organ even if a fetus dies in the process.

Unfortunately, this theological response to the problem of ectopic pregnancies is not a reasonable solution. While it saves the woman's life, it also causes her unnecessary harm in most cases. Surgically removing the site of the ectopic pregnancy permanently damages the woman's reproductive system. In fact, terminating an ectopic pregnancy by removing the site, when there is no medical need to do so, is simply bad medicine. It is hard to see how it would not be medical malpractice; it is also hard to see how it is a morally reasonable response to the pregnancy.

Selective abortion

Sometimes, perhaps as the result of fertility drugs or a fertility procedure such as IVF, a woman may become pregnant with more than one fetus, perhaps as many as six or more. The risks to the woman and to the fetuses increase with the number of fetuses in the pregnancy. Most people think that five or more fetuses is a matter of serious risk for the woman and for the fetuses themselves. One persistent problem in multiple pregnancies is premature birth and the many problems associated with it.

An ethics that cherishes life, especially human life, will do everything possible to prevent multiple pregnancies with five or more fetuses. But when it happens, the woman and the physicians are presented with a moral dilemma. The dilemma is compounded by the fact that it happens so rarely that we do not have good information about outcomes involving five or more fetuses. Thus our analysis has to be speculative.

Let us consider the rare pregnancy of five or more fetuses. We want to salvage as much human life as possible. We certainly want to preserve the woman's life, and we also want to take reasonable care of the fetuses. As soon as we begin to think the many fetuses in the uterus are setting up a situation where great damage will be done to the woman and to the fetuses themselves, we have to ask how we might reduce this damage. One obvious option is to abort some of the fetuses. This can be achieved by injecting potassium chloride into some of the fetuses at about the twelfth week of gestation. They will die, and the remains will be absorbed by the mother's body. The abortion of selected fetuses is intended to give the other fetuses, and the mother, a more realistic chance of survival.

In these situations, the intent is not really to terminate a pregnancy (the woman remains pregnant), but to increase the chances of a healthy pregnancy and the birth of healthy babies. To accomplish this, some fetuses have to be destroyed. It is truly a conflict situation, but an ethics of right reason or prudence indicates that life can be better cherished in such a situation by selective abortion. The deliberate abortion of some fetuses is tragic, but less tragic than (1) losing all of them, or losing some and leaving the others terribly impaired and (2) undermining the health and well-being of the mother, and perhaps losing her life itself.

Although many people, including those ordinarily opposed to abortion, would agree that reducing multiple pregnancies with five or more fetuses is the best we can do in the unfortunate situation, the moral perplexity increases when the number decreases. What are we to think when a woman with triplets wants the pregnancy reduced? Certainly, triplets are a burdensome pregnancy, and it often does more damage to a woman's body than a pregnancy of one or two babies. But are the burdens of carrying triplets sufficient to justify the destruction of one of them? In an ethics of prudence that cherishes human life, such a reduction, assuming there are no other complications with the pregnancy, is suspect because the reasons for destroying human life in the case of triplets are weaker than they are in pregnancies with a higher number of fetuses.

Seriously defective fetuses

Once we discover early in a pregnancy that a fetus is seriously defective the question of abortion arises, and with good reason. Terminating an early pregnancy when the fetus is expected to die later in the pregnancy or shortly after birth, especially if it is known that the fetus or newborn will suffer significantly in its brief life, can be defended as reasonable. There is little point in continuing a pregnancy for months once we know that little more than suffering and an early death awaits the fetus. We can give good reasons why we should not kill a mature fetus or a newborn infant, no matter how short the life expectancy, but it is much more difficult to say that the abortion of a grossly defective human fetus in the early stages of development undermines the human good.

How defective must a fetus be before an ethics that cherishes life can acknowledge the cogency of the reasons for aborting it? Obviously, the defects must be serious. Anencephaly is one such serious defect. The afflicted child, who lacks a brain, or most of it, has a high chance of being born dead; even if he or she is born alive, death usually follows in a matter of hours. The defect is so devastating that everyone agrees most life-sustaining treatments are not appropriate for the unfortunate neonate. Other examples of seriously defective fetuses include those with the genetic defects known as trisomy 13 or trisomy 18. If born, these babies will suffer significantly from the genetic defects and from the interventions often employed to sustain their lives, yet they seldom survive beyond the first year of life. It is at least arguable that the reasons supporting early abortion of these defective fetuses are plausible.

It is not possible to say exactly which prenatal defects are serious enough to justify an early abortion. In an ethics dedicated to the affirmation of life, they would be few. An ethics that cherishes life will generally find abortion unreasonable, and the more mature the fetus, the stronger the objections. Exceptions occur when the failure to abort will do more harm to the human good than the abortion. Before an exception can be made, however, moral reasoning must clearly establish the justification for destroying the prenatal life. Human life, even prenatal human life, is a fundamental good deserving of great protection, and its destruction should always be an exception. Good reasons exist for making such exceptions when the pregnancy is ectopic or involves five or more fetuses. It can be reasonably argued that good reasons exist in other tragic situations as well.

The central question in the abortion controversy is not whether the fetus is a person or has rights, or whether the pregnant woman has the right to choose whether she will continue the pregnancy or abort the fetus. Rather, the central question is: "What reasons in what circumstances justify destroying prenatal human life?" To put it another way: "What values can possibly outweigh the destruction of prenatal human life?" Unfortunately, the central question is seldom debated because so much of the literature on abortion is taken up by the vocal minority of people who tolerate no exceptions to their dogmatic positions.

RU 486

In the late 1950s researchers developed contraceptive pills. These pills introduce enough estrogen—a hormone associated with pregnancy—into a woman's body to block ovulation. Over the years the pills were refined, and today they are widely accepted as a reliable and relatively safe means of birth control.

More recently, researchers have developed what some now call the abortion pill. These pills introduce an agent into the woman's body that attacks progesterone, another hormone associated with pregnancy. Progesterone prepares the lining of the uterus to receive a fertilized ovum during each menstrual cycle. If that function can be thwarted, the fertilized ovum or embryo will not implant or, if it is implanted, it will be dislodged.

In 1980 scientists working at the French firm of Roussel Uclaf synthesized an antagonist of progesterone called mifepristone or, as it is more widely known, RU 486. Tests in women soon showed that this antiprogestin drug could both prevent implantation and dislodge an implanted fetus. The abortive function of RU 486 is highly effective when its ingestion is followed in 48 hours by a low dose of a prostaglandin analogue. Until recently, the prostaglandin was given by injection or by vaginal insertion, but oral intake is now possible. The prostaglandin causes the uterus to contract, and the contractions expel the dislodged fetus.

Over one hundred thousand women have used RU 486 in France since its approval in 1988. It is also widely used in Great Britain and China. At first Great Britain restricted its use to residents. Beginning in 1994, however, it allowed visitors to receive RU 486, and women began traveling to England for medical abortions. Other countries, most notably Sweden and Germany, are in the process of approving the drug.

In the United States, the process of approval has been slowed. The Food and Drug Administration (FDA) must approve all new drugs, and this requires research and testing in accord with FDA standards. Roussel Uclaf has been in no hurry to seek FDA approval. The reason is at least partly political. Opponents of legalized abortion, alarmed by the possibility that abortion could be made so simple and private, have mounted a strong campaign in this country against the drug, and they found a sympathetic ear in the Bush administration. In 1988 the FDA took the rather unusual step of issuing an "import alert" prohibiting people from bringing the drug into the country.

This led to a well-publicized case in July 1992. Leona Benten, claiming she was pregnant, announced that she was bringing some RU 486 back from Europe. Since the pills violated the FDA import ban, U.S. Customs confiscated the pills in New York. Ms. Benten's lawyers took the case to federal district court and won—the court ordered immediate release of her pills. But the order of the federal district court was stayed by the federal court of appeals, and this prevented release of the drug. Her lawyers filed an application with the U.S. Supreme Court, asking it to lift the stay, but the Supreme Court declined in a 7–2 opinion. Thus Ms. Benten's pills were not released.

Actually, the FDA "import alert" was not as ominous as it sounds; it applied only to the importation of unauthorized drugs into the country; that is, drugs not approved by the FDA. Roussel Uclaf, the company with the worldwide patent for RU 486, could have imported the drug for purposes of testing, but had decided against seeking FDA approval for testing in the United States because it feared any efforts to test and market the drug would result in antiabortion protests. The potential profits from RU 486 are slight—only one pill is needed for an abortion—and Roussel Uclaf is concerned that opponents of abortion will encourage the boycott of all their products in the United States if they introduce RU 486.

The climate in Washington changed when the Clinton administration took office in 1993. Within months, Roussel Uclaf made preliminary agreements for clinical trials in the United States with a nonprofit agency known as the Population Council. In May 1994 the firm released the patent for the pill, free of charge, to the council. The testing necessary for FDA approval began in late 1994 at abortion clinics around the country. At the same time, an organization known as Abortion Rights Mobilization announced it had signed an agreement with an unnamed overseas manufacturer to begin testing a generic version of the drug in this country. The National Right to Life Committee and other abortion opponents responded by announcing in July 1994 that they will campaign for people to boycott products made by subsidiaries of Roussel Uclaf in the United States. Testing, however, is expected to proceed and RU 486, or its generic equivalent, may be available for domestic use as early as late 1995. If approved, an abortion by RU 486 is expected to cost as much as a surgical abortion, about $400.

Contrary to some superficial perceptions, the use of RU 486 for abortion is not as simple as taking a "morning-after" pill. A review of how RU 486 is currently used in France will be informative.

Early abortion is legal in France, but the philosophy behind the legalization differs from the prevailing view in the United States, where abortion is justified by the rights of privacy and choice. The French legislation acknowledges the importance of choice, but also the importance of fetal life. It allows abortion before the end of the tenth week, but only in cases of distress.

A woman in early pregnancy seeking a nontherapeutic abortion in France must first visit a physician to receive a brochure printed by the government; it reminds her that the law limits abortion to cases of distress. The brochure also contains information about public benefits and programs helpful to mothers and children, and about adoption. The physician is also required to inform her of the medical risks and of the seriousness of the abortion.

Next, the pregnant woman must visit an approved counseling service to discuss her distress and the alternative ways to resolve it short of having the abortion. This agency will give her a certificate verifying that she has had the consultation.

If she still desires the abortion, she must confirm this in writing to her physician no sooner than one week after her initial visit to the physician. The one-week waiting period is designed to give her a chance to reflect on the seriousness of the abortion.

These procedures are required for all abortions in France, not just abortions using RU 486. Underlying the entire process is the understanding that fetal life is valuable, that abortion is not a simple choice but a decision forced by distress and necessity, and that the decision is a very serious one that must not be rushed or made without adequate information and consultation. All of this conveys a message about the value of human life and about the distress pregnancy can cause a woman, a message that is almost totally absent in both the extreme pro-choice and pro-life positions found in the United States.

RU 486 will undoubtedly become more of an issue in the future. Drugs inducing abortions introduce a new kind of abortion, medical abortion. Unlike the surgical abortion, where a physician aborts the fetus, the woman taking RU 486 performs the abortion herself. Medical abortions are also more private than surgical abortions, more difficult for antiabortion groups to protest, and more difficult for the law to control. The medical abortions may also become more simple, and may soon not require the medical supervision now needed.

Although RU 486 is a new kind of abortion, it does not introduce any new dimensions to the moral reasoning about abortion. It matters little from the ethical point of view whether fetal life is destroyed by a drug that dislodges it from the endometrial lining of the uterus or by a vacuum device that sucks it out. In both procedures fetal life is being destroyed, and that is not a good thing. In the ethical framework we have been using, it is immoral to destroy human life unless there is an adequate reason to justify doing it.

RU 486 will, however, introduce some new subsidiary moral dilemmas. For example, consider the moral dilemma of a pharmacist opposed to abortion who is asked to fill a prescription for RU 486. We are aware that doctors and nurses opposed to abortion routinely refuse to participate in them for reasons of conscience, and that this refusal is accepted behavior. Now that drugs can cause abortions, may pharmacists opposed to abortion refuse to fill prescriptions for the antiprogestins that will be used to destroy fetal life? If they provide the drugs for abortion, are they accomplices in what they feel is immoral? Some would argue that the pharmacist providing the drug for a medical abortion is involved in the abortion no less than a person assisting in a surgical abortion, but that seems a little unreasonable.

MATERNAL–FETAL CONFLICTS

For a very long time physicians did not care for pregnant women unless they were sick, and they did not assist at births. Most births did not occur in hospitals. Pregnancy and birth, after all, are not illnesses, and doctors and hospitals are for sick people. There was little prenatal care, and most deliveries were assisted by midwives.

All that began to change a century or so ago. Physicians took over the delivery of babies, and midwifery all but disappeared. Physicians soon realized that prenatal medical care was important, so they began to offer this as well. In this way, both birth and pregnancy became medical concerns, and the hospital became the place where most babies are born.

Until recently, the prenatal care was directed almost exclusively toward the woman. Not much could be directly known about the fetus. The physician's knowledge could only come from such practices as palpitating it and by inference from laboratory analyses of the woman's urine and blood. In short, prenatal medical care was the care of one patient—the woman who was pregnant.

The development of techniques and technology to diagnose fetal health changed this. Ultrasound, alpha-fetoprotein screening, chorionic villi sampling, and amniocentesis are now often used, along with other diagnostic interventions, to detect fetal abnormalities. Once problems are diagnosed, the obvious next step is to see whether they can be treated. In recent years, for example, physicians have begun operating on fetuses during the pregnancy. Although still in its infancy, fetal surgery has been used to correct urinary obstructions, diaphragmatic hernias, and hydrocephalus. Results range from poor to modest; surgery for hydrocephalus has had poor results, while surgery to repair the hernias and urinary problems has been more promising.

Once the fetus is viewed as a human subject worthy of medical intervention for its own sake, a drastic change occurs in the physician–pregnant woman relationship. The pregnant woman is now no longer the only patient—the fetus also becomes a patient needing treatment, perhaps even surgery. This raises complex ethical issues because (1) we have to consider whether the treatment is reasonable not simply for the fetus, but also for the woman who will be affected by an intervention of no direct biological benefit to her, and (2) we have to consider what is the right thing to do when the fetus needs treatment, but the woman declines to give informed consent for the intervention into her body. While society can take custody of a child whose parents refuse to provide proper medical care, it cannot take custody of a fetus or unborn child when the woman refuses medical care for it.

Some, however, suggest that interventions to aid the fetus without the woman's permission are justified in some situations. Perhaps the most dramatic examples of this are the few cases where physicians successfully convinced courts to allow invasive medical interventions, usually cesarean sections, against the woman's wishes. In 1987, for example, a nineteen-year-old Washington, D.C., woman named Ayesha Madyun arrived at the hospital after two days of labor. Eighteen hours later she still had not delivered, and there were signs of fetal distress. Physicians recommended a cesarean section, but she refused consent. Protected by a court order, they forced the surgery on her and saved the baby.

However, not all courts have responded this way. In New York, a judge refused to order a cesarean section on a thirty-five-year-old woman with ten children, despite the physicians' predictions that the cord wrapped around the baby's neck would strangle the baby if a vaginal birth was attempted. The judge, a woman, said no one can be forced to have surgery for the benefit of another person, even if the other person is her child. More recently, other courts have followed this reasoning.

These cases highlight a new kind of moral dilemma that arises for physicians when a fetal problem is diagnosed and a treatment is available. What does a physician do when a pregnant woman refuses medical treatment for her fetus or unborn child? The more the fetus is viewed as a patient, the more difficult it is for the physician to be comfortable doing nothing when something helpful can be reasonably done. It is somewhat ironic that about the same time that *Roe v. Wade* viewed abortion in terms of a right to privacy and neglected to consider the value of prenatal life, medicine was elevating the hitherto inaccessible fetus to the status of a patient worthy of diagnosis and treatment.

To illustrate the complexity of maternal–fetal conflicts, we turn to a well-publicized case.

THE CASE OF ANGIE

The Story

Angela Carder was approximately twenty-six weeks into her pregnancy when a routine checkup uncovered a large malignant tumor in her lung. She had already battled bone cancer for almost ten years and had been in remission for the previous two years. She was admitted to George Washington University Hospital in the District of Columbia, and her condition rapidly deteriorated. It soon became clear that she was dying. She was heavily sedated, and her physician thought it was likely she would die within twenty-four hours. A priest administered the last rites as her family prayed with her.

She had consented to treatments that might prolong her life in order to give her fetus a better chance at survival, but her primary concern, which was echoed by her husband and parents and supported by her physicians, was the comfort care she needed in her dying. She had previously agreed that a cesarean could be performed if her life could be extended another two weeks, but she did not want a cesarean section before twenty-eight weeks because she thought that the risks to the child resulting from a delivery before that time were too great.

Hospital administrators questioned her decision, and they sought legal advice. The attorneys, in turn, sought a judicial opinion. In other words, they wanted a judge to tell the hospital whether or not the physicians should intervene to save the fetus. A neonatologist who supported immediate intervention predicted a 50 to 60 percent chance of survival for the child, and a better than 80 percent chance a surviving baby would not be handicapped. At this point, Angie's mother reported that her daughter remained opposed to the delivery at twenty-six weeks. Her only wish was "I only want to die, just give me something to get me out of this pain."

Ethical Analysis

Situational awareness

We are aware of the following facts in Angie's story.

1. Angie was imminently dying and in need of comfort care.

2. If a cesarean section were performed, the premature baby would have about 50 to 60 percent chance of surviving; if it did survive, there would be about one chance in five it would be handicapped.

3. Angie had refused consent for a cesarean section before the twenty-eighth week of her pregnancy.

We are also aware of these bad features:

1. The cesarean section would add more pain and suffering to a dying woman.

2. Given her current position, any surgical intervention would be without informed consent; indeed, it would be forced on her against her wishes.

3. Angie was not expected to live until the twenty-eighth week. If she died while pregnant, the unborn child would almost certainly die also. If the surgery was done at once, there would be about an even chance a new life could be saved.

Prudential reasoning in the story of Angie

Patient's perspective. Note, first, that we are concerned with two patients here, Angie and her twenty-six-week possibly viable fetus. This complicates things immensely, especially since Angie's life is ending. We begin by considering the moral question from Angie's perspective. The surgery is of no benefit to her, will cause her significant additional pain, and will actually contribute to her death. Of course, the surgery could well save her fetus or unborn child, and this is a circumstance the pregnant woman has to consider if her refusal of surgery is to be morally justified. This is so because her refusal of the surgery means almost certain death for a possibly viable twenty-six-week fetus.

What the patient has to weigh in a situation such as this is her pain and suffering against the possible life of her fetus. Was she reasonable in declining surgery at this point? It certainly seems so. She had determined that she did not want to give birth before twenty-eight weeks. Before that point, she felt the chances of a good outcome for the fetus did not outweigh the risks to the fetus and the pain and suffering she would experience. That is a reasonable position. On the other hand, had she decided to take a chance and have the cesarean, that choice also seems morally justified.

Suppose her fetus was not at twenty-six weeks but at thirty-six weeks—would she still be morally justified in refusing surgery? This would be much harder to justify in an ethics of reason that cherishes life. Many, of course, would argue that a woman's choice over her fetus is absolute and thus, if she chose to decline the surgery at thirty-six weeks, then that is her choice. Indeed it is, and if that is her choice then it should be respected because the alternative—forcing surgery on an unwilling human being—is wrong. But the real question here is whether the decision to decline surgery to save a thirty-six-week fetus would be a morally justified decision.

Providers' perspective. The second stage of the ethical problem began when Angie declined the surgery. In such a case, should the hospital, judge, obstetrician, neonatologist, and attorneys try to force the surgery in order to save the other patient, the twenty-six-week fetus that could be viable? Certainly the death of the fetus is a bad thing that the hospital should try to avoid, although in this case there is about a 40 or 50 percent chance death will occur even if the surgery is done.

Is it reasonable for providers to force treatment on a woman in order to save, or in this case to try and save, her fetus? It seems not. Forcing surgery on someone who does not want it is itself a terrible evil. It is an assault that violates the dignity and bodily integrity of the human being who becomes no longer a patient but a victim. Certainly the intention—to save the fetus— is good, but good intentions by themselves do not justify the morality of our actions or, in more traditional language, the end does not justify the means. Even if one is convinced a woman is acting immorally toward her fetus, that still does not justify another immoral action—operating on her against her will. Forced interventions are not ethical interventions; they are not reasonable treatments, but immoral assaults.

The Court Decisions

Judge Emmett Sullivan of the District of Columbia Superior Court rushed to the hospital with a police escort on the morning of June 16, 1987. He was to spend most of the day there, conducting hearings to decide what medical care should be provided for the fetus. Those advocating the surgery argued that Angie was going to die anyway, so we might as well try to save the fetus. Angie's family and the lawyer representing her argued that we cannot do the surgery against her will, and that the surgery would in effect kill her since she was so weak at this point. During the rushed hearings, the hospital started prepping Angie for the cesarean section.

The judge heard the arguments of both sides, and then concluded: "It's not an easy decision to make, but given the choices, the court is of the view the fetus should be given an opportunity to live."

It was a little after four o'clock in the afternoon when the obstetrician told Angie of the judge's decision. Although she was on a respirator, she indicated her agreement with it. Then, a little later, the chief of obstetrics reminded her that Dr. Hamner, her obstetrician, would do the cesarean section only if she consented to it. Then she very clearly mouthed "I don't want it" several times. The chief of obstetrics immediately reported her refusal of consent to the judge. An attorney pressing for the surgery argued that her refusal made no difference because the assumption of the entire hearing was that she was refusing consent. He pointed out that if she had given consent, there would have been no need for the judicial intervention.

The surgery was scheduled for six-thirty that evening. Meanwhile, the attorney for Angie had appealed the judge's decision, and the surgery was delayed while a hastily assembled panel of three judges heard the appeal over the telephone. The arguments were of necessity brief. After a short consultation the three judge panel declined to stay the first judge's order. In effect, this gave the green light for the surgery.

Angie was taken to the operating room and, since her obstetrician refused to operate without her consent, another physician willing to do the cesarean had to be found. The cesarean section was done, and a premature infant of twenty-six weeks was delivered. Despite extensive treatment in the neonatal intensive care unit of the university hospital, the baby died in two hours. Two days later, Angie died. Her death certificate listed several causes of death—one of them was the surgery.

In November 1987 the panel of three judges who had heard the appeal over the telephone issued their written opinion, giving the reasons for the decision they had made the previous June. Their arguments were weak. One of them, for example, was that, although Angie could have aborted her third trimester fetus under *Roe v. Wade* if it was threatening her life, this did not give her the right to deny the fetus proper care once she decided not to abort it. Hence, they claimed that she should have consented to the cesarean section. Another argument centered on an analogy: just as a parent cannot refuse treatment necessary to save a child, so a woman cannot refuse treatment necessary to save her fetus.

The opinion of the three judge panel upholding the order for the surgery was then remanded for further consideration by the full court of appeals. Finally, in April 1990, almost three years after the incident, the District of Columbia Court of Appeals, in a decision known as *In Re: A.C.*, reversed the 1987 decisions: "We hold that in virtually all cases the question of what is to be done is to be decided by the patient—the pregnant woman—on behalf of herself and the fetus." The court of appeals recognized that the previous judges should not have ordered the surgery against Angie's will.

In an interesting footnote, the court noted that judges should not be called into hospitals to decide issues of life and death: "We observe nevertheless that it would be far better if judges were not called to patients' bedsides and required to make quick decisions on issues of life and death."

Ethical Reflection

There are two major ethical questions in this case. First, was Angie's decision to decline surgery designed to save her child before the twenty-eighth week morally reasonable and, second, were the decisions of the judges, attorneys, and physicians to force the surgery on her against her will in order to save the unborn child morally reasonable? We have already tried to show that Angie's decision, given the burden to her and the uncertain outcome, was reasonable. That leaves the second question, the prudential judgment of those who pushed for the surgery. Can this be justified? It seems not. We have no convincing reason for forcing surgery on a dying person to save a possibly viable fetus.

Part of the temptation to see the surgery as morally justified comes from a failure to distinguish the unborn from the born. The crucial distinction between the fetus an hour before birth and an hour after birth does not hinge on the physical structure of the fetus—the body of a newborn is pretty much the same as it was an hour before birth—but on the circumstances. The fetus is inside another human being, and we cannot claim custody of the unborn child without invading her body. All that changes at birth. If a mother refuses proper medical care for her neonate, we can take custody of the child without invading her body against her wishes, and that is the crucial difference.

The debate over the conflict between respecting the woman's control of her body during pregnancy and providing appropriate care for her fetus is far from over. The final court of appeals decision in Angie's case is more easily justified morally than was the attempt by the hospital to force surgery on a dying woman in an effort to save a premature unborn baby. Nonetheless, this decision left the door open for exceptions. What might they be? It is difficult to say, but surveys of obstetricians point to the following situations where some argue that interventions to save an unborn baby near term could be undertaken against the woman's wishes: (1) the head is clearly too large for the birth canal, (2) the placenta has detached from the uterine wall, and (3) the placenta is blocking the birth canal.

Professional organizations have tried to resolve these difficult dilemmas. The American College of Obstetrics and Gynecology (ACOG) issued an ethical statement entitled "Patient's Choice: Maternal–Fetal Conflict" in 1987, and the American Academy of Pediatricians (AAP) followed with an ethical statement entitled "Fetal Therapy: Ethical Considerations" in 1988. As the titles suggest, the ACOG statement tends to support the wishes of the woman, while the AAP statement underlines the potential benefits to the fetus.

Both statements, however, try to overcome the woman's refusal of treatment beneficial to her fetus by education and persuasion rather than by coercion. Both statements discourage appeals to the judicial system in an effort to force treatment on unwilling patients, but neither rules it out altogether. Finally, both statements reflect a wide ethical consensus that everything possible should be done to prevent providers from making the patient an adversary. Providers do not make the patient, or the proxy, an adversary when they disagree with the patient or proxy on a moral issue and communicate the reasons for that disagreement. But providers do make patients adversaries when they try to coerce them by using the power of the law to force invasive medical interventions on them against their wishes. The woman's choice may not be morally justified, but neither is it morally justified to force medical interventions on unwilling patients.

USING FETAL TISSUE

In the past decade we have become aware of the possible benefits fetal brain tissue may have for the treatment of certain diseases such as parkinsonism (an incurable and degenerative neurological disease) and some types of diabetes. Thousands of fetal tissue transplantations have been made in Europe, China, and Mexico, along with a hundred or so in the United States. The results have not been impressive, although recent studies show a definite, albeit limited, benefit from the procedure.

The attempts to reverse certain diseases by transplanting living cells from a dead fetus to a patient would not of themselves cause a major ethical dilemma as long as the ethical parameters guiding both experimental therapy on human subjects and transplantation are observed. The use of fetal brain tissue, however, becomes complicated because most of the fetal tissue comes from elective abortions. Many are concerned that the donation of fetal tissue will mask the morally problematic aspects of some abortions, and perhaps even encourage them. Hence fetal tissue transplantation has been inextricably linked with the abortion controversy in our country.

The Political Scene

The political struggle over the use of fetal tissue in our country has been intense. When it became apparent that fetal brain tissue might help people with parkinsonism, the National Institutes of Health (NIH) sought approval in

1987 from the Department of Health and Human Services to fund transplants, noting that the research was politically sensitive since it might give the appearance that funding the research was encouraging abortions.

The Assistant Secretary of Health, Robert Windom, directed NIH to establish an external committee to study the matter. The Human Fetal Tissue Transplantation Research Panel was composed of 21 people, including several people known to be opposed to abortion, most notably attorney James Bopp, general counsel for the National Right to Life Committee, and Rev. James Burtchaell, then a professor of theology at Notre Dame and author of several articles and a book opposing abortion.

In 1988 the panel recommended by a vote of 18–3 that, with certain restrictions, federal funding of fetal tissue transplantation would be appropriate. The advisory committee of the NIH director unanimously accepted this recommendation in December of the same year. Nonetheless, the administration continued a moratorium against federal funding of fetal tissue transplantation research. It feared that the beneficial use of fetal tissue would encourage abortions, and both the Reagan and Bush administrations had adopted a strong political stance against abortion.

Congress tried to overcome the moratorium on federal funding, but its efforts were vetoed by the President. In May 1992, an election year, President Bush did soften the moratorium somewhat by allowing NIH to fund research if the fetal tissue was obtained from spontaneous abortions (miscarriages) and from abortions of ectopic pregnancies. His executive order also established a fetal tissue bank to collect and distribute tissue drawn from these sources. Under the Clinton adminstration the Department of Health and Human Services (HHS) withdrew support for the fetal tissue bank and the project was cancelled in 1993.

Unfortunately, evidence suggests that ectopic and spontaneous abortions cannot supply sufficient fetal tissue for transplantations and for other promising programs of fetal research. In 1987 there were about eighty-eight thousand ectopic pregnancies in the United States. About 60 percent of ectopic pregnancies abort spontaneously, and studies show well over half of the remaining ones are defective fetuses. Thus the amount of tissue obtained from surgical abortions of healthy ectopic fetuses will be relatively small.

Spontaneously aborted fetuses from uterine pregnancies are also not a promising source of fetal tissue. Many of them are defective; chromosomal abnormalities alone count for about 60 percent of the defective uterine fetuses aborted. Moreover, nearly all spontaneously aborted fetuses are unsuitable for transplantation because they have actually died two or three weeks before the miscarriage. And many of those few fetuses that are living when the miscarriage occurs are expelled outside a health care setting and become too contaminated for use. The idea that ectopic pregnancies and miscarriages can provide an adequate source of fetal tissue for transplantation and other research is simply not realistic.

In 1993 the Clinton Administration relaxed the ban on fetal tissue research, and limited federally-funded studies began in order to ascertain the benefits of fetal tissue transplantation. This brings us back to the moral problem of obtaining tissue that could benefit sick people from elective abortions.

Ethical Issues

Much of the literature favoring the recovery of fetal tissue from aborted fetuses is content to argue that, since abortion is legal and a woman's right, using the tissue that would otherwise be discarded presents no ethical problem. The authors usually insist on certain safeguards such as (1) the woman must consent to the transplantation and she must not be asked for this consent until after she has decided on abortion, (2) no money is involved, and (3) the woman cannot designate the recipient of the fetal tissue. These restrictions, however, seem motivated more by political expediency than ethical cogency. If a woman has a right to destroy a fetus until the third trimester, then it seems she also has the right to donate the "products of conception," or even sell them, to whomever she wishes. If abortion in the first two trimesters is ethical simply because the woman chooses to have it, then it is not clear why it would not be ethical for her to dispose of the remains as she chooses.

But if one rejects the idea that abortions can be justified by simple choice or by a right and approaches the problem with an ethics that cherishes life and sees all abortions as bad—and therefore immoral unless serious reasons can justify the loss of human life—then it is not easy to justify retrieving fetal tissue from abortions unless it can be first established that the abortion was justified by adequate moral reasons. The moral danger in using fetal tissue from abortions is that the beneficial use of the tissue could make the woman less sensitive to the destruction of human life that occurs in every abortion. The use of aborted tissue to benefit other people can easily mask the ideal of preserving fetal human life unless there are overriding reasons to destroy it.

It is sometimes suggested that those harvesting fetal tissue need not be concerned with the morality of the abortion, and that it could be moral to use fetal tissue derived from immoral abortions. It is argued that this would be no different from using the bodies of murdered people for medical research and organ transplantation. Just as it is appropriate to accept the body and the organs of a murder victim without in any way condoning the murder, so we should be able to accept the fetal tissue of an aborted fetus even if we consider the abortion immoral.

But this analogy limps badly. Despite the superficial similarity between the situations, there are crucial differences. First, everyone recognizes that murder is immoral and illegal, but the morality and proper legal status of abortion is a matter of intense debate. There is no chance that using the organs of a murdered victim will blind us to the immorality of murder; there is the chance that using fetal tissue will blind us to the immorality of some abortions.

Second, there is little likelihood that people contemplating murder will be influenced by the benefits that can be derived from the victim's body, but there is a strong likelihood that people contemplating abortion will be influenced by the benefits that can be derived from the destroyed fetus.

Third, people ordinarily commit murder for rather base motives well known to homicide detectives—motives such as hate, rage, jealously, greed, passion, power, etc.—but most women having abortions do not have the motivations of a murderer, and thus abortion is seldom the same as murder, despite extreme pro-life rhetoric to the contrary.

It is also sometimes suggested that rules can be put in place to ensure that fetal tissue retrieval will not increase the number of abortions. Undoubtedly this is true, but it misses the point. For the majority of those opposed to fetal tissue transplantation, the issue is not primarily whether the procedure will increase abortions, but their conviction that many abortions are simply immoral. Hence it is *not* helpful to argue this way: "The crucial ethical issue is whether the medical use of fetal tissue encourages induced abortions; if it does not, the propriety of the abortion itself seems irrelevant to the subsequent use of the fetal tissue." The crucial ethical issues are the ethics of the abortion itself, and the complicity of those using tissue from morally problematic abortions.

There are some plausible reasons for arguing in favor of fetal tissue transplantation, and for federal funding of the research to study it. First, the tissue may well help people suffering from several serious problems. This factor alone, of course, does not justify aborting fetuses in order to obtain the tissue. Destroying human life to get tissues or organs helpful to others may be expedient, but it is not ethical.

Second, the ban on federal funding for fetal tissue transplantation did not stop all the use of fetal tissue for research—private monies were funding some programs. But, and this is the negative side of the government's decision to refuse funding for the research, the privately-funded research was not overseen by institutional review boards. These review boards are required by law in institutions accepting federally-funded medical research in order to protect the "human subjects" involved in the research, and the law defines a fetus as a human subject. With no federal support for fetal tissue research, the only research being done was privately funded, and thus the research escaped oversight by institutional review boards.

Researchers using private funds have realized the need for ethical oversight. In January 1991 two medical societies, the American College of Obstetricians and Gynecologists (ACOG) and the American Fertility Society (AFS), established their own National Advisory Board of Ethics in Reproduction (NABER). The board is charged with developing ethical standards for the use of fetal tissue and for the new reproductive technologies. NABER is now supported by private foundations and functions independently of ACOG and AFS. Many feel that this is a step in the right direction, but it still falls short of federally-sponsored panels and boards.

An ethics that cherishes life cannot condone destroying fetal life in order to get fetal tissue. Nor can it condone using fetal tissue obtained from abortions that are considered morally unjustified if such use makes the user an accomplice in the immoral abortion. The real moral question is the question of complicity—if someone else is doing something I consider wrong, in what circumstances, if any, can I derive something beneficial from the wrongdoing without becoming implicated in the wrongdoing? At what point does the use of tissue from abortions that I consider immoral make me an accomplice in the immorality, and therefore become something I cannot do in good conscience?

Moral complicity can be difficult to establish. We all know that if we hold someone so another person can shoot him, then our complicity in the murder is so significant that we are as guilty as the murderer who pulled the trigger. On the other hand, we all know that we cannot live in the world without "dirty hands." Some states, for examples, use tax dollars to pay for abortions. Many citizens believe at least some of these abortions are immoral, yet they continue to pay tax dollars that provide that welfare service. They are thus accomplices in the abortions that they consider immoral, but it is difficult to judge this complicity immoral because it is so remote from their personal lives. So the question about using fetal tissue is: is it morally justified for a person to use the tissue from what she considers immoral abortions for research and transplantation?

It is a delicate question. Once we say abortion is bad and therefore try to reduce the number of abortions by various ways, it is difficult to say we are justified in advocating any use of the fetal tissue. In effect, we are, on the one hand, trying to reduce abortions and, on the other, trying to get tissue from them for the medical research we want to do and for the therapy we want to provide. Such a position obviously involves us in a conflict of interest.

An Ethical Position

What follows is an attempt to work out an ethically responsible position in the complex issue of abortion and fetal tissue transplantation. A reasonable position will avoid the two extremes that do not do justice to the complexity of the situation. One of these extremes takes the position that induced abortion is such a terrible evil that the destroyed fetuses—considered by some to be murdered unborn children—should never be used in a way that might encourage abortion or undermine the campaign designed to stop all elective abortions in our country. The other extreme takes the position that, since abortion is legal, the use of destroyed fetuses is justified simply by the utilitarian argument that it will benefit sick people with tissue that would otherwise simply be discarded. This position, of course, begs the fundamental question: Are all the legally allowed abortions morally justified and, if they are not, how can one morally justify transplanting the fetal tissue harvested from immoral abortions?

A more reasonable position, one that avoids these extremes, might proceed as follows:

1. Consider the fetus a human subject. This is the position taken by the National Commission for the Protection of Human Subjects of Biomedical and Behavioral Research in 1975. It is a sound position because it recognizes that the fetus is human life, yet avoids controversial terms such as "person" or "baby." Because the fetus is a human subject, it deserves protection. Among the protections is the stipulation that someone must give informed consent for what happens to it.

2. Next, consider dead fetuses, and ask whether using tissue from them can be morally justified.

a) If the abortion was spontaneous, using tissue from a dead fetus presents no moral problem if the woman consents to it. Unfortunately, these abortions or miscarriages are not a promising source of sufficient fetal tissue for therapy.

b) If the abortion was induced, we have to distinguish between moral and immoral abortions:

1. If the induced abortion was morally justified, the use of fetal tissue presents no moral problem if the woman consents to it. For example, a woman about to undergo the abortion of an ectopic pregnancy could easily justify donating the fetal tissue for research or transplantation and give the appropriate informed consent.

2. If the induced abortion is not morally justified, and some of the 1.5 million abortions in the United States are morally suspect, the situation is much more conflicted. There are two major questions: first, who will give consent and, second, how can one justify complicity in using tissue for transplantation obtained from abortions thought to be immoral? If we can give morally respectable answers to these questions, then we can tentatively justify fetal tissue transplants from these fetuses.

    First, the question of informed consent. It is an issue because the consent for transplantation from a human subject who never had decision-making capacity must be given by a proxy. The natural proxy for a fetus is, of course, the pregnant woman. However, if the woman has decided to act immorally toward the fetus, as is the case when the abortion is not morally justified, some argue that she no longer is concerned with the best interests of the fetus and is disqualified from giving informed consent for research on it.

    If the woman seeking an immoral abortion is not the one to give consent for the use of its tissue, who is in a position to give consent? Some suggest the law could give consent in these cases, much the way British law currently provides consent for organ retrieval from children, subject to parental veto. Others propose that the consent could be obtained from a disinterested third party, perhaps a hospital committee such as the institutional review board (IRB) or institutional ethics committee (IEC). The important thing is to obtain consent for the transplantation from someone who is not behaving immorally toward the fetus and who is beyond any conflict of interest in the situation.

    Second, the question of complicity. Once the fetus is dead, it seems reasonable to say the tissue obtained from an abortion considered morally unjustified could be used, provided complicity in the abortion is removed or at least so reduced that it becomes morally insignificant. Complicity in retrieving fetal tissue from dead fetuses after morally unjustified abortions can be reduced if a physician other than the one harvesting the tissue makes the determination that the fetus is dead and if the recipient is anonymous. And a woman should not provide fetal tissue for someone she knows. This reduces the chance a woman would deliberately become pregnant or seek an abortion in order to harvest tissue from the fetus. These planned abortions are clearly inconsistent with due respect for fetuses and their status as human subjects. One way to separate those donating fetal tissue from those using it is by reestablishing the fetal tissue bank to control the collection and distribution of the tissue.

Moreover, the donation of fetal tissue should be a donation in the true sense of the word. No one should receive compensation for fetal tissue. And physicians providing it should not be promised any other benefits such as getting their name on the article that reports the research done with the tissue, etc.

3. Finally, consider living fetuses, and ask whether using tissue from them can be morally justified. The drive for fresh fetal brain tissue will inevitably encourage some abortionists to attempt removal of living fetuses so living tissue can be harvested from the brains. Thus the abortion procedure will be designed to deliver a live fetus, and the immediate cause of its death will be the subsequent removal of its brain tissue. This changes the whole picture of complicity because now it is no longer a question of using tissue from a dead human subject, but of harvesting tissue from a living subject and destroying the subject's life in the process.

In this kind of situation, the people involved in tissue transplantation are deeply implicated in the action destroying human life. And if the abortion itself is considered immoral, then harvesting tissue from the still living fetus clearly shares deeply in that immorality. It is a little more complicated if the abortion is morally justified. Consider a morally reasonable abortion where the physician tries to remove a fetus whole to enhance its transplantation potential. Would it be moral to harvest tissue from such a dying, but not yet dead, fetus? Perhaps. There are some good reasons for proceeding this way, but there are also good reasons for saying we should not remove brain tissue or vital organs from human subjects while they are still alive. This is especially true if the fetus has developed awareness—that is, is one of us. The retrieval of brain tissue from a living fetus not yet one of us remains an open question.

This ethical analysis is only a sketch of the complicated ethical dilemmas surrounding the use of fetal tissue, and many questions remain unanswered. The sketch is intended primarily to stimulate discussion and debate about an issue that will become more prominent in the near future if fetal tissue proves to be of significant therapeutic value. The position sketched here is tentative and has much in common with the recommendations of the NIH panel on tissue transplantation. Since the use of fetal tissue in research and therapy may result in much that is good but can also undermine our valuation of prenatal human life, moral reflection and dialogue are crucial.

Underlying this entire chapter is the awareness that prenatal life is human life, and that an ethics of the good tries to enhance life whenever possible and never damages or destroys human life without a sufficiently strong reason to balance the bad inherent in every destruction of life. Medical interventions now extend to the fetal patient. Whether these interventions are designed to destroy fetuses or to treat fetuses, they raise important moral issues, and we have considered but a few of them.

SUGGESTED READINGS

For the history of abortion, see John Noonan. 1979. "An Almost Absolute Value in History," *The Morality of Abortion: Legal and Historical Perspectives*, ed. John Noonan. Cambridge: Harvard University Press. pp. 1–59. For the history of the abortion controversy in America, see Laurence Tribe. 1990. *Abortion: the Clash of Absolutes*. New York: W. W. Norton & Company; John Noonan. 1979. *A Private Choice: Abortion in America in the Seventies*. New York: The Free Press; Gilbert Steiner, ed. 1983. *The Abortion Dispute and the American System*. Washington: Brookings Institution; Sidney Callahan and Daniel Callahan, eds. 1984. *Abortion: Understanding the Differences*. New York: Plenum Press.

The major legal turning point in the United States came on January 22, 1973, in *Roe v. Wade*, 410 U.S. 113 (1973). The court decided a second abortion case the same day—*Doe v. Bolton*, 410 U.S. 179 (1973). Mary Doe, a pseudonym, was a twenty-two year old married woman living in Georgia and pregnant with her fourth child. A former mental patient in a state hospital, she was impoverished and unable to care for her children. The two older ones were in a foster home, and the third had been placed for adoption. Her husband had abandoned her, forcing her to live with her indigent parents and their eight children, but she and her husband had recently reconciled. Unlike the Texas law at issue in *Roe v. Wade*, a law dating back to the middle of the nineteenth century that forbade all abortions except those to save the life of the mother, the nineteenth century Georgia laws had been revised in 1968 to allow abortions of pregnancies that would seriously and permanently injure the woman's health, or that involved a seriously defective fetus, or that were the result of rape. In *Doe. v. Bolton*, the court, consistent with its findings in *Roe v. Wade*, found that limiting abortions to these situations was unconstitutional.

The Supreme Court, however, did let some parts of the Georgia law stand, among them an important provision that allows physicians and nurses to refuse participation in abortions and that protects them from any retaliation if they do refuse. This is the legal basis that protects physicians and nurses who work in organizations such as a hospital or a health maintenance organization (HMO) and decline to participate in abortions.

For an extensive historical and legal account of the cultural and legal developments leading to *Roe v. Wade*, see David Garrow. 1994. *Liberty and Sexuality: The Right to Privacy and the Making of Roe v. Wade*. New York: Macmillan Publishing Co. For the sad and difficult real life of "Jane Roe," see Norma McCorvey with Andy Meisler. 1994. *My Life, Roe v. Wade, and Freedom of Choice*. New York: HarperCollins. After an abusive marriage and giving up her three children by three different fathers, Norma now supports herself by cleaning houses in Dallas.

Citations for the other Supreme Court cases relevant to abortion and mentioned in the text are: *Maher v. Roe*, 432 U.S. 464 (1977); *Harris v. McRae* 448 U.S. 297 (1980); *Planned Parenthood v. Danforth*, 428 U.S. 52 (1976); *City of Akron v. Akron Center for Reproductive Health*, 462 U.S. 416 (1983); *Thornburgh v. American College of Obstetricians and Gynecologists*, 476 U.S. 747 (1986); *Webster v. Reproductive Health Services*, 492 U.S. 490 (1989); and *Planned Parenthood Association of Southeastern Pennsylvania v. Casey*, 112 S. Ct. 2791 (1992).

For commentaries on the Supreme Court decisions, see George Annas. "The Supreme Court, Privacy, and Abortion." *NEJM* **1989,** *321,* 1200–03; and "The Supreme Court, Liberty, and Abortion. *NEJM* **1992,** *327,* 651–54; Claudia Mangel. "Legal Abortion: The Impending Obsolescence of the Trimester Framework." *American Journal of Law and Medicine* **1988,** *14,* 69–108; Tara Koslov. "Abortion on the

Supreme Court Agenda: *Planned Parenthood v. Casey* and its Possible Consequences." *Law, Medicine & Health Care* **1992**, *20*, 243–48; and Patricia Martin. "The Role of Women in Abortion Jurisprudence: From Roe to Casey and Beyond." *Cambridge Quarterly of Healthcare Ethics* **1993**, *2*, 309–19. This issue (pp. 327–30) also contains a helpful bibliography on the ethical issues surrounding prenatal and neonatal life. Also helpful is *Roe v. Wade*, annotated by Bo Schambelan (Philadelphia: Running Press, 1992), which has the complete texts of *Roe v. Wade* and *Doe v. Bolton*, as well as a postscript summarizing the relevant Supreme Court decisions since *Roe v. Wade*.

Although the Supreme Court has been the prime mover in the effort to liberalize the restrictive abortion laws inherited in most states from the nineteenth century, it need not have happened this way. All the Western European countries but one (Ireland) also abandoned their strict abortion laws in the latter half of the twentieth century, but in a different way. Instead of judicial fiat, they changed their laws in a process of parliamentary debate. Moreover, the new laws allowing abortion often begin by affirming the value of fetal life and the responsibility to protect it, and only then allow exceptions for grave reasons. This differs greatly from the decisions of our Supreme Court, which begin by affirming the right of the woman to destroy fetal life and then restrict this right for the sake of the fetus only in the third trimester. For an important essay on this difference between the American and European liberalization of abortion laws, see Mary Glendon. 1987. *Abortion and Divorce in Western Law*. Cambridge: Harvard University Press, chapters 1 and 3.

The Catholic moral position on terminating ectopic pregnancy by the often medically unnecessary procedure of removing the fallopian tube or other affected site is summed up in the *Ethical and Religious Directives for Catholic Health Facilities*. 1971. Washington: United States Catholic Conference. Directive 19 reads:

> "In extrauterine pregnancy the dangerously affected part of the mother (e.g., cervix, ovary, or fallopian tube) may be removed, even though fetal death is foreseen, provided that: a. the affected part is presumed already to be so damaged and dangerously affected as to warrant its removal, and that b. the operation is not just a separation of the embryo or fetus from its site within the part (which would be a direct abortion from a uterine appendage); and that c. the operation cannot be postponed without notably increasing the danger to the mother."

This directive represents the "solution" to the problem of ectopic pregnancy advanced by T. Lincoln Bouscaren in 1933. The Catholic Church had forbidden ectopic abortions, and the women who obeyed the proscription were dying. Bouscaren found a clever way around the Vatican condemnation—he said physicians could operate to remove the site, not the embryo, and hence the surgery would not be a direct abortion. See T. Lincoln Bouscaren. 1933. *Ethics of Ectopic Pregnancy*. Chicago: Loyola University Press. Today some theologians find Bouscaren's approach to ectopic pregnancies inadequate. See, for example, James Keenan. "The Function of the Principle of Double Effect." *Theological Studies* **1993**, *54*, 294–315. Nonetheless, Directive 48 of the new *Ethical and Religious Directives* approved in late 1994 still forbids direct abortion of an ectopic fetus. See *Origins* **1994**, 27 (December 15, 1994), 458.

For a discussion of selective abortion, see Richard Berkowitz. "Selective Reduction of Multifetal Pregnancy in the First Trimester." *NEJM* **1988**, *318*, 1043–47; and Richard Layzer. "Selective Reduction—A Perinatal Necessity?" *NEJM* **1988**, *318*, 1062–63. Another kind of case where selective abortion is an issue is the rare situation where one twin is so defective it cannot live outside the uterus and its continued presence in the uterus constitutes a threat to the healthy twin. If nothing is done while the seriously deformed twin is living, the healthy twin may also be lost; if the deformed twin is removed, then an abortion occurs. In such a situation, the deformed twin is threatening not the life of the mother, but the life of the healthy twin. See George Robie. "Selective Delivery of an Acardiac, Acephalic Twin." *NEJM* **1989,** *320,* 512–13.

For the medical aspects of RU 486 see Beatrice Couzinet et al. "Termination of Early Pregnancy by the Progesterone Antagonist RU 486 (Mifepristone)." *NEJM* **1986,** *315,* 1565–79; Etienne-Emile Baulieu. "RU 486 as an Antiprogesterone Steroid: From Receptor to Contragestion and Beyond." *JAMA* **1989,** *262,* 1808–14; and "Updating RU 486 Development." *Law, Medicine & Health Care* **1992,** *20,* 154–56. Baulieu also published, with M. Rosenblum. 1991. *The "Abortion Pill;"* RU 486: *A Woman's Choice.* New York: Simon & Schuster. Etienne-Emile Baulieu played a major role in the development of RU 486. Volume 20 (1992) of *Law, Medicine & Health Care* is devoted to articles on the ethical, legal, and medical issues associated with the drug. See especially Judith Senderowitz, "Are Adolescents Good Candidates for RU 486 as an Abortion Method?" (pp. 209–14); and Ruth Macklin, "Antiprogestin Drugs: Ethical Issues," (pp. 215–19). See also Lisa Cahill. "'Abortion Pill' RU 486: Ethics, Rhetoric, and Social Practice." *Hastings Center Report* **1987,** *17* (October–November), 5–8. For the political pressures operating until recently against efforts to license the drug in this country, see Lawrence Lader. 1991. *RU 486: The Pill That Could End the Abortion Wars and Why American Women Don't Have It.* New York: Addison-Wesley.

The case of Angie is taken from *In Re A.C.,* 573 A.2d 1235 (1990). For commentaries on this and similar cases see William Curran. "Court-Ordered Cesarean Sections Receive Judicial Defeat." *NEJM* **1990,** *323,* 489–92; George Annas. "She's Going to Die: The Case of Angela C." *Hastings Center Report* **1988,** *18* (February–March), 23–25 and "Foreclosing the Use of Force: A.C. Reversed." *Hastings Center Report* **1990,** *20* (July–August), 27–29. See also: Martha Field. "Controlling the Woman to Protect the Fetus." *Law, Medicine & Health Care* **1989,** *17,* 14–29; Lawrence Nelson and Nancy Milliken. "Compelled Medical Treatment of Pregnant Women." *JAMA* **1988,** *259,* 1060–66; Veronika Kolder et al. "Court Ordered Obstetrical Interventions." *NEJM* **1987,** *316,* 1192–96; and Thomas Elkins et al. "Maternal-Fetal Conflict: A Survey of Physicians' Concerns in Court-Ordered Cesarean Sections." *Journal of Clinical Ethics* **1990,** *1,* 316–19.

For a brief summary of the political controversy surrounding the transplantation of fetal tissue, see George Annas and Sherman Elias. "The Politics of Transplantation of Human Fetal Tissue." *NEJM* **1989,** *320,* 1079–82; Jerome Kassdirer and Marcia Angell. "The Use of Fetal Tissue in Research on Parkinson's Disease." *NEJM* **1992,** *327,* 1591–93; and Daniel Garry et al. "Are There Really Alternatives to the Use of Fetal Tissue from Elective Abortions in Transplantation Research?" *NEJM* **1992,** *327,* 1592–95. For a thoughtful criticism of using fetal tissue from elective abortion, see James Burtchaell. "University Policy on Experimental Use of Aborted Fetal Tissue." *IRB: A Review of Human Subjects Research* **1988,** *10,* 7–11, reprinted in James Burtchaell. 1989. *The Giving and Taking of Life.* Notre Dame: University of Notre Dame Press, pp. 155–87. For an opposing view, see Henry Greely et al. "The Ethical Use of Human Fetal Tissue in Medicine." *NEJM* **1989,** *320,* 1093–96. A good overview of the issue is an extensive bibliographic note by Mary Coutts. "Fetal Tissue Research." *Kennedy Institute of Ethics Journal* **1993,** *3,* 81–100. The position of the National Advisory Board on Ethics in Reproduction (NABER) can be found in Cynthia Cohen and Albert Jonsen. "The Future of the Fetal Tissue Bank." *Science* **1993,** *262* (10 December), 1663–65.

12

Neonatal Life

There is a myth about babies and, like most myths, it is not totally realistic. The myth is that all babies are healthy and beautiful; the reality is that some babies are born diseased, seriously defective, or too early. Deciding how to treat these babies is one of the more difficult challenges parents and physicians face in health care ethics.

Until a half-century ago, there was not much to decide. Neither neonatologists nor neonatal intensive care units (NICUs) existed. Their absence meant fewer ethical dilemmas because many impaired infants did not survive with the simple treatments that were available. Today we can save many neonates who would have died a few decades ago, but the interventions can be painful, and they often provide only limited lives marked by significant suffering. And so we have to ask about the morality of invasive treatments: when are they prudent and when are they unreasonable? Or, to put it another way, when do the medical interventions contribute to the infant's overall well-being despite the discomfort they cause, and when do they cause so much pain for so little benefit that it would be unreasonable to use them? These questions are especially important when, due to a terrible genetic defect or other problem, we know the infant is doomed to a short life of considerable suffering.

In this chapter we will proceed as follows. First, we will make a few remarks about the history of neonatal medical care; second, we will review some of the more common problems affecting neonates; third, we will consider two special difficulties in making moral decisions about neonatal treatment; fourth, we will examine what are called the Baby Doe rules; and fifth, we will examine three cases, including the famous Baby Doe case.

HISTORICAL BACKGROUND

Today most pregnant women seek medical care during their pregnancy, plan on delivering their babies in a hospital with the help of physicians or midwives and nurses, and expect to receive some postnatal care for themselves and their babies. Moreover, if the baby is impaired in any way, most parents expect the physicians and nurses to provide treatment.

These are relatively new expectations. For most of human history physicians did not provide prenatal care, most women did not deliver in a hospital, and little or nothing was done—because there was little that could be done—for infants who did not thrive. In the United States, for example, only 5 percent of babies were born in hospitals at the beginning of this century. Forty years later it had climbed to a national average of 50 percent, and to 75 percent in urban areas, where hospitals were more accessible. Today almost all births in the United States occur under medical supervision.

Moving births into the hospital and under the care of doctors meant all babies automatically became hospital patients and received medical treatment if they needed it. As a result, more and more children survived the early days, months, and years of life, and more and more parents came to expect that medicine could save their children despite impairments.

Parents of earlier generations had no such expectation. They expected to lose some of their children in the early years, and often did. In the first half of the eighteenth century in London, for example, three out of every four babies died before the age of five. The frequent deaths of babies and young children led to a kind of fatalism about infant mortality. People simply took it for granted that many newborns and infants would die in the early years of life.

Coupled with the great natural loss of babies and infants was the practice of infanticide, the killing of unwanted babies. It is difficult to know just how widespread this practice was in the societies that preceded us in our cultural tradition. Ethicists supporting the euthanasia of defective infants tend to see infanticide as quite widespread in our history, while those against the killing of defective babies suggest the practice was more rare and, when it did occur, was tolerated rather than praised as a noble and good thing to do.

The general Hebrew, Christian, and Stoic attitudes against abortion would have set the stage in the ancient Judaic–Christian and Greek–Roman worlds for a stand against infanticide. Moreover, the ancient practice of "exposure" of unwanted infants, usually defective ones, was not always a death sentence. Babies being abandoned by "exposure" were often left where others would likely find them. Some were picked up and raised by adoptive parents, as the famous and tragic drama of Oedipus reminds us. Abandoned by his parents Jocasta and Laos, he was raised by another couple, thus setting the stage for him to kill, unknowingly, the man who was his father, and then to marry, again unknowingly, the woman who was his mother.

On the other hand, Plato (*Republic* 460c) wanted defective babies set aside to die in hidden places, and Aristotle (*Politics* 1335b20) advocated laws against raising them. The famous Twelve Tablets of Roman law ordered defective babies to be killed quickly and Seneca, a Roman philosopher and political leader of the first century, clearly condoned infanticide (*De Ira* 1.15).

The killing and abandonment of impaired infants has now been condemned for centuries. The current emphasis is on saving them, an attitude reinforced by the medical setting where most infants are born. Some survivors, however, cannot live long or fare well even with the miracles of modern medicine, and this creates the moral dilemmas. Parents and physicians wonder whether great effort should always be made to keep severely handicapped babies alive when the most that can be expected is a short life of frequent surgeries and hospital admissions, or a longer life of significant suffering and little chance of engaging in simple human activities.

In October 1973 an English physician named John Lorber published a landmark article describing how aggressive treatment was withheld from some infants with spina bifida. In his cohort of thirty-seven babies in a twenty-one-month period, twelve were selected for aggressive treatment and the remaining twenty-five were considered so compromised by paralysis, large lesions, reverse spine curvature, multiple congenital defects, or a grossly enlarged head that they received comfort treatment but no oxygen, tubal nourishment, antibiotics, or cardiopulmonary resuscitation. Nor were they subjected to any invasive medical tests. All twenty-five died within nine months, as did one of the twelve selected for aggressive treatment. Three of those aggressively treated were fully normal, seven survived with slight paralysis and some of these were incontinent, and one survived with severe paralysis, kidney problems, lateral spine curvature, and incontinence. The article forced many people to question the prevailing expectation that every neonate should be given maximum treatment.

At almost the same time, Raymond Duff and A. G. M. Campbell reported on a thirty-month period in which 1,615 babies entered the Yale–New Haven Hospital by birth and another 556 were accepted in transfer. Of the 299 who died, 256 had been treated aggressively; parents and physicians had made decisions to forego life-sustaining treatment for the remaining forty-three. Again, the article forced readers to face the question of when to treat, and when not to treat, seriously deformed and critically ill infants.

Unlike John Lorber, who took a strong stand against euthanasia and infanticide, Duff and Campbell recognized in their article "a growing tendency to seek early death as a management option, to avoid that cruel choice of gradual, often slow, but progressive deterioration of the child who was required under these circumstances in effect to kill himself."

Seeking "early death as a management option" suggests, of course, infanticide or the euthanasia of seriously impaired infants. Today a number of ethicists support this option. The important thing, they argue, is good comfort care; once we decide unreasonable life-sustaining medical treatment will be withheld or withdrawn, then we should recognize that killing these infants is better than allowing them to die slowly. Others oppose it, arguing that euthanasia of children lacks a key element every serious proposal for euthanasia contains—the patient does not voluntarily request it. Euthanasia of infants is always involuntary euthanasia.

The articles by Lorber and by Duff and Campbell, along with a host of others that rapidly followed in the next decade, set the stage for the moral debate about treating infants. The ethical issue is simple: When is it better for an infant to bear the many burdens of interventions such as the long-term use of ventilators, multiple surgeries, and frequent cardiopulmonary resuscitations when the most that can be hoped for is a shortened life of considerable suffering? Before considering some of the moral aspects of this question, we will look at a few of the major problems afflicting newborns.

A SAMPLING OF NEONATAL ABNORMALITIES

Low Birth Weight (LBW)

Babies weighing less than 2,500 grams (about five-and-one-half pounds) are considered LBW infants. Most of them are premature, and many weighing near 2,500 grams do well with some supportive care. Others, especially those closer to the 500 gram mark, do poorly if they survive. About 75 percent of babies under 1,000 grams (about two pounds, three ounces) will experience bleeding in the brain, and one in four of these will suffer severe impairments such as mental retardation with an IQ below seventy or cerebral palsy.

Most low-birth-weight babies are premature and suffer from the common problems of prematurity. Often their lungs are not sufficiently developed, and resuscitation and ventilators are frequently needed. Unfortunately, these interventions can cause additional harm to the delicate premature lungs. Moreover, extremely premature infants often have feeding problems. Their gastrointestinal tracts cannot handle adequate nutritional intake, and both sucking and swallowing reflexes are not fully developed. Nourishment by IV lines can help, but it is often difficult to find sites for insertion, and sometimes the kidneys are not yet able to handle the fluids being provided. Finally, premature infants are susceptible to infections since their immune systems are immature.

Spina Bifida

This congenital problem results from the failure of the spine to fuse properly, leaving a section of the spinal cord exposed. Sometimes the membrane with its spinal fluid and nerve tissue bulges outward, creating a more serious problem.

While the severity of spina bifida varies greatly from patient to patient, most victims suffer additional damage. They are at risk for infection, and they frequently suffer some paralysis and nerve damage in the lower extremities, causing loss of bowel and bladder control. Many also have fluid in the brain because the cerebrospinal fluid cannot circulate well in the spinal column. A surgically implanted shunt can drain the fluid into the abdomen where it can be absorbed, but the operation is delicate and carries some risk both of physical and mental damage.

The history of treating infants with spina bifida has been one of changing attitudes. During some periods it was thought aggressive surgical, medical, and rehabilitative interventions should be employed for every infant; at other times less aggressive treatment, more in line with the approach of Dr. Lorber, was thought best.

Anencephaly

This condition is a more severe problem of the neural tube—the neocortex or cerebral hemispheres of the brain simply do not develop. Although anencephaly admits of some variation, the basic diagnosis is the absence of almost all the brain except the brain stem. Some anencephalic infants look normal and can breathe on their own. Today, the number of anencephalic infants is dropping because many women elect to abort once prenatal diagnosis confirms the problem. Of those not aborted, many are stillborn, and the remainder die within hours because they are seldom fed or treated. If fed, a few anencephalics can live for months or even a year or more, but they can never develop normally because they have little or no brain tissue within their skulls.

In some ways, an anencephalic infant resembles what some call neocorti-cally dead persons and, as was mentioned in chapter six, some people would like to equate the two. But the neocortically dead and the anencephalic infant differ in several crucial ways. First, the neocortically dead person once had a living neocortex and the brain tissue then died, while the anencephalic never had a living neocortex and therefore no brain tissues ever died. The anencephalic suffers from the lack of a brain, not the death of the brain. Death implies something was living and then ceased to live, but the anencephalic child never had a brain. This difference undermines the efforts to draw an analogy between neocortical death and anencephaly.

Second, the best evidence available today indicates that older children and adults suffering from neocortical death have lost all capability of aware-ness. They cannot, and will never again, feel anything. There is some evidence, however, that anencephalic infants can feel at birth. While destruction of the neocortex in an older child or in an adult precludes awareness, this is not so certain in the case of infants, where the brain stem may support primitive awareness. We cannot call a human being neocortically dead as long as the possibility of awareness is present.

The traditional therapeutic response of the obstetrical team to an anence-phalic infant was to do nothing except provide basic comfort care until the infant died. Nobody seriously considered treatment because treatment cannot restore a missing brain. If the anencephalic neonate did have awareness, it would soon be lost, and infants with irreversible loss of awareness have no interests. It cannot be said, then, that treatment would be in their best interests. For most people, withholding treatment from anencephalic infants was mor-ally incontrovertible.

More recently, however, several ethical controversies have arisen con-cerning anencephalic infants. First, some ethicists suggest aggressive interven-tions to keep them alive are justified to preserve their organs for transplanta-tion. In such cases, the life-support equipment will keep the baby alive until the recipients are ready, then the life support will be withdrawn, the baby will die, and the fresh organs will be immediately harvested.

Second, some suggest these infants should be considered brain-dead. The idea behind this move is the desire to harvest their organs while they are still breathing, much as organs can be harvested from a brain-dead patient breathing on a ventilator. A few years ago, some physicians in Germany were actually taking organs from anencephalic infants, but legal authorities put an end to the practice.

Third, some are beginning to suggest that infants with anencephaly should be given sedatives to ease their dying, even though even the smallest dose of a sedative carries a high risk of being lethal. These people are not arguing for euthanasia; they advocate only the lightest dose of sedation to relieve distress, although they do recognize it might also be lethal.

Fourth, some do advocate euthanasia for anencephalic infants. They argue that the baby is dying anyway and that treatments are not going to be provided, so the most humane thing is to kill them with a lethal injection, especially if there are signs of suffering.

Fifth, some parents are now insisting that physicians treat their anencephalic baby with medical nutrition and life-sustaining treatments. In 1993 one such case involving a child known as "Baby K" received widespread publicity; we will describe the circumstances later in the chapter.

Trisomy

Normally the chromosomes of a human being are found in twenty-three pairs, but occasionally one of the pairs is really a triplet—it carries an extra chromosome. The condition is known as trisomy. Trisomy 21 means the twenty-first chromosome is not a pair but a triplet, trisomy 18 means the eighteenth chromosome is a triplet, etc. Some of the more important abnormalities involving trisomy are as follows.

1. *Trisomy 13:* This chromosomal abnormality causes facial distortions, including widely spaced small eyes with abnormal retinas, low-set ears, and poorly formed lower jaw. The infants are severely retarded, and they often suffer congenital heart disease and central nervous system disorders. Life expectancy is short; almost half die the first month, and the fewer than 20 percent that do survive the first year suffer mental defects, seizures, and failure to thrive. Physicians and parents often wonder whether it is reasonable to use aggressive life-sustaining treatment since the long term prognosis is so poor.

2. *Trisomy 18:* This abnormality also causes physical deformities and mental retardation. The skull is narrow and elongated with poorly formed ears placed lower than normal, hands are clenched with overlapping fingers and malformed thumbs, and the feet bulge outward on the bottom. Most of the infants have congenital heart disease and significant gastrointestinal and renal problems. About half the infants will die in the first two months; only 10 percent survive the first year. With aggressive treatment and institutionalization, about 1 percent will reach the age of ten. Again, people naturally wonder whether the burdens of treatment to the child are justified in light of such a poor prognosis.

3. *Trisomy 21:* This is perhaps the best known trisomy problem. The more popular name is Down's syndrome. It is marked by a sloping forehead and low-set ears. The eyes are almond-shaped and have gray or yellow spots. Mental retardation ranges from severe to moderate, and life expectancy can often be measured in decades. Babies with Down's syndrome do not normally present moral dilemmas because they are not suffering and do not need special medical attention. With supportive care they can easily enjoy limited thriving, and some suggest their mental retardation is such that they are not fully aware of their condition and may actually live rather happy lives.

Many babies with Down's syndrome, however, have some additional physical problems. Blockages (atresias) in the intestine or the esophagus are common, as are openings (fistulas) between the esophagus and the trachea. Attempting to feed babies with these problems, of course, is out of the question. Luckily the blockages and the openings can usually be corrected with relatively simple surgery, and the infants can then be fed normally.

However, several notable cases have arisen where the parents refused consent for the surgery to correct these physical problems. Without informed consent the surgeons could not operate, and without the operation the babies could not be fed. We will read the story of one of these babies, the baby known as "Baby Doe," and we will review the history of the "Baby Doe" regulations this famous case produced.

Significant Intestinal Loss

Some infants develop problems before or after birth that destroy large segments of their intestines. Perhaps the intestines became so twisted that the blood supply was cut off and the tissue died, or perhaps an infection caused the damage. The loss is life-threatening if the remaining functioning intestine is so short that the absorption of food necessary for life cannot occur. Tubal feeding is of no help since the intestines cannot absorb the nutrients.

Recently, the TPN (total parenteral nutrition) feeding techniques we explained earlier have been used with some success. Nutrition by IV lines has its problems, however, because infection often sets in, and finding new sites on a baby's body for the insertion of IV lines is a challenge. An ethical dilemma, therefore, centers on whether to start these infants on TPN, knowing that they will probably never be able to eat or drink and will probably need TPN for the rest of their lives. This dilemma may disappear in the future, however, if the transplantation of intestines from infant cadavers (now being tried) ever becomes a reliable surgical response to the problem.

Conjoined Twins

Some babies born joined together can be surgically separated so both can live individual lives despite the handicaps resulting from the conjoining. Others cannot be separated, but they can live joined lives. Still others cannot be separated and cannot live joined lives; if left joined both will soon die, but if they are separated the stronger might live. This last situation presents a formidable ethical dilemma that, mercifully, happens only rarely.

Consider, for example, conjoined twins sharing the same heart mass, and the cardiac mass cannot be divided so each will have enough of a heart to survive. If the twins are not surgically separated, both will soon die because the heart mass cannot support two growing bodies. If the twins are separated, the surgery will, in effect, kill the weaker twin but enable the other to live longer with the heart that will now provide for only one body. Sometimes most of the heart mass is located more in the weaker twin's chest. In this case the surgical separation becomes a kind of heart transplant—the heart mass located mostly in the weaker twin is removed and placed in the chest of the stronger. A heart is thus transplanted from a living human being so that the sibling can live. One brother or sister is killed so that the other brother or sister can survive.

In August 1993 there was widespread publicity about just such a case. Surgeons at the Children's Hospital in Philadelphia separated the Lakeberg twins of Wheatfield, Indiana, after they were flown in from a hospital in Chicago where they were born. The parents and surgeons knew the operation would kill one twin, but they hoped to save the other. Although the chances of survival were slim, one baby, Angela, did survive the operation.

Angela never left the ICU and needed continuous ventilation most of the time. Ten months after the separation she developed a bacterial infection and died in June 1994. Dr. Russell Raphaely, a physician at the hospital, reported that a medical team had resuscitated her two or three times in the three hours preceding her death. Her parents were not with her when she died. Her father, who had admitted using some of the money donated to the family by sympathetic people for cocaine, was back in jail hours after her death on charges of auto theft.

As often happens, the ethical issues in this case are many. The surgery that saved Angela killed her sister, was unlikely to benefit her significantly, caused her pain and suffering during the ten months it prolonged her mostly ventilator-dependent life in the ICU, and cost over a million dollars, some of which Indiana Medicaid has agreed to pay. Moreover, physicians responded with CPR several times when she suffered cardiopulmonary arrests in the last few hours of her life.

Although these cases of conjoined twins are rare, the problem is worth noting because it creates such an important ethical dilemma: doing nothing means both babies will die, but saving one will kill the other. If the prohibition against directly killing the innocent allows no exceptions, nothing can be done. In an ethics of right reason, however, there is a way to justify the surgery. This ethics recognizes that the situation is truly tragic: Either both will shortly die, or one will die and the other will have a chance at life. It is at least arguable that letting both die is less reasonable than taking the drastic step of separating the twins in a desperate effort to save one. Such a move, however, challenges the important claim made by many people that "directly killing an innocent person is always wrong." It shows once again how difficult it is to formulate an ethics in terms of absolute prohibitions that admit of no exceptions.

Of course, other ethical issues surround this kind of case, not the least of which are the slim chance that the survivor would live well for more than a few months or years and the immense costs of treatment. In the minds of many ethicists, these factors indicate that the surgery is rarely reasonable and should not have been attempted in the Lakeberg case.

Diaphragmatic Hernias

As a fetus develops, the diaphragm normally closes the opening between the abdominal and chest cavities. When it does not, the intestines migrate into the chest cavity and prevent lung development. About one in four thousand babies suffers from this defect, and many need ventilator support until surgery to repair the hernia. For some babies, however, ventilator support is not enough; they need extracorporeal membrane oxygenation (ECMO) if they are to survive. ECMO is a machine that draws blood from the baby's jugular vein, enriches it with oxygen, then returns the oxygenated blood to the carotid artery. It provides what the lungs cannot provide even when assisted by mechanical ventilation.

The babies needing ECMO can be roughly divided into two groups. Half of them are so sick that only 10 percent will survive after surgery; the remaining half are strong enough that 80 percent of them will survive. The ethical dilemmas center on the group with only a 10 percent survival rate. We have to ask whether it is reasonable to subject the newborn infants in this group to the discomforts of the ECMO technology and of the multiple surgeries that are usually required, when 90 percent of the time these burdens result in little but suffering for a dying infant. For each success story in this group, nine other infants were aggressively and painfully treated when it was of no benefit to them. The problem, of course, is that we do not know beforehand which baby will, and which nine will not, benefit from ECMO and the surgery.

SPECIAL DIFFICULTIES IN DECIDING FOR NEONATES AND SMALL CHILDREN

Two special difficulties occur in making decisions about treatment for very young children. First, the best interests standard is enormously complicated and at times not relevant for infants and, second, the baby's parents are not always able to function as reliable proxies for their children.

Problems with the Best Interest Standard

Babies and young children clearly cannot make their own decisions—they need a proxy. And proxies clearly cannot make the decisions for the infants based on the preferred standard, substituted judgment, because the infants never had the opportunity to form their own wishes and preferences. Hence the proxy for an infant has to rely on the best interests standard.

But making decisions on the basis of best interests is more difficult for babies than it is for adults. The proxy has some information about an adult's attitudes and interests in life, and this can be a big help in figuring out what is in the adult patient's best interest. But babies have not yet developed any life of their own, so the proxy is working in a kind of vacuum.

Moreover, it is difficult to assess how the burdens caused by congenital impairments and by treatments affect babies. In general, many impairments seem less burdensome for children than they would be for comprehending adults, and many treatments seem more burdensome.

Congenital impairments may be less burdensome for some infants because their perspective is different. We may not think it is in our best interests to live with the impairments of some infants, but the person born in such a condition may well have a different view. If we imagine, for example, an infant born blind, deaf, and missing a limb, we might be tempted to think that his life is not worth living and to withdraw treatment. But we are thinking from our point of view, as someone who knows what it is to have sight, hearing, and a whole body, and then to lose them. A child who never enjoyed these might not think the same way. What we would consider a terrible loss may not be experienced as such a loss by him because he never had what he now lacks.

On the other hand, treatments may be more burdensome for babies because the neonatal body is so small and fragile. Of course, we can only guess at the suffering medical interventions cause infants. We can get a pretty good idea of how much discomfort medical interventions cause adults from their reactions, but babies do not react to pain as do adults. And we cannot simply extrapolate from the discomfort a ventilator, an IV, a feeding tube, CPR efforts, or surgery causes adults to the discomfort these same interventions cause babies. Nonetheless, it does seem that an IV in the arm, for example, would be less of a burden to a one hundred pound patient than it would be to a four pound premature infant.

The best interests standard in relation to infants is further undermined by the high level of prognostic uncertainty endemic to neonatology. In the Baby Jane Doe case (1984) that we will consider, for example, the experts at a renowned facility predicted early death without surgery to correct a spina bifida problem. However, the surgery was not performed, and the infant has lived for years and now attends a school for the developmentally disabled.

Finally, in some situations the best interests standard for infants becomes suspect because it leads to unreasonable conclusions. Best interests centers on an analysis of benefits and burdens—a decision is in someone's best interest if the benefits outweigh the burdens; that is, if the good outweighs the bad. Life itself is an important good, and sometimes it can be sustained with little or no burden to the infant. Ventilation, for example, can prolong the life of some newborn anencephalic infants who may have some awareness and be of little burden for them. Thus the best interests standard suggests using these treatments, yet most everyone agrees that ventilators are unreasonable for anencephalic infants.

Before leaving our consideration of the difficulties in using the best interests standard for infants, we should mention an additional factor that some people believe is relevant to an infant's best interests. They say that best interests embraces the kind of social life that the baby will have if he or she survives. If the impaired baby happens to be born in unfortunate circumstances, then they suggest it might not be in the child's best interests to be treated aggressively because follow-up care at home would not be available. For example, if an impaired baby is delivered by a woman with a long history of dysfunctional mothering, then saving the baby now might be doing little more than setting the child up for more suffering in a unsuitable home situation, a terrible burden for any child. According to this argument, treatment might be in the infant's best interests if the child was part of a loving, mature, and supportive family, but would not be in the child's best interests if the child is a member of a dysfunctional family that obviously could not, and perhaps would not, provide needed support for the impaired child.

There are good reasons for thinking this approach is profoundly discriminatory and therefore immoral. Moreover, interpreting the best interests standard this way undermines the efforts of society to care for sick people of any age who do not happen to have family support. We do not become good and noble people by declining treatment because babies lack family support. Socially induced burdens are truly burdens for a child, especially one suffering from serious impairments, and some home situations are definitely not beneficial for children. But these social burdens are peripheral to our consideration of the benefits and burdens of the child's treatment, and this is what we evaluate in the best interests standard. The ethical response to unfortunate social burdens faced by the infant is not to withhold treatment, but to provide whatever treatment is medically appropriate and then to make efforts toward correcting the wider social problem.

Problems with Parental Proxies

The second special difficulty associated with making treatment decisions for infants is that the customary proxies for infants, the parents, may not always make good judgments about what is truly in their child's best interests. This can be so for two reasons: some parents find it so difficult to accept the birth of a defective child that they decline reasonable treatment, and some parents find it so difficult to accept the death of a child that they insist on unreasonable treatment. The actual cases at the end of this chapter illustrate both of these positions.

Parental distress upon the discovery of a seriously impaired or deformed infant is understandable, especially if it comes as a surprise. The distress increases as the future impact on their lives, and on the lives of the children they may already have, begins to sink in. If parental consent for life-sustaining treatment is needed, parents are sometimes tempted to see withholding consent as a way to resolve the tragedy that could affect them and their other children for years. Once this thought begins to take hold, the parental proxies are enmeshed in a conflict of interest that can easily undermine their ability to make decisions based on the child's best interests. Many see the Baby Doe case as an example of this.

Some parents tend to be unreasonable in the other direction; that is, they insist that everything possible be done for their baby, even when the burdens of "everything" obviously outweigh whatever slim and dubious benefits the infant might gain. Parents sometimes demand treatments that, because of circumstances, amount to little more than child abuse, although they do not see it that way. They sometimes insist on invasive and painful therapies that do little more than prolong a life of misery because they believe life, no matter how painful, limited, and short, is always in the child's best interest. Parents unable to decline unreasonable life-sustaining treatment for their child are not really able to act well as proxies, and their insistence on treatment can do more harm than good. Many see the stories of Danielle and Baby K as examples of this tendency.

THE BABY DOE REGULATIONS

In 1982 what was to become one of the most highly publicized cases involving medical treatment for infants unfolded in Bloomington, Indiana. The baby was known as Baby Doe, and in the next section we will provide an ethical analysis of the case. In this section, however, we want to review the regulations and legal requirements generated by the case. In a modified form, these regulations, often called the Baby Doe regulations, are still in effect. Many people find some aspects of them morally suspect, so it is well to know something about them and their history.

History of the Baby Doe Regulations

In April 1982 parents in Bloomington, Indiana, refused consent for relatively simple life-saving surgery on their baby. The baby suffered from Down's syndrome and an additional life-threatening disorder. Without the surgery the baby could not be fed, and the child soon died despite the efforts of providers to obtain court authorization for the surgery.

In May 1982, acting on President Reagan's instructions, the Department of Health and Human Services (HHS) responded by issuing a notice affecting every hospital receiving federal funds. It stated:

> Under section 504 it is unlawful for a recipient of federal assistance to withhold from a handicapped infant nutritional sustenance or medical or surgical treatment required to correct a life-threatening condition if: (1) the withholding is based on the fact that the infant is handicapped; (2) the handicap does not render the treatment or nutritional sustenance medically contraindicated.

Section 504 of the 1973 Rehabilitation Act outlaws discrimination against people on the basis of handicap. The notice from HHS was an attempt to extend the Rehabilitation Act to the medical treatment of defective infants.

In March 1983 HHS published an interim rule requiring hospitals to display posters informing everyone that treatment cannot be withheld from infants with handicaps. Any person having knowledge "that a handicapped infant is being discriminatorily denied food or customary medical care" was urged to call the 'Handicapped Infant Hotline' (1–800–368–1019) at HHS to report violations. Callers could remain anonymous, and reports of serious infractions would trigger investigations.

In April 1983 a federal court struck down this interim rule on the grounds that it was "arbitrary and capricious," and that the usual opportunity for public comment about a proposed rule was waived by HHS without justification. The hotline, however, stayed open and calls continued to come in. The government investigated over forty complaints in the next six months. Some people called the teams of government investigators "Baby Doe Squads."

Here are two examples of what happened. On the morning of March 29, 1983, an anonymous caller reported a case in the Strong Memorial Hospital in Rochester, New York, involving conjoined twins. Two investigators from the New York Office of Civil Rights rushed to Rochester, arriving by late afternoon. They were joined by a third investigator who had flown in from Washington. They met for three hours with a hospital administrator and the attending physician, and reviewed the medical records. The physician informed the investigators that the parents were worried about publicity.

The investigators met with the neonatologist the government had hired as a consultant when he arrived in Rochester after nine o'clock in the evening. When this physician discovered the parents had not consented to the investigation, he declined to review the records or visit the hospital.

The next morning the hospital administrator asked the federal investigators to stay away from the hospital because the case was receiving publicity in the media and the parents were upset. Unwelcome at the hospital and lacking the cooperation of its medical consultant, the team left Rochester without further action. More than nine months later, HHS acknowledged it had not yet completed its review. After nothing ever came of the investigation, people were left wondering why the investigators from New York and Washington had rushed to Rochester to investigate the treatment of the babies.

Another investigation occurred at Vanderbilt University Hospital in Nashville. Just before noon on March 23, 1983 the hotline received a call reporting that ten infants were not receiving proper treatment or nourishment. Less than ten hours later, two investigators from the Atlanta Office of Civil Rights and one from Washington were on the scene, along with a medical consultant the government had retained. They worked at the hospital until after midnight, then returned the next morning at eight o'clock to continue their investigations until late afternoon. Then they left without telling the worried physicians and nurses what they had found. Only some time later did the Office of Civil Rights inform the hospital that it had found no violations of the HHS regulations.

Between March and the end of November that year, the Office of Civil Rights received over 1500 calls on the hotline and investigated forty-nine of them. HHS acknowledged in January 1984 that none of the forty-nine investigations resulted "in a finding of discriminatory withholding of medical care." The federal investigations, of course, were upsetting for the already distressed parents and for the physicians as well.

In July 1983 HHS issued a more carefully crafted proposed interim rule to replace the one the federal judge had struck down in April. Notice of this rule did allow for public comment, and almost 17,000 reactions were received, most of them in favor of it as the result of an intense campaign by groups convinced that most cases of withholding treatment from impaired infants violates their right to life. HHS made some modifications in light of these comments and published its final rules in January 1984.

In June 1984 a federal court struck down these rules on the grounds that section 504 of the Rehabilitation Act was never intended by Congress to apply to health care decisions for impaired infants. The court also said that the investigations by the Office of Civil Rights must stop. HHS appealed this ruling, and the case went all the way to the United States Supreme Court. In June 1986 the Supreme Court upheld the lower court ruling, thus affirming that section 504 of the 1973 Rehabilitation Act does not apply to health care for impaired infants. This ended the government's efforts to mandate the medical care of infants under the Rehabilitation Act.

Meanwhile, proponents of the Baby Doe regulations had initiated another approach. They successfully lobbied Congress to include laws requiring treatment of impaired infants in amendments to the Child Abuse Prevention and Treatment Act. This act authorizes federal grants to help states prevent and treat child abuse. The amendments expand the definition of medical neglect to include the "withholding of medically indicated treatment." The amendments further mandated that, in order to qualify for federal grants under the act, states must have programs or procedures in place to respond to reports of such medical neglect. The amendments to the Child Abuse Act were signed into law by President Reagan on October 9, 1984.

This means that the legal basis for the Baby Doe rules now in effect are amendments to a public law enacted by Congress. The public law, however, does not contain provisions for a hotline or for any "Baby Doe Squads" to investigate reported noncompliance. In fact, the Congressional Record for July 26, 1984, reveals that one of the six senate sponsors of the Baby Doe amendments, Senator Kassebaum, said for the record that she was deeply troubled by the aggressive enforcement actions HHS had taken in this matter.

The Substance of the Current Baby Doe Regulations

The amendments to the Child Abuse Prevention and Treatment Act define "medical neglect" to include "withholding of medically indicated treatment." The key issue, then, is: What is "medically indicated treatment"? In response, the amendments define three interventions as *always* "medically indicated." These are: nutrition, hydration, and medication. In addition, all other interventions "most likely to be effective in ameliorating or correcting" the infant's life-threatening conditions are also "medically indicated," except in three situations designated by A, B, and C in the following section. The most important paragraph in the regulations reads as follows:

> The term "withholding of medically indicated treatment" means the failure to respond to the infant's life-threatening conditions by providing treatment (including appropriate nutrition, hydration, and medication) which, in the treating physician's or physicians' reasonable medical judgment, will be most likely to be effective in ameliorating or correcting all such conditions, except that the term does not include the failure to provide treatment (other than appropriate nutrition, hydration, or medication) to an infant when, in the treating physician's or physicians' reasonable medical judgment, (A) the infant is chronically and irreversibly comatose; (B) the provision of such treatment would merely (*i*) prolong dying, (*ii*) not be effective in ameliorating or correcting all of the infant's life-threatening conditions, or (*iii*) otherwise be futile in terms of the survival of the infant; or (C) the provision of such treatment would be virtually futile in terms of the survival of the infant and the treatment itself under such circumstances would be inhumane.

What can be said about these regulations that require nutrition, hydration, and medication in all cases, and all other treatment thought to ameliorate or correct life-threatening conditions in all but three narrowly defined exceptional circumstances? A great deal, but we will confine our commentary to several remarks.

First, as you can see, the definition of medically indicated treatment is not presented very clearly in these regulations, and people still disagree on what the regulations mean by it.

Second, they seem to require medical nutrition for babies in persistent vegetative state. These babies are not comatose, and hence do not fall under the first exception. This leaves us in a strange situation because it does not make much sense to allow withdrawal of feeding tubes from comatose infants, but not from those in PVS.

Third, if the infant is not irreversibly comatose and is not dying, and if the treatment is effective in ameliorating or correcting the life-threatening conditions and not futile in terms of survival, then the regulations seem to require that treatment must be given . . . unless it is "virtually futile *and* inhumane" (emphasis added). Now, suppose the treatment is not actually or virtually futile, but is nonetheless inhumane because it is so painful and will leave the baby in great pain. For example, if it is possible to keep a badly burned baby who might survive alive for months with life support, the treatment is not virtually futile. In some cases, however, due to great suffering and a poor prognosis, it could be considered inhumane to subject the burn victim to this life-sustaining treatment. Yet the treatment is required by the Baby Doe regulations because, while inhumane, it would not also be virtually futile.

Many ethicists understandably have a strong objection to federal rules that require physicians and nurses to provide any inhumane treatments. If the rule said an exception could be made for treatment that was virtually futile or inhumane, this problem would not exist. But the regulations allow treatment to be withheld only if it would be *both* virtually futile *and* inhumane. Thus inhumane treatments that are not virtually futile, and there are some, must be given according to the current Baby Doe regulations.

Fourth, the Baby Doe rules require medication at all times without exception. While some medication is for pain relief, and this should always be given where appropriate, other medications are directed toward curing illness, and there are times when it makes no sense to give these medications. Consider a suffering, dying child who develops pneumonia. Since the Baby Doe regulations require medication for illness at all times, the physician must treat the pneumonia with antibiotics. Insisting that the pneumonia of every suffering, dying child must be treated strikes many people as morally unreasonable.

Reaction to the Baby Doe Regulations

Many people disagree with the Baby Doe regulations. They argue that the regulations undermine the parents' prerogative to decide what is in the best interests of their baby and, in some cases, actually mandate treatment that is at least arguably not in the best interests of the child.

A survey that received 494 responses from members of the Perinatal Pediatrics Section of the American Academy of Pediatrics showed 76 percent believed the regulations were unnecessary, 66 percent believed they interfered with parents' ability to determine what is in the best interests of their children, and 60 percent believed the regulations did not adequately consider the suffering caused by treatments prompted by the regulations. The survey article summarized many of the arguments against the Baby Doe regulations, including the following points.

1. The regulations are not needed. The U.S. Supreme Court had found that no evidence supported HHS's claim that such regulations were needed

when it struck down the Baby Doe regulations that the Department of Health and Human Services had tried to impose under section 504 of the Rehabilitation Act.

2. The regulations ignore what the Supreme Court had called "the decisional responsibility" of the parents.

3. The regulations cause a misuse of scarce resources.

4. The regulations exert undue pressure on state agencies and physicians.

5. The regulations are not clear; the survey showed many perinatal physicians disagreed about what was required in specific cases. The lack of clarity is obvious in the paragraph quoted above.

6. The regulations sometimes require treatment so burdensome that it is not in the child's best interests and is therefore unethical.

Enforcement of the Baby Doe Rules

As ominous as the Baby Doe regulations seem, their actual impact on parents and physicians is not, or should not be, as great as some would have us believe. What happens to someone who ignores the rules and is "caught"? The short answer is: nothing that would not have happened under the state laws already in existence before the Baby Doe rules were passed by Congress. The only federal penalty for violation of the federal Baby Doe rules affects the states, not individuals. And the penalty is not for any violation of the treatment regulations but for the state's failure to have programs and procedures in place for investigating complaints about violations of the regulations. And the penalty for this failure does not affect any person directly—if a state does not have programs and procedures to investigate violations of the Baby Doe regulations, the only thing that happens is that it may suffer the loss of future federal grant money for its child protection agency. Violations of the Baby Doe rules do not subject any parent, physician, or nurse to any penalty; the only penalty is a loss to the state of federal grant money.

We should note that some states (Alaska, Arizona, Indiana, Oregon, and Pennsylvania, for example) choose not to apply for the these federal grants, and thus are not directly affected by the Baby Doe rules at all. Other states have elected to establish procedures to enforce the Baby Doe regulations in order to maintain eligibility for federal grants. Massachusetts is one such state, and a look at its procedures for investigating Baby Doe complaints will be helpful in understanding how reported violations of the Baby Doe regulations are handled.

In Massachusetts, responsibility for child abuse violations rests with the Department of Social Services (DSS), the Commonwealth's child protection agency. If it receives a report that the Baby Doe regulations are being violated, it assigns a social worker to investigate the complaint. The social worker must then obtain signed consent from the parents permitting the hospital to discuss the medical record of its patient and permitting the social worker to review a patient's medical record. Among other things, the social worker will ascertain whether there was a consensus about treatment among physicians and nurses, and whether the case was already reviewed by a committee at the hospital. (An ethics committee is helpful here.)

If the parents decline to give consent for the social worker to look at their child's medical records, or if the hospital declines to let the social worker talk to people or see the infant, the social worker reports this to DSS authorities, who will attempt to resolve the issue of access. If necessary, they can seek court action.

If the parents do give consent, the social worker investigates the complaint and makes a report. The report is reviewed by the social worker's supervisor, the area or regional director, and, if appropriate, a DSS attorney. If these people determine that the parents gave informed consent for the treatment of their child that is consistent with the definition of "medically indicated treatment," then they will dismiss the complaint. If they think the treatment is not consistent with "medically indicated treatment," then "a decision is made as to how to proceed with the case." What does this mean? The Massachusetts policy and procedures say only that the DSS will inform the parents and hospital of its decision and, if necessary, seek temporary custody of the infant to obtain the "medically indicated treatment." The DSS policy also states: "Department staff are not expected to make decisions about the care or treatment of a child or to 'second guess reasonable medical judgment.'"

From this account we can see that the Baby Doe regulations do not become an issue in Massachusetts until somebody complains to the state child protection agency, the DSS. If this agency finds the regulations are being violated, it can seek temporary custody of the infant to ensure that medically indicated treatment is provided. The important point is that the DSS has no authority to assess any penalties against physicians or parents for violations of the Baby Doe rules. If the DSS discovers parents are not giving proper medical care to a child, it simply seeks legal custody of the child so a guardian can give consent for appropriate treatment.

This is not a very threatening situation for a physician. Yet, as the survey of physicians indicated, many perinatologists feel forced to treat excessively as a result of the Baby Doe regulations. In view of the very limited state and federal reactions if an investigation does show the regulations were not followed, the fears of parents and physicians about exposure to serious penalties for making decisions outside the scope of the Baby Doe regulations seem more imaginative than realistic.

THE CASE OF BABY DOE

The Story

The story behind the Baby Doe regulations is a brief and tragic one. The infant who was to become known as the famous Baby Doe was born with both Down's syndrome and a life-threatening defect on April 9, 1982, at the Bloomington Hospital. The esophagus was not open to the stomach and had a fistula allowing nourishment to pass into the lungs, where it would cause pneumonia and other problems. Physicians wanted to correct the problem with surgery. When the parents refused to give informed consent, the hospital sought a court order for the surgery. A judge held a hearing at the hospital with the baby's father and with the physicians involved with the delivery and pediatric care of the infant. Some physicians thought the child should have the surgery, others did not. The father, who had worked with children suffering from Down's syndrome in his job as a school teacher, and the mother decided not to give consent for the surgery.

The judge ruled that Mr. and Mrs. Doe had the right to choose a medically recommended course of treatment for their child in the present circumstances; that is, they could follow the recommendation of those physicians who thought it would be appropriate to withhold surgery. The hospital appealed the judge's decision, but the order was upheld by the supreme court of Indiana. Lawyers representing the hospital were on the way to Washington to seek a review by the U.S. Supreme Court when the baby died. Later efforts to have the Supreme Court review the case failed.

The complete story of Baby Doe will never be known because the courts have sealed the records to protect the family. Press reports indicate that the family lawyer said the baby had additional problems and would have needed multiple surgeries with only a 50 percent chance of survival. A consulting pediatrician, on the other hand, was reported as saying that there were no other problems and gave the infant a 90 percent chance of survival. The autopsy report did not mention any life-threatening defects except those connected with the esophagus.

The death of Baby Doe caused a national reaction. Critical editorials appeared in the *New York Times* and *Washington Post*. George Will, the parent of a child with Down's syndrome, wrote: "The baby was killed because it was retarded."

Ethical Analysis

Situational awareness

We are aware of the following facts in the Baby Doe story.

1. Baby Doe had Down's syndrome. In addition, the baby had a tracheo-esophageal fistula and may have had other problems as well.

2. Down's syndrome is not physically painful and, despite the handicaps obvious to observers, seems not to be a serious emotional burden for the victim of this genetic disorder. Most people with Down's syndrome manifest a contentment that we find somewhat baffling.

3. The esophageal problems can be successfully corrected by surgery most of the time, and parents would be expected to give consent for the necessary operation if the child were otherwise normal.

4. The parents refused consent for the life-saving surgery, and the child died in several days because it could not be fed.

We are also aware of these good and bad possibilities in the case.

1. The life of a person with Down's syndrome is a good; the person does not have the longevity of other people, but can live for decades without evident distress.

2. The surgery will cause some discomfort but save the infant's life.

3. Withholding surgery will result in the loss of the infant's life.

4. Raising a child with Down's syndrome is a significant burden for the parents and usually becomes something of a burden for the community as well.

Prudential reasoning in the Baby Doe story

We are handicapped in this case because the court records containing the facts were sealed, but let us suppose the situation is one that happens with some frequency: a baby is born with Down's syndrome and also suffers from a life-threatening but correctable defect. What response does prudential reasoning suggest for the parents and for the physicians?

Proxies' perspective.   The answer in most cases is clear: Unless there are other, more serious, complications, we have every reason to think the surgery to correct the life-threatening problem is in the baby's best interest. The surgery will be a minor burden for the baby but provide a great benefit—it will save a life that can be lived without undue suffering and with a considerable degree of contentment. The fact that the child happens to suffer also from Down's syndrome is not a reason to decline medical care, especially life-saving surgery with a high degree of success.

The reasonableness of this view becomes more clear if we imaginatively vary the story a little. Think of a ten-year-old child with Down's syndrome and also life-threatening appendicitis, and imagine that the parents, not wanting such a child, refuse consent for the surgery and the child dies. Most people could easily see that it is not reasonable to let a ten-year-old child with Down's syndrome die when surgery could correct the life-threatening problem. Yet, except for the difference in years, the case of Baby Doe is not significantly different from that of an older child with Down's syndrome who needs an appendectomy.

Providers' position.   News stories indicated that physicians were divided about what to do when the parents declined consent for the surgery. Reports indicate that the obstetrician thought foregoing surgery was an acceptable option, while those caring for the baby thought that providing it was a moral responsibility. The Indiana courts, perhaps overemphasizing parental autonomy and rights in the matter of health care decisions for children, sided with the parents.

It is impossible to see how any physician or court could support the parents' position in this case. Certainly, parents are the proper proxies for their children, but simply because they decide on something does not make it right for the providers to go along with it. Neither the self-determination of a patient, nor the determination of a proxy for a patient, is ever sufficient to establish the moral reasonableness of what is decided; we always have to ask whether the decision of the patient or proxy, especially if it is to decline life-saving treatment, is morally justified. In this case there is no reason strong enough to justify withholding the surgery from the infant who will die without it. No provider would hesitate to recommend this surgery for an older child or adult with Down's syndrome, and none should hesitate to recommend it for an infant with the same condition. On the other hand, those providers fighting to treat the infant had good reason for doing so—the surgery would significantly benefit the child with very little burden.

Ethical Reflection

No parent wants to cope with a baby suffering from Down's syndrome, but this is not a reason to refuse normal medical care to keep the baby alive. The primary criterion for moral judgment centers on what is in the baby's best interest. There is almost universal agreement among ethicists that a baby with Down's syndrome suffering from a rather common life-threatening problem with his esophagus or intestines should be treated so he can live.

A year before Baby Doe was born, a similar case involving a baby with Down's syndrome and also a life-threatening intestinal problem came before the courts in England. There the Lord Justice concluded, correctly I believe, that parents' wishes are very important, but not necessarily the views that must prevail in treatment decisions for their children. The Lord Justice decided that, since a Down's syndrome person is not living a life full of pain and suffering, the surgery that would be performed without question on anyone else with this intestinal problem must be performed on infants with Down's syndrome as well.

Despite the moral lapse that happened in the Baby Doe case, the reactions of the Reagan Administration and of the Department of Health and Human Services are very difficult to justify morally. It is not helpful to have a federal department or even a public law setting forth rules and regulations for the medical treatment of impaired infants. These situations are often very ambiguous and call for a very nuanced prudential reasoning. When there are clear cases of providing treatment, such as surgery for infants with Down's syndrome to correct life-threatening defects, laws and procedures already exist whereby the parents' unreasonable refusals can be overridden. Long before the Baby Doe regulations were formalized as amendments to the federal Child Abuse Act, state courts had the authority to remove children, temporarily or permanently, from the custody of their parents in order to arrange for their proper medical care.

Unquestionably, life-and-death decisions affecting vulnerable persons are not simply matters of private decision—they fall under public morality and eventually the law itself. But laws protecting children have existed for a long time—the child abuse and neglect statutes in every state make parental failure to provide adequate medical care for their children a criminal offense. Courts have consistently held that normal treatment for children must be provided over the objections of the parents, if necessary. No new Baby Doe regulations, let alone on-site investigations by teams from the Office of Civil Rights, were needed.

The Reagan Administration and HHS were on solid moral ground when they said Baby Doe should have been treated. But they were not on solid moral ground when they tried to regulate health care for infants under section 504 of the Rehabilitation Act. And Congress was not on solid moral ground when it incorporated the Baby Doe regulations in amendments to the child abuse law. Trying to regulate medical and surgical care by federal regulations or law creates more burdens than benefits. The Baby Doe regulations have caused unnecessary upset in many people's lives, intruded on the parent–physician relationship, wasted tax money, caused some infants to be over-treated and to suffer unnecessarily from medical interventions that good ethics would not require, and they have brought little, if any, benefit to impaired infants.

The "Handicapped Infant Hotline" is gone, as are the "Baby Doe Squads," but the Baby Doe regulations still linger. In reality, they are not a serious threat because enforcement is left to the states and no penalty is levied against parents or providers for lack of compliance. Nonetheless, the shadow of these regulations still looms large over many who care for infants and, unfortunately, still has a chilling effect that undermines good medical and moral reasoning.

THE CASE OF BABY JANE DOE

The Story

Baby Jane Doe was born on October 11, 1983, at St. Charles Hospital in Port Jefferson on Long Island, and then transferred for intensive care to the NICU of the State University of New York Hospital at Stony Brook. She suffered from spina bifida, hydrocephalus (excessive cerebrospinal fluid in the brain), and microcephaly (a small head). She could not close her eyes, was unable to suck effectively, had a malformed brain stem and hand, and was prone to spasticity in her upper extremities. Her parents were told she needed surgery to close the opening on her back and to drain the fluid from her brain. With surgery, she was expected to survive twenty years but would be severely retarded, paralyzed, bedridden, epileptic, and susceptible to constant urinary tract and bladder infections. Without surgery, she was expected to live any-where from a few weeks to two years.

After discussing the situation at length with physicians, nurses, social workers, and a priest, the parents decided against surgery on her back. They did, however, consent to other treatments, including antibiotics to fight the inevitable infections.

Ethical Analysis

Situational awareness

We are aware of the following facts in the Baby Jane Doe case.

1. Baby Jane had a serious problem with spina bifida. Surgeries to close the opening on her back and to drain fluid from her skull could help but, if she lived, her life would probably last less than 20 years and she would have serious and chronic medical problems. She would also suffer significant mental retardation. Yet prognosis is very difficult in these cases, so great uncertainty existed about just what kind of a life she would have. Her pediatrician at Stony Brook did predict, however, that it would not be very good and that she would not live long without the surgeries.

2. Her parents declined the surgery to close the lesion on her back, but readily gave consent for other treatments. Baby Jane Doe was all too typical of the dilemmas parents and physicians face in the NICU—she needed surgery to live, but the most it was expected to provide would be a limited life of considerable suffering and discomfort.

We are also aware of these good and bad features in the Baby Jane case.

1. Her life was a good, and her death would be unfortunate.

2. The pain and suffering from the surgery, and from the chronic medical problems that would haunt her life, were bad.

3. A child with spina bifida is a serious burden for parents to bear. Seriously impaired infants require a great deal of care and support.

Prudential reasoning in the Baby Jane Doe case

Proxies' position.   The parents were in a real dilemma because it is impossible to know just how much the child would suffer with the spina bifida and the associated problems. No loving parent wants to give consent for several surgeries if the outcome is only a short life of misery for the child. And no loving parent wants to decline surgeries that would, all things considered, bring more benefits than burdens to their child.

The parents' decision making was made more complicated by the conflicting views they received from the pediatricians. One physician thought the surgeries should be done, another thought the problems were so serious it made little sense to try to keep Baby Jane alive. Dr. George Newman, a pediatrician who did not think the surgeries were indicated, testified that the parents made their decision "on the basis of the combination of malformations that are present in this child," which are such that "she is not likely to ever achieve any meaningful interaction with her environment, nor ever achieve any interpersonal relationships . . ." Another physician at Stony Brook, Dr. Albert Butler, also later testified he thought the parents were making a reasonable choice.

People can only make decisions on what they know and believe at the time. If the parents thought Baby Jane could never interact with her environment, then her life would have been of little benefit to her. No meaningful interaction is a life without meaning, and it is at least arguable that an ethics based on right reason does not require proxies to give consent for painful interventions and surgeries that do no more than keep a meaningless, and painful, life going. The proxies may well have thought this at the time after discussion with Dr. Newman, although the encouragement of other providers to treat the infant should have suggested that Newman's opinion was just that—an opinion.

Providers' position.   The providers advocating treatment were on the stronger moral ground here. They felt this baby's life was worth saving with the surgery, despite the unresolved chronic problems. Undoubtedly Baby Jane would bear exceptional burdens in life, as would her parents, but they did not think those burdens clearly indicated that people should refuse to treat her at this point.

Ethical Reflection

Prudence often suggests we should provide most treatments when we think they might be helpful. This gives us a chance to see how the situation evolves. If the treatments bring little benefit and cause significantly disproportionate burdens, then they can be stopped. Knowing how uncertain the prognosis for infants is, the prudent response may be to give most infants suffering from spina bifida a chance by treating and then reevaluating the interventions as time goes on, knowing that clearly unreasonable treatments can always be stopped.

There are exceptions. It does not make sense to use medical treatments to prolong an infant's life when there is no possibility of human interaction with the world. And it would be cruel to use medical interventions to maintain an infant whose life is and will continue to be afflicted with chronic and intense pain and suffering. But things have to be pretty bad before we can justify foregoing life-sustaining treatment for infants expected to live through childhood, as was the case with Baby Jane Doe. Many spina bifida children do have meaningful interactions with people, and their pain can be made tolerable.

Looking on this case from the perspective of an ethics based on prudential reasoning, the right thing would have been to operate on her back to close the spina bifida lesion and to insert a shunt to drain the excess fluid from the brain and thereby minimize brain damage. Then, as future problems developed, the reasonableness of any additional treatments would have to be weighed anew.

Baby Jane Doe and the Courts

Although the matter would probably have ended if the medical staff had simply gone along with the parents' decision to decline the surgery, it did not. A lawyer long active in the right-to-life movement, Lawrence Washburn, a resident of Vermont but affiliated with firms in New York, was tipped off by someone in the hospital about the parents' decision to decline surgery. Without seeing Baby Jane or her medical records, or talking with her parents, he brought a suit against the parents in a New York state court. At the initial hearing on October 20, a Judge Tanebaum presided. In the previous year this judge had run for public office as a nominee of the New York Right-to-Life Party.

When Washburn's right to intervene in the case was challenged in court, Judge Tanebaum appointed a local attorney, William Weber, to be the guardian *ad litem* for Baby Jane. After his report and two days of hearings, the judge ruled that Baby Jane needed surgery and authorized Weber to give consent for it.

When Weber had first talked with the parents and Dr. Newman, he was inclined to agree with them that surgery was not indicated. But when he read the medical record, he noticed things were not as bleak as Dr. Newman was telling the parents. Thus he felt it was right for him to give consent for the surgery.

The attorney for Baby Jane's parents appealed Tanebaum's finding and Weber's consent for surgery. The New York Appellate Division reversed Tanebaum's ruling and supported the parents' right to make the decision declining the surgical intervention. Now it was the guardian's turn to appeal, and he took the case to the highest court in New York, the state court of appeals.

In a unanimous decision on October 28, 1983, this court affirmed the right of the parents to make the decision about surgery for their child. The court noted that the proper agency to bring court proceedings in cases of the mistreatment or neglect of children is not an individual citizen but the state child welfare agency, and that this agency had investigated and found no cause for complaint. The court was critical of those who would displace parental responsibilities and engage in "unusual, and sometimes offensive, activities and proceedings." These remarks were obviously directed against attorney Washburn, the stranger whose action brought everyone into court.

Guardian Weber, however, still thought the surgery should be done, and he appealed the decision of the New York Court of Appeals to the U.S. Supreme Court. On December 12, 1983, the U.S. Supreme Court refused to review the case, thereby allowing the ruling of the New York high court to stand.

Meanwhile the case got into the federal court system in two separate actions. First, after the New York Court of Appeals ruling, Lawrence Washburn asked the federal district court in New York to appoint another guardian for Baby Jane. The court's response of January 20, 1984, must have startled him. Not only did the federal court refuse his request, but fined him $500 under a federal law allowing penalties against lawyers who "harass, cause unnecessary delay or needlessly increase the cost of litigation." The federal judge also called Washburn an "interloper" and said that the State of New York could make a legal effort to recover its legal costs in the case from Washburn.

The other federal court involvement actually began earlier. Investigators from the Office of Civil Rights, a "Baby Doe Squad," were sent to Stony Brook on October 19 to see whether discrimination against the handicapped under Section 504 of the 1973 Rehabilitation Act was involved. When investigators asked to see the medical records, the hospital refused on the grounds of patient confidentiality. HHS asked the Department of Justice to intervene, and Attorney General Edwin Meese gave the green light for the government to sue the hospital in federal court for the medical records. The Justice Department filed suit on November 2, arguing that government investigators should have access to the records to see whether Baby Jane's civil rights were being violated under the Baby Doe regulations.

Since the New York courts had already resolved the case in favor of the parents, the Attorney General of New York now represented the hospital against the U.S. Department of Justice. He, together with the lawyers for the parents, argued that section 504 of the Rehabilitation Act (the law forbidding discrimination on the basis of handicap) was never intended by Congress to apply to treatment decisions for impaired children and, therefore, did not give the federal investigators authorization to inspect a patient's medical records. He also argued that the investigators were violating the family's constitutional right of privacy.

On November 16 the federal district court judge denied the request of the Department of Justice to allow federal investigators access to the medical records. The Department of Justice appealed this decision. On February 23, 1984, the federal court of appeals upheld the district court. The Department of Justice then appealed this decision, this time to the U.S. Supreme Court. The Supreme Court upheld the federal court of appeals in June 1986. This is the U.S. Supreme Court case that finally stopped the government's attempt to base Baby Doe regulations on section 504 of the Rehabilitation Act.

From this review, you can see how complicated these cases can become, and how tragic they are for the family. It is somewhat ironic that William Weber and Lawrence Washburn were probably right to think the surgery was morally indicated. Baby Jane Doe, whose real name is Keri-Lynn, was not as ill as her physicians thought. While the court proceedings were under way, her parents had quietly given consent for the shunt to drain fluid from her skull and for other treatment, but not for the surgery on the spine. The spinal lesion healed by itself, and Keri-Lynn has been living at home and has done better than many of her doctors expected. She interacts in a meaningful way with her environment, she talks and she attends a school for the handicapped. She cannot walk, but she has some mobility in a wheelchair.

This shows how hard it is to predict just how well an infant with spina bifida will manage and suggests the prudent response is treatment unless the treatment is clearly unreasonable.

The story of the original Baby Doe was a story of parents refusing life-sustaining treatment for their child. There are other stories that run in the opposite direction: some parents insist on unreasonable treatment for their children. The tragic stories of Danielle and Baby K are two such stories.

THE CASE OF DANIELLE

The Story

Danielle was born prematurely on March 26, 1985, at Brigham and Women's Hospital in Boston. She weighed less than four-and-a-half pounds and had some serious problems: anoxic encephalopathy (lack of oxygen to the brain), severe retardation with seizures, a strong possibility of developing pneumonia and pulmonary edema (fluid in the lungs), and spastic quadriplegia (paralysis with spasms of all four extremities and extending into the trunk). Physicians discussed various treatment options with Barbara, her mother. She told them she wanted everything possible done for her child.

Danielle was transferred to neighboring Children's Hospital for a week, then moved back to the NICU at Brigham and Women's, then to a long-term care rehabilitative facility. In July she was transferred back to Children's Hospital, where she remained through the following winter. It looked as if

Danielle would be spending her life in an institution, but Barbara had other ideas. She persuaded the staff at Children's Hospital to train her so she could care for Danielle at home.

At the end of February, Danielle suffered a serious setback, and again needed hospital care, including a ventilator. Physicians and nurses at Children's Hospital began to think that the burdens of all the medical interventions were outweighing any benefits a baby with such a poor prognosis could ever hope to receive. Barbara disagreed. Treatment continued, Danielle did improve somewhat, and in April 1986, thirteen months after she was born, she was able to return home, breathing on her own.

Two weeks later, she was back at Children's Hospital with pneumonia. It was quickly controlled, and she returned home once more. In early May she was back in the hospital for six weeks, then home for a month. In the following seven months she was readmitted three more times, and in February 1987 she was again admitted, this time with serious respiratory problems that would require a ventilator.

At this point, a large group that included eight physicians, five nurses, a social worker, and a hospital attorney discussed Danielle's deteriorating condition. Some of the people were members of the hospital ethics committee and questions about the ethics of using a ventilator on such a sick infant were raised. The group unanimously agreed that such invasive treatment was not in the best interests of the child, and that they could not in good conscience provide it. Barbara did not agree. The hospital stabilized Danielle without ventilation and then began seeking a facility that would accept Barbara's decision to use a ventilator that would likely be needed. Meanwhile, Barbara contacted an attorney at the Disability Law Center. This began a legal process that we will return to later.

Barbara's insistence on ventilation, despite the physicians' belief that it was not in the best interest of Danielle, created a concrete moral dilemma at the hospital. The hospital ethics committee convened a meeting on short notice to consider the problem. With but one exception, members of the ethics committee thought that it would be ethical to withhold further advanced life-support interventions because they would cause too much suffering with too little benefit. The handwritten notes of its meeting included the following points:

- mechanical ventilation would be inhumane in view of the pain and suffering it would cause Danielle, with no expectation it would reverse her acute deterioration.
- mechanical ventilation was so unreasonable that it would, in effect, be medical abuse.
- the desired benefit from ventilation is so doubtful and limited that the invasive and painful life-support procedures cannot be justified. Hence, providers felt that their position against using mechanical ventilation "could be supported by moral arguments."

The next day, Massachusetts General Hospital accepted Danielle as a patient. Less than a month later, she was well enough to go home again.

Since that time she has stabilized and has needed fewer days in the hospital. Court findings in 1993 indicate that Danielle "is blind, deaf, profoundly re-tarded, unable to eat or swallow, has almost no use of her arms or legs, cannot speak or communicate in any clear way and needs round-the-clock acute nursing care." She is nourished by a gastrostomy tube and suctioned frequently to keep her breathing passage opened. She has constant seizures. Her pulmonary status has improved but she still requires supplementary oxygen. Her mental status will remain that of a three-month-old infant.

Estimates for the costs of Danielle's care range between one and two million dollars for the first two years of her life. Now that she is cared for at home, and thanks to the dedicated efforts of her mother, her expenses have declined, but a 1987 published report stated that the home nursing care alone was then costing $84,000 a year. When Danielle was about seven, a jury returned a verdict of negligence against several obstetricians attending Barbara during her delivery and awarded 20 million dollars, of which 11.5 million was designated for Danielle's future medical expenses over the next twenty-five years she is expected to live. The total cost for treatments prolonging the life of this profoundly retarded, blind, deaf, almost immobile human being needing constant acute nursing care, therefore, could run close to 15 million dollars.

Ethical Analysis

Situational awareness

We are aware of the following facts in the story of Danielle.

1. Danielle was severely retarded and paralyzed. Her ability to interact with her environment was very limited and she had no potential for significant improvement.

2. She has needed a ventilator several times in the past, and may well need it again if respiratory crises develop.

3. Her life expectancy was, as is so often the case with infants, uncertain. Physicians at Children's Hospital were convinced Danielle was inexorably sliding toward death when they objected to starting the ventilator in March 1987, but the pediatricians at Massachusetts General Hospital were not so sure, and they were right when they said she was not necessarily dying at that time. Court findings when she was about seven indicated she could live another twenty-five years.

4. Her mother wanted everything done; some providers thought future attempts at resuscitation and use of a ventilator had become unreasonable in view of her condition and the suffering the interventions caused.

We are also aware of these good and bad features in the case.

1. The preservation of Danielle's life is a good; human life is always a good, even if minimal.

2. The pain and discomfort caused by the continual treatment, some of it invasive, are unfortunate.

3. The burden of care on Danielle's mother was also great, although interviews with her imply she has no second thoughts or regrets about her decision to have everything done for Danielle. Private nurses usually cover two shifts a day, and Danielle's mother provides care at other times. Barbara stated in an interview: "I no longer play tennis. I don't go to movies or dinner.

I'm in this house twenty-four hours a day. But look at what my staying in has accomplished."

4. The financial burden, already immense and continuing as long as Danielle lives, is also significant. Although it is covered by a health insurance plan, the millions of dollars needed for treatment that cannot cure but merely preserve the status quo obviously burden others in the plan.

Prudential reasoning in the story of Danielle

Proxy's position.   Barbara deserves the greatest empathy. Every parent naturally wants to save his or her child's life. Her sincerity is unquestioned—she has sacrificed much to care for her daughter. Her dedication to her child, and the sacrifices she has made, attest to the generosity of her spirit.

The difficulty, of course, is for parents to adjust to the new era of advanced life-support systems. In principle, everyone knows their use is sometimes unreasonable and even inhumane. Unless a parent is ready to admit that advanced and invasive medical interventions are sometimes *not* in the infant's best interest, no real moral reasoning can occur. The imperative "Do everything to keep my baby alive" is not always morally justified because "everything" can sometimes be unreasonable or even cruel for the child.

An ethics of right reason would certainly support a parent who decided at some point that resuscitation and ventilation were not in the best interests of a child in this condition. It is more difficult, however, to determine when providing these interventions becomes unreasonable and therefore unethical. Yet reasons are not easily found that justify the extensive, and sometimes painful, treatments for such a damaged child. It simply is not always good to keep some human beings alive as long as possible with modern techniques and technology, and this may well be one of those cases where the better parental decision would have favored a more modest treatment protocol.

We should also note that the wishes of Danielle's father, Frank Hall, are conspicuously absent from the published report of this case. His silence is as noteworthy as Barbara's intense involvement. Normally, both parents would be functioning as proxies for their child, but there is no evidence of that in this case. It would be very helpful to know what Danielle's other proxy, her father, thought was in her best interests.

Providers' position.   Once providers are convinced the treatment has degenerated into what is tantamount to bad medicine or even child abuse, they have little choice but to refuse to perform it and to seek a transfer of the patient. Sound morality does not allow anyone to do what they think is not right, and neither does the law. In a 1986 case involving withdrawal of medical nutrition and hydration from a PVS patient named Paul Brophy, the Massachusetts Supreme Court reminded providers that the law does not compel medical professionals to "take active measures which are contrary to their view of their ethical duty toward their patients." And more than a decade ago, the President's Commission report *Deciding to Forego Life-Sustaining Treatment* stated: "Health care professionals or institutions may decline to provide a particular option because that choice would violate their conscience or professional judgment though, in doing so, they may not abandon a patient."

The fact that the physicians at Children's Hospital incorrectly thought that Danielle would not overcome the crisis that hit her in February 1987, when she was about two years old, is not relevant to an ethical evaluation of their position. People can only respond as they honestly see the situation at the time, and that is what they did. They thought her decline had become inevitable even if ventilation were used, and therefore they thought it unreasonable to subject her to the ventilator. As it turned out, Danielle was not as sick as they thought, but that is irrelevant when we evaluate the morality of their decision. People can only decide on what they truly think will happen and, given their diagnosis and prognosis at that time, their decision was ethical.

Physicians at Massachusetts General arrived at a different prognosis and, on the basis of this more optimistic prediction, had a slightly better reason to treat Danielle. However, the fact that they managed to keep Danielle alive and get her home does not automatically mean that they made the right moral decision. For an infant such as Danielle, the primary moral challenge is to know when the aggressive treatment is not in her best interests. This, of course, is not an easy thing to do, and thus the decision by physicians at Massachusetts General was not necessarily unethical, especially in view of the fact the baby's mother was convinced aggressive treatment should be given.

Ethical Reflection

This was a truly ambiguous situation, and one without an ethically satisfactory answer. There are many reasons for thinking the burdens caused by the lengthy and aggressive treatments that included ventilator support and several emergency resuscitations could not be justified in view of the little benefit the life they saved could offer Danielle. On the other hand, not everyone involved in the case agreed with this. Barbara Hall certainly did not, but neither did everyone on the ethics committee at Children's Hospital and neither did some pediatricians at Massachusetts General Hospital. For some providers, the ventilator did seem ethically justified. Perhaps what can be said is this:

1. It is fairly easy to justify morally the decision of a proxy to forego a ventilator in a situation such as this; it is much more difficult, but not impossible, to justify the decision of a proxy to insist on the ventilator.

2. It is also fairly easy to justify morally the decision of providers not to provide such extensive treatment; it is much more difficult, but not impossible, to justify the decision of providers to treat, especially if that is what both parents want, and if the child's suffering is not intense and unremitting.

The reason for leaving the door for treatment open a crack is based on a wider consideration than the simple best interests of the child. Prudential reasoning makes an effort to consider seriously a wide range of circumstances, and one salient circumstance in the treatment of infants is the wishes of the parents. Now this is not a *carte blanche*—parents certainly cannot demand what are unquestionably unreasonable and clearly abusive treatments. But, given the difficulty of prognosis in the care of infants, it is seldom easy to know what constitutes abusive treatments.

One very important feature of this case is that the mother wanted this treatment, and some people at both hospitals, as well as a judge who examined the situation, were not convinced her request was unreasonable. In cases such as these, where providers and others involved in the situation disagree about what is the right thing to do, the parents' desire that their child be treated counts for something in resolving the issue. Certainly, providers who believe the parents' request is unquestionably immoral should not violate their ethical integrity and provide it. But their conscientious objection to treatment is not necessarily the only morally justified answer.

Thus one can argue that foregoing aggressive treatment such as ventilators and CPR is the right thing to do in this case; one can also argue that, given the mother's insistence and deep personal involvement, following her request is also not unreasonable. Unless we are prepared to condemn Barbara's decision as patently immoral, then we cannot absolutely exclude a moral ground for providing treatment at her request. And although the reasonableness of her decision is not apparent to many, her demand for treatment is an informed one and there is no reason to question her love for Danielle. The very fact that a parent wants treatment counts for something; it is an important circumstance in the case. It is a terrible thing to stop treatment against a parent's wishes. Sometimes it is clearly justified and has to be done, but it is not clear that this was one of those times.

The bond between parent and child is not totally captured in the medical and moral judgments of best interests. Parents not actually neglecting or abusing their infants need a little extra margin of leeway that we might not grant to any other proxy decision maker. If they truly care for their children, they are in the best position to know what is right for their infants. They may make the wrong decision, as anybody acting in good conscience may do, but unless we are willing to accuse them of neglect and child abuse, the less worse position may be that we have to allow this parental responsibility for infants to play itself out in the decisions they make, provided it is not obvious to everyone that these decisions are causing unjustified suffering for the children.

The immense costs of the treatments and the little benefit they produce beyond the prolongation of a terribly impaired life is another important ethical issue in this case. But it is an issue on another level, a social level. If Frank and Barbara Hall had to bankrupt their family and deprive the other children of life's necessities, then Barbara's decision would be more difficult to defend. But this is not the case, and it is not the case that welfare funds are being used, so the cost of the treatment is not a major issue for the parents or the hospitals.

Cost is, however, a major ethical issue for society and third party payers. We do have to ask how many millions of dollars should be spent to provide aggressive treatment for a paralyzed child unable to eat, subject to respiratory arrest and seizures, and whose mental development will remain about that of a three month old infant. Maybe several million is reasonable, maybe a billion is reasonable, but at some point the sheer cost of such treatment for such a damaged life is unreasonable in a society where so many children lack adequate primary care.

The Legal Proceedings

The attorney whom Barbara contacted on March 5, 1987, obtained a probate court hearing that very day. Judge Mary Muse immediately issued a temporary restraining order preventing the hospital from entering a DNR order. Then she appointed a guardian *ad litem* to discover the facts in the case for the court, and a second guardian to represent Danielle. After his discovery process, the guardian *ad litem*, fearing Danielle was getting worse, asked the judge to hold an immediate hearing in a hospital conference room. The judge agreed and it got under way about ten o'clock that night.

Dr. Robert Crone of Harvard Medical School and Children's Hospital explained the providers' position: putting Danielle back on the ventilator would not reverse her deteriorating condition and yet would cause more pain and suffering since, in addition to the mechanical ventilation through the tracheotomy, new monitoring catheters would have to be inserted in her veins. The lawyers for Barbara Hall and the guardians appointed by the court argued for treatment. It was well past midnight when the judge suspended the hearing until the next morning.

The next day the guardian *ad litem* arranged for a pediatrician from Massachusetts General Hospital to examine Danielle and make a recommendation to the court. Dr. Eileen Ouellette examined Danielle and reported to Judge Muse in the afternoon. Dr. Ouellette testified that Danielle was capable of experiencing pain and so sick she might not survive even with mechanical ventilation. Nonetheless, she said her hospital, Massachusetts General, would provide treatment at the mother's request. The transfer was arranged that very day. When Danielle left Children's Hospital the legal dispute ended.

Judge Muse, however, realized that the case was extremely complex and difficult. She suggested that it might be worthwhile for the parties to appeal it to the appellate level, perhaps even to the Massachusetts Supreme Court, so a precedent-setting ruling could be made that might prevent such unfortunate conflicts in the future. The lawyers for Barbara Hall agreed. So did the court-appointed guardians who were also attorneys. But the attorneys for Children's Hospital were not interested in pursuing the matter further, so an appeal was never made.

Given the helpful contributions of many court decisions, including major Massachusetts decisions involving DNR orders and withdrawing medical nutrition from PVS patients, it is unfortunate the issue was not argued in court. This is so because it is absurd to force physicians always to do "everything possible" whenever parents or families request it, since "everything" can be very bad medicine indeed. It is also a very difficult and touchy situation to forego life-sustaining treatment when the parents are requesting it. Since both the legal and ethical responses in this kind of case are unclear, some legal direction from a state supreme court would have been helpful to physicians and hospitals.

Although it does not directly concern our ethical analysis of how Danielle should have been treated, there is a legal footnote worth noting in this case.

Attorneys for the Halls brought a medical malpractice suit against three physicians involved in Danielle's delivery. They claimed that the physicians had been negligent and had failed to inform Barbara adequately about Danielle's fetal distress and the risks of a vaginal delivery. The jury agreed, and awarded the 20 million dollars mentioned above. The exceptionally high award was 1.6 million dollars more than attorneys for the Halls had sought. It was appealed, but in 1993 a state superior court ruled that the 20 million dollar award was not excessive and noted that juries are allowed some latitude in the calculation of damage awards.

THE CASE OF BABY K

The Story

Ms. H delivered Baby K by cesarean section on October 13, 1992, at Fairfax Hospital in Falls Church, Virginia. During the pregnancy, Ms. H was told her fetus was anencephalic and that abortion was an option, but she decided to continue the pregnancy. Immediately after delivery, Baby K experienced respiratory distress and was placed on a ventilator. After several days, physicians informed Ms. H that no treatment could help her anencephalic infant, and that the ventilator should be withdrawn because it was medically inappropriate. Ms. H insisted on retaining the ventilator. A three person subcommittee from the hospital ethics committee was consulted; they concluded that the ventilator should be discontinued because it was "futile" and recommended legal recourse if the mother refused to allow its withdrawal. By this time, it was clear that Baby K was permanently unconscious.

By the end of November 1992, Baby K was able to breathe without the ventilator. The hospital transferred her to a nursing home with the understanding that it would accept her again as a patient if ventilator support was needed in the future. Baby K was back in the hospital on January 15, 1993, for ventilation, but returned to the nursing home on February 12. Then she was admitted again for ventilation on March 3 and remained a patient until April 13.

The hospital sought a ruling in federal court allowing it to withhold ventilation if Baby K was brought back to the emergency department in respiratory distress. It argued that the ventilation was medically and ethically inappropriate for permanently unconscious anencephalic infants. The court appointed a guardian *ad litem* to represent Baby K; the guardian agreed that the ventilator was truly inappropriate treatment for Baby K. Mr. K, Baby K's father who has never been married to Ms. H, also believed that his baby should not receive ventilator support.

Ms. H, however, insists her baby should be placed on a ventilator whenever she needs it. According to court documents, her position stems from her "firm Christian faith" that all life should be protected. She believes "that God will work a miracle if that is his will." Otherwise, she believes, "God, and not other humans, should decide the moment of her daughter's death."

Ethical Analysis

Situational awareness

We are aware of the following facts in the story of Baby K.

1. Baby K is an irreversibly unconscious anencephalic infant. There is no chance of improvement—she has no brain. She will live in a vegetative state until she dies.

2. She has needed a ventilator several times in the past and may well need it again.

3. Her father, her physicians, and the guardian *ad litem* do not think a ventilator is an appropriate medical treatment in her situation. Ms. H, her mother, insists on using it. Her position is based on her religious faith—she believes it would be contrary to her Christian beliefs to withhold a ventilator from her baby.

4. The hospital is so disturbed over the mother's demand for what it perceives as unreasonable medical treatment that it has petitioned the federal district court for relief.

We are also aware of these good and bad features in the story.

1. If Baby K does not receive ventilation when she needs it, she will die, and death is always bad. The death of a persistently vegetative body, however, is not nearly as bad as the death of a psychic body (that is, a body with the capacity for awareness). The vegetative body has already suffered almost total neurological damage. The end of the vegetative life will simply be the last stage in the loss of human life that has already occurred.

2. Not using the ventilator will cause distress to Ms. H; using the ventilator will cause distress to Mr. K, her father, and to the caregivers forced to provide a treatment they believe is not medically indicated.

3. While ventilation provides nothing beneficial for Baby K, nor harms her in any way, it does require considerable financial support. Someone is paying for expensive medical support that is of no benefit to the baby, and this is bad.

Prudential reasoning in the story of Baby K

Patient's perspective. Baby K obviously had no prior wishes about anything. She is not a moral agent in the story. Nor does she have any interests. Since nothing matters to her, not even whether she lives or dies, neither providing nor withholding treatment can be said to be in her "best interests."

Proxies' perspectives. Her parents are her proxies, and they are unable to use either the substituted judgment or the best interests standards of proxy decision making. They can only rely on our third standard in cases such as this, the reasonable treatment standard. Since a ventilator is of no benefit to a permanently unconscious anencephalic infant, there is no reason to provide it except to fulfill Ms. H's desires. And there are several reasons for not providing the unreasonable treatment, among them irrational expenditure of money and the distress of caregivers asked to provide medically inappropriate treatments.

Ms. H's position, however, is not grounded in reasons, but on her religious faith. As we pointed out in the Wanglie case (chapter 7), religious beliefs are notoriously hard to critique. While some important religious thinkers—the thirteenth-century theologian Thomas Aquinas was one of them— insist that no moral position derived from the Christian faith could ever conflict with reason, not every Christian believer embraces this position. Many claim that what is unreasonable or foolish in the eyes of the moral philosopher is not always foolish in the eyes of God. For these believers, the religious belief becomes a trump card; once played, no reasoning can undermine it. The religious belief, no matter how unreasonable, becomes, in the mind of the believer, the reason for the decision.

Providers' perspective.   Providers and the guardian *ad litem* agree with the father that the ventilator should not be used. Their position is the only reasonable one when the status of the patient is considered.

But the providers have another problem, a problem similar to the one that the providers faced in the Wanglie story. A proxy is demanding treatment for a patient on religious grounds. Refusal of the life-support therapy will be viewed by the mother as contrary to her religious beliefs.

If the medically inappropriate use of the ventilator was causing the baby any burden, then the providers' primary responsibility to protect the patient from unreasonable medical treatment would lead them to reject the proxy's demands. But the ventilator does not cause any burden to Baby K; she is irreversibly unconscious. This suggests, as it did in the Wanglie case, that it could be reasonable, given the mother's religious position that cannot be touched by any reasoning, to continue to provide ventilation when needed. The treatment makes no sense, but it causes no harm to the patient. And, as was pointed out in the Wanglie case, the idea that vegetative life is valuable is recognized in our culture. As evidence of this, we need only remind ourselves that a person coming into the ICU and shooting Baby K would be charged with murder, something that reminds us of the importance of vegetative life in law.

In a pluralistic society, respect has to be given to the religious beliefs of others whenever possible. Since the ventilator causes no harm to the patient, a case can be made that the unreasonable medical treatment can be provided by the physicians and nurses out of respect for the mother's religious convictions.

However, the unreasonable medical treatment does cause other harms, and these have to be considered. Providing treatment of no benefit a patient can experience can be distressing. Those paying for the useless life-sustaining treatments are also being harmed. They might well argue that the burdens they are forced to undergo as the result of the inappropriate treatment outweigh the mother's unreasonable demands and decline to finance it. In other words, while the providers, once they realize that the treatment does not harm the patient, may decide to stop short of opposing the mother's wishes, those paying for the treatment might well feel that it is their responsibility to decline payment for expensive and unreasonable treatment. In practice, however, this is difficult to accomplish in the current political climate and unlikely to help in this particular case.

The Court Decision

On July 7, 1993, Judge Claude Hilton of the federal district court issued his opinion. He noted that the parents disagreed on what should be done, but accepted Ms. H's contention that she has the right to decide what is in her child's best interests since she was more involved in her care than the baby's father. Moreover, he asserted: "When one parent asserts the child's explicit constitutional right to life as the basis for continuing medical treatment and the other is asserting the nebulous liberty interest in refusing life-saving treatment on behalf of the minor child, the explicit right to life must prevail."

This sentence captures the essence, and the inherent weakness, of rights-based arguments in complex moral dilemmas. In the extreme form exemplified in this case, the mother's right-to-life position is coupled with her right-to-decide position; and both are then used to demand that all requested life-sustaining medical treatments must be provided for her irreversibly unconscious anencephalic infant, regardless of how unreasonable they are or how much burden they cause others. Extreme rights-based positions, whether they advocate the right to life or the right to choose, simply fail to function well in complex situations involving life and death.

The judge also noted that Ms. H appealed not only to the right to life, but to a religious argument, and that this has constitutional implications, specifically those under the First Amendment, which allows people the free exercise of their religion. Obviously, we cannot harm others in the name of religion—human sacrifice, once accepted by many religions, would not be tolerated by the First Amendment—but here the ventilation causes the patient no harm. Whenever it is a matter of practicing religion, the government needs "clear and compelling" interests to violate a person's First Amendment religious rights, and the court did not think such compelling interests were present in this case. The judge also noted, correctly, that providing ventilation for Baby K whenever it was needed "is not so unreasonably harmful as to constitute child abuse or neglect." Thus, in its own way, the court recognized the religious "trump card" that we mentioned above and acknowledged that the mother's religious convictions played a role in its decision, something it could allow especially since the treatment caused no harm to the unconscious baby.

The decision of the federal district court was appealed. On February 10, 1994, a three-judge panel of the Fourth Circuit upheld, by a 2–1 decision, Judge Hilton's ruling. Unlike Judge Hilton, who argued on the basis of several conclusions of law, among them the Emergency Medical Treatment and Active Labor Act (EMTALA), section 504 of the Rehabilitation Act, section 302 of the Americans with Disabilities Act, and the 1984 amendments to the Child Abuse Act, as well as other constitutional and common law issues, the appeals court considered only the provisions of EMTALA.

This legislation is designed to prevent "patient-dumping," a practice whereby patients without financial resources were turned away from emergency departments despite being in serious trouble or in active labor. The law requires the hospitals to accept the patients or at least to stabilize them before transfer. Attorneys for Ms. H argued that the EMTALA requires ventilation for Baby K if she arrives at the hospital in respiratory distress. And once she is on ventilation, the hospital will have to continue her care (no one else is anxious to accept her in transfer) until she can once again breathe on her own.

Efforts to argue that the EMTALA was never intended for treatment of anencephalic infants in persistent vegetative state convinced only the dissenting judge. The other two judges found no such exception in the wording of the law, and therefore concluded that everybody coming to the hospital and needing emergency life-sustaining interventions must be treated. They noted that the only recourse is for Congress to amend the law. They also acknowledged "the dilemma facing physicians who are requested to provide treatment they consider morally and ethically inappropriate," but insisted a court cannot ignore the plain language of a statute and stated it was "beyond the limits of our judicial function to address the moral or ethical propriety of providing emergency stabilizing medical treatment to anencephalic infants."

A petition was made requesting a review of the case by the full panel of judges on the federal appellate court, but the petition for a rehearing was denied by the court in March 1994. In October 1994 the United States Supreme Court refused to review the ruling of the Fourth Circuit, so its decision stands.

Baby K, now known as Stephanie, reached her second birthday in October 1994. She was still in a persistent vegetative state, totally unaware of herself and of her surroundings. Her mother's insurance company has paid almost $250,000 in hospital bills and Medicaid is paying the nursing home for the care of her vegetative body. Her mother, now identified as Contrenia Harrell, visits her daily. Physicians have told her that Stephanie's brain will never develop, but a story in *USA Today* (October 13, 1994) reported that Contrenia is not convinced. "I believe in God for a total miracle . . . that she'll be a living testimony to the world," she said.

SUGGESTED READINGS

For a brief introduction to infanticide, see Stephen Post. "History, Infanticide, and Imperiled Newborns." *Hastings Center Report* **1988**, *18* (August–September), 14–17. John Lorber's article on withholding treatment from infants with spina bifida appeared as "Early Results of Selective Treatment of Spina Bifida Cystica" in the *British Medical Journal* **1973**, *4*, 201–04. Raymond Duff and A. G. M. Campbell's article appeared as "Moral and Ethical Dilemmas in the Special-Care Nursery." *NEJM* **1973**, *289*, 890–94. See also John Lorber. "Results of Treatment of Myelomeningocele: An Analysis of 524 Unselected Cases with Special References to Special Selection for Treatment." *Developmental Medicine and Child Neurology* **1971**, *13*, 279–303; John Freeman. "The Shortsighted Treatment of Myelomeningocele: A Long-Term Case Report." *Pediatrics* **1974**, *53*, 311–13; and "To Treat or Not to Treat: Ethical Dilemmas of the Infant with a Myelomeningocele. *Clinical Neurosurgery* **1973**, *20*, 134–46.

The harvesting of organs from living anencephalic infants in Germany was reported by Wolfgang Holzgreve et al. in "Kidney Transplantation from Anencephalic Donors." *NEJM* **1987**, *316*, 1069–70.

For ethical reflections on defective newborns in general, see Earl Shelp. 1986. *Born to Die? Deciding the Fate of Critically Ill Newborns*. New York: Free Press; Robert Weir. 1984. *Selective Nontreatment of Handicapped Newborns: Moral Dilemmas in*

Neonatal Medicine. New York: Oxford University Press; Allan Buchanan and Dan Brock. 1989. *Deciding for Others: The Ethics of Surrogate Decision Making*. Cambridge: Cambridge University Press, chapter 5; Helga Kuhse and Peter Singer. 1985. *Should the Baby Live? The Problem of Handicapped Infants*. New York: Oxford University Press; Thomas Murray and Arthur Caplan, eds. 1985. *Which Babies Shall Live? Humanistic Dimensions of the Care of Imperiled Newborns*. Clifton, N.J.: Humana Press; Richard McCormick. "To Save or Let Die: The Dilemma of Modern Medicine." *JAMA* **1974**, *229*, 172–76; Anthony Shaw. "Dilemmas of 'Informed Consent' in Children." *NEJM* **1973**, *289*, 885–90; Albert Jonsen et al. "Critical Issues in Newborn Intensive Care: A Conference and Policy Proposal." *Pediatrics* **1975**, *55*, 756–68; Nancy King. "Transparency in Neonatal Intensive Care." *Hastings Center Report* **1992**, *22* (May–June), 18–25; Andrew Whitelaw. "Death as an Option in Neonatal Intensive Care." *Lancet* **1986**, *2*, 328–31; John Arras. "Toward an Ethic of Ambiguity." *Hastings Center Report* **1984**, *14* (April), 25–33; Nancy Rhoden. "Treating Baby Doe: The Ethics of Uncertainty." *Hastings Center Report* **1986**, *16* (August), 35–42; and William Silverman. "Overtreatment of Neonates? A Personal Retrospective." *Pediatrics* **1992**, *90*, 971–76.

Several of these authors advocate involuntary euthanasia for severely impaired infants (Weir, Shelp, Singer, and Kuhse, for example) as does H. Tristram Engelhardt. 1986. *The Foundations of Bioethics*. New York: Oxford University Press, pp. 228–36. On the question of euthanasia for infants, see also Richard McMillan et al., eds. 1986. *Euthanasia and the Newborn*. Dordrecht: Reidel.

The current Baby Doe regulations were published in the *Federal Register* 50 (15 April 1985), 14878–901. The account includes brief summaries of the on-site investigations triggered in response to calls received on the hotline. The Massachusetts response to the Baby Doe regulations is found in the Department of Social Services Policy #86–010 entitled "Policy and Procedures for the Receipt and Investigation of Reports of Medical Neglect Alleging that Medically Indicated Treatment is Being Withheld from Disabled Infants with Life-Threatening Conditions," revised 7/1/89.

Among the many commentaries on the Baby Doe case itself and on its associated legal and political controversies are: Dixie Huefner. "Severely Handicapped Infants with Life-Threatening Conditions: Federal Intrusions Into the Decision Not To Treat." *American Journal of Law and Medicine* **1986**, *12*, 171–205; Nelson Lund. "Infanticide, Physicians, and the Law: The 'Baby Doe' Amendments to the Child Abuse Prevention and Treatment Act." *American Journal of Law and Medicine* **1985**, *11*, 1–29; Stephen Newman. "Baby Doe, Congress and the States: Challenging the Federal Treatment Standards for Impaired Infants." *American Journal of Law and Medicine* **1989**, *15*, 1–60; Thomas Murray. "The Final, Anticlimactic Rule on Baby Doe." *Hastings Center Report* **1985**, *15* (June), 5–9; John Moskop and Rita Saldanha. "The Baby Doe Rule: Still a Threat." *Hastings Center Report* **1986**, *16* (April), 8–14; and John Lantos. "Baby Doe Five Years Later: Implications for Child Health." *NEJM* **1987**, *317*, 444–47.

For the survey of the members of the Perinatal Pediatrics Section of the American Academy of Pediatrics mentioned in the text, see Loretta Kopelman et al. "Neonatologists Judge the 'Baby Doe' Regulations." *NEJM* **1988**, *318*, 677–83. For the remark of George Will and the decision of the English court favoring treatment for a baby with Down's syndrome and also a life-threatening defect, see Richard McCormick. 1981. "Saving Defective Infants: Options for Life or Death." In *How Brave a New World?* Washington: Georgetown University Press, chapter 18.

The Baby Jane Doe story is taken from Kathleen Kerr. "An Issue of Law and Ethics." *Newsday*, October 26, 1983. Ms. Kerr was the lead reporter on the team that won a Pulitzer Prize for the reporting of the Baby Jane Doe story. See also Kathleen

Kerr. "Reporting the Case of Baby Jane Doe." *Hastings Center Report* **1984,** *14* (August), 7–9; Bonnie Steinbock. "Baby Jane Doe in the Court." *Hastings Center Report* **1984,** *14* (February), 13–19; and "The Baby Jane Doe Case" in Pence, *Classic Cases,* chapter 7.

The story of Danielle is based on Seth Rolbein. "A Matter of Life and Death." *Boston Magazine,* October 1987; and John Paris, Robert Crone, and Frank Reardon. "Physicians' Refusal of Requested Treatment: The Case of Baby L." *NEJM* **1990,** *322,* 1012–15. The story of Baby K is taken from *In the Matter of Baby "K,"* No. CIV. A. 93–104–A, U.S. District Court, E.D. Virginia (1993), and *In the Matter of Baby K,* 16 F.3d 590 (4th Cir 1994). For a commentary, see George Annas. "Asking the Courts to Set the Standard of Emergency Care—the Case of Baby K." *NEJM* **1994,** *330,* 1542–45.

13

Euthanasia and Physician-Assisted Suicide

The word euthanasia means "good death." If that were all it meant, it would not be controversial. We all hope for a good death, a death without pain and suffering. In some religious traditions, people pray for a "happy death" and call it a "blessing" when someone dies after a painful terminal illness. In current usage, however, euthanasia means something more than a good death or dying well. When people speak of euthanasia today, they mean causing a patient's quick and painless death, usually by lethal injection or drug overdose. Euthanasia is the intentional killing of a patient in response to her informed and voluntary request. Physician-assisted suicide is also the killing of a patient—a patient killing herself with a physician's help.

Euthanasia and physician-assisted suicide are major issues in health care ethics for two reasons. First, those seeking to be killed are patients, usually very ill patients and, second, the people currently giving the lethal injections or prescribing the lethal drugs are physicians. Thus euthanasia and assisted suicide have become issues in the ethics of patient–physician relationships.

Euthanasia and physician-assisted suicide have also become the center of intense public controversy in our country, and in other countries as well. This was perhaps an inevitable development. In the 1970s the great debate was whether physicians could ever withdraw life-sustaining treatments—most notably respirators. In the 1980s the debate was whether physicians could ever withdraw medical nutrition and hydration. Now, in the 1990s, the central public controversy is whether physicians can ever help patients to commit suicide or even put them to death.

HISTORICAL OVERVIEW

In recent centuries most people, including physicians, were unalterably opposed to physicians killing their patients or helping them kill themselves. So strong was this opposition that euthanasia and suicide were not even considered topics for serious moral discussion. This is no longer true; these topics are now the subject of serious debate and, in some places, political action.

The debate is really an ancient one. In the classical world of Greece and Rome (ca. 500 B.C.E. to 350 C.E.), many thought euthanasia and suicide were morally acceptable in appropriate circumstances. One group of people was a notable exception—the Pythagoreans. They developed a strong tradition in medicine, one devoted to the ethical formation as well as to the medical education of their physicians. Hippocrates was a physician in the Pythagorean tradition, and many people still appeal to the Hippocratic Oath for moral guidance in medicine.

The Pythagoreans in general, and the Hippocratic medical tradition in particular, were opposed to euthanasia. The reason is not hard to find. Pythagorean religious beliefs included two important doctrines—the kinship of all life and the transmigration of souls. Pythagoras believed that life was somehow a single reality shared by all living things; there was no such thing as "my" life or "your" life, but simply life. Our souls recycle through life in different forms many times over until they finally attain some form of purified reincarnation. The Pythagoreans thought great care must be taken not to disrupt or destroy this cycle of life. Deliberately bringing about any death, even the death of animals, was considered wrong.

Most other people in classical Greece, however, accepted euthanasia and suicide in extenuating circumstances. Aristotle, for example, thought it ethical to end the life of defective infants. His view on suicide was somewhat complex. He argued against it whenever it violated any of the virtues. For example, a person committing suicide to escape from the troubles and sufferings of life acts cowardly and thus fails the virtue of courage. And a person committing suicide in a city-state where it was prohibited by law, as it was in Athens, violates the virtue of justice by breaking the law. But there is no blanket condemnation of suicide in Aristotle's teaching. If a suicide did not conflict with any virtues, there would be no reason to consider it immoral. In fact, it might even be an act of courage and love, as would be a suicide for the sake of saving the lives of others.

Other Greek philosophers actually advocated suicide. Epicurus encouraged hedonism, and made seeking pleasure and avoiding pain the norm of living. Once the pain of living overwhelms the pleasures one can hope for, he thought suicide was an appropriate moral response. Stoicism, the philosophy that dominated the Greek and Roman classical worlds for centuries after 300 B.C.E., also advocated suicide at the end of life. Stoic philosophy advocated living "according to nature," and many Stoics did not hesitate to kill themselves when the struggle to live became an unreasonable effort to prevent death. For them, death was natural, and so helping it come at the end was reasonable and virtuous. And, since they thought that exercising the virtues constituted a good life, suicide becomes reasonable whenever illness, poverty, or pain so overwhelms a person that living virtuously is no longer possible.

The Hebrew culture, another great tradition shaping our moral consciousness, was more conservative than the Stoics about suicide. Undoubtedly this stemmed, in great measure, from the Biblical belief that human life was created by Jahweh or God, a belief that implies we should be careful about destroying what God has created. Thanks to this belief in divine creation, and the later Christian acceptance of it, the Mosaic commandment "Thou shalt not kill" has played a powerful role in our culture's prohibition of suicide.

For centuries, the Biblical commandment "Thou shalt not kill" has been understood to forbid all intentional taking of innocent life, including my own life, and therefore to prohibit euthanasia and suicide. A careful reading of the Hebrew Bible, however, reveals that this conclusion is a misunderstanding. While the Bible does show a strong respect for life, it does not set forth absolute prohibitions against killing the innocent or committing suicide. The killing of the first-born child in every Egyptian family during the night of the original Passover is not seen as immoral (*Exodus* 11). In fact, the killing of the Egyptian children during the exodus from Egypt, as well as the terrible damage to the crops and marine life inflicted by the plagues, were remembered by the Hebrews as great deeds of the Lord (*Deuteronomy* 11).

The Bible also commands the Israelites to kill innocent people in military campaigns. It depicts God commanding his people to kill all the children and women, as well as the men, whenever their army has conquered a nearby enemy city (*Deuteronomy* 20). The deliberate killing of all the inhabitants in the captured cities is particularly disturbing from a moral point of view because the Bible depicts the Hebrews as the invaders; they were moving in from the desert to take the already occupied land and cities for themselves.

The Bible does not restrict the killing of children to the enemies' children; it commands the Israelite parents of a stubborn and rebellious son to have him apprehended and brought to the elders so the parents can testify against him. If their testimony is convincing, the townspeople will then gather round and stone the young man to death (*Deuteronomy* 22).

It is, of course, impossible to know how often the Biblical commandments authorizing such killings were actually carried out. Records dating back to the Mosaic era are practically nonexistent, and it may be that many of the killings sanctioned by the early Biblical texts seldom occurred in practice.

We also read about suicide in the Bible. King Saul killed himself. Badly wounded, he had asked his armor bearer to kill him, but the man refused, so Saul killed himself with his own sword. Later, a member of Saul's camp told David that Saul had asked to be killed and claimed he had killed him. Far from being shocked at the report of King Saul's request for euthanasia, David laments him as an honorable and illustrious man (1 *Samuel* 31 and 2 *Samuel* 1).

The Biblical story of Samson's suicide is also well known. His enemies bribed his mistress, Delilah, to find out the secret of his great strength. Three times he lied to her, but finally admitted it was his long hair. While he was sleeping, she cut off his hair. Now powerless, he was captured, blinded, and forced to work as a slave. Some time later he was dragged before his captors during a celebration in some sort of large building, and they mocked him. By this time, enough of his hair had grown back to restore his incredible strength. In anger, he managed to pull down the two main columns supporting the roof, killing himself and thousands of his enemies. His last words were: "Let me die with the Philistines!" (*Judges* 16:30).

The fact that Samson killed himself did not prevent St. Paul from considering him one of the heroes of the Hebrew faith, along with David, Samuel, and the prophets (*Hebrews* 12:32). And there is no doubt Samson's action was understood as a suicide. With his strength restored, he could have escaped, but he chose to die. So clearly is this a suicide that St. Augustine thought it necessary to claim that God himself must have made an exception to the moral law forbidding all suicide and secretly ordered Samson to pull the building down on himself (*City of God*, I:21).

Given the commandments both for and against killing in the Hebrew Bible, it is unwise to use Biblical texts as arguments for or against killing, even killing the innocent. Biblical quotations are not good arguments for or against abortion, or killing the innocent, or euthanasia, or suicide, or capital punishment. The texts are not consistent, and therefore not conclusive. What does seem clear, however, is that the people of the Biblical tradition, as time went on, tended more and more to kill less and less, and that this tendency to avoid killing is a major factor behind our culture's traditional stand against euthanasia and suicide.

Another strong cultural factor against euthanasia and suicide is Christianity. Christians were deeply moved by the example of their founder, who refused to allow the use of weapons to defend his life, and who accepted his rigged trial and execution without a struggle. They took a strong stand against killing, and most of them considered late abortions, infanticide, capital punishment, warfare, and suicide immoral homicides.

At the end of the fourth century, when the Romans made Christianity the official religion of the Empire, political realities intruded and forced the Christians to reconsider their earlier doctrines of nonviolence. Soon they began allowing exceptions to their prohibition against killing. The most notable exception was in response to the need to defend the Empire, chiefly from the barbarians coming down from northern Europe. Christian theologians set forth what became known as the "just war" doctrine. This doctrine, developed in great detail by St. Augustine (354–431), allowed unjustly attacked people to defend their empire or country with lethal force if necessary.

Christians accepted the morality of capital punishment at about the same time. The Empire had to be protected against criminals, and the death penalty was seen as a powerful deterrent to criminal activity. The list of crimes subject to the death penalty varied from time to time and place to place. In the Middle Ages, Christians expanded it to include the ecclesiastical crime of heresy. People refusing to give up theological doctrines condemned by the Roman Catholic authorities were killed, usually by being burned alive.

These exceptions to the prohibition "thou shall not kill" were all "official" killings, that is, killings sanctioned by civil or religious authorities. The authorities sent soldiers into battle, and the civil or religious courts and tribunals condemned the criminals and heretics to death. But medieval Christians introduced another exception for killing, one that did not need official approval; they allowed killing in self-defense. In self-defense, the person attacked, a private citizen, is the one deciding to use lethal force, not the public authorities. Some Christians found it rather difficult to justify killing in self-defense because it contradicted the example of Jesus—when his enemies came to kill him he made no defense—but eventually killing in self-defense became as morally acceptable as killing in war and killing those condemned by civil or religious tribunals.

All the killings that the Christians considered exceptions to the prohibition against killing shared a common theme: the person killed was somehow not innocent. According to the just war theory, the enemy was not justified in attacking, so the enemy soldiers are not innocent. And criminals and heretics are not innocent, nor is the person assaulting someone. All these people are guilty of serious crimes and can be killed if necessary.

Thus, what began for Christians as a universal prohibition against all killing became in time a more narrow prohibition: do not deliberately kill innocent people. This remains a central Christian position today. We should note, however, that a few Christians continue to reject the exceptions to the original prohibition against killing and remain convinced that any killing is contrary to Christian morality. They are called "pacifists." They oppose all capital punishment and killing in self-defense, and adopt a pacifist stance on questions of war. Although these Christians are a small minority of Christians in the world today, their doctrine was the one embraced by the majority of early Christians and is actually more easily reconciled with the teachings of Christ and the Gospel than the later Christian moralities of war, capital punishment, and self-defense.

The religious prohibition against killing the innocent has received strong philosophical support in the past few centuries. When the political theories centered on natural rights blossomed in the seventeenth century, the primary right, the right to life, was obviously a move to protect every human being against being killed. The development of the right to life in political and moral philosophy provided a strong basis for protecting the lives of the innocent.

Yet, in a somewhat ironic way, the rights movement that originally protected human life is now used to justify destroying it. This happens in one of two ways. First, if life is understood as a right of mine, it can be argued that I should be able to waive that right and kill myself or ask someone to kill me. Second, if I have rights other than the right to life, and the right to die is one of them, then I should be able to kill myself or have someone kill me. Both of these rights-based arguments are now used to defend euthanasia and physician-assisted suicide.

Immanuel Kant developed another influential modern philosophy with a strong prohibition against killing the innocent, and his moral philosophy remains very influential today. He wrote that suicide is a horrible violation of our duty toward ourselves and "nothing more terrible can be imagined." We are "horrified at the very thought of suicide; by it man sinks lower than the beasts . . ." He went on to say that "moral philosophers must, therefore, first and foremost show that suicide is abominable."

In another work, however, Kant raised questions about specific cases that cannot but make us wonder whether or not he would allow exceptions to his apparently absolute prohibition of suicide. Kant knew that his king, Frederick the Great, carried lethal poison into battle so he could kill himself rather than be captured and held for ransom that would bleed his country. Kant hesitated to condemn the king's plan as immoral. And he also wondered whether it would really be unethical for a person, suffering from an incurable disease that would cause him to go mad, to commit suicide lest his madness cause harm to others.

From this brief overview, we can see an almost unanimous long-standing religious and philosophical position against private decisions to kill. The one exception was lethal force as a last resort in self-defense. In the past few decades, however, the movement to expand acceptable killings to include "rational" suicide and active euthanasia has been growing stronger in an ever-intensifying movement to legalize euthanasia and physician-assisted suicide.

In 1988 the *Journal of the American Medical Association* published an anonymous account of a doctor, still in residency, killing a young woman suffering from cancer. The piece, entitled "It's All Over, Debbie," aroused widespread and heated reactions. In 1989 *The New England Journal of Medicine* published an article by twelve respected physicians on caring for hopelessly ill patients. Ten of them concluded that it was not immoral for a physician to assist in the rational suicide of a terminally ill patient. Less than a year later, a physician in Michigan, Dr. Jack Kevorkian, designed a "suicide machine." A woman in the early stages of Alzheimer's disease used it, with his help, to kill herself. That suicide, and more than a dozen others that he also helped arrange, received widespread publicity and resulted in his arrest. In 1991 Dr. Timothy Quill of New York wrote an article in *The New England Journal of Medicine* describing how he helped a patient with incurable leukemia kill herself with an overdose of barbiturates. And that same year, Derek Humphrey's book, *Final Exit: The Practicalities of Self-Deliverance and Assisted Suicide for the Dying*, appeared. It advocated assisted suicide and euthanasia for dying patients who wanted it. The book sold well despite its lack of thoughtful reasoning and misleading statements about the rights people already have under present law to stop treatments.

Advocacy for euthanasia has increased on political and legal fronts as well. It is most advanced in Holland, where euthanasia has been practiced without legal intervention for years. Although the Dutch Penal Code still considers euthanasia a crime punishable by up to 12 years in prison or by a fine of up to about $60,000, both trial courts and the Dutch Supreme Court have been consistently excusing physicians practicing euthanasia since 1973. Physicians escape prosecution by showing that their duty to alleviate suffering prevailed over the duty to preserve life.

The courts do expect physicians to limit euthanasia to cases where these three conditions exist: (1) voluntary and persistent request by the patient, (2) unbearable suffering, and (3) the physician must consult with a colleague about the patient's condition and about the appropriateness of the patient's request to be killed, and must report the euthanasia to civil authorities. In 1993 both the Dutch Parliament and Senate began the process to legalize euthanasia and physician-assisted suicide.

In the United States, efforts are also underway to make euthanasia and physician-assisted suicide legal. Many states permit voters to change state laws by voting for initiative petitions, so one strategy for change consists of putting the issue on the ballot as a referendum question. In 1991 the Hemlock Society proposed a series of amendments to Washington's 1979 living-will law that would allow euthanasia and physician-assisted suicide. The proposal, known as Initiative 119, failed but received 46 percent of the votes. Another group, known as Compassion in Dying, then challenged in federal court Washington's law prohibiting assisted suicide. In May 1994 the judge ruled that the law against suicide was indeed unconstitutional.

How could this be? The judge argued as follows. First, the decision to commit suicide is deserving of the same constitutional protection as the decision of a woman to have an abortion. Since the U.S. Supreme Court has ruled that state law cannot interfere with the right of a woman to destroy her fetus, it follows that it should not interfere with the right of a person to destroy herself. Second, dying patients receiving life-sustaining treatment can choose death by refusing the treatment, but dying patients not receiving life-sustaining treatment have no such option unless the law allows them to kill themselves. Since the Fourteenth Amendment guarantees equal protection under the law, state laws against suicide are unconstitutional.

The court's questionable position stems from a common failure in reasoning—the failure to make distinctions. In both legal and moral reasoning there are clear distinctions between destroying a fetus before viability and destroying someone after birth and between removing life-sustaining treatment and helping someone commit suicide. The decision of the federal district court has been appealed.

In November 1992 Proposition 161 appeared on the ballot in California. It would have allowed both euthanasia and physician-assisted suicide, but it was defeated, although it also received 46 percent of the vote.

In November 1994 the Hemlock Society sponsored Measure 16 on the Oregon ballot. It was narrowly drafted, allowing only physician-assisted suicide and not euthanasia. Moreover, the physicians would be able to help patients kill themselves only by prescribing lethal drugs and not by other means such as the carbon monoxide poisoning favored by the well-known Dr. Jack Kevorkian. The measure included other restrictions as well. Two physicians must agree that death is expected within six months, the patient must be competent, two requests (at least fifteen days apart) for the lethal overdose must be made, and then a waiting period of forty-eight hours must pass before the prescription can be written. This ballot measure passed, and Oregon thus became the first state to legalize physician-assisted suicide. Almost immediately the constitutionality of the new law, scheduled to take effect on December 8, 1994, was challenged in court.

Before we examine the ethical arguments for and against euthanasia and physician-assisted suicide, a review of some relevant distinctions will be helpful.

RELEVANT DISTINCTIONS

Most discussions of euthanasia and assisted suicide include at least some of the following distinctions.

Euthanasia and Assisted Suicide

This seems like a very clear and sharp distinction, most notably because the physician does the killing in euthanasia and the patient does it in suicide. Yet the distinction between euthanasia and assisted suicide is weaker than it might first appear. In both cases, the physician plays an important role in the killing. In euthanasia, the physician alone causes the death, and in physician-assisted suicide both the physician and the patient cause the death. By providing the lethal overdose and the proper instructions for suicide, the physician is very much an active participant in the killing that occurs in the physician-assisted suicide. For this reason it may be helpful to think of physician-assisted suicide as "medical suicide" and euthanasia as "medical killing."

We can see the physician's role in physician-assisted suicide more clearly if we imagine that a man wanted to kill his wife, told his physician about it, and asked the physician to provide the lethal overdose and instructions on how to use it to kill. Here we have no trouble recognizing that the physician is very much an active participant in the subsequent killing. The physician's role is no less active if the man wanted the overdose to kill himself.

Thus euthanasia and physician-assisted suicide are similar in a crucial way. In both, the physician is a moral agent deeply involved in causing the death of a patient. In the case of suicide, of course, there is a second moral agent active in causing death, the patient, but the physician is still playing a major causal role. Teaching a person how to kill someone, whether that someone is the person to be killed or another, and providing them with the poison to do it, is simply not that different from actually injecting the lethal dose. Efforts to consider physicians helping people commit suicide as only "indirectly" involved in the killing are suspect; the law and common sense have always recognized that people providing poisons for a planned killing are directly implicated in that killing.

Moral reasoning about euthanasia and physician-assisted suicide, as well as debates about whether these should be public policy and legally allowed for those who want to die this way, should recognize the strong similarity between euthanasia and physician-assisted suicide. While there are differences between medical killing and medical suicide, the similarity between the two is so strong that they stand or fall together. In euthanasia the physician does the killing; in physician-assisted suicide the physician and the patient form a team to do the killing.

Active and Passive Euthanasia

This widely used distinction echoes the killing–letting die distinction discussed earlier. Sometimes it is clear. If a person is dying and I do absolutely nothing, then I am letting the person die and we could call it passive euthanasia. Most often, however, people use the active–passive euthanasia distinction in a questionable way. They want to call removing life support or medical nutrition from a dying patient "passive" euthanasia. But "passive" is not the proper word here because the actual removals of life-sustaining treatments are activities.

Even if the distinction between active and passive euthanasia is used correctly, however, it is not really morally helpful. It does not tell us whether something is moral or immoral. Being passive in the face of a death does not necessarily absolve one of responsibility for that death. Parents neglecting their infant are passive in regard to the infant's death, but their behavior is still immoral. And necessary pain medications may actually cause death, but providing them in appropriate circumstances is still moral. It would be well if we could drop the phrase "passive euthanasia," and use the word euthanasia to designate the intentional killing of a patient (medical killing) and not treatment withdrawals or medications intended to mask pain. Unfortunately, "passive euthanasia" seems so firmly entrenched in people's minds that it will be with us for a long time.

Voluntary, Involuntary, and Nonvoluntary Euthanasia

Voluntary euthanasia occurs when the patient voluntarily asks to be killed. It presupposes all the requirements for informed consent are met. These include: (1) the patient has the capacity to understand, reason, and communicate; (2) the patient has sufficient information about diagnosis, prognosis, treatment options, etc.; and (3) the patient is not coerced or manipulated into giving consent. If these requirements are met and the patient wants to be killed, then it is a matter of voluntary euthanasia. Proponents of euthanasia usually begin by supporting only voluntary euthanasia.

Nonvoluntary euthanasia occurs when any of these requirements is missing. The patient may never have had the capacity to make such a decision or, if she had the capacity, never have made the decision. Or, perhaps, the patient may not have all the information, or was depressed by her suffering, or was so distressed by the burden she was causing the family and providers that she felt obligated to request euthanasia.

Most moralists reject nonvoluntary euthanasia in their writings, but this rejection does not always follow in practice. As we shall see, there is now convincing evidence from Holland, where only voluntary euthanasia is permitted under the guidelines, that a considerable number of patients have been killed who could not have given voluntary consent. The extension of euthanasia from cases where the patient voluntarily requests it to those not requesting it is logical in one sense—if the rationale for euthanasia is relief of suffering, then it follows that we should relieve the suffering of all, even those without the capacity to request euthanasia. Thus, while in theory only voluntary euthanasia is advocated by supporters of euthanasia, in practice the Dutch experience reveals how easily voluntary euthanasia leads to nonvoluntary euthanasia and how, once voluntary euthanasia is accepted, some physicians do begin killing people without their consent and feel justified in so doing.

Involuntary euthanasia occurs when a patient is opposed to being killed. No moralist of any stature sees any justification for this. Most simply, and correctly, consider it murder.

Ethics and Public Policy

Sometimes it is argued that a distinction should be made between personal morality and public policy. The main idea driving this move is the recognition that irresolvable conflicts on some basic moral issues exist in our pluralistic society, so some matters are better ignored by public policy. Abortion is given as one example of this. Some argue that public policy should recognize that abortion is a private matter between a woman and her physician. Thus it should allow those believing abortion is morally justified to have an abortion and allow those believing it is not morally good to avoid involvement. In somewhat the same way, some argue that euthanasia should be recognized as a private matter between a suffering patient and his physician, and thus public policy should allow those believing euthanasia is morally justified to practice it and allow those not believing it is morally good to avoid involvement.

A second idea underlying the effort to distinguish personal ethics and public policy goes in the opposite direction. It envisions a public policy forbidding euthanasia in order to prevent abuse, but making no effort to prosecute it when physicians follow acceptable guidelines. This is the current situation in Holland; the law forbids euthanasia, but prosecutors do not prosecute as long as physicians follow the guidelines.

The distinction between ethics and public policy has its advantages. On some issues, there are essential differences between public policy and the moral values one personally embraces. Yet there are serious dangers with such a distinction when it is a matter of ending human life. Morality is seldom purely private; it almost always affects the common good, the good of the society. The virtues are not simply personal, but public. The public good is undermined when many private individuals become lazy, promiscuous, cowardly, rash, or selfish. Private vices undermine both private lives and the public good. Thus Aristotle recognized that there is no sharp distinction between ethics and politics; in fact, for him ethics is merely the private side of what he called politics—the seeking of the public good.

While the distinction between public policy and private ethics has some merit, it would only be a temporary stopgap. Sooner or later a society must reach some consensus on when human life can be destroyed, or the dissent festers and eventually surfaces. The history of the abortion controversy reminds us of this. In 1973 the Supreme Court made it a matter of personal choice until the third trimester of the pregnancy. This approach has not worked, and the socially disruptive controversy about abortion continues.

MORAL REASONING AND EUTHANASIA

Before we turn to the arguments for and against euthanasia, six remarks will be helpful.

1. "Killing" and "kill" are the appropriate words to use in discussions of euthanasia and assisted suicide. Euthanasia and suicide are killings, and we should not conceal that reality by calling these actions by any other name. In euthanasia, physicians kill their patients; in assisted suicide, physicians help patients to kill themselves. The moral question is whether physicians and patients can morally justify these killings when they are voluntary and motivated by compassion and mercy.

2. In euthanasia and assisted suicide, the person killed is "innocent." This means euthanasia and assisted suicide are not akin to the usual exceptions we make for killing (namely, just war, capital punishment, and self-defense). In these cases, the person killed was an enemy, a criminal, or an attacker, and therefore not considered "innocent."

3. In euthanasia and assisted suicide, the innocent person is not giving up his life to save the life of others. Therefore we cannot use any argument based on heroic self-sacrifice to justify the loss of life.

4. It is impossible to deliberate morally about euthanasia if we begin by saying "intentionally killing the innocent" is "always and everywhere wrong" or "intrinsically evil" or "immoral without exception." In most cases, intentionally killing an innocent person is immoral, but there are exceptions. For exam-

ple, suppose a well-armed severely ill mental patient is on a rampage killing people. He is, morally and legally, innocent. The person who had no choice but to kill him to stop the rampage has killed an innocent man, but few would say the killing is immoral. Tragic yes, but not immoral. Again, suppose a captured spy commits suicide to avoid revealing under torture the identity of other spies; few would say his suicide is immoral, although he does kill a person he considers innocent—himself.

What is always and everywhere wrong is not "intentionally killing the innocent," but intentionally killing without adequate reasons to justify the loss of human life. The issue is whether or not the killing of the innocent in euthanasia and assisted suicide is morally justified by sufficient reasons. If the reasons for the killing are not adequate, then the killing is not morally justified.

5. Voluntary euthanasia and assisted suicide are, in effect, team killings. Both the patient and the physician are deeply involved, and hence both are moral agents. The specific moral question is: When, if ever, is it morally good for physicians to kill patients who request it, or to help patients kill themselves? To morally justify the killings, both the physician and the patient must show how the killing makes their lives good, or at least avoids the less worse. Patients thinking of killing themselves must show how the killing will contribute to their good or avoid the less worse, and physicians thinking of killing patients must likewise show how the killing will contribute to their personal good or avoid the less worse. It is never enough for a physician to justify his role in the killing by saying that it was the patient's request or that it was good for the patient.

6. We must keep in mind that there are various degrees of causing death, and that we consider some of them morally good in appropriate circumstances. In chapter three we listed the five major ways physicians' actions have a causal impact on the patient's death. They were:

- active euthanasia
- assisted suicide
- pain medication so heavy it shortens life
- withdrawal of needed life-sustaining treatment
- withdrawal of medical nutrition and hydration

As we discuss euthanasia and physician-assisted suicide, then, we have to acknowledge that the question is not whether it is ethical for physicians to play any causal role in patients' deaths; we already know that they do, and we can morally justify it in appropriate circumstances. The question is whether we should limit the physicians' causal roles in death to treatment withdrawals and medications intended to mask pain, or whether we should allow physicians to kill by lethal injections and to help patients kill themselves. The central issue in the euthanasia debate is whether we can morally justify extending the physician's causal impact on a patient's death from the already accepted cases of withdrawing life support and using necessary pain medication to the stronger causal actions of assisting in suicide and giving lethal injections.

We turn now to this central moral question: can the killing called euthanasia and physician-assisted suicide be morally justified? We will consider first the reasons advanced by proponents of euthanasia and assisted suicide, then some criticisms of those reasons, and finally the reasons advanced by opponents of these practices.

REASONS FOR EUTHANASIA AND PHYSICIAN-ASSISTED SUICIDE

There are three main reasons advanced to justify the intentional killing of willing patients by physicians.

Respect for Patient Self-Determination

The idea that people should decide for themselves how they want to live and die is central to most arguments favoring euthanasia and suicide. In the early 1970s, in one of the first major ethical documents in the young field of medical ethics, the *National Commission for the Protection of Human Subjects* proposed three ethical principles; one of them was patient autonomy. A decade later the *President's Commission for the Study of Ethical Problems in Medicine and Biomedical and Behavioral Research* proposed three similar underlying values; one of them was patient self-determination. The reliance of these two landmark reports on the principles and values of autonomy and self-determination underlined the growing importance of patient control in medical ethics.

At first, the notions of autonomy and self-determination were employed solely to justify withdrawal of unwanted life-sustaining treatments. Soon, however, autonomy and self-determination were being used in another way. Some patients began insisting that self-determination enabled them to have physicians kill them or at least help them to kill themselves.

If autonomy and self-determination are accepted as fundamental moral principles or moral values, then voluntary requests for assistance in suicide or for lethal injections will seem morally justified to some. If autonomy is understood as a principle whereby whatever I choose is thereby morally right, then it can be argued that my choice to be killed is moral and that I can ask my physician to help me.

Closely associated with the argument for euthanasia based on self-determination are arguments from rights. For centuries our culture has championed liberty, the right to choose, as a fundamental right. If liberty is a human right, there seems no reason why a person cannot freely choose to kill herself or ask someone else to do it for her. Some people also create an additional right, the right to die, and argue that this right justifies suicide and euthanasia. In a culture sensitive to rights, no one wants to violate a patient's rights, and this makes the rights-based arguments for euthanasia and suicide appear plausible.

People relying on rights-based ethics, of course, do advocate another fundamental natural or human right, the right to life. The right to life is obviously contrary both to the right to choose death and to the right to die. A chronic conflict haunts moralities based on rights as they try to harmonize a right to life with the rights to choose death and to die. The paradox is most often solved by claiming that rights can be overridden or waived. In cases of suicide and euthanasia, the strategy is to say that the patient voluntarily waives the right to life. Once the right to life is waived, the rights to choose and to die can prevail. These rights, it is claimed, justify the collaboration of the patient and the physician in the killing.

Relief of Suffering

Some people suffer terribly before they die. Advocates of euthanasia argue that the pain of dying is sometimes uncontrollable, and that a quick merciful death is morally justified in these cases. Opponents of euthanasia claim most, if not all, suffering can be controlled by medication, although sometimes this means so heavily sedating dying patients that they are "snowed"—that is, pretty much unconscious. Advocates of euthanasia claim this makes no sense; if dying people are suffering terrible intractable pain and want to die, they say it is more humane to honor requests for euthanasia than to induce somnolence by drugs while awaiting inevitable death.

The argument here is a powerful one because it is based on two of the noblest human feelings: compassion and mercy in the face of another's suffering. The relief of suffering has long been one of the primary goals of medicine, and good physicians are always eager to alleviate pain. For some, this is reason enough to argue that physicians should respond to the pleas for euthanasia or assistance in suicide. If a suffering patient believes with good reason that he will be better off dead, then the physician refusing to help can appear to be lacking mercy and compassion if she refuses to kill him or help him commit suicide.

Proponents of this argument for euthanasia are usually quick to say the suffering need not be physical; it could be psychological. The fear of losing control or dignity at the end as the result of diseases such as Huntington's, amyotrophic lateral sclerosis (ALS), Alzheimer's, etc., can cause great distress and can also be, some say, a reason for euthanasia or assistance in suicide when the final disintegration sets in.

Normal Medical Practice

The third argument for medical aid in euthanasia and assisted suicide is rooted in the claim that these actions are no more than a normal evolution in modern medicine faced with three changing circumstances. First, thanks to medical research and better diagnosis, we now know more about the inexorable and painful degeneration of certain diseases. The certainty of what will be a painful dying suggests to some that we might try to make the inevitable death easier for the patient. Second, although many people influenced by Christianity once saw meaning and value in suffering, fewer do today. They see no reason for enduring a miserable end and seek euthanasia to avoid it. Finally, now that a widespread consensus exists about withdrawing life-support treatments—what some call passive euthanasia—the move to active euthanasia seems to some a reasonable next step for medicine at the end of life.

It is true that medical practice evolves, and significant stages in this evolution are apparent. From a widespread conviction that death was an enemy that must be kept at bay because its victory would be a defeat for the physician and his craft, medicine has developed the more mature idea that the physician, with his equipment and remedies, should retreat in some cases. In the medical ethos now developing, the physician often welcomes death and sometimes helps it arrive by withdrawing treatment.

For some, there is little difference between these withdrawals and lethal injections or between heavy sedation for pain and deliberate lethal overdoses. They view euthanasia and assistance in suicide as consistent with the legitimate medical desire to prevent the indignity of personal disintegration that accompanies some deaths, as an extension of normal caring for a patient who does not want the suffering and indignity of a terrible and messy death. Dying patients, after all, desire only what everyone wants: a good death. If a good death is a blessing, as so many have said for so long, then medical assistance in dying is an act of beneficence, a part of the total care a physician provides for her patient. In this way, euthanasia and physician-assisted suicide can appear compatible with the noble aims of medical practice.

Moreover, polls indicate that assistance in dying is now what many people want from their physicians. Recent efforts to place euthanasia and assisted suicide on state ballots have succeeded, and the ballot questions have drawn an impressive percentage of the vote. More and more people, it seems, are considering the options of euthanasia and assisted suicide normal parts of medical practice.

REASONS AGAINST EUTHANASIA AND PHYSICIAN-ASSISTED SUICIDE

Killing a human being is a momentous act, and our history reveals a tendency to limit the scope of morally acceptable killing. The killing of enemy prisoners, once practiced by such great European heroes as Charlemagne and the Crusaders, is now widely condemned. Public executions are also a thing of the past and, in fact, most countries in our cultural tradition have abolished capital punishment. Infanticide is no longer tolerated, and people killing their own babies are now prosecuted as murderers, something unheard of in earlier times. Weapons of mass killing have been built and were used twice at the end of World War II, but many have raised strong moral objections to any future use of strategic nuclear weapons.

In all this we can see the effort to reduce killing, to narrow down the range of morally and legally acceptable killings to the point where killing is morally suspect unless authorized by political or judicial authorities (war and capital punishment) or undertaken privately as a last resort to save a life. This suggests that a strong *prima facie* case exists against killing. The burden of proof in the question of euthanasia and assisted suicide, therefore, rests with the advocates of change, with those desiring to establish the legal and moral validity of these private killings.

The reasons for not killing patients and for not helping them kill themselves fall into two groups. The first group comprise attempts to refute the arguments used to justify euthanasia and physician-assisted suicide. If the reasons used to justify euthanasia and physician-assisted suicide are not sufficiently convincing to overcome the traditional cultural stance against the private killing of innocent people, then the traditional stance against euthanasia and physician-assisted suicide should prevail.

The second group of arguments against euthanasia and assisted suicide focus on the reasons why it is not good for physicians to kill patients, nor good for patients to kill themselves, nor good for society to have physicians killing patients or helping them kill themselves. In tragic situations where no option the patient chooses will promote a good life in any meaningful sense, these arguments focus on showing that there are less worse alternatives than euthanasia or physician-assisted suicide. In other words, the second class of arguments are substantive arguments designed to show why euthanasia and physician-assisted suicide are not morally justified.

Critiques of the Arguments Favoring Euthanasia

Critique of the patient self-determination argument

Arguments for euthanasia and physician-assisted suicide based on patient autonomy, patient self-determination, or the right to choose all contain a major limitation: they cannot by themselves establish what is morally right or wrong. Saying something is morally right simply because it is autonomously and freely chosen is missing the whole point of ethics. The task of ethics is to determine that what is freely chosen is morally good; that is, that it will truly contribute to the agent's good. The agent may think the killing is good, and freely choose it, but that is not enough. Ethical reasoning must show the killing will be truly good, or the less worse, for those engaging in it.

Certainly patients should be responsible for their lives and make the important choices, but no choice becomes morally justified simply because it is chosen. Few people think those who freely choose to play Russian roulette or take part in a duel are doing something morally good. And few think that slavery is moral for those who freely choose to enslave themselves to slave owners. Self-determination, choice, and personal responsibility are important moral notions, but they are not moral reasonings. Unfortunately, the tendency in the United States to consider autonomy or patient self-determination a fundamental moral principle from which we can deduce moral judgments about particular actions has led some to think whatever a patient chooses is morally justified.

Moreover, even if we accepted the argument from self-determination, it would justify euthanasia and assisted suicide only for those people with the capacity to request it. Just as not everyone has the capacity to give informed consent for treatment, so not everyone has the capacity to request voluntary euthanasia or assistance with suicide. The requirements for recognizing the validity of self-determination when euthanasia is the issue will have to be at least as stringent as the requirements for informed consent when accepting or rejecting life-sustaining treatment is the issue.

In fact, a good case can be made that informed consent requirements for euthanasia and suicide should be more stringent than for treatment refusals. We would hesitate, for example, to let suicidal persons make major decisions affecting their lives; how much the more should we hesitate to let them make a decision about being killed or killing themselves. People who are suicidal are not always in the best frame of mind to make good decisions about important issues of life and death. And we should keep in mind that we have very little knowledge about how illness, especially painful and lengthy illness, affects the reasonableness and voluntariness of decision making.

It should be a matter of concern that those proposing euthanasia and assisted suicide have not yet developed anything as advanced as the widely accepted doctrine of informed consent for accepting and declining treatment. This doctrine sets forth, as we saw in chapter four, important requirements for determining the capacity of the patient to make decisions, for the extensive information that must be provided, and for avoiding any manipulation that would undermine the voluntary aspect of the decision. These requirements cannot be met in situations involving many severely sick and dying patients.

It is somewhat ironic that so many who invoke patient self-determination as a justification for euthanasia have thus far failed to insist on full-fledged informed consent for the lethal injection. One important aspect of informed consent, as we saw, is providing the person with information about all the alternative treatments that could be employed, but some supporters of euthanasia spend little time explaining the alternative approaches available to control their patients' suffering. Without a good grasp of what alternatives such as hospice care can do, the patient's request for euthanasia or physician-assisted suicide is not a truly informed request.

Finally, ethicists supporting euthanasia invariably acknowledge that the argument from self-determination alone is not strong enough to justify suicide and euthanasia. Their argument is never that the simple desire to be killed is sufficient to justify the killing, but that other realities such as actual or expected suffering, approaching death, or permanent loss of awareness must be present. Thus self-determination is not really an adequate argument or a sufficient reason justifying euthanasia and physician-assisted suicide. It is, rather, a condition that most advocates of euthanasia insist must be met before the killing can be considered morally justified. Advocates of euthanasia or physician-assisted suicide do not claim it is right to kill people, or to help them kill themselves, simply because they want to be killed; they always give another reason to show why the killing is the right thing to do. And that other reason is rooted in compassion for the patient's suffering.

Critique of the argument based on relief of suffering

Long before autonomy or patient self-determination became a paramount concept in health care ethics, those advocating euthanasia relied on this argument, and it is a strong one. Relief of suffering has always been a goal of morally good people and of medicine itself. The argument claims physicians should, in cases where the suffering is intractable and death inevitable, respond in a spirit of mercy and compassion to a patient's desire for euthanasia or assistance in suicide.

Stated this way, the argument prompted by mercy is clearly a limited one. Euthanasia and physician-assisted suicide are moral options only when patients are experiencing, or expect to experience, severe intractable suffering that cannot be otherwise controlled. This means patients in an indefinite coma or persistent vegetative state are not candidates for euthanasia, even if their advance directives indicate this is what they would want. They are not candidates for euthanasia because they are not suffering and no merciful act can benefit them.

The relief of suffering argument, however, is even more limited than this because suffering can almost always be relieved without killing the person. It is possible to medicate patients so heavily that they are beyond awareness. This, of course, creates a very unsatisfactory situation in that sometimes it means patients are so drugged or "snowed" that their existence is reduced to a vegetative state.

Nobody really wants to live in such a state, but this is not the point. The point is whether it is morally less worse to relieve suffering by killing when we can relieve it short of killing the person. In other words, medicating patients into oblivion as they are dying may well be the worst thing we can do to them except for the other alternative—killing them. If we can relieve pain and suffering with medications, then no matter how unsatisfactory the situation, it is at least arguable that this route is less worse than killing them. Given our cultural tradition against private killing, the only situation where euthanasia would be justified by the relief of suffering argument, then, is a situation where the suffering can be relieved by no other way than by killing the patient. There may be such situations (on the battlefield, for example), but they are almost inconceivable in a normal health care setting.

Ironically, the argument for euthanasia based on relieving suffering was much stronger before anesthesia and pain medication became so effective. Until this century, the suffering of some patients was truly intense and intractable, but now massive medication to reduce or even eliminate awareness is available. Knowing a heavy dose of pain medication might in fact kill the person does not make giving it an action akin to euthanasia because the intention is radically different. The intention—and intentions are important in ethics—in giving medication for pain is fundamentally different from the intention in giving a lethal injection. It is one kind of moral action to give drugs in order to mask pain; it is quite another kind of moral action to give drugs in order to kill.

Critique of the argument based on normal medical practice

Arguments derived from the idea of "normal practice" are never persuasive in ethics. While normal practice is a good starting point for moral reflection, the rightfulness of conduct is not established by it, but by reasons. The moral philosopher must show not that something is considered normal, but that what is considered normal will actually contribute to the good.

In ancient Greece, the Sophists had argued that custom or personal preference established moral goodness. Socrates, Plato, Aristotle, and the Stoics all argued that something more was needed for virtue. In some societies cannibalism was normal practice; in others, polygamy, infanticide, torture, and slavery were normal practices. Few today claim these practices are morally right. It was once normal medical practice to operate and to do medical research without informed consent, to conceal a grim diagnosis and prognosis from patients, and to discard defective newborns, but few today claim these practices are morally sound.

Furthermore, it is not at all clear that responding to the desire to be killed with euthanasia or assistance in suicide is truly a part of medical practice. The decision of a person to be killed, or to kill herself, is much more than a medical decision—it is a fundamental decision about a person's whole life and how it should end. It is not a clinical decision involving treatment of disease or of pain, but an existential decision involving the destruction of human life. Physicians and nurses have no special training or expertise whereby they can join in decisions about ending someone's life. This is not a professional or clinical decision. Killing people, and helping them kill themselves, is a social issue of immense consequence. Killing innocent people has never been, and is not now, normal practice for any segment of our society.

Substantive Arguments Claiming Euthanasia and Assisted Suicide Are Immoral

Since there is a cultural presumption against killing innocent people even when they request it, criticisms of the arguments favoring euthanasia constitute a good reason for not accepting euthanasia and physician-assisted suicide. Opponents of euthanasia and physician-assisted suicide, however, have also offered more positive arguments designed to show that euthanasia and assistance in suicide are immoral behaviors. What follows are some of the more popular arguments against euthanasia and physician-assisted suicide.

The religious argument against euthanasia and suicide

There is first the familiar biblical injunction "Thou shalt not kill." Despite the references indicating that the Bible sanctions various killings, including the killing of the enemy's women and children and of one's own unruly sons, a consensus has emerged that the Bible takes a strong stand against most intentional killing of innocent people. Thus, for those accepting a moral tradition rooted in the Bible, the prohibition "doctors must not kill" seems to be well-grounded.

A second aspect of the religious argument against euthanasia and assisted suicide rests on the doctrine of creation. According to this doctrine, God created the world out of nothing and continues His creative involvement to this day. For believers, God is the lord and giver of life; that is, He gives life as a gift and remains lord of it. Killing, therefore, is a rejection of the gift of life and of God's sovereignty over it. By killing, people assume a power over life and death that belongs not to them but to God. God decides who are to be born, and when and how they are to die. People act immorally if they usurp God's sovereignty over life and begin "to play God." As *Deuteronomy* 32:39 says: "Learn that I, I alone, am God, and there is no God besides me. It is I who bring both death and life."

The religious argument has great appeal for many, especially those influenced by the Biblical doctrine of creation. Its use is not confined to theologians. Kant, for example, was a philosopher who argued at great length that morality is an affair of reason, not religious revelation, but he employed a religious argument against suicide. He believed we were placed in this world by God for specific purposes, and that people committing suicide desert their posts and are rebelling against God. John Locke, a major architect of the theory that every human being has natural rights, among them the rights to life and liberty, also argued against suicide by claiming God sent us into the world to be about His business, and thus we are bound to preserve ourselves and not quit our station willfully.

While the religious arguments against euthanasia and physician-assisted suicide will be important for many believers, they obviously presuppose certain beliefs about the Biblical commandments and creation. For those not believing in divine laws or creation, they carry no weight. Thus the religious arguments against suicide are limited because they are based on religious beliefs not shared by all.

The argument from nature against euthanasia and suicide

Some philosophers claim killing ourselves, or asking others to kill us, is immoral because it runs counter to the natural impulse for self-preservation and is thus against human nature. Certainly, asking someone to kill us, or doing it ourselves, does seem to go against the natural desire to live, but the argument from nature is actually a weak one. The natural desire for self-preservation can be overridden two ways: by great and hopeless suffering, and by the choice to sacrifice our lives for a cause, perhaps religious martyrdom or heroic self-sacrifice whereby we give up our lives that others may live.

The weakness of the argument from nature against euthanasia also arises from the ease with which it can be turned into a reason for euthanasia or suicide. The Stoics, for example, the original proponents of a morality based on "acting according to nature," were comfortable with suicide. They thought death is "according to nature," and thus we can bring it about at the proper time. And if one accepts Freud's analysis of human nature, then the natural instinct to survive and thrive is accompanied by an equally natural instinct for self-destruction. For the Freudian, the drive to self-destruction is as natural, though normally not as powerful, as the drive for self-preservation. The often repeated story of how Freud asked his physician for a lethal overdose at the end of his life adds an interesting footnote to his theory of the interplay of *eros* and *thanatos*, the natural instincts for life and death in all of us.

The social argument against euthanasia and suicide

As far back as Aristotle, the argument was made that suicide was an act of injustice against society. Whatever might be the advantages of suicide from the individual's point of view, others will be hurt, most notably the society. Suicide is wrong when it undermines the common good, the good shared by the many now weakened by the death of one who killed himself or requested that he be killed. Certainly there are situations where this is true. The death of contributors to the common good will weaken that good, much as the death of a parent in a family of small children brings great distress to the family.

But this is also a weak argument against euthanasia and physician-assisted suicide. By far, the usual candidates for euthanasia or assisted suicide in medical settings are already beyond contributing much to the common good. Those closest to them, and others in the community as well, may already be praying for their happy death and will consider that death, when it comes, a blessing and not a detriment to society.

The argument against a public policy of euthanasia and suicide

Proponents of this argument often prescind from whether or not euthanasia and assisted suicide are morally right or wrong, and focus instead on the public policy level. Their position is that, regardless of whether you think euthanasia is moral or immoral, it would not be moral to institute a public policy of euthanasia and physician-assisted suicide because such a public policy would do more harm than good. They advance several reasons to show why this is so.

The possibility of mistakes.   Most proponents of euthanasia insist they are advocating only voluntary euthanasia. No one will be killed unless he requests it.

But the notion of "voluntary" is problematic here. We can never be sure the request to be killed, given the fact we consider most killings tragic, is truly voluntary. The more the patients are suffering, the more likely they will be candidates for euthanasia, and the less likely they will be free of depression, weariness, and the influence of medications. Illness distorts judgment and can make us less able to act in a truly voluntary way. The last thing a physician wants to do is kill somebody as the result of a misunderstanding, but unless we can say for sure that the sick, suffering, medicated person's request for euthanasia or assistance in suicide is truly well-informed and voluntary, then the risk of killing someone by mistake—that is, killing a patient who is not fully informed (including all alternatives) and freely choosing to be killed—remains such a strong possibility that no public policy should allow an environment where it might occur. It is a function of public policy to forbid situations where there is reason to believe inappropriate or accidental death might happen.

Morally sensitive physicians, of course, will make every effort to determine whether the person asking to be killed is suffering from any pain or depression that would affect judgment or undermine the ability to choose freely, but determining whether or not the decisions of sick, suffering, and dying patients are truly informed and voluntary is a most difficult task. The decision to be killed is a major decision, and major decisions are often not well-made when people are besieged by pain and suffering. There is some merit, then, in a public policy that will not allow physicians to kill or help to kill patients.

Undesirable consequences of legalizing euthanasia.   Many fear that legalization of voluntary euthanasia and physician-assisted suicide will lead to various undesirable consequences for medical practice, among them the following:

- Legalization of euthanasia will, or at least could, undermine the trust that some suffering patients would have in their physician once they know the physician is willing to kill them if they give the word. And some of these patients may feel very vulnerable because they are not insured and are incapable of paying for care. In a society that accepts euthanasia, these patients cannot help but worry about the financial pressure their medical treatment and hospitalization places on physicians and institutions. And they know that once the deed is done, the person killed cannot complain that it was done without voluntary consent.

Physicians have awesome power. They have ready access to lethal drugs; many know how to kill quickly and quietly, and how to enter the proper cause of death in the records. Unlike the rest of us, people die around them all the time, so no one suspects anything is amiss when another sick person dies. Medical examiners seldom look carefully at deaths of sick people that occur in a hospital or nursing home. In a society that rejects euthanasia, abuses are few and far between because they amount to murder. At the present time, our doctors are well aware it is illegal to kill, and few want to risk prosecution for murder. But in a society that accepts euthanasia, this protection is lost. It will become much more difficult to prevent killing that is not within the guidelines, as the experience in Holland shows. The physician–patient relationship is based on trust, and the trust will erode in the minds of some, perhaps many, if any killing by physicians is socially authorized.

- Legalization of euthanasia will, or at least could, also undermine our commitment to provide the best of care to those dying patients who decline to choose suicide or euthanasia. In a society where other patients in similar circumstances generously exercise their "right to die," and thereby cease to be a drain on personnel and resources, it is easy to consider those refusing to step out of the way selfish and their demand for care inappropriate.
- Legalization of euthanasia will, or at least could, put additional burdens on sick patients because it presents them with another choice, and a most serious one. At the present time, patients do not have to make any decision about euthanasia; if it becomes legal, then it will become an option for them. They may do nothing about it, but doing nothing will then be a choice not to accept the legal option of euthanasia or assistance in suicide.
- Legalization of euthanasia will, or at least could, be divisive for physicians who still think of themselves in some ways as colleagues, and who often call their organizations "colleges." With euthanasia as a social policy, a divide will inevitably exist between physicians who consider the killing immoral and those who do not, between those willing to kill their patients and those scandalized by the very thought of doing it. Hospitals and nursing homes will also be divided along these lines because in our country many of these institutions are operated by church-affiliated groups whose religious traditions consider suicide and euthanasia immoral, and they will steadfastly oppose it. And a divide will open up between some physicians and some

institutions because hospitals and nursing homes opposed to euthanasia will hesitate to admit physicians known to practice it in an effort to avoid, on their premises, what they consider murder.

- Legalization of euthanasia will, or at least could, change the face of medicine in a way that will be disconcerting to many. For centuries, the primary goal of medicine has been to cure, not to kill. Medicine has also tried to comfort, but the idea that physicians should comfort some people by killing them has not been a major part of medicine's ethos. Physicians have been trained to diagnose illness and then to treat it if possible and to comfort where necessary, but they have not been trained to kill patients or to help them kill themselves. The goal of medicine has never been to destroy life. Introducing euthanasia and assisted suicide will change all that by introducing a second and conflicting goal in medicine. Medicine would now have three goals: most of the time its goal will be saving and improving life, some of the time it will be comforting the dying, and some of the time it will be killing. Instead of cherishing life always, the ideal will now include destroying life sometimes. The thought of such a change in the goals of medicine causes many people, including some physicians, great distress, because it is such a radical departure from the traditional view of what physicians do when they practice medicine.

- Legalization of euthanasia will, or at least could, undermine the delicate relation between the law and medical decisions to forego life-sustaining treatment. Prosecutors and judges have come to recognize that there is an area at the end or at the edge of life where decisions to forego treatment supporting life, including medical nutrition, do not normally require judicial oversight. One reason why courts have been comfortable doing this, despite their traditional concern for the protection of innocent human life, has been the existence of the clear line between withdrawing life-sustaining treatment and giving lethal injections or overdoses to bring about death. Prosecutors and judges do not have to worry whether doctors are killing patients inappropriately since all killing is now illegal. At the present time, the central question is never whether a lethal injection or overdose to end life should be given, but whether treatment should be withdrawn. The courts have tended, with some notable exceptions, to leave treatment decisions to medical expertise.

This respect for medical decisions at the end of life will change if we expand medical decision-making to include euthanasia and assistance in suicide. If some deliberate killing (euthanasia and physician-assisted suicide) is legally allowed, we can expect intense scrutiny by prosecutors and judges because society has a great interest in monitoring killing. The prosecutors and courts that tended to leave treatment decisions to physicians will not feel the same about euthanasia and assisted suicide. These actions are not about withdrawing treatments but about killing, and any killing invites close legal scrutiny by law enforcement personnel.

The long struggle to have the courts leave medical decisions to forego life-sustaining treatment to the patient and physician will thus be undermined if medical practice is expanded to include euthanasia. Once physicians begin to kill, the law will move to the bedside. There will have to be legal guidelines for euthanasia, and those charged with enforcement will want to be sure they are followed exactly. Put simply, physicians can expect prosecutors and courts in our country to be much more concerned about euthanasia than they have been about withdrawals of life-sustaining treatments and medical nutrition.

Legalization of euthanasia will be a "slippery slope." Many argue that a public policy accepting voluntary euthanasia for the suffering and hopelessly ill patient can easily serve as a wedge to dislodge traditional barriers against other kinds of killing. If we legalize voluntary euthanasia, then involuntary euthanasia is likely to follow. Proxies, not knowing for sure what an incapacitated patient wants, will decide it is in the patient's best interest to be put to death quietly and quickly, and will expect the decision to be carried out as any other health care decision made by a proxy. Parents and physicians will decide euthanasia is best for their defective children; children and physicians will decide euthanasia is best for aging parents who have lost decision-making capacity. People will argue that those human beings so mentally compromised that they were never capable of making health care decisions should not be deprived of compassion when they are suffering, and thus euthanasia should be available for them. Accepting voluntary euthanasia will quickly lead to the acceptance of nonvoluntary euthanasia.

And, if we legalize euthanasia for the terminally ill, euthanasia for those not terminally ill will likely follow. Some will see no reason why the self-determination of patients, which now enables them to refuse life-sustaining treatments even when they are not hopelessly ill, should not extend to requests for euthanasia and assistance in suicide. It will be argued that the refusal of treatment necessary for life is equivalent to a decision to die, and once patients have decided to die, they should be able to choose the manner of their death and to be helped by their compassionate physicians to achieve it.

And, if we legalize euthanasia to relieve suffering, then euthanasia for those not suffering will inevitably follow. Some already see no reason why people in a permanent coma or a persistent vegetative state should not be killed, yet these patients are not suffering. Once we accept euthanasia for these permanently unconscious patients, it will likely spread to other cases where suffering is not an issue.

Thus, the argument runs, a public policy of voluntary euthanasia will likely lead to public acceptance of involuntary euthanasia, a public policy of euthanasia for the hopelessly ill will likely lead to public acceptance of euthanasia for those not hopelessly ill, and a public policy of euthanasia for people suffering severe pain will likely lead to public acceptance of euthanasia for people not suffering pain.

In short, once we legalize euthanasia and assisted suicide for the patient most often mentioned as appropriate—the person with a hopeless disease suffering unbearable pain who requests it—we can expect the practice to spread to other situations. Physicians will likely begin killing, or helping to kill, people who never said they wanted it, or who are not suffering, or who are not terminally ill.

This is what is widely known as the "slippery-slope" argument against euthanasia and physician-assisted suicide. In essence, it is an argument that concentrates on the undesirable consequences the legalization of euthanasia will likely generate. Some proponents of this slippery-slope argument think euthanasia itself is immoral; other proponents think it could be morally justified, at least in some extreme cases. But both groups argue that legalizing euthanasia or physician-assisted suicide for any reason, no matter how sound, will lead to situations where it is not morally defensible. They feel there is no way to control the killing once it starts, and that it will expand to infanticide and other forms of killing people without their consent or for reasons other than those that might be prescribed by the legal guidelines.

Some presentations of the slippery-slope argument against euthanasia invoke the chilling history of Nazi Germany, where euthanasia was accepted years before the death camps became a reality. The progression from euthanasia to wholesale killing in Nazi Germany is a powerful version of the slippery-slope argument because many older Americans remember World War II and the great military effort to defeat Germany. That war was followed by the famous trials of Nazi leaders in Nuremberg, where shocking evidence of forced euthanasia and other medical abuses by German physicians emerged.

In the minds of many, the road to abuse in Germany began when a few physicians adopted the attitude that some people—those who were severely or chronically ill—were living lives not worthy to be lived. Once this attitude set in, it was a small step to accept ending such worthless lives. Then the category of people living unworthy lives was expanded to include those not contributing to society, and then to those not wanted in the society because of their ideological views or racial identity.

Eventually, some say inevitably, what began as a modest euthanasia movement in the 1920s became the Holocaust of the 1940s, where 8 million innocent people were murdered. This shows, some say, that once we begin killing innocent people, especially if physicians do it, terrible evils will follow. The only way to prevent the abuse is to draw a strong line against all killing, including euthanasia.

Today's proponents of euthanasia, of course, disagree with such a conclusion. They sometimes attack the validity of the slippery-slope argument by saying enough protection can be built into the legalization of physician-assisted suicide and euthanasia that the slide into immoral killing will not occur. The defeated referendum known as Initiative 119 on the 1991 ballot in the state of Washington stipulated, for example, that the proposed legalization of euthanasia would apply only when the patient was (1) competent, (2) voluntarily requesting it, and (3) terminally ill with less than six months to live. The 1992 referendum in California, also defeated, added still more protections by including the qualifications that the voluntary request must be "enduring" and communicated in a revocable written directive signed by two unrelated witnesses, and that the physicians carrying out the killing must report euthanasia and the circumstances to appropriate authorities. The 1994 referendum in Oregon, which was successful, was even more restrictive, allowing only physician-assisted suicide. Putting such protections in place, it is argued, will prevent any slide down a slippery slope.

Moreover, proponents of euthanasia argue that the situation in Germany earlier in the century, especially during the Nazi years, bears so little resemblance to Europe and to the United States at this time that no significant comparisons can be drawn between that society and our own. And, in many ways, they are right.

There is, however, the more recent example of euthanasia in Europe that strengthens the slippery-slope argument. As we noted earlier, although the Dutch Penal Code makes euthanasia a criminal offense, for more than twenty years prosecutors in Holland have made it clear that euthanasia in cases of necessity will not be prosecuted provided physicians follow the guidelines or rules proposed by the Royal Dutch Medical Association, the State Commission on Euthanasia, and the Dutch government. The key points in the Dutch guidelines are as follows.

- The patient must have the capacity to make decisions, have an irreversible disease, be experiencing unbearable suffering, and be well-informed about euthanasia and about alternative ways of controlling suffering.
- The patient's request must be voluntary and persistent; it must reflect an enduring longing for death.
- The physician must consult at least one colleague with experience in euthanasia and, after the killing, provide a written report to the coroner explaining the disease and how the guidelines were followed.

These requirements, designed to prevent the slide down a slippery slope by restricting euthanasia to situations where both patient self-determination and the case for compassion are clear, are essentially the same as those in place for the past twenty years in Holland. Have they been successful in holding the line on euthanasia?

The simple answer is no. A 1991 Dutch report, authorized by the Committee on the Study of Medical Practice Concerning Euthanasia (also called the Remmelink Committee because its president was the attorney general of the Supreme Court, J. Remmelink), acknowledged that there have been hundreds of cases of nonvoluntary euthanasia and defended these cases even though they violated the published guidelines. The report analyzed the 129,000 deaths in Holland during 1990 and found that 2,300 of them were reported as euthanasia. In more than a third of these cases (about 1,000), a crucial guideline accepted by the Dutch Medical Association was violated: the patients killed had made no clear request for euthanasia. A few of those patients were children.

The high number of outlaw cases of euthanasia is disturbing. Moreover, to make matters worse, it was reported that some Dutch physicians declined to acknowledge every case of euthanasia. Obviously, some would be inclined to report a natural cause for the death whenever the euthanasia was not in accord with the guidelines. Hence, the number of patients actually killed without requesting it was undoubtedly higher than the 1,000 reported that year.

Advocates of euthanasia point out that those killed without having clearly requested it were in terrible condition and unable to request euthanasia. While interviews suggest that this was undoubtedly true in most cases, it is not relevant to a very important question in the debate about the legalization of euthanasia. That question is: Can we rely on physicians to adhere to the publicly accepted guidelines? The evidence from Holland is that we cannot.

In reality, then, proponents of the slippery-slope argument against legalizing euthanasia find strong support for their position in the Dutch experience, where it has not been possible to restrict euthanasia to the established guidelines. The evidence from Holland also raises questions about how honest physicians will be when it comes to reporting truthfully, in accord with guidelines, their practice of euthanasia. Of course, some proponents of euthanasia argue that the Dutch slide down the slippery slope is not inevitable, and that better safeguards could have prevented it. One wonders just what those effective safeguards could be.

It is also disturbing that the proponents of euthanasia in Holland have tended to ignore the illegal acts of euthanasia. Instead of calling for legal action against the physicians who violated the guidelines, the attitude seems to be that the guidelines are too conservative, and that the guidelines should be expanded to include the euthanasia of people who have not requested it and of children when parents and physicians think it is appropriate. This attitude tends to confirm the suspicion of many that legalizing voluntary euthanasia is only the first step down the slippery slope to nonvoluntary euthanasia.

We should note, however, that slippery-slope arguments are never conclusive. A slippery-slope or "wedge" argument can never prove absolutely that terrible consequences will follow if a certain line is crossed. A slippery-slope argument does not enjoy logical necessity; the first steps are not premises leading necessarily to the next steps in the argument. The power of slippery-slope arguments derives from experience and history; if we eat the first peanut, we may well eat a few more.

The slippery-slope argument in euthanasia has some plausibility because, to this point in history, no society has yet demonstrated just what set of guidelines and protections will be effective in preventing a slide from voluntary euthanasia of the suffering, irreversibly ill to other forms of killing. The slippery-slope argument can never prove that unwanted abuses will occur once we accept euthanasia, only that they might occur. But the argument remains thought provoking because the practice of euthanasia in Holland, the one modern example we have, has shown how quickly acceptance of voluntary euthanasia for the hopelessly ill and suffering patient is followed by other forms of killing.

We turn next to a widely noted account of a physician-assisted suicide written by a physician and published in a major medical journal. It is a case that will reveal how complex the issue truly is, and how good people disagree on how physicians should act.

THE CASE OF DIANE

The Story

Diane, a middle-aged woman, presented with a rash and a chronic tired feeling. Her blood count was suspicious, and a bone marrow biopsy confirmed the worst: an acute form of leukemia. Without treatment, she would die within a few months.

The treatment is not pleasant. It begins with three weeks of induction chemotherapy in the hospital that helps three out of four patients. If she is one of the three, she will receive additional chemotherapy with a two out of three chance it will benefit her. If it does, she will then undergo a two month hospitalization for a bone marrow transplantation with a 50 percent chance it will be effective for her. The bottom line is that her chance of survival is zero with no treatment and about one in four (25 percent) with the difficult chemotherapy treatments and bone marrow transplantation.

Her husband and college-age son wanted her to start the treatments, as did her physician, Dr. Timothy Quill, but she refused. Dr. Quill was bothered by her decision, since he knew her as a fighter, but he respected it.

Diane then made a disturbing request. She told Dr. Quill that she wanted to kill herself when she could no longer maintain control of herself and her dignity as she died. Dr. Quill, a former hospice physician, assured her that he could keep her comfortable, but she wanted no part of lingering in the relative comfort of heavy medication as she died.

A week later she requested barbiturates to help her sleep. Subsequent conversation with Dr. Quill revealed she was having trouble sleeping, but it was also clear that she wanted to have enough barbiturates to commit suicide. After assuring himself that she was not despondent and that she was truly making an informed decision, Dr. Quill prescribed the barbiturates, making sure that she knew how to use them for sleep and how many to take for suicide.

In three-and-a-half months bone pain, weakness, fatigue, and fevers began to dominate her life. Time was rapidly running out. She told her friends that she would be leaving soon and said a tearful good-bye to Dr. Quill. Two days later, after her final good-byes to her husband and son, she asked to be alone for an hour. They found her on the couch, covered by her favorite shawl.

Dr. Quill went to the house. He called the medical examiner, telling him the cause of death was "acute leukemia" to avoid any investigation a suicide might have triggered. He then wrote a moving account of the story for a respected and widely read medical journal, *The New England Journal of Medicine*, and many of the letters published in response to his article were favorable.

His account helped stimulate the public debate on euthanasia and physician-assisted suicide in a thoughtful and sensitive way. For this we should be grateful, because intelligent and graceful discussion is the only way a society can resolve these issues.

Ethical Analysis

Situational awareness

We are aware of these facts in Diane's story.

1. Diane had terminal leukemia. With no treatment, she would die in a matter of months; with difficult treatment, she had one chance in four of surviving. She decided to decline treatment.

2. Dr. Quill, a physician with hospice experience, assured Diane that he knew "how to use pain medicines to keep patients comfortable and lessen suffering."

3. "It was extraordinarily important to Diane to maintain control of herself and her own dignity during the time remaining to her." If she could not maintain this control, she wanted to kill herself.

4. When she requested barbiturates from Dr. Quill, he prescribed them and made sure she knew how to kill herself with them. "Knowing of her desire for independence and her decision to stay in control, I thought this request made perfect sense."

5. Diane committed suicide.

We are also aware of the following good and bad features in the story.

1. Diane's acute leukemia and the dim prospects of cure despite very difficult treatment were terrible realities for her, her family, and her physician.

2. Once she had declined treatment, her impending suffering and death were also significantly bad features. And for her, the inevitable loss of control at the end was a most upsetting aspect of what would be her final days.

3. The distress her physician, who had known her for eight years, would experience if he did not help her fulfill her last important wish was another bad feature in this case.

4. One good feature of the situation was that, unlike earlier times, the medications and knowledge to keep her comfortable to the very end were available.

5. Another good feature was that, judging from the written account, her physician was a caring and compassionate man. Convinced he was giving her "the best care possible," he was nonetheless honest enough to acknowledge: "I am not sure the law, society, or the medical profession would agree" with his assistance in her suicide.

Prudential reasoning in the story of Diane

Here we look at the story from the perspectives of the moral agents in this case, the patient and the physician. We ask how moral agents in such a situation might behave to achieve their personal good.

Patient's perspective: Once her leukemia was diagnosed, Diane was faced with several difficult decisions. The first was whether or not to accept treatment. If she declined treatment, she could avoid the side effects and discomfort of chemotherapy and transplantation, but it meant certain death in a matter of months. If she underwent treatment, the chance of failure would be 75 percent, and she might experience the burdens of treatment for nothing. Prudence suggests that this is one of those situations where either decision is morally justified. A patient deciding to seek the chance of survival has good reasons for so acting, but so does a patient deciding to decline the burdensome treatment when history shows it fails most of the time. In an ethics of prudence, either decision of the patient in this situation can easily be justified from a moral point of view.

Once she decided to decline treatment, she was faced with a second major decision: whether to endure her dying or, at some point, to kill herself. Neither of these decisions would lead to a good life in any meaningful sense of the term. Heavy medication is not good, and suicide ends life. Diane was in a tragic situation where no option would bring what we call happiness and fulfillment in life. Her situation was analogous to Aristotle's soldier whose post is being overrun: he can stand firm and be killed, or he can desert and become a coward. In such a situation, the moral person can only choose the less worse. According to Aristotle, it is less worse for the soldier to fight courageously than to desert. Which choice is less worse for a person in Diane's tragic position—killing herself or accepting comfort care as she dies?

Her decision to kill herself is not easily justified in an ethics of prudence. The killing of a human being, even a human being dying of leukemia, is a momentous action. Whenever we deliberately kill, we need forceful reasons to justify it. The reasons that justify killing must be cogent reasons because destroying human life, even human life ravaged by final illness, is such a serious move that society has struggled to avoid it.

What reasons might justify suicide in a situation such as this? None are offered in the account of Diane's final months written by her physician. We do know that it was "extraordinarily important to her to maintain control of herself" and that she had a "desire for independence." These are important factors, but they are not pieces of moral reasoning. In ethics, when the issue is damage to life, what someone desires or thinks important is not always the same as what is morally reasonable. The morally reasonable is determined by asking whether what we desire or think important is truly good for us, or at least the less worse option. And, since our good is inextricably linked with others, we have to ask as well how what we do affects them and the community.

In this case, it is difficult to think of any reason to justify the suicide. The suicide would not save the lives of others, nor was it necessary to avoid severe uncontrollable pain. It might be argued that the thought of losing control caused her unbearable suffering, and that this suffering could only be avoided by the suicide. There is some merit to this reasoning, and the account indicates Diane may well have felt this way, but such reasoning is questionable. In logical form the reasoning would look like this:

- Losing control as I die is bad (I view the loss of control as a terrible suffering);
- I am about to lose control;

- Therefore, I have a sufficient reason to kill myself. The bad features of killing myself are less important than the bad features of losing control as the disease advances and I need stronger medication for pain.

Most would agree that losing control is bad, but it is at least arguable that it less worse than destroying a human life, even a human life that is almost over. The fear of losing control hardly seems a morally sufficient reason for killing a human being, even a dying human being. Losing control is terribly unfortunate, but not so unfortunate in these circumstances that it justifies killing in order to prevent it from happening.

The patient made a third major decision in this case: she decided to ask another human being, her physician, to help her kill herself. This adds another moral dimension to the case. Most people would find it an emotional burden to help someone kill herself, especially if the assistance were not really necessary. While it is sometimes true that a person is unable to commit suicide without help, this was not the case here. At the time she killed herself, Diane could easily have done it without any help from her physician.

People find all sorts of ways to kill themselves without assistance in relatively painless ways. Everyone is familiar with the tragic newspaper accounts of people sitting in parked cars, with the windows up and motor running for warmth, who are found dead of accidental carbon monoxide poisoning. Apparently the passage from life to death is so painless they are not stimulated by discomfort to do the one simple thing that could save their lives—open the door and get out. The most recent physician-assisted suicides of Dr. Kevorkian remind us of how painless these deaths are; his "patients" kill themselves by putting a simple plastic mask over their faces and then breathe carbon monoxide from a canister.

For patients with as much mobility as Diane had, painless suicide is an action they can accomplish all by themselves, without any assistance from anybody. Why, then, do so many still able-bodied patients seek assistance from their physicians? Some suspect it may well be an inarticulate desire to have approval for the suicide. Physician assistance in suicide gives it an approval in the eyes of some patients that it might not otherwise have. It reminds one of a case reported by the media where a man insisted that he wanted his respirator withdrawn. The court approved his request, but told him he would have to shut it off himself. He declined.

It may well be that some people want to commit suicide, but do not want to do it themselves; they want their physician to do it with them. This not only places an awful burden on the physician, but makes one wonder whether the unnecessary assistance of a physician in their suicide is at least partially motivated by the need to have an authority figure endorse the suicide and share the responsibility. If a person could easily commit suicide without physician assistance, but nonetheless seeks it, we have to wonder why. And we have to guard against the perception that killing and assisting in suicide by physicians are somehow more easily justified morally than killings and assistance in suicides by those who are not physicians.

Physician's perspective.   What is the moral response of a physician when a patient planning on suicide requests a prescription for barbiturates and for instructions on how to kill herself with them? Giving someone intent on killing a poison and teaching her how to use it in a lethal way makes the physician an accomplice in the killing that follows. He will need convincing moral reasons to justify his participation in the suicide.

In the original published account of this case, the physician did not provide any moral reasoning for his decision to help Diane kill herself. Although he acknowledged he had an uneasy feeling about the "spiritual, legal, professional, and personal" boundaries he was exploring, neither ethics nor morality were mentioned. Several of his remarks suggested moral reasoning, but they remained undeveloped.

For example, Dr. Quill's account speaks of his being an advocate of a patient's right to die with as much control and dignity as possible. The mention of a "right" suggests moral reasoning because some moralists argue that we have a moral obligation to respect another's rights. But the assertion of a right is not a substitute for moral reasoning. Before I can use a right in moral reasoning, I must show the claimed right exists and contributes to the human good, something many deny about the "right to die." And if I can show the "right to die" exists and is something morally good, I must still give reasons for extending the "right to die" to the "right to kill oneself," and then for extending it again to the "right to receive physician assistance" when the patient could do it herself. And if I can show all this, then I must also show that the exercise of that "right to die," so understood, indicates, at this time and in these circumstances, that assisting in this suicide is morally reasonable behavior.

In other words, before a physician can use the "right to die" as a moral reason for helping a patient kill herself, he has to show (1) that the right to die is truly a right, (2) how the right to die can be expanded into a right to kill oneself, and (3) how the right to kill oneself justifies the physician helping someone kill herself when no help is necessary. None of this appears in the analysis we have of Diane's suicide.

Another example of inchoate moral reasoning appears when Dr. Quill identified several bad features that may develop if he does not help Diane kill herself. He feared the effects of a violent death on her family, the consequences if her suicide attempt was unsuccessful and left her damaged, and the possibility that a family member might try to help her and would suffer legal and personal repercussions. Identifying the bad features that might happen if I choose not to act in a situation is an important first step in moral reasoning, but only that. Moral reasoning will also consider the bad features that will happen if I do choose to act in the situation. Helping someone kill is a notable bad feature. Good people do not kill or help others kill, unless they can justify it with reasons sufficiently strong to justify the destruction of human life.

The lack of an effort to develop moral reasoning that would justify helping someone kill herself may be the result of how the physician viewed his participation in the killing. He wrote: "Although I did not assist in her suicide directly, I helped indirectly to make it possible."

The distinction between direct and indirect roles in killing needs to be approached with care. In ethics, some have made a distinction between direct and indirect killing. They say that a pilot dropping a bomb on a military target in a city kills the soldiers directly but kills the civilians indirectly. Here direct and indirect killing depends on intention. The bombing pilot may intend to kill the enemy soldiers, but not the civilians. Their deaths are foreseen but unintended side effects. It is clear, however, that this traditional use of direct and indirect killing is not what the physician is appealing to in this case.

Nonetheless, the physician believes his help was indirect. For the sake of argument, let us assume that this is so. This still leaves us with the major moral question: Was it moral for him to participate "indirectly" in the suicide? Describing a participation in a killing as indirect does not imply the participant escapes responsibility for the killing.

To see this clearly, imagine the following. A neighbor tells you he wants to kill himself. He wants to borrow your gun and have you show him how to use it. You loan him your gun, making sure he knows how to use it to kill himself. Some time later, he shoots himself with your gun, in just the way you instructed him. Obviously, your "indirect" assistance does not absolve you of your responsibility for your role in the suicide. To see this, it is important not to camouflage your role. Call your role indirect if you will, but acknowledge that your role in the killing was so significant that your assistance is immoral unless offset by compelling moral reasons.

The Legal Aftermath

This case happened in New York, at that time one of the twenty-six states with laws making it a crime to help people kill themselves. The district attorney, however, decided not to prosecute Dr. Quill. He explained that "Diane" was never identified and that there was no evidence of a crime because there was no body to examine for possible evidence that would indicate a crime.

He was forced to change his mind and call for a grand jury investigation after a reporter identified Diane and located her body in a laboratory. Forensic investigation revealed the barbiturates in Diane's body, but the grand jury declined to indict Dr. Quill for assisting in the suicide. The disciplinary board of the New York State Health Department also investigated the incident and decided Dr. Quill was not guilty of misconduct since he did not "directly" participate in the suicide.

Ethical Reflections

Our desire for independence as we die is understandable, but it is a desire, not a reason. Maintaining control of ourselves is also important, very important for people such as Diane, but this importance does not automatically justify everything we can do to maintain control. Not every action designed to fulfill our desires or to achieve what is important to us can be morally justified. Whenever it is a question of damaging or destroying human life, something more is needed, and what is needed are reasons to justify the destruction.

In our culture there is a tendency to think we are authentically human only if we are in control. But that is not a realistic reaction to the human condition. At some time or other, everyone is vulnerable and needs others.

The desire to remain in control no matter what is not a reasonable desire because it is incompatible with the human condition. Only an almighty being could always be in control, and we are not almighty but vulnerable. We can, and should, control much in our lives, but it is unreasonable to think we can control everything. There are times when it is reasonable to place our lives in the hands of others, to let go, to acknowledge our humanity. In a cultural milieu that prizes control and autonomy, this can be difficult.

It is with great hesitation that we attempt to judge the dead, especially those who have died by their own hand. There is something almost disrespectful about it, and we should not do it unless we have a good reason. But we can learn from the dead. We learn from autopsy and the dissection of cadavers in medical school, and there is something almost disrespectful about this as well. So too, we can learn from published accounts of suicides. We can perform a postmortem moral examination, not to criticize the dead or embarrass their families, but to work our way through the difficult moral issue of physician-assisted suicide. Unless we analyze the actions of people such as Diane and those associated with Dr. Kevorkian, our moral discourse about suicide will remain totally theoretical.

If we accept the idea that the taking of human life is such a serious personal and social event that it should be a last resort, then an ethics of prudence is hard pressed to justify this suicide and the physician's assistance in the suicide. This is not to say that suicide and assistance in suicide could never be morally justified, but simply that this does not seem to be one of those cases. The main reasons why the moral arguments allowing suicide fail here are that Diane was not suffering uncontrollable pain, and that her desire for control is not enough to justify killing a human being—herself. There is no question that she wanted to kill herself, but the ultimate moral issue when the destruction of human life is involved is not what one wants but whether what one wants is reasonable; that is, whether it contributes to the human good, or at least is the less worse option.

This case is most difficult because we have every reason to believe that Diane and Dr. Quill were sensitive human beings doing what they thought was best. To disagree with what they thought is not in any way to imply a pejorative judgment about them as human beings. And we must acknowledge two things. First, their moral judgments may have been the right ones, and the position presented here the wrong one. Second, their good intentions and personal beliefs are not sufficient to establish the morality of what was done—people with the best of intentions have often done what is not good.

CONCLUDING REFLECTIONS

Since we can expect the intense public debate about euthanasia and assisted suicide to continue, the following remarks may be helpful.

First, deliberately killing another human being is a very serious action. Our first reaction should be to avoid it and not allow it to happen except as a last resort. This is the thrust of our tradition in recent centuries.

Second, the burden of proof in the moral argument about euthanasia, therefore, rests on those proposing the moral rightness of these killings. They must establish the morality of euthanasia and show the wisdom of making it legal.

Third, opponents of euthanasia who argue that euthanasia is wrong because intentionally killing innocent people is always wrong are begging the question. They must show why it is immoral to kill suffering hopelessly ill people who request it. It is not enough to state the absolute moral prohibition "do not deliberately kill innocent people," and ignore the very complicated circumstances surrounding euthanasia.

Fourth, since an individual good is not always a social good, and therefore may not be morally justified, an exclusive focus on a patient-centered ethics in medicine is misleading. Any adequate ethics embraces both individual and social consequences of behavior. Physicians killing patients is not a private medical matter—people killing other people has always been a matter of great social and legal concern. Hence no individual stories that seem to cry out for euthanasia or assisted suicide are ever, of themselves, sufficient arguments for allowing a social practice of euthanasia and assisted suicide. Since killing is involved, it is never a matter of purely private ethics; there is an important social dimension to it as well.

Fifth, the unfortunate publicity surrounding Dr. Jack Kevorkian's assisted suicides can all too easily blind opponents of euthanasia and physician-assisted suicide to the valid concerns of those proposing the legalization of these options. Dr. Kevorkian's behavior does not easily fit into what Aristotle would call good and noble behavior, or virtuous activity. Most of the suicides he has assisted would fall outside the carefully crafted guidelines used in Holland, and many proponents of physician-assisted suicide have no support for the way he helps people end their lives.

Sixth, the most prominent movement to eliminate the suffering of the dying, which reduces the need for physicians to kill them or help them kill themselves, is hospice care. The first hospice in America was opened in 1924; in 1992 there were 1700 of them caring for 200,000 patients each year. Hospice studies show most patients can be kept comfortable as they die, although some do require heavy sedation, usually only in the last few days of life. It is somewhat ironic that great improvements in hospice and palliative care in the last two decades in the United States have been matched by a growing movement to allow physicians to kill patients, or help them kill themselves, lest they suffer from somatic pain or psychological distress as they die.

Seventh, in the last analysis, the ironic simultaneous growth of the hospice and euthanasia movements may well be partially generated by two different views of ethics. The action-guides of modern ethics—the right to choose, the right to die, the right of privacy, the principle of autonomy, and the principle of beneficence—can all be used to justify euthanasia and physician-assisted suicide. An ethics of prudential reasoning aiming at living well, however, is hard pressed to find reasons for euthanasia and physician-assisted suicide now that pain management and palliative care can ease the suffering confronting some at the end of life. Even when the situation becomes truly tragic, and the only choice is between the less worse and the more worse, prudence directs one toward the less worse. And sedation is always less worse than killing.

SUGGESTED READINGS

For the history of attitudes toward euthanasia and physician-assisted suicide, see Paul Carrick. 1985. *Medical Ethics in Antiquity*. Boston: D. Reidel Publishing Company. Two papers by Ludwig Edelstein are especially helpful in understanding the limited role of Hippocratic medicine and morality in the classical world. See "The Hippocratic Oath: Text, Translation and Interpretation," and "The Professional Ethics of the Greek Physician," in Ludwig Edelstein. 1987. *Ancient Medicine*. ed. Owsei Temkin and C. Lilian Temkin. Baltimore: Johns Hopkins University Press, pp. 3–63 and 319–48.

Aristotle's remarks on infanticide are in the *Politics* 1335b2-0 and his remarks on suicide are in the *Eudemian Ethics* 1230a1–4 (suicide to escape from trouble or pain shows a lack of courage) and in the *Nicomachean Ethics* 1138a6–14 (suicide that violates the civil law is an act of injustice against the city-state). A helpful collection on the various views of suicide in our cultural tradition is Baruch Brody, ed. 1989. *Suicide and Euthanasia: Historical and Contemporary Themes*. Dordrecht: Kluwer Academic Publishers.

Kant's stand against suicide is from his *Lectures on Ethics*, pp. 148–54. His question about whether Frederick the Great harbored an intention contrary to the moral law when he carried poison into battle lest he be captured is found in his *The Metaphysical Principles of Virtue in Ethical Philosophy*, James Ellington, trans. Indianapolis: Hackett, 1983, pp. 84–5. Here Kant also asks whether it is immoral for a person bitten by a mad dog to kill himself lest his incurable madness from the bite lead him to harm others.

"It's All Over, Debbie" appeared in *JAMA* **1988,** *259,* 272. The particular author of this piece in the weekly column entitled "A Piece of My Mind" was not identified. A year earlier, the same column had published an opposing view. See Carl Kjellstrand. "The Impossible Choice." *JAMA* **1987,** *257,* 233. The article by twelve physicians, ten of whom thought it would be ethical for physicians to help patients kill themselves in certain situations, is Sidney Wanzer et al. "The Physician's Responsibility Toward Hopelessly Ill Patients: A Second Look." *NEJM* **1989,** *320,* 844–49. Derek Humphrey's book *Final Exit* was published in 1991 by the National Hemlock Society. The federal court ruling that Washington's statute prohibiting assisted suicide is unconstitutional is *Compassion in Dying v. Washington*, 850F. Supp. 1454 (D.C. Wash. 1994).

Among the many helpful articles on euthanasia and physician-assisted suicide are: Dan Brock. "Voluntary Active Euthanasia." *Hastings Center Report* **1992,** 22 (March–April), 10–22; Daniel Callahan. "When Self-Determination Runs Amok." *Hastings Center Report* **1992,** 22 (March–April), 52–5; Willard Gaylin et al. "Doctors Must Not Kill." *JAMA* **1988,** *259,* 2139–40; David Orentlicher. "Physician Participation in Assisted Suicide." *JAMA* **1989,** *262,* 1844–45; Marcia Angell. "Euthanasia." *NEJM* **1988,** *319,* 1348–50; Christine Cassel and Diane Meier. "Morals and Moralism in the Debate Over Euthanasia and Assisted Suicide." *NEJM* **1990,** *323,* 750–52; Timothy Quill, Christine Cassel, and Diane Meier. "Care of the Hopelessly Ill: Proposed Clinical Criteria for Physician-Assisted Suicide." *NEJM* **1992,** *327,* 1380–84; Howard Brody. "Assisted Death—A Compassionate Response to a Medical Failure." *NEJM* **1992,** *327,* 1384–88; Robert Miller. "Hospice Care as an Alternative to Euthanasia." *Law, Medicine & Health Care* **1992,** *20,* 127–

32; Susan Wolf. "Holding the Line on Euthanasia." *Hastings Center Report* **1989,** *19* (January–February), supplement, pp. 13–15; Lisa Cahill. "Bioethical Decisions to End Life." *Theological Studies* **1991,** *52,* 107–25; and John Paris. "Active Euthanasia." *Theological Studies* **1992,** *53,* 113–26.

For a classic article reprinted in many anthologies see Yale Kamisar. "Some Non-religious Views against Proposed 'Mercy-killing' Legislation." *Minnesota Law Review* **1958,** *42,* 969–1042. On the difficulty of knowing just what motivates a person's desire for euthanasia or suicide, the view of psychiatrists is important. See Yeates Conwell and Eric Caine. "Rational Suicide and the Right to Die: Reality and Myth." *NEJM* **1991,** *325,* 1100–02. For the impact of suicide assistance on physicians, see Steven Miles. "Physicians and Their Patients' Suicides." *JAMA* **1994,** *271,* 1786–88. See also Thomas Preston. "Professional Norms and Physician Attitudes Toward Euthanasia." *Journal of Law, Medicine and Ethics* **1994,** *22,* 36–40.

Among the many books wherein euthanasia is discussed at some length are Germain Grisez and Joseph Boyle. 1979. *Life and Death with Liberty and Justice: A Contribution to the Euthanasia Debate.* Notre Dame: University of Notre Dame Press; James Rachels. 1986. *The End of Life: Euthanasia and Morality.* New York: Oxford University Press; Timothy Quill. 1993. *Death and Dignity: Making Choices and Taking Charge.* New York: Norton; and Margaret Battin. 1994. *The Least Worse Death: Essays in Bioethics on the End of Life.* New York: Oxford University Press. The New York State Task Force on Life and the Law has taken a strong stand against legalizing euthanasia and physician-assisted suicide. See its report entitled *When Death is Sought: Assisted Suicide and Euthanasia in the Medical Context.* 1994. Albany: Health Education Services.

The controversial Dutch experience with euthanasia is described and debated in Carlos Gomez. 1991. *Regulating Death: Euthanasia and the Case of the Netherlands.* New York: The Free Press; Maurice de Wachter. "Active Euthanasia in the Netherlands." *JAMA* **1989,** *262,* 3216–19 and "Euthanasia in the Netherlands." *Hastings Center Report* **1992,** *22* (March–April), 23–30; Alexander Capron. "Euthanasia in the Netherlands: American Observations." *Hastings Center Report* **1992,** *22* (March–April), 30–33; Henk ten Have and Jos Welie. "Euthanasia: Normal Medical Practice?" *Hastings Center Report* **1992,** *22* (March–April), 34–38; John Keown. "On Regulating Death." *Hastings Center Report* **1992,** *22* (March–April), 39–43; Margaret Battin. "Voluntary Euthanasia and the Risks of Abuse: Can We Learn Anything from the Netherlands?" *Law, Medicine & Health Care* **1992,** *20,* 133–43 and "Euthanasia: The Way We Do It, The Way They Do It." *Journal of Pain and Symptom Management* **1991,** *6,* 298–305; Paul Van der Mass et al. "Euthanasia and Other Medical Decisions Concerning the End of Life." *Lancet* **1991,** *338,* 669–74; Johannes van Delden et al. "The Remmelink Study: Two Years Later." *Hastings Center Report* **1993,** *23* (November–December), 24–27; and Gerrit Kimsma and Evert van Leeuwen. "Dutch Euthanasia: Background, Practice, and Present Justifications." *Cambridge Quarterly of Healthcare Ethics* **1993,** *2,* 19–31.

For an example of the sometimes heated debate about euthanasia see Daniel Callahan. "When Self-Determination Runs Amok." *Hastings Center Report* **1992,** *22* (March–April), 52–55 and a response by John Lachs. "When Abstract Moralizing Runs Amok." *Journal of Clinical Ethics* **1994,** *5,* 10–13, with a response by Daniel Callahan. "*Ad Hominem* Run Amok: A Response to John Lachs." *Journal of Clinical Ethics* **1994,** *5,* 13–15. A 1993 survey in Washington State, where voters defeated a proposal allowing euthanasia and physician-assisted suicide known as Initiative 119 in 1991, revealed that physicians were sharply polarized on the issue. See Jonathan Cohen et al. "Attitudes Toward Assisted Suicide and Euthanasia

Among Physicians in Washington State." *NEJM* **1994**, *331*, 89–94. For a review of the recent referenda questions in Washington, California, and Oregon see George Annas. "Death by Prescription." *NEJM* **1994, 331**, 1240–43.

The growing public debate about euthanasia is hampered by controversies over terminology and the moral implications of the distinctions employed in the debate. See, for example, James Rachels. "Active and Passive Euthanasia." *NEJM* **1975,** *292*, 78–80; Dan Brock. "Taking Human Life." *Ethics* **1985**, *95*, 851–65; Bonnie Steinbock. 1980. *Killing and Allowing to Die.* Englewood Cliffs: Prentice Hall; Raymond Devettere. "The Imprecise Language of Euthanasia and Causing Death." *Journal of Clinical Ethics* **1990**, *1*, 268–74 and "Reconceptualizing the Euthanasia Debate." *Law, Medicine & Health Care* **1989,** *17*, 145–55; Howard Brody. "Causing, Intending, and Assisting Death." *Journal of Clinical Ethics* **1993,** *4*, 112–17; Joseph Lombardi. "Killing and Letting Die: What is the Moral Difference?" *New Scholasticism* **1980,** *54*, 200–12; Gilbert Meilaender. "The Distinction between Killing and Allowing to Die." *Theological Studies* **1976**, *37*, 467–70; Raanan Gillon. "Euthanasia, Withholding Life-Prolonging Treatment, and Moral Differences between Killing and Letting Die." *Journal of Medical Ethics* **1988,** *14*, 115–17; and Lawrence Gostin. "Drawing a Line Between Killing and Letting Die: The Law, and Law Reform, on Medically Assisted Dying." *Journal of Law, Medicine & Ethics* **1993,** *21*, 94–101.

For an example of a carefully crafted policy proposal that would allow voluntary euthanasia and physician-assisted suicide as a last resort when palliative and supportive treatments are inadequate see Franklin Miller et al. "Regulating Physician-Assisted Death." *NEJM* **1994**, *331*, 119–123. The choice of language in this article is not without interest. There is a growing tendency by those favoring legalization of euthanasia and physician-assisted suicide to speak of it as "physician-assisted death." If this language is accepted, the debate about euthanasia will then center on whether physicians should offer assistance when their patients are dying. This is not a debate at all; of course physicians, as well as nurses, family, and friends, should help dying people die. The death of a hospice patient receiving palliative care is a physician-assisted death—the death is made easier by the interventions of the physician and nurses. The soothing language of "physician-assisted death" misleads us about the crucial ethical question: Do physicians ever behave in a good and noble way by killing their patients or helping them kill themselves; that is, is killing ever the less worse option for relieving suffering? Recourse to soothing language undermines the arguments of those proposing the legalization of euthanasia and physician-assisted suicide by suggesting their proposal cannot withstand debate if direct and realistic language is employed. The ethical problem is not selling euthanasia to physicians and the public but figuring out what is the less worse option for society—killing or sedation—in the tragic cases where euthanasia can be considered a possible option.

For the value of the slippery-slope argument, an argument used by many opposed to euthanasia and physician-assisted suicide, see Douglas Walton. 1992. *Slippery Slope Arguments.* New York: Oxford University Press; Wilbren van der Berg. "The Slippery-Slope Argument." *Ethics* **1992**, *102*, 42–65 (a condensed version appeared in the *Journal of Clinical Ethics* **1992**, *3*, 256–68 with commentaries by Benjamin Freedman, Raymond Devettere, and David Ozar); Bernard Williams. "Which Slopes are Slippery?" in Michael Lockwood, ed., *Moral Dilemmas in Modern Medicine.* 1985. Oxford: Oxford University Press, pp. 126–37; and Bruce Jennings. "Active Euthanasia and Forgoing Life-Sustaining Treatment: Can We Hold the Line?" *Journal of Pain and Symptom Management* **1991,** *6*, 312–16.

Dr. Quill's article on the suicide of Diane and his role in it is "Death and Dignity: A Case of Individualized Decision Making." *NEJM* **1991,** *324,* 691–94. For a sympathetic account of this suicide and a critical account of Dr. Kevorkian's assisted suicides, see Robert Weir. "The Morality of Physician-Assisted Suicide." *Law, Medicine & Health Care* **1992,** *20,* 116–26. See also Timothy Quill. "Doctor, I Want to Die. Will You Help Me?" *JAMA* **1993,** *270,* 870–73 and "The Ambiguity of Clinical Intentions." *NEJM* **1993,** *329,* 1039–40.

For the background and efficacy of hospice care, see Vincent Mor, David Greer, and Robert Kastenbaum. *The Hospice Experiment.* 1988. Baltimore: Johns Hopkins University Press; Robin Fainsinger et al. "Symptom Control During the Last Week of Life on a Palliative Care Unit." *Journal of Palliative Care* **1990,** *6,* 5–11; and Robert Miller. "Hospice Care as an Alternative to Euthanasia." *Law, Medicine & Health Care* **1992,** *20,* 127–132.

The Department of HHS' Agency for Health Care Policy and Research (AHCPR) has published an extensive (257-page) clinical guideline on pain management developed by an interdisciplinary panel of clinicians, patients, and others. The guideline includes a section on pain management for AIDS patients, since the suffering associated with AIDS is similar to that of many cancers. The panel acknowledges that not all pain can always be eliminated, but that available palliative care "can effectively relieve pain in most patients" (p. 2). See *Management of Cancer Pain.* 1994. U.S. Government Printing Office.

14

Medical Research

Research involving animals and human subjects is an important part of modern medicine. New techniques and technologies, as well as new drugs, are routinely tested on animals and humans before physicians use them in normal clinical practice. Since the tests can cause harm to the animals and humans, they pose ethical concerns. We have to ask whether the actual or potential harms caused by the research are reasonable; that is, whether they are consistent with living well. Patients and researchers undermine their own good when they do things that could cause suffering or damage life without sufficient reasons.

The primary ethical concern in medical research centers on what it does to the people who are the subjects of the testing. Of concern also is what the research does to human embryos and fetuses, and to animals. Embryos and fetuses are human life, and damaging human life without sufficient reason is immoral. Animals suffer and die, and causing them to suffer or to die needlessly is also immoral.

A distinction is frequently made between therapeutic and nontherapeutic research. In therapeutic research the subjects are sick, and the hope is that the research will both benefit them and provide knowledge of benefit to others. In nontherapeutic research the subjects are not sick or, if they are sick, there is no real expectation of any benefit to them from the research. Nontherapeutic research is entirely for the benefit of people other than the subjects of the research.

The distinction between therapeutic and nontherapeutic research is not really helpful in ethical deliberation for several reasons. First, although the distinction is sometimes clear, it can be ambiguous. Many research protocols for drugs, for example, involve random clinical trials with sick people. Some patients receive the drug and others, a control group, receive placebos. For the patients actually receiving the drug, the research will be, or at least might be, therapeutic, but for those not receiving it, the research will be nontherapeutic. Thus, the same drug trial is both therapeutic and nontherapeutic. Of course, the reverse could also be true—the study could be countertherapeutic by harming the patients receiving it, as sometimes happens.

Furthermore, even when the distinction is not ambiguous, it contributes little to ethical reasoning. The moral deliberations about the possible bad effects of the medical research, and the reasons that justify risking them, are the same whether the research is therapeutic or nontherapeutic. The balance between the expected benefits and burdens is what matters, not whether the research is therapeutic or not. In fact, the distinction between therapeutic and nontherapeutic research can obscure good moral reasoning by suggesting that we can tolerate unreasonably high levels of harm and risks of harm as long as the intervention might help the patient. It can lead to the attitude that a dying patient has nothing to lose and can try anything. This is not good ethics—some medical research and unproven drugs are not good for dying patients.

Sometimes the words "experimentation" and "experiment" are used to describe medical research. Although literally correct, the word is not a happy choice. The idea of "experimenting" with human beings is not a comfortable one. It is too close to the notion of experiments in the natural sciences, where the researchers manipulate nature to produce desired results. Medical research involving human subjects differs so greatly from scientific research in biology or physics that it seems best to avoid the term, except in situations such as concentration camps, where physicians did experiment on people as if they were things.

In this chapter we will avoid both the distinction between therapeutic and nontherapeutic research, and the word experimentation. We will use the term medical research to designate any medical or psychological interventions on human subjects or animals, including drug trials, that are not yet established as standard clinical practice. And we will use the term "human subject" to designate not only children and adults, but human embryos and fetuses as well.

The current moral awareness about medical research, and the various laws and regulations governing its practice, developed in large measure as a reaction against earlier mistreatment of human beings in research projects. There is much to be learned from remembering how medical research became unethical when the desire to achieve scientific and medical progress overshadowed moral sensitivity to the well-being of the patients involved.

NOTORIOUS EXAMPLES OF QUESTIONABLE ETHICS IN RESEARCH

A brief look at several well-known abuses in research is valuable for understanding current concerns in the ethics of medical research.

The Tuskegee Syphilis Study (1932–1972)

When this study began in 1932, injection of various heavy metals, especially mercury and various arsenicals, was a standard treatment for syphilis. The treatment was controversial. There were some indications that the treatment helped patients with syphilis, but it also seemed to cause other problems and symptoms. Moreover, a Norwegian study dating from 1891 suggested that some people with syphilis had survived for decades with no treatment, sometimes without symptoms. This suggested that the disease was not always fatal, and that populations without treatment might actually do better than those treated, and weakened, by the standard injections.

The U.S. Public Health Service wanted to find out just how lethal syphilis was if not treated. The Public Health Service could do this by studying the natural course of the disease over a long period of time in a rather large population. The study would compare the health and longevity of people infected with the disease with those not infected. The infected group, of course, would not be treated because treatments would interfere with the natural course of the disease.

The Public Health Service soon found a ready-made group for its syphilis study. In 1929 the Julius Rosenweld Foundation had funded an effort to eradicate syphilis in Macon County, Alabama, where about 40 percent of the men were infected. The foundation's effort to eradicate the disease ended when its endowment shrank during the Great Depression a few years later. The U.S. Public Health Service decided to conduct its study of syphilis with the same population. It selected about 600 adult males for the research. About 400 had syphilis, and the remaining 200 served as a control group. The research was centered in Tuskegee, and hence the project became known as the Tuskegee Syphilis Study.

The infected men were not informed about the nature of the research. They did not receive any treatment for their syphilis, although researchers sometimes told them that the procedure was a "treatment" when they wanted spinal taps for analysis. During the study, some men in the control group contracted the disease. They were transferred to the infected group but never told of their syphilis, thus exposing their sexual partners to it.

The study continued long after the early 1940s, when it became known that penicillin was successful in treating syphilis. At this point there was no need to continue the study—the success of penicillin left the researchers with no reason for studying how syphilis develops in humans when it is not treated. But the research continued. Researchers were able to prevent the infected men from being drafted for military service in World War II, lest military physicians discover their syphilis and treat it with penicillin. And the researchers provided local physicians with the names of those infected and asked them not to give these men antibiotics for any reason, lest the medications undermine the study. Thus, bacterial infections unrelated to syphilis were not treated.

Finally, in the late 1960s Peter Buxton, a researcher working for the U.S. Public Health Service, complained about the morality of the ongoing research project, which was now under the auspices of the Centers for Disease Control in Atlanta. After several years, when the CDC made no move to stop the study, Buxton told his story to a reporter. In July 1972 the *New York Times* ran the story on the front page, and other newspapers soon picked it up. CDC officials tried to defend the study, but public outrage was strong. One cartoon in a newspaper showed a dead patient, covered by a sheet, and a nurse, holding a syringe of penicillin, asking the physician: "Now can we give him the penicillin?"

In February and March of 1973, Senator Kennedy of Massachusetts chaired a highly visible congressional hearing on the research as public criticism grew. Many citizens were shocked that the Centers for Disease Control and the U.S. Public Health Service were involved in research involving deceit and the denial of treatment in order to obtain useless information about the natural development of syphilis without treatment. And many could not help but notice that all the subjects in the study were poor black men. The fact that many of the physicians in Macon County collecting data in the later years of the study were also black did little to erase the idea that the decision not to offer treatment had racial overtones.

Once the terrible history was exposed, survivors and families sought damages in federal court. In July 1973 they accepted an out-of-court settlement. The compensation, considering the personal damage and the risks to the men, was not much. Infected survivors received $37,500 and control group survivors received $16,000. Families of the men involved in the study who had died before 1973 also received compensation. If the deceased man had been infected, his family received $15,000; if he had not been infected, $5,000.

Although most people learning of the research in 1972 had no problem seeing how immoral it was, physicians who had known of the study for years apparently never saw how wrong it was. The research had never been a secret. Between 1936 and 1973 at least thirteen articles reported findings of the study in journals such as the *Archives of Internal Medicine* and the *Journal of Chronic Diseases*. The articles in the professional journals, unlike those in the press, expressed no moral discomfort about the poor men selected for the research and left without treatment long after the cure for the disease was developed.

This bit of history shows how easily sensitivity to moral issues can diminish when groups with special interests are not sufficiently self-critical about the morality of what they do. It shows as well the need for public and professional scrutiny of medical research.

Experiments in Nazi Germany (1942–1945)

During World War II, prisoners and other detained people were forced into dangerous and painful medical experiments. Japanese physicians, for example, injected Chinese prisoners with syphilis, cholera, plague, and other diseases in order to observe how the illnesses progressed.

The most upsetting events, however, occurred in Europe under Nazi Germany. As is well known, about 8 million people lost their lives in the death camps during the war, about 6 million of them Jews. At some of the camps, Buchenwald and Auschwitz for example, people were also used for crude medical experiments. Subjects were deliberately infected with diseases to test the efficacy of vaccines and treatments, placed in altitude chambers to gather data affecting air crews at high altitudes, exposed to cold so the revival of extremely chilled bodies could be studied, shot so treatment for gunshot wounds could be improved, given electric shocks to see how much electricity people could survive, and exposed to radiation in experiments designed to sterilize them. Some subjects died from the experiments; others suffered terribly. Many of these were later killed when they were no longer useful to the experiment.

Physicians designed and conducted these experiments. Perhaps the most widely known of them was Dr. Josef Mengele. He not only selected those to be killed as the trains arrived at the camp, and killed some himself, but also conducted extensive medical experiments. Of special interest to him were twins, and he experimented with many pairs of twins, sometimes killing them in order to dissect their bodies.

All of the medical experiments conducted in the camps were clearly immoral, not only according to standards widely accepted today, but according to official German regulations governing novel treatments and medical research that had been in place since 1931. The German regulations governing medical research were very advanced for the time, and they required voluntary consent from the subjects of the research before it could begin. Physicians conducting research in the camps simply ignored the regulations of their country, especially the requirement for voluntary consent.

After the Allied victory over Nazi Germany in 1945, trials of war criminals were held in the German city of Nuremberg, the site of huge Nazi rallies in the 1930s. The Nuremberg Military Tribunal indicted twenty German physicians and convicted fifteen of performing medical experiments without the subjects' consent. Seven of these were hanged; the other eight received long prison terms. Dr. Mengele, however, as so many others, had escaped to South America before the trials. Despite efforts to capture him, he remained free. It is thought that he died in Brazil years later.

As the result of international outrage over the Nazi medical experiments, the judges at Nuremberg set forth certain basic principles for medical research. The first of these ten principles, known as the Nuremberg Code, says: "The voluntary consent of the human subject is absolutely essential." Other principles allow the subject to withdraw at any time, and they remind the physician that he must terminate the experiment if it is likely to injure or kill the subject, and that he must avoid all unnecessary physical and mental suffering and injury.

The famous Nuremberg Code was published, along with accounts of the trials, by the U.S. Government Printing Office in 1949. One might assume that medical researchers in the United States would abide by the Nuremberg Code from that time onward. Unfortunately, they sometimes did not.

Hepatitis at the Willowbrook State School (1956–1970)

The Willowbrook State School on Staten Island was an institution for retarded children. When the research on hepatitis started in 1956, it had a population of about 4,500 and a staff of about 1,000. Since a large number of the children were not toilet trained, most of them became infected with hepatitis, usually a mild variety, within a year of admission. Wanting to study the disease and to develop an effective immunization to eradicate it, two researchers from the New York University School of Medicine, Saul Krugman and Joan Giles, conducted various trials. One of them consisted of inoculating newly admitted children with gamma globulin, then dividing them into two groups. Children in one group were then deliberately infected with hepatitis to learn how effective the inoculations were.

Researchers obtained the consent of parents before enrolling children in the study. However, the validity of this consent can be questioned. By 1964 Willowbrook was overcrowded, with about 5,000 children in a facility designed for 3,000. Long waiting lists developed, but immediate placement was available if parents agreed to enroll their children in the hepatitis study. The inducement of immediate placement for children hard to manage at home undermined the validity of the parents' consent to the research.

After papers based on the study were published in respected medical journals, some people questioned the ethics of the research. Perhaps the most notable criticism was a letter by Dr. Stephen Goldby published in the prestigious British medical journal *The Lancet* on April 10, 1971. In an editorial remark, the editors of the journal agreed with his criticisms of the research despite their earlier editorial support of the study. Goldby claimed the study was "quite unjustifiable," and that it was not right to experiment on children when it is of no benefit to them.

Goldby's criticisms were vigorously denied by the researchers at Willowbrook. They were only partially successful, however, in defending their research. A rather general consensus arose that adequate information had not been provided to the parents, and that the consent in many cases was not truly voluntary due to the pressures on the parents to enroll their retarded children, many of whom were difficult to care for at home, in the study in order to gain admission to the school. Moreover, some found it difficult to think the parents' consent could have considered the best interests of their child. Deliberately infecting a healthy child with hepatitis is hardly in the best interests of the child.

The research eventually ceased after the objections surfaced, but not everyone was convinced it was all that immoral. When the *The New England Journal of Medicine* published a report on the study in 1973, for example, the editor reminded readers that the *Journal* does not publish unethical research, thus reassuring them of his opinion that the research was morally acceptable. Nonetheless, many others were upset that a vulnerable population of retarded children in a state school could be deliberately infected with hepatitis, and the highly publicized incident served to raise consciousness about medical research in the early 1970s.

Cancer Research at the Jewish Chronic Disease Hospital (1963)

In 1963 Dr. Chester Southam, a physician at the Sloan–Kettering Institute for Cancer Research in New York, organized a study at the JCDH facility that involved injecting live cancer cells into twenty-two patients. Dr. Southam was doing research on the ability of the body's immune system to fight cancer. He knew that cancer patients were less able to fight cancer cells than healthy people, but he did not know why this was so. Was the weakened immune system caused by the cancer already in the body or was it caused by the general debilitation experienced by people suffering from cancer?

He thought that the injection of cancer cells into debilitated patients would provide him with the answer. If they became less able to fight cancer after the injections, it would indicate that the cancer was the cause of the weakened immune system. If, on the other hand, they did not become less able to fight cancer after the injections, then general debilitation, and not cancer, was the reason cancer patients were less able to fight cancer. The research was funded in part by Sloan–Kettering, the U.S. Public Health Service, and the American Cancer Society.

The consent process in the study was terribly flawed. Some patients did not have decision-making capacity. Others had it, but were not told they were being given injections of cancer cells. No written records of the consent process were kept.

An attorney on the JCDH's Board of Directors became concerned about the hospital's exposure to liability for injecting patients with cancer cells, and about the possible moral abuse of the patients. The research was then investigated, and Dr. Southam, along with the medical director at JCDH, who had approved of the study without submitting it to his hospital's research committee, were placed on probation for a year. The Board of Regents of the State University of New York found the physicians guilty of fraud, deceit, and unprofessional conduct. The involvement of the U.S. Public Health Service in the obviously unethical study helped alert it and other government agencies to the need for ethical guidelines governing federally funded research.

Obedience Tests at Yale University (1960–1963)

Behavioral research is also an issue for health care ethics, and in the 1960s and early 1970s attention was drawn to several ethically questionable studies in this field. A widely publicized case was the studies on obedience conducted at Yale University by Stanley Milgram. Milgram was interested in learning about how human beings react to a person in authority, even when he directs them to do things against their better judgment.

Subjects for the study were recruited by newspaper advertisements and were paid a nominal fee for their participation. Eventually, they numbered over a thousand. Researchers told the participants that the study was designed to determine how punishment might stimulate memory. They were then put at the controls of a device that generated electric shocks ranging from 15 volts ("slight shock") to 450 volts (a stage beyond "Danger—Severe Shock"). The person whose memory was being tested was strapped in a chair with electric wires from the device attached to his wrists. He was given lists of word pairs to memorize. Each time he failed to memorize the words, the person at the controls was ordered to apply an electric shock, and to increase the voltage by 15 volts after each failure. The person at the controls had been given a sample of a 45-volt shock before the experiment started—it caused a mild jolt.

As the memory failures multiplied, the people receiving the shocks of increasing intensity began to manifest distress. They groaned at 75 volts, complained of pain at 120 volts, demanded to be released at 150 volts, and screamed in agony at 285 volts. By 300 volts they were speechless. Naturally, the people applying the shocks began to hesitate as they saw the distress, and questioned the researcher about continuing. The researcher assured them that the experiment must go on for the advancement of science, that the shocks were painful but not really dangerous, and that the researcher would accept full responsibility for whatever happened.

People giving the shocks expressed serious reservations. Some said they did not want to continue but they did give additional shocks after the researcher adamantly ordered them to continue. The test ended either when the person giving the electric shocks disobeyed the researcher and refused to continue, or when the person failing to memorize the word pairs received the maximum shock—450 volts.

Researchers conducting the study were surprised by what happened. Even though no nobody at the controls really wanted to give the full shock treatment, almost two out of three (62 percent) went all the way to 450 volts. In other words, most people obeyed the authority figures even though they were not threatened with any punishment for disobedience, and even though they were convinced that they were inflicting pain on a screaming human being begging to be released from the experiment.

Of course, there were no shocks. The screaming "victims" were acting— they were not receiving any electrical charges. They were not being tested for memory or for anything else. It was the people giving the shocks who were being tested, and the results were upsetting. Researchers found that if people in authority give orders, many will follow them even though they feel what they are doing is wrong.

As the research became known, criticism grew. Critics pointed out that the subjects could not have given informed consent for the research project because they had been deceived about its true nature, and that the researchers had not explained all the risks to them. Indeed, a number of subjects did become upset when they realized how weak they were, and how easily they obeyed orders to harm others. The experiment truly harmed them, yet they had not been warned of any risks when they agreed to take part, and information about risks is crucial to informed consent.

REACTIONS TO THE QUESTIONABLE MEDICAL RESEARCH

By the 1960s a growing sense of discomfort about these and other studies led to several important initiatives that have raised the moral level of medical research. The major stages in that story are as follows.

The Work of Henry Beecher

A major turning point came in 1966 when Henry Beecher published an article in *The New England Journal of Medicine* entitled "Ethics and Clinical Research." Beecher, a distinguished professor of research in anesthesia at Harvard Medical School, reported twenty-two research projects where he felt the researchers failed to provide the subjects with adequate information or to obtain truly voluntary consent. Although the article did not identify the research projects (he did, however, identify the research for the editors of the *Journal*, and they verified that the facts were true), Beecher claimed they represented mainstream research in the past 15 years.

In almost every study, the subjects selected were in situations where truly voluntary consent would be impossible or difficult to obtain. Many were military personnel, charity patients, newly born or retarded children (Willowbrook was one of Beecher's examples), very elderly, terminally ill, or alcoholics with advanced cirrhosis of the liver. One of Beecher's conclusions was that ethically questionable medical research was the rule, and not the exception. He also believed that investigators failed to disclose risks fully, or to seek true consent, because they were under such intense pressure to achieve tenure on the faculties of medical schools and to advance their careers.

The research cited by Beecher was indeed mainstream. Published reports of the studies he identified had appeared in such journals as the *Journal of the American Medical Association*, *The New England Journal of Medicine*, *Circulation*, and the *Journal of Clinical Investigation*. Fourteen of the twenty-two protocols were in university medical schools and hospitals, including Harvard Medical School, the University of Pennsylvania, Georgetown University, Ohio State, New York University, Northwestern University, Emory, and Duke. Three of the studies were conducted at the National Institutes of Health (NIH). Funding for the research came from such sources as the Armed Forces Epidemiology Board, the National Institutes of Health, the U.S. Public Health Service, the Atomic Energy Commission, and large drug companies including Parke-Davis and Merck. Beecher also reported that these twenty-two cases were not the only problems he found. He had identified another twenty-eight instances of ethically suspicious research but did not include them in the article for lack of space.

It is of interest to note, in passing, that Beecher did not believe rules and regulations, while necessary, could solve the problem of unethical research. He argued that rules often do more harm than good, and they never curb the unscrupulous. Ethical abuses in medical research, he felt, will be eliminated only if researchers actually become good and decent people—that is, virtuous. His conviction that ethics is more a matter of being good, of being virtuous, rather than a matter of following rules and regulations (or principles or laws) echoes, of course, a fundamental theme of this book.

As we will see, however, government regulations did play a major role in elevating the moral level of medical research after Beecher's report. This history suggests that rules and regulations do play an important role in an ethics of virtue. While following rules and regulations is not the essence of ethics, the rules and regulations can be very helpful in guiding people to a good life.

Beecher's work made an immediate impact. He enjoyed a reputation as a respected researcher himself and had previously published a book, entitled *Experimentation in Man*, where he tried to increase awareness about the complex moral issues involved in research on human subjects. Once his 1966 article broke the ice by pointing out the widespread lack of ethical concern in many cases of medical research, other literature about questionable research soon followed. M. H. Pappworth's *Human Guinea Pigs: Experimentation on Man* appeared in 1967, Beecher's own *Research and the Individual* in 1970, and Jay Katz's *Experimentation with Human Beings* in 1972. Pappworth listed over 500 papers where he found the research questionable from a moral point of view, and Katz presented a wide-ranging collection of materials from psychology and law, as well as medicine, that revealed the tension between protecting the humanity of the subject and advancing medical research to benefit humankind.

Early Federal Initiatives

Even before Beecher's article, some federal efforts to establish ethical guidelines for research had begun in the United States. In 1953, for example, a National Institutes of Health policy called for peer review of research at the

NIH to protect the human subjects from undue risks. In 1966, the Surgeon General, William Stewart, issued a *Statement of Policy* on clinical investigations using human subjects. It required approval of research funded by the Public Health Service by a committee of the principal investigator's "institutional associates." The committee was to review three things: (1) the subject's rights and welfare, (2) the methods of obtaining informed consent, and (3) the risks and potential medical benefits.

After Beecher's revelations, the Department of Health, Education and Welfare (the predecessor of the Department of Health and Human Services) issued *The Institutional Guide to DHEW Policy on Protection of Human Subjects* (1971). This guide also emphasized both institutional review and informed consent in medical research. By this time, the committees reviewing research proposals were being called "institutional review boards;" this phrase, sometimes shortened to IRB, remains popular today.

After the Tuskegee study became public in 1972, the Department of Health, Education and Welfare (HEW) appointed a panel to review that case, as well as the current policies for the protection of research subjects. In 1973 the panel recommended the immediate termination of the Tuskegee study and noted that sound policies for the protection of human subjects simply did not exist. That same year the American Psychological Association adopted a code of research ethics entitled "Ethical Principles in the Conduct of Research with Human Participants." And from February to July 1973, the Congressional committee chaired by Senator Kennedy continued to examine now-well-known cases such as Willowbrook and Tuskegee, and to hear testimony from Jay Katz and others on the lack of protection for human subjects in many research protocols, most of them funded by federal money.

The National Commission

The time was ripe for legislative action, and Congress responded by passing the National Research Act in July 1974. This act created the *National Commission for the Protection of Human Subjects of Biomedical and Behavioral Research* (henceforth the "National Commission"). This commission existed until 1978 and was one of the most influential factors in the development of medical ethics during that decade.

When Congress set up the National Commission, it directed the members to "conduct a comprehensive investigation and study to identify *the basic ethical principles* which should underlie the conduct of biomedical and behavioral research involving human subjects" and to "develop guidelines which should be followed in such research to assure that it is conducted *in accordance with such principles. . .*" [Sec. 202 (a)(1)(A), emphasis added]. In effect, Congress directed the National Commission to develop not simply an ethics of medical and behavioral research, but a particular kind of ethics, an ethics based on principles. Beecher's plea for an ethics of virtue was forgotten.

Yet it is doubtful that anything but federal guidelines would have been effective in the climate of that time. A virtue ethics, after all, takes a long time to develop in a moral agent. It assumes a period of moral education and requires a maturity that comes only with experience. Given the abuses and the pressing questions about new medical research, something was needed immediately. Regulations and rules were the answer, and it was assumed that principles were needed to justify the rules.

Prompted by Congress, the eleven members of the National Commission set out to identify the basic ethical principles of medical research and to develop effective mechanisms for their implementation. Their work lasted four years (1974–1978) and resulted in two major reports. The first is known as *The Belmont Report: Ethical Principles and Guidelines for the Protection of Human Subjects of Research* and the second is *Institutional Review Boards: Report and Recommendations*. It will be helpful to comment briefly on both of these reports.

The *Belmont Report* endorsed a model of ethics known as "applied normative ethics," sometimes called "principlism" today. According to this model, ethics begins with a few basic principles. The commissioners defined a basic ethical principle as a "general judgement that serves as a basic justification for the many particular prescriptions for and evaluations of human actions." The report identified three such principles: autonomy, beneficence, and justice. These principles serve as the basis for developing more precise second-order norms or rules. The rules are then applied to individual cases to determine what actions are ethical.

The National Commission's approach followed closely the model of ethics advocated by an influential moral philosopher of that time, William Frankena. Earlier in the century, much of the work in normative ethics in England and the United States had been following two major but incompatible traditions of moral philosophy, each grounded on one basic principle. One tradition emphasized justice as the basic principle. Justice was understood as equality—the obligation to treat everyone equally (that is, fairly). The modern inspiration for this tradition was Immanuel Kant, an eighteenth-century German philosopher. The second tradition emphasized *beneficence* as the basic principle. Beneficence was understood as the general good—the greatest good for the greatest number. The modern inspiration for this tradition was John Stuart Mill, a nineteenth-century English philosopher.

Unfortunately, the moralities of justice and of beneficence often collide. Treating each person equally sometimes undermines the general good, and acting for the general good is often unfair for some.

Frankena's creative solution was to suggest that the normative basis for determining the rules of morality must embrace both basic principles: equality or justice and the general good or beneficence. He thus proposed that the rules of morality rest on not one but two principles—the principle of justice and the principle of beneficence. Frankena thought these two principles were "in some sense ultimately consistent." He summarized his model of principles and rules as follows:

> Thus, in such expressions as "the principles of morality" . . . what is ordinarily referred to may be defined as . . . the moral action-guide that everyone who looks at the world clear-headedly and informedly from that point of view will eventually agree on . . . In short, our moral discourse . . . involves the concept of an objectively or absolutely valid moral action-guide, and our moral judgments and decisions claim to be parts or applications of such an action-guide.

The National Commission adopted this model of applied ethics, and to the two principles of justice and beneficence it added a third: the principle of autonomy or respect for patient self-determination. This principle reflected the growing movement of patients' rights, especially the right to choose, and the several landmark legal cases establishing requirements for informed consent that we reviewed in chapter four.

Although the National Commission was concerned with medical research, the model of ethics whereby principles provide an "objectively or absolutely valid moral action-guide" was appealing to many people struggling to develop a coherent ethics for all medical practice in an age of rapidly developing new techniques and technologies. More recently, however, some ethicists are becoming uncomfortable with an ethics grounded on objectively or absolutely valid principles and their derived rules. Among the critics is a former member of the National Commission itself, Albert Jonsen:

> As a Commissioner, I participated in the formulation of that (Belmont) Report . . . Today I am skeptical of its status as a serious ethical analysis. I suspect that it is, in effect, a product of American moralism, prompted by the desire of Congressmen and of the public to see the chaotic world of biomedical research reduced to order by clear and unambiguous principles.

The model of applied normative ethics wherein principles and rules are applied to particular cases is not, of course, the model we are using in this text. Here the model is an ethics based not on principles, but on the natural inclination of each moral agent to seek what is truly good for herself. Whatever contributes to this good, rightly understood, is considered ethical. Principles and rules remain important, but they do not determine in the last analysis how a moral agent behaves morally well. This is determined by prudence, and any principles or rules in an ethics of prudential reasoning are derivative guidelines, not foundational norms or absolutely valid action-guides.

The second report of the National Commission, *Institutional Review Boards*, was every bit as important as the *Belmont Report*. It recommended oversight of all proposed medical research by an institutional committee responsible for protecting human subjects. These institutional review boards (IRBs) are required by the Department of Health and Human Services (HHS) in all institutions receiving federal money for research. The actual name of the board varies from facility to facility, but institutional review board (IRB) is the generic title of these boards.

The primary purpose of the IRB is to balance protection of human subjects with the need for research on human subjects. Hence, a major responsibility of the IRB is to ensure that the subjects of research, or their appropriate proxies, receive adequate information and are able to give truly voluntary consent. Among the things a subject or proxy must know are: the purpose of the study, that it involves research, the foreseeable risks or discomfort that may be experienced, benefits the subjects or others might receive, alternative treatments available, and, if the risk is more than minimal, whether or not compensation and medical care for injuries is available. Subjects must also be told that their participation is voluntary, that they may withdraw at any time, and that their refusal to participate or their decision to withdraw will not penalize them or detract from their proper medical care in any way.

The IRB is typically composed of physicians, nurses, social workers, chaplains, pharmacists, and administrators from the institution. It also includes several representatives from the community, people not affiliated with the institution. The federally mandated institutional review boards have been able to maintain a high level of ethical integrity in medical research.

The major reason for the lasting impact of the National Commission is the fact that many of its recommendations became the basis for regulations promulgated by the Department of Health, Education and Welfare (HEW), later the Department of Health and Human Services (HHS), and by the Food and Drug Administration (FDA). These agencies instituted an extensive set of regulations for research on human subjects in 1981, and have since added important amendments, most notably in 1991. The federal regulations are taken seriously because most hospitals conducting research receive federal funding (chiefly research grants, Medicare, and Medicaid) and are therefore required to follow them.

The President's Commission

The *President's Commission for the Study of Ethical Problems in Medicine and Biomedical and Behavioral Research*, which met from 1980 to 1983, issued a number of reports pertaining to research on human subjects. The President's Commission supported the National Commission's insistence on informed consent, the institutional review boards, and the use of ethical principles (sometimes it called them "values") as norms for making ethical judgments. The final report of the President's Commission acknowledged how the National Commission had appealed to the now familiar ethical principles of autonomy, beneficence, and justice. It stated that these principles "are a basic part of the Western cultural and philosophical traditions," and cited both the National Commission's *Belmont Report* and an important text entitled *Principles of Biomedical Ethics*, written by two leading ethicists, Tom Beauchamp and James Childress, as evidence that these principles have "special importance in evaluating the ethical implications of decisions, actions, and policies in medicine and biomedical and behavioral research."

The reactions to the morally questionable research of several decades ago led to many positive developments in the ethics of research involving human subjects. Thanks to increased moral awareness, the federal requirements of informed and voluntary consent, and oversight by institutional review boards, a high level of moral responsibility has now been achieved in medical research.

Nonetheless, problem cases continue to be reported. Toward the end of 1993, for example, three cases of questionable moral procedures emerged. First, three prominent cancer researchers at the Montefiore Medical Center in New York admitted in statements to the U.S. Attorney that they had used an unapproved drug on sixteen patients with brain cancer in 1987. The FDA had approved the experimental drug for kidney cancer, but not for brain cancer. When the project was investigated by the FDA, the NIH, and the FBI, the physicians involved, according to press reports, lied in an effort to cover up the unapproved use of the drug.

It was also reported that five of fifteen subjects in an NIH trial of a new drug (Fialuridine or FIAU), designed to combat hepatitis B, died as a result of taking the drug. The consent form indicated that subjects had been told of six specific risks (fatigue, nausea, rashes, bone marrow suppression, seizures, and pains or numbness in the arms and legs), but not that the drug might be lethal. The consent form also said that "FIAU is a new medication, and its side effects have not been completely described." While the researchers did not expect any deaths to result from the research, some ethicists felt that the IRB review of the research proposal was not adequate because the information given the subjects was vague, incomplete, and somewhat misleading, especially for sick patients looking for a cure after they had not benefited from the standard treatment for hepatitis B.

Finally, it was reported at this time that one of the world's largest manufacturers of medical devices, C. R. Bard of New Jersey, agreed to plead guilty to 391 counts, including the shipping of adulterated products for human experimentation. The company agreed to pay a fine of $61 million, the largest penalty for health care fraud in history. The chairman of the company and five former executives also face criminal charges.

What had happened? One of Bard's divisions manufactured catheters that are used in balloon angioplasty, a procedure designed to open blocked arteries. The procedure was first used in 1980 and is now performed about 400,000 times per year. In February 1988 Bard was aware that one of its catheter designs sometimes failed to deflate, but it concealed this information when it sought FDA approval for the product. Once approved, some of these catheters did fail to deflate, and a few people died as a result. Bard hastily redesigned the catheter, and then sold the modified design without proper FDA approval. When the FDA finally caught up with the company, the FDA Commissioner was quoted as saying that Bard was "using unsuspecting patients as guinea pigs and operating rooms as laboratories for unapproved products."

Stories such as these still appear all too frequently. They remind us of the ongoing vigilance needed to ensure the protection of human subjects in contemporary medical research and in the development of new medical techniques and technologies. And a series of disclosures in 1994 of earlier questionable government research involving radiation studies years ago also reminds us of how important moral oversight is in medical research.

The task of moral awareness and oversight in research is made all the more difficult because some populations of human subjects present unique and complicated problems for ethical consideration. We will now consider several such populations.

RESEARCH ON EMBRYOS AND FETUSES

The 1974 public law authorizing the National Commission contained two important items affecting research on the fetus: it directed the commission to produce a report on fetal research within four months after it began work, and it imposed a moratorium on federally funded fetal research while that report was being prepared. There were several reasons why Congress wanted immediate action on questions of fetal research. In January 1973 the *Roe v. Wade* decision had struck down all state laws protecting fetuses in the first two trimesters.

The *Roe v. Wade* decision offered no protection to the fetus in the first six months of its life. Some felt that this lack of protection might encourage some scientists to do research on living fetuses destined for abortion, as well as on dying aborted fetuses. The great fear was that the worthwhile goals of fetal research would actually encourage the abortion of healthy fetuses for the wrong reasons and would not respect fetal human life.

At the same time, some upsetting reports of research on live fetuses both before and after abortions resulted in public demonstrations at NIH headquarters, although NIH had not been involved in the research. Then, in Boston, a grand jury indicted four physicians for allegedly violating an 1814 statute forbidding "grave-robbing," a law originally designed to prevent stealing from cemeteries. The physicians were conducting research to learn whether antibiotics given to a pregnant woman would also affect the fetus. Several women planning an abortion at Boston City Hospital agreed to take the antibiotics, and the physicians retrieved their fetuses after their abortions for examination. The District Attorney claimed the women had given consent for the medications, but not for the postmortem examinations of the fetuses. Hence, he accused the physicians of "grave-robbing." Although the charges were eventually dropped, the case made a significant impact on medical researchers.

More than a dozen state legislatures, no longer able to restrict abortions in the first two trimesters after *Roe v. Wade*, reacted by passing laws designed to prevent the use of aborted, or about to be aborted, fetuses in medical research. Some national guidelines were obviously needed, and this explains why the Congress pressed the National Commission for an early report on fetal research.

The National Commission produced its report in record time. Its *Research on the Fetus* appeared in April 1975, and its recommendations became the basis for federal regulations promulgated the following July. These regulations, with some changes and additional amendments over the years, are the regulations governing fetal research today.

The Federal Regulations on Fetal Research

Some of the important highlights as found in Title 45, Code of Federal Regulations, Part 46 (45 CFR 46) are:

1. The fetus is a human subject deserving of care and respect. A fetus begins at implantation and continues for the duration of the pregnancy. Once expelled or extracted, the living human subject is still considered a fetus unless it is mature enough to survive outside the uterus, in which case it is no longer a fetus but an infant (46.203).

2. Although an embryo created by fertilizing an ovum in a laboratory (IVF) does not fall under the definition of a fetus, the regulations also cover research on embryos produced by IVF. The regulations disallow funding of IVF research unless it has been found ethically acceptable by an "Ethics Advisory

Board" (EAB) that would be established by the secretary of the Department of Health, Education, and Welfare (HEW) (46.205). As we will see, the EAB existed only for a brief time (1978–1980), and no IVF research proposals were supported with federal funds until 1994. (An EAB did approve an IVF research proposal in 1979, but its recommendations were never accepted by HEW or its successor, the Department of Health and Human Services [HHS], so federal support of that IVF research project never did occur.)

3. The federal regulations are not concerned with research on dead fetuses, or on fetal parts taken from them. Regulations for research on dead fetuses or on fetal materials (cells, tissue, etc.) are determined by state or local laws (46.210). Many states do have laws governing research on dead fetuses.

4. No research can be carried out on fetuses—even fetuses destined for legal abortions—unless first tried on animals (46.206).

5. No research can be carried out on pregnant women—even on women planning legal abortions—until experiments have also been conducted on women who are not pregnant (46.206). This is to ensure that the research on the woman will not put her fetus at risk.

6. Strict limitations govern research on fetuses during pregnancy, regardless of whether the woman desires a healthy birth or an abortion. The regulations allow research on a fetus in only two cases: (1) if its purpose is the health needs of the fetus or (2) if its purpose is important biomedical knowledge that cannot otherwise be obtained, and the risk to the fetus is "minimal" (46.208). Both parents must give consent for the research, although the man's consent is not necessary under certain specified conditions.

The definition of "minimal risk" to a fetus for research undertaken not for its health needs, but for general scientific knowledge, is difficult to determine. Some have suggested that "minimal risk" should be a variable notion tied to the age of the fetus. Thus researchers should be very careful about harming a thirty-eight week fetus, but need not be so careful about harming a six week fetus. In other words, the protection of immature fetuses in research need not be as great as the protection of mature fetuses. Hence "minimal risk" for a mature fetus would not be the same as "minimal risk" for an early fetus.

Many object to this approach, claiming that the same level of protection should apply to fetuses of any age. Their position seems reasonable. It certainly is reasonable if the woman is hoping to give birth, but it also seems reasonable if she is planning on an abortion. Fetuses are defined as human subjects, and it is at least arguable that subjecting human subjects destined for destruction to risky research does not enhance but undermines the moral character of the researcher. Some, of course, will argue the other way, and claim that it makes no sense to protect fetuses destined for abortion from research risks.

7. The regulations for research on fetuses after the pregnancy is ended are more complicated (46.209). The regulations envision three situations.

The fetus is living but not viable. Research is permitted only if (1) the purpose is obtaining important biomedical knowledge not otherwise available, (2) the interventions will not cause cardiopulmonary arrest, and (3) the vital functions of the fetus will not be artificially maintained.

The fetus is viable. The regulations are not concerned with research on a viable fetus. A viable fetus outside the uterus is an infant, and it is thus subject to the regulations governing research on children.

The fetus may be viable. When it is not known whether or not the fetus is viable, no research is permitted unless (1) the purpose is to enhance the chances of its survival to viability or (2) the purpose is important biomedical knowledge not otherwise available and the research presents no risk to the fetus.

8. The regulations also direct the secretary of Health, Education and Welfare to establish one or more ethics advisory boards (EAB) to deal with the ethical, legal, social, and medical issues of fetal research (46.204). The EAB would be made up of people not employed by HEW and would include ethicists as well as representatives of the professions and of the general public. With the approval of the EAB, the secretary may waive or modify the regulations. The EAB would also offer advice on the ethical issues of fetal research and, if requested, on HEW's general policies, guidelines, and procedures. Finally, the EAB would approve all research on IVF. Unfortunately, the EAB has not functioned for years. Its story is an interesting one.

The Ethics Advisory Board

The federal regulations, following the recommendations of the National Commission, clearly envisioned both local and national ethical review boards for reviewing proposals seeking federal funding for research on embryos and fetuses. According to the regulations, the local institutional review boards (IRBs) review each proposal at the institutional level, and an ethics advisory board (EAB) would review the research at the national level.

Unfortunately, the EAB does not exist. The EAB was established in 1978 but it reviewed only two proposals. The first was for the IVF study mentioned above. An EAB approved the study under specified conditions, but its recommendations were never accepted by HEW, and the research was never funded. The second proposal was a request for a waiver to the "minimal risk" rule in a study involving fetoscopy where some fetal loss was expected. An EAB again approved the research and this time HEW Secretary Califano did grant a waiver for study in 1979.

In 1980 Ronald Reagan became president and appointed a new secretary of HEW. Secretary Harris declined to renew funding for the EAB when its original charter expired on September 30, 1980, and the board dissolved. Since that time, there has been no national EAB to review these research proposals. Under the regulations this meant that no federal funds could support (1) any research on IVF or (2) any research on fetuses that would impose more than a "minimal risk," unless the research is directed to the health of that particular fetus.

Since few procedures of research on embryos or fetuses can be shown to have only minimal risk for the subject, the absence of an EAB disallowed federal funding for many IVF and fetal research projects. Responsible research that could have been federally funded after a favorable review by an EAB could not be federally funded because the EAB did not exist. This meant that most of the IVF and fetal research in the United States had to seek private funding. The problem with this is that the privately funded research escapes review by an official national ethics commission.

The government's discouragement of fetal research intensified in 1988. The assistant secretary of HHS, Dr. Robert Windom, imposed a moratorium on funding for any fetal research involving the transplantation of fetal tissue derived from elective abortions. Windom then appointed a panel—the Human Fetal Tissue Transplantation Research Panel or HFTTR—to study the issue. As we saw in chapter eleven, the panel recommended that the research on fetal tissue transplantation be funded, provided certain ethical restrictions were observed. The NIH accepted the HFTTR panel's recommendations, but HHS continued the moratorium against funding fetal transplantation research.

When President Clinton took office in 1993, the climate for research on fetal tissue and IVF improved. The moratorium on fetal tissue research was lifted, and in January 1994 the National Institute of Neurological Disorders and Stroke provided the first federal funding for fetal tissue research. It awarded 4.5 million dollars to three institutions for research in transplanting fetal tissue from elective abortions to patients with Parkinson's disease.

The door was also opened for federally funded IVF research, although in a rather unfortunate way. The federal regulations (45 CFR 46.204(d)) state that no IVF research can be funded until the proposal has been reviewed by the Ethics Advisory Board—the board that has not existed since 1980. Instead of reconstituting the EAB to review IVF proposals—a potentially delicate exercise, given the national sensitivity about abortion—NIH officials added an unobtrusive sentence to the 1993 NIH Revitalization Act. This sentence simply states that the provisions of 45 CFR 46.204(d) "shall not have any legal effect." This means that review by a national EAB is no longer necessary before proposals for IVF research can be federally funded.

Since IVF has been a lucrative medical intervention for both nonprofit and for-profit facilities, this move was welcomed by many in the field. And it comes as no surprise that one group lobbying for this change in the regulations was the American Fertility Society.

From an ethical viewpoint, however, the move is regrettable. Review by a national ethics board, something most countries have, would be a valuable complement to the local institutional review boards. Sensing that some kind of ethical oversight is needed on the national level, the NIH did convene a Human Embryo Research Panel in January 1994 to recommend guidelines for the federal funding of research involving embryos. In September 1994 this panel recommended allowing federal support for laboratory research on embryos in the first fourteen days of development (until the formation of the primitive streak) under yet to be developed guidelines. If the provisions of this report are accepted by NIH and guidelines put in place, federally funded research on embryos for IVF and other purposes could begin as early as 1995.

Ethical Reflections Relevant to Research on Embryos and Fetuses

Research on embryos and fetuses is morally sensitive for the following reasons. First, an embryo or fetus is human life, and whenever there is a question of real or possible damage to human life, moral deliberation and judgment are required. Damage to embryonic or fetal human life is something bad, and we cannot pursue behavior entailing bad features unless we can show reasons that will justify the harm we cause or could cause. Our first ethical responsibility, then, is to ascertain whether and when we can endanger embryonic and fetal human life by medical research, especially medical research that will damage or destroy the human subject.

Everyone realizes that embryonic and fetal research leads to medical benefits. Research on human subjects is the only way we can learn some things, and some of these things have led, and will continue to lead, to the better care and treatment of human life, including fetal human life. Moral reasoning about embryonic and fetal research is an effort to strike a delicate balance between the risks imposed on the embryo and the benefits expected from the study.

Second, research requires informed consent. When the human subject is still a minor (under eighteen), the parents would normally be the ones to give consent for the research. In consenting to research affecting their children, parents are expected to protect their children from undue risks and harms.

When the human subject is still a fetus, the woman would normally be the one to give consent for the research. In consenting to research affecting her fetus, she is expected to protect it from undue risks and harm. While she certainly is motivated to protect the fetus if she intends to give birth, she has no reason to protect it if she intends to abort it.

This creates a serious problem about the legitimacy of her giving consent for research on her fetus. The main purpose of informed consent in medical research is to protect the human subject, in this case the fetus. This purpose is lost if the woman giving the consent has already decided to destroy the fetus in an abortion. This is why some ethicists insist that a woman who has decided to abort a fetus is not the proper person to give consent for research on it, at least while it is alive.

Third, fetal research is often associated with abortion, and abortion is a highly controversial issue. Some researchers see great advantages for fetal research in legal abortion. First, once a woman has decided to abort her fetus, there is an opportunity to do research on drugs or diagnostic interventions that would be too dangerous for the fetus if she was intending to give birth. Second, since legal abortions are performed in medical settings, they provide a rich source of clean fetal remains for research.

Other people take a different view. They fear that the use of fetuses for medical research will encourage more abortions. They argue that the promise of making a contribution to medical science will overshadow the moral issues involved in the abortion itself. Some of them fear that desperate women may even become pregnant for the purpose of selling their fetuses for research, just as some women now take money (usually about $10,000) for carrying a fetus that they will give to others at birth, and just as some women now sell their eggs, often for several thousand dollars.

Fourth, the risks of fetal research are difficult to establish. We simply do not know as much about risks to the fetus as we do about risks to adults or children. For example, many fetuses (some say more than 15 percent) are spontaneously aborted after the pregnancy has begun. If these fetuses were the subjects of research, it would be difficult to know whether the research or some other factor was the cause of the miscarriage. The difficulty in assessing risks to fetuses makes moral judgments about fetal research difficult.

Fifth, the father's role in giving consent for the research is a sensitive issue. Some say that the father should assume some responsibility for the pregnancy he caused, and this implies that he should share in making decisions about medical interventions on the fetus. Others see the man's participation in decisions about the fetus an intrusion into the control a woman should have over what happens inside her body. The issue remains a troubling one.

For these five reasons, then, research on fetuses is a very complicated moral issue. Given the sensitive nature of fetal research and the undeniable medical benefits that can accrue from it, what might be a reasonable ethical approach to the issue?

The recommendations of the National Commission and the subsequent federal regulations based on them, which we outlined above, are a good starting point. The commission insisted that the fetus is a human subject from the time of implantation and thus deserves protection, as does any human subject of medical research. Unlike the *Roe v. Wade* decision, which offers no protection for a fetus before viability, the federal regulations governing fetal research do protect fetuses, and this is a positive first step.

The current guidelines of the American Fertility Society and the proposals in the September 1994 report of the NIH Human Embryo Research Panel are also a starting point for reasoning about research on embryos. The AFS guidelines call for informed consent and respect for the human life of the embryo. Both reports allow some research on embryos and are generally consistent with the guidelines recommended by national commissions in other countries. Nonetheless, some people strongly object to any research on human embryos.

In any moral evaluation of research on fetuses or embryos, there are three major ethical concerns. First, it is important to recognize that embryos and fetuses are living human beings and therefore must be treated with respect. It is incomprehensible to argue that we can achieve a good life by treating human life with disrespect.

Research and respect for human life, however, are not incompatible. Medical research on human beings for good reasons and with due respect for their humanity is morally justified. Given the need to respect and to protect human life, however, it is also reasonable to insist that any research on living embryos and fetuses, as well as on children, must be a last resort. This means that the research on animal embryos and fetuses, and on defective embryos and dead human fetuses, has gone as far as it can go in providing the data sought by researchers.

Second, it is important to recognize that informed consent is crucial for research on all human beings. Embryos and fetuses cannot give informed consent, but somebody with a relationship to them must give it. Researchers cannot just take the embryos and fetuses, and do whatever they want with them. Normally parents give consent for medical research on their children, and women give consent for research on their embryos and fetuses. In such cases the parents of the child, or the pregnant woman, are presumed to have the best interests of their offspring at heart.

If a parent has decided to destroy an embryo or a fetus, however, the issue of informed consent becomes complicated. As we have pointed out, the purpose of informed consent in medical research is to protect the human subject. Hence, some argue that the person intending to discard an embryo or destroy a fetus is no longer interested in protecting the human subject, and therefore cannot give legitimate consent for research on it.

Others argue that, although parents intending to destroy a fetus or discard an embryo may not be the appropriate people to give consent, other parties could provide the informed consent so important to medical research. They suggest that the IRB, the hospital ethics committee, or some other panel could give consent for research after ascertaining that the research would not cause suffering or treat the embryo or fetus in a disrespectful way.

The issue of informed consent for research on embryos and fetuses destined for deliberate destruction remains one of the most difficult of ethical problems. It is not easy to determine a reasonable response, that is, a response that will respect human life. A first step toward resolving the dilemma, however, can be taken if we distinguish between the morally justified destructions of embryos or fetuses and the destructions that are not morally justified. If the destruction of the embryo or fetus is morally justified, then there are reasons for saying that the parents of the embryo, or the woman carrying the fetus, can give consent for the research. If, on the other hand, the destruction of the embryo or fetus is not morally justified, then there are reasons for saying that the parents of the embryo, or the woman carrying the fetus, are not the proper people to give consent for the research.

Consider, for example, a morally justified destruction of an embryo. After years of infertility, a married couple turns to IVF in an effort to have their child. Embryos are created in vitro, and testing reveals that one of them is so genetically defective that embryo transfer into the woman would be unreasonable. There are good reasons for saying that discarding the defective embryo is morally justified in such a case. Once the moral justification of discarding the embryo is established, the parents should be able to give consent for research on it. Their consent is not incompatible with the assumption that they should protect the embryo and preserve its life—protection and preservation no longer make sense in this case. The major moral issue remaining is one of human dignity and respect for life in the research. This dignity and respect is preserved in many ways, among them: the embryo will not be sold, it will not be allowed to develop beyond 14 days, and it will not be treated simply as cells or tissue, but as a new human being resulting from the union of egg and spermatozoon.

Consider, as another example, a morally justified abortion. We cannot repeat here what was said about abortion in chapter eleven, but most people agree that some abortions are morally justified. An easy example is an ectopic pregnancy. There are good reasons for saying that abortion of an ectopic fetus is morally justified. Once the moral justification for the abortion is established, the woman should be able to to give consent for research on it, provided steps are taken to respect its human life. Her consent in the case of a morally justified abortion of an ectopic fetus is not incompatible with the assumption that we should protect and preserve fetal life—protection and preservation of fetal life no longer makes sense if the fetus is ectopic.

On the other hand, if the abortion is not morally justified, there are good reasons for saying that the woman is not the appropriate person to give consent for research on it. To say an abortion is not morally justified is to say that the fetus should be protected, and it would be inconsistent to accept informed consent from the person who should be protecting the fetus but decided to destroy it.

Some, of course, do not see the moral problem here. They say that abortion is legal, that it is a matter of choice in the first two trimesters, and that no moral problem exists about using those fetuses before, during, or after legal abortions. However, the moral issues are not so easily dismissed. The central question is not whether the abortion is legal but whether it is morally justified. Under present law, it is perfectly legal, for example, for a woman to have an abortion because she has discovered her healthy five-month fetus is female, and she wants a boy. Such an abortion, though legal, is hardly moral. Most ethicists would consider it immoral for at least two reasons: (1) the sex of a healthy fetus is not a morally cogent reason for destroying it, especially at 20 weeks, and (2) sexual discrimination, always immoral, is embedded in the woman's decision.

Certainly, people disagree on what reasons justify an abortion, but most admit that some of the 1.5 million abortions in the United States are justified. Others, however, are not.

Hence the third major ethical concern: It is important to recognize that one can all too easily become an accomplice in immoral abortions by using fetuses produced by them for medical research.

Using fetuses from immoral abortions is somewhat analogous to using stolen animals in research. When laboratories use stolen dogs and cats—family pets—for research, they are accomplices in the immorality of the original theft. In a similar way, using tissue from immoral abortions makes the researchers accomplices in the immorality of the abortion.

This problem has long been recognized by ethicists, and they take one of two general positions. Some say researchers could never morally use any tissue from immoral abortions. Others claim the research and the abortion can be sufficiently separated to eliminate the researcher's cooperation in the immoral abortion.

One thing that would help here is the national Ethics Advisory Board. Its review of proposals could include insistence on the distance between abortion and fetal research, a distance that is crucial given the intense abortion controversy in the United States and the immorality of some abortions.

In summary, the main considerations in embryonic and fetal research center on three major concerns. First, we want to protect human life and human subjects from harm, yet acknowledge the benefits of research on embryos and fetal human subjects. Second, we want to acknowledge the importance of informed consent and insist on a proper place for it in embryonic and fetal research. Third, we want to separate fetal research from abortions that are not morally justified. If we can adequately respond to these concerns with intelligent guidelines and, in addition, if we can avoid causing suffering in a fetus that has developed awareness, there are reasons for saying some embryonic and fetal research is morally reasonable as a last resort to acquire information of medical benefit.

RESEARCH ON MINORS

In 1983 the Department of Health and Human Services issued specific regulations governing research on children. The regulations (45 C.F.R. 46, Subpart D) allow four kinds of research on children:

> Research with no more than minimal risk is permitted.
> Research with more than minimal risk is permitted if it is intended to benefit the child.
> Research with a "minor increase" over minimal risk is permitted if it is likely to yield "generalizable knowledge" about the child's condition; that is, knowledge of benefit to others.
> Research not meeting these three conditions but which a "panel of experts" determines will present a reasonable opportunity to understand, prevent, or alleviate serious problems affecting the health and welfare of children, and which will be conducted in accord with sound ethical principles and the assent of the children, is also permitted.

Unfortunately, these categories are open to a rather wide range of different interpretations by the local IRBs reviewing the research proposals. The regulations governing research on adults (45 C.F.R. 46 Subpart A) do define "minimal risk" as a risk not greater than what a person encounters in routine physical or psychological tests, but no definition is given of a "minor increase" over minimal risk.

A major controversy has existed for years over the issue of informed consent for research on children. Parents or guardians normally give informed consent for medical interventions on children, unless the child is emancipated or the treatment is covered by one of the "minor treatment statutes" discussed in chapter five. Informed consent given on behalf of people without decision-making capacity, however, normally follows the "best interests" standard; that is, parents should only consent to what is in the best interests of the child. Some research will be of no benefit to the child; in fact, it might even pose some risk or actually cause harm.

Some ethicists have argued that no parent or guardian can give consent for any intervention that is not for the benefit of the child. One well-known health care ethicist, Paul Ramsey, held just such a position. Ramsey argued from a moral principle known as "respect for persons." According to this principle, unless a person consents, we cannot use him for any experiments not directly beneficial to him, even if there is no risk involved. Since young children cannot give valid informed consent, no research involving them is morally justified.

Others disagree. Richard McCormick, for example, has argued that we can presume children would, if they could, consent to research posing no more than slight risk, even if it is of no benefit to them. While McCormick's position appears reasonable, his reasoning in defense of it may not be the best. It is open to the same criticisms directed against the Massachusetts Supreme Court and its use of substituted judgment in cases involving children; namely, we have no reason for saying we know what never-competent children would want if they were competent.

We can, however, morally justify limited research on children another way. In our discussion of permanently unconsciousness patients whose wishes are not known, we acknowledged that the two usual standards of proxy decision making—substituted judgment and best interests—do not apply. We appealed to a third standard—reasonable treatment—to decide whether to continue treatment or medical nutrition. We could appeal to the same standard here for research on children not able to give consent. The general reasonableness standard, for example, would allow parents to consent to something like drawing blood from a five-year-old child for research, even if the research would be of no conceivable benefit to the child. This reasonableness standard is consistent with the federal regulations allowing research of no benefit to the child, provided it creates no more than minimal risk for the child.

The federal regulations governing research on children introduce an important consideration relevant to informed consent. They acknowledge that children usually cannot give informed consent, but they specify that something called "assent" is often possible. Under the regulations, the local IRB determines whether or not the child incapable of giving informed consent can nonetheless give or withhold assent to the research. In making the determination, the IRB considers the age, maturity, and psychological state of the child. In effect, the child's assent to the research means that she agrees to the procedures even though she is not yet capable of giving a truly informed and voluntary consent.

OTHER SPECIAL POPULATIONS IN RESEARCH

We note, in passing, that other populations pose particular problems for medical research. Most of the ethical problems arise because these populations do not have sufficient capacity to give informed consent or, if they do have decision-making capacity, are in a position where the voluntariness of their consent may be easily undermined. Prisoners, for example, are in a vulnerable position and could easily be exploited. Special regulations exist to protect them.

The mentally ill, the handicapped, and the disabled are also vulnerable, and special care must be taken so they will not be exploited. Care must also be taken that the elderly are not coerced or unduly influenced to participate in research protocols.

Military personnel represent another vulnerable population. During Operation Desert Storm in 1991, unapproved drugs were used on soldiers without their informed consent. Since the drugs had not been fully tested and approved by the FDA, their use was not medical but experimental. The FDA did issue an interim regulation allowing the military to use the unapproved drugs. A serviceman challenged the FDA ruling in federal court but lost. The court said that the FDA could issue an interim regulation allowing the use of unapproved drugs without informed consent, if those administering the drugs believed obtaining informed consent from the recipients was not feasible. This decision (*Doe v. Sullivan*, 938 F.2d 1370 [1991]) is notable in that it runs counter to the careful protection of human subjects found in most government regulations and court decisions. Its impact is undoubtedly limited by the special circumstances of military personnel preparing for combat and by the reasonable belief that the drug would benefit most of the military people going into combat in the Persian Gulf area.

Still another special population presenting unique problems for research comprises those with AIDS. Many people suffering from this disease are well informed, and some are anxious to use unapproved drugs in the chance that they, or others, might benefit from them. Given the predicament faced by people with AIDS, their requests are easily justified morally, provided there is a plausible reason to believe the drugs might benefit them. People facing certain death have good reasons for taking chances with unapproved drugs that would be unreasonable for others to try. At the same time, these requests are not so easily justified when there is little or no reason to believe the drugs will benefit them. The following case highlights the dilemma.

THE CASE OF COMPOUND Q

The Story

Compound Q is a drug extracted from Chinese cucumber roots. In the late 1980s laboratory tests indicated that it attacked the HIV in cell cultures, so it looked promising as a treatment for AIDS. To know for sure, of course, additional study and controlled clinical trials would have to be conducted. Only then could the FDA approve the drug for use.

For Project Inform, an AIDS advocacy group, this would take too long. AIDS was a crisis for many people it represented, and help was needed immediately. Martin Delaney, the head of Project Inform, led efforts to conduct quick clinical trials of Compound Q. He enlisted physicians in several cities with high populations of patients suffering from AIDS who agreed to give volunteer patients Compound Q. The physicians would arrange blood tests to check the efficacy of the drug and observe any side effects that might develop.

His first practical problem was obtaining supplies of the drug. He solved this by recruiting a nurse named James Corti, who had been smuggling drugs into the United States for AIDS patients for several years. Corti managed to obtain several hundred doses of Compound Q in Shanghai and get them into the country. Nine physicians began telling AIDS patients about the unapproved drug and giving it to those who wanted it. About one hundred eventually took Compound Q during its brief trial in 1989.

The secret study ended when three patients participating in the study died rather quickly. The death of Scott Sheaffer received the most attention.

He was HIV positive but was not very sick until he took Compound Q. Then he deteriorated rapidly. Physicians treating him at two hospitals did not know he had taken Compound Q. They could not reverse his decline, and he soon died. His rapid fatal decline was not typical of how other people with AIDS died. The role of Compound Q in his death is unknown; it might not have played any role.

Ethical Analysis

Situational awareness: We are aware of the following facts in the story of Compound Q.

1. People with AIDS are dying; there is no known cure.

2. Compound Q did attack the HIV in cell cultures; it might help patients with AIDS.

3. The FDA requires careful clinical trials before it approves new drugs for clinical use. Some people with AIDS who might be helped will die before these clinical trials can be completed. Some people with AIDS were willing to take a chance with Compound Q before it was approved.

4. The Project Inform clinical trials were not well-conducted. The study did not divide the patients into two cohorts, and give some people the drug and others a placebo. Only in this way can reliable information emerge. Moreover, no preliminary studies were conducted in animals, no institutional review board reviewed the study, and no acceptable provision was made for monitoring possible side effects.

Prudential reasoning in the story of Compound Q

Patients' perspective.   People with AIDS are in a tragic situation. They are going to die if they rely on accepted therapies. Some of them are willing to try any promising drug to escape death. They are no longer very concerned about the risks and possible harms of the unproven drugs; these concerns have faded in the face of their fatal disease. Given their desperate plight, it is not surprising that some of them think it is reasonable to try unproven drugs such as Compound Q. The chance of success is slim, but it is their only hope.

Providers' perspective.   Physicians treating many people suffering from AIDS are also influenced by the tragedy of the disease. It is not surprising that some of them find it reasonable to cooperate with the decisions of their informed patients and use unproven drugs that might be helpful.

Researchers' perspective.   Most people interested in research to find a therapy or vaccine for AIDS find a secret drug study totally unreasonable. Researchers criticized this study for its lack of scientific standards. They were also concerned that the unproven drugs could harm, or even kill, those taking them. Perhaps most importantly, however, they were concerned that this kind of clinical trial makes it practically impossible for them to conduct their studies. Most clinical studies of drugs are random clinical trials and double blinded; that is, neither the researchers nor the patients know who is receiving the drug and who is receiving the placebo. If no one knows who is in the treatment group and who is in the control group, researchers are in a better position to infer that improvements noted in the treatment group are due to the drug and not some other factor.

But few people with AIDS are willing to volunteer for this kind of study, where they might be randomly selected for the control group and not receive any drug that could be helping them for the duration of the study. Those already sick with AIDS would rather participate in the type of study conducted by Project Inform, where everybody receives the promising drug (in this case, Compound Q). Given this tendency, it is not hard to understand why researchers find these outlaw trials with smuggled drugs harmful in the long run—they undermine their ability to conduct random clinical trials of what could be a helpful drug in the fight against AIDS.

The FDA Action

When publicity surfaced about the deaths of three patients taking Compound Q, the FDA ordered the trial stopped. After reviewing the data, however, it allowed the Project Inform study to continue with important modifications. Sandoz Pharmaceuticals developed a synthetic form of the drug for the new trials. Preliminary reports have not shown that Compound Q is effective in the treatment of AIDS.

Ethical Reflection

This kind of case reveals how the phrase medical research is something of an oxymoron. The goal of clinical medicine is the health and comfort of a particular patient now; the goal of clinical research is gaining knowledge for the health and comfort of many patients, mostly in the future. The perspectives of patients and of the physicians caring for them differ from the perspectives of researchers and of the FDA. These differing perspectives lead, as can be expected, to different judgments about what is morally reasonable.

The case of Compound Q is a dramatic example of the frequent conflict between the different legitimate goals of medical care and medical research. In an effort to reduce this conflict, the NIH and the FDA established a "parallel track" strategy soon after the Compound Q controversy emerged. One track will subject the promising drug to the usual random clinical trials. A second track will allow certain patients—those not eligible for clinical trials or not helped by approved drugs—to receive the unapproved drug. DDI (dideoxyinosine), another drug showing some promise against AIDS, was the first drug placed on a parallel track.

The parallel track approach has merit but is not without its problems. First, there is the practical problem of payment. Most third-party payers will not pay for unproven therapies. While drugs being tested in a clinical trial are usually provided free, this is not the case for drugs distributed outside the trial track. Many AIDS patients are not able to pay privately for DDI.

Second, researchers found it difficult to enroll AIDS patients in random clinical trials once DDI was available outside the research track. Put simply, it was a promising drug and patients did not want to chance being placed in the control group and not receiving it. The parallel track approach thus hinders researchers from finding a proven therapy for AIDS.

The case of Compound Q also highlights the conflict between different ethical attitudes currently dominating American health care ethics. If one begins with a rights-based approach, or the principle of autonomy, or the principle of justice understood as treating each individual equally, then one can conclude AIDS patients should have access to promising but unapproved drugs. One can argue they have a right to choose them, that they are well-informed and can determine for themselves what is right, and that if some patients in a random clinical trial receive them, then it is only fair that everybody can have them.

On the other hand, if one begins with a utilitarian approach that considers the greatest good for the greatest number, or the principle of beneficence, then one can conclude that AIDS patients should have access only to approved drugs. One can argue that the dispensation of unproved drugs disrupts random clinical trials and thereby harms others by delaying research into what might be helpful, and that it would be contrary to beneficence to give a potentially harmful unproven drug to patients simply because they wanted it.

What might an ethic of prudential reasoning work out in such a dilemma? It will begin by acknowledging several new factors in medical research related to AIDS. First, the use of unproven drugs cannot be stopped. AIDS advocates have been obtaining them, and people with AIDS have been using them, for years. Second, many people with AIDS are not ignorant of how dangerous unproven drugs can be. Unlike many patients of the past, patients with AIDS do not need an overly paternalistic government to protect them from the unknown. They are often very knowledgeable about drugs and about their disease. Third, the traditional protocols long employed by the FDA to approve new drugs are cumbersome, as the FDA itself has acknowledged. Finally, cooperation between AIDS advocates and the FDA has been absent too often.

Prudential reasoning will move, as it often does, toward a middle ground. The patient with AIDS must be helped, but at some point what might be good for her will disrupt the common good that requires a sound approval process and will thereby undermine the good of others. Sound medical research must proceed, but at some point it blinds us to the needs of the individual patient suffering now, who is well informed and willing to take the risks of using promising but unapproved drugs. In some cases prudence will find the drug sufficiently promising that it would not be good to deny it to those wanting it; in other cases prudence will find the trials sufficiently promising that it would not be good to undermine them. In all cases, prudence will urge greater dialogue and cooperation between patients suffering from AIDS and people dedicated to sound medical research and to the protection of human subjects.

ANIMALS AND MEDICAL RESEARCH

The last special population we want to mention is composed of research subjects who are not human—animals. Many therapies are first tested on animals before they are tested on human subjects, and this research on animals has contributed to important developments in human health care. Experiments on dogs helped isolate insulin in 1921, and this led to the development of insulin therapy that has been so beneficial for many people suffering from diabetes. Research on animal primates was a key factor in the 1953 development of polio vaccines. So many other examples of beneficial research using animals could be given that it is impossible to deny the value for humans of biomedical research using animals.

Until recently, many people were unaware that the use of animals in medical research involved any moral issues. In most cultural traditions, people simply assumed that they could use animals for their own purposes. They hunted them down and killed them, sometimes for food, sometimes for clothing, sometimes for decoration, sometimes for sport. They used them for work, for transportation, and for amusement. They domesticated some of them and made others into personal pets.

The roots of this attitude run deep. The book of *Genesis* 3:28 depicts God giving humans dominion over all other living things—the fish in the sea, the birds of the air, and the animals of the earth—implying that people can use these creatures as they see fit. Jewish and Christian theology emphasized the disparity between humans and animals by insisting that God created only humans in his "image and likeness," and that this gives them a dignity not shared by animals. The Bible shows little concern for animal life.

Nor is there much respect for animals in Greek thought. The early Pythagoreans did respect animals because they thought that an animal might embody a reincarnated human soul, but Socrates and Plato rejected this idea. They taught that once the human soul leaves the body at death, it never returns to another body. The Pythagorean reason for respecting animal life was thus lost when its doctrine of reincarnation was superseded by the Platonic and later Christian teachings of an immaterial human soul living after death in a disembodied state.

René Descartes, known as the "father of modern philosophy," is a more modern example of one who did not accord any moral standing to animals. He compared them to machines. If someone designed a clever machine, he said, that looked like a human being, we would not be fooled for long that it really was a human being. In particular, we would notice two things. First, even though the machine may have been programmed to make the sounds of words, it would be incapable of participating in a meaningful conversation. Second, even though the machine may have been programmed to act in many different ways, it would be unable to learn how to act in all sorts of circumstances as humans can, thanks to their ability to reason. On the other hand, if someone designed a clever machine that looked and acted like a monkey, we would never be able to tell the difference between the machine and the monkey. The implication of Descartes' argument is obvious: if animals are like machines, and may one day be indistinguishable from them, they have no important moral standing.

It is not surprising, then, that ethical concerns for animals are almost totally absent from the major works of moral theology and moral philosophy in our cultural traditions. Ethics centered on how we treat ourselves and other human beings, but not on how we treat animals or the environment. In the past few decades, however, concern for our treatment of animals and for our relationship with the environment has been growing as more and more people become aware of the ethical issues in these areas of life.

Of the three main modern approaches to ethics—natural rights, the Kantian moral law, and utilitarianism—two (natural rights and utilitarianism) offer some support for the ethical treatment of animals. Moral theories based on rights can be expanded to include an ethics about animals by simply extending the notion of natural rights to animals. Once we claim animals have rights, especially the right to live naturally, we have given animals a moral standing that we must respect. The attribution of rights to animals reminds us that they are not there simply for our purposes.

The second major moral theory, utilitarianism, can also be extended to provide a moral standing for animals. The fundamental moral principle of utilitarianism is the "greatest happiness principle"—the action or the rule that brings the greatest happiness or pleasure to the greatest number is what is morally required. Now, since higher animals obviously experience pleasure and pain, they can easily be counted among the "greatest number" who will be affected by our actions. The utilitarian obligation to increase pleasure and reduce pain can easily be extended to include the pleasure and pain of animals. One of the founders of utilitarianism, Jeremy Bentham, took issue with Descartes on this very point. Descartes had thought that animals are like machines because they cannot speak or reason. Bentham countered: "The question is not Can they *reason*? nor Can they *talk*? but Can they *suffer*?"

Unfortunately, the third major moral theory, that of Kant, offers little to support the moral standing of animals. His ethics centered exclusively on respect for humanity. One version of his fundamental moral principle was: Act in such a way that you treat humanity, whether in your own person or in the person of another, always at the same time as an end and never simply as a means. Since he derived all moral laws from this fundamental moral principle, his moral laws pertain only to humanity, not to animals. Kant did suggest that mistreatment of animals is wrong, but it is wrong not because it is bad for the animals or because animals have moral worth, but because the mistreatment undermines the humanity of those tormenting the animals.

Today, considerable debate swirls around the ethics of our relationships with animals. As we have noted, this is a new moral concern since the older religious, theological, and philosophical ethics of our tradition all but ignored moral questions about the welfare of animals. And, as we might expect, the debate about the morality of behavior toward animals embraces a wide range of positions. At one extreme are those who argue against almost all use of animals for human purposes. They say it is immoral to use animals for medical research, to hunt, to use animals for work or transportation, to breed animals for food, to eat animals, to confine them as pets, etc. At the other extreme are those who maintain the more traditional position. They say almost any use of animals is morally acceptable as long as it contributes to human well-being. They have no problem using animals for medical research, or hunting them for sport, or plowing fields with them, or trapping them for fur, or raising them for food, or confining them in cages.

The debate over the ethics of how we should relate to animals will undoubtedly continue for some time. It is a whole new area for moral philosophy and moral theology, and it will take time to develop. In the meantime, by following the ethics of prudence and the human good that we have been developing in this book, several helpful points can be made about the use of animals in medical research.

First, deliberately doing anything that causes suffering or damage to life does not contribute to our good, unless we have cogent reasons to offset the bad things resulting from our actions. This ethics of right reason demands good reasons for research that will hurt or kill animals.

Second, this ethics encourages us to cherish, and not damage, all life— human life as well as the life of all living things, including animals and the environment. Yet it acknowledges the morality of employing living beings (including human beings) as the subjects of medical research even though no benefit, and some pain or damage, may ensue in their lives, provided certain moral safeguards are in place to prevent exploitation and provided beneficial advances in medicine are anticipated.

Third, biomedical research on animals is important, and sometimes crucial, for understanding and treating some human diseases. Research using computer models, plants, and live cultures can only go so far. Often the research must involve animals (and humans) before the therapeutic intervention or drug can be accepted as normal medical practice. Hence, there are good reasons for some animal research. The moral debate in this ethics of the good, then, centers on what reasons are strong enough to justify the suffering, damage, and death of animals used in research.

Fourth, undoubtedly, some animal research today is morally questionable. Better efforts are needed to reduce unnecessary pain and suffering. One thing we need is more explicit federal regulations, analogous to those developed in the past few decades for research on human subjects, guiding research on animals. These regulations would not require that animals be treated the same as human subjects in research, but would protect them from morally unreasonable treatment by requiring convincing reasons for any harmful experimentation.

Another way to prevent immoral animal research is by requiring approval by the local IRB operating under appropriate guidelines. By way of example, we can look at the review process used at Stanford University Medical Center to prevent the abuse, inappropriate use, or neglect of animals in research.

All the animal research at Stanford must be approved by the university's Panel on Laboratory Animal Care. Among recent members of the panel were a hospital chaplain and several veterinarians from the community with no other relationship with the university. Before beginning research involving animals, the investigator must give reasons why the animals have to be used and explain all the procedures that will involve them. He must also show how any pain or distress greater than that caused by a routine injection will be minimized, and list the anesthetics and pain-killing drugs that will be used. If surgery is involved, the preoperative, surgical, and postoperative interventions must be outlined in detail.

Perhaps the best way to prevent immoral animal research is to increase the effort aimed at reminding researchers of two things. First, the traditional ethics of our culture, both religious and philosophical, failed to acknowledge our moral relationship with animals. This failure has left us with a sort of moral vacuum where animals are concerned, so our traditional attitudes of dominion over them are not morally well-founded and cannot be trusted.

Second, an ethics based on the human good recognizes that our good is not achieved by causing unnecessary suffering and death in this world. This recognition serves as the basis for the humane treatment of all animals, including laboratory animals. The day may come when none of us will kill and eat animals or use them in research, but that day is not now realistic. Our immediate moral concerns, then, center on providing humane care for the animals we use, with good reasons, for nourishment and research.

SUGGESTED READINGS

The Tuskegee study is treated at length in James Jones. 1981. *Bad Blood: The Tuskegee Syphilis Experiment*. New York: The Free Press; and Pence, *Classic Cases*, chapter 9. See also articles by Arthur Caplan, Harold Edgar, Patricia King, and James Jones in a special section entitled "Twenty Years After: The Legacy of the Tuskegee Syphilis Study." *Hastings Center Report* **1992**, 22 (November–December), 29–40; William Curran. "The Tuskegee Syphilis Study." *NEJM* **1973**, *289*, 730–32; and Allan Brandt. "Racism and Research: the Case of the Tuskegee Syphilis Study." *Hastings Center Report* **1978**, 8 (December), 21–29.

Among the many treatments of the Nazi medical experiments are George Annas and Michael Grodin, eds. 1992. *The Nazi Doctors and the Nuremberg Code: Human Rights in Human Experimentation*. New York: Oxford University Press; Robert Jay Lifton. 1986. *The Nazi Doctors: Medical Killing and the Psychology of Genocide*. New York: Basic Books, chapters 15 and 17; Jay Katz. 1972. *Experimentation with Human Beings*. New York: Russell Sage Foundation, chapter 1; and Leo Alexander. "Medical Science Under Dictatorship." *NEJM* **1949**, *249*, 39–47. Alexander was a psychiatrist who served as a consultant to the American Chief of Counsel for War Crimes at the Nuremberg trials. The Nuremburg Code is frequently reprinted in books on medical research. Cf. for example Ronald Munson, *Intervention and Reflection: Basic Issues in Medical Ethics*, 4th ed., p. 392; Thomas Mappes and Jane Zembatty, *Biomedical Ethics*, 3rd ed., p. 210; and Robert Levine. 1981. *Ethics and the Regulation of Clinical Research*. Baltimore: Urban & Schwarzenberg, pp. 285f. The first principle ("The voluntary consent of the human subject is absolutely essential") is not always easy to arrange in practice. Recently physicians were testing a hand pump in St. Paul, Minnesota, that both compressed and then decompressed the chest of a person in cardiac arrest outside the hospital. Emergency medical technicians and paramedics were using the pump in some sections of the city in an effort to determine whether it was more effective than the standard CPR used in other sections. Of course, a person in cardiac arrest cannot give informed consent for the experimental pump, so the FDA (which approves medical devices) stopped the trial. Unfortunately, it is very difficult to see how one could ever obtain informed consent for trials involving resuscitation equipment designed for use by emergency medical personnel in cases of unexpected cardiopulmonary arrest outside a medical setting. Prudential reasoning suggests, therefore, that there may be cases (cardiac arrest, for example) where the informed consent of the subject for some unapproved equipment is not absolutely essential. See Keith Lurie et al, "Evaluation of Active Compression-Decompression CPR in Victims of Out-of-Hospital Cardiac Arrest," *JAMA* **1994,**

271, 1405–1411; and Carin Olson, "The Letter or the Spirit: Consent for Research in CPR," *JAMA* **1994,** *271,* 1445–1447.

Paul Ramsey's criticism of Willowbrook is found in *The Patient as Person.* 1970. New Haven: Yale University Press, pp. 47–56. The editorial defense of Willowbrook as "not unethical" is by Franz Ingelfinger. "Ethics of Experiments on Children." *NEJM* **1973,** *288,* 791–92. An excellent summary of the cancer research at the Jewish Chronic Disease Hospital can be found in Katz, *Experimentation,* chapter 1.

Accounts of the obedience studies can be found in Stanley Milgram. 1974. *Obedience to Authority: An Experimental View.* New York: Harper & Row Publishers; Sissela Bok. 1979. *Lying: Moral Choice in Public and Private Life.* New York: Random House, pp. 193–95; and Ruth Faden and Tom Beauchamp. 1986. *A History and Theory of Informed Consent.* New York: Oxford University Press, pp. 174–77. Milgram defended the ethics of his research—see, for example, his "Subject Reaction: The Neglected Factor in the Ethics of Experimentation." *Hastings Center Report* **1977,** 7 (October), 19–23. Here he argues that misinformation has a place in behavioral research if it is unavoidable, and that almost no subjects in his experiments were harmed since questionnaires returned after the tests showed over 98 percent of the people were "glad" or "very glad" they participated in the experiment.

Among the articles and books sparking the public reaction to the questionable morality prevailing in medical research were: Henry Beecher. "Ethics and Clinical Research." *NEJM* **1966,** *274,* 1354–60; M.H. Pappworth. 1967. *Human Guinea Pigs: Experimentation on Man.* Boston: Beacon Press, 1967; Henry Beecher. 1970. *Research and the Individual.* Boston: Little, Brown and Co.; and Jay Katz, *Experimentation.* See also David Rothman. "Ethics and Human Experimentation: Henry Beecher Revisited." *NEJM* **1987,** *317,* 1195–99; Jay Katz. "Reflections on Unethical Experiments and the Beginnings of Bioethics in the United States." *Kennedy Institute of Ethics Journal* **1994,** *4,* 85–92; and Jay Katz. "'Ethics and Clinical Research' Revisited: A Tribute to Henry K. Beecher." *Hastings Center Report* **1993,** *23* (September–October), 31–39.

The quotation from William Frankena is from "the principles of morality" in Kenneth Goodpaster, ed. 1976. *Perspectives on Morality: Essays of William Frankena.* Notre Dame: Notre Dame University Press, p. 174. The essay originally appeared in C. L. Carter, ed. 1973. *Skepticism and Moral Principles.* Chicago: New University Press. The influential textbook that helped establish the ethical model of principles in medical ethics was Beauchamp and Childress, *Principles of Biomedical Ethics,* 1979 (first edition), 1982 (second edition), 1989 (third edition), and 1994 (fourth edition). Commissioner Albert Jonsen's criticism of the principlism found in the National Commission's *Belmont Report* can be found in his "American Moralism and the Origin of Bioethics in the United States." *Journal of Medicine and Philosophy* **1991,** *16,* 115–29; the quotation is from p. 125.

For the HHS and FDA regulations influenced by the reports of the National Commission, see 46 *Fed. Reg.* 8,366 (January 26, 1981) and 46 *Fed. Reg.* 8,942 (January 27, 1981). See also the 56 *Fed. Reg.* 28,003 (June 18, 1991) for later modifications to the regulations. Press reports of the recent morally questionable research incidents are taken from the *New York Times,* October 5, 1993, p. C 3, and October 28, 1993, p. B 5, and from the *Boston Globe,* October 31, 1993, pp. 1 and 28.

The President's Commission reports on research are: *Protecting Human Subjects* (1981), *Whistleblowing in Biomedical Research* (1981), *Compensating for Research Injuries* (1982), and *Implementing Human Research Regulations* (1983). They were originally published by the U.S. Government Printing Office and later by Indiana University

Press. The quotations showing the central role played by the three principles in the commission's work are from the final report, *Summing Up* (1983), p. 67.

Among the many articles on embryonic and fetal research are Leon Kass. 1985. *Toward a More Natural Science*. New York: The Free Press, especially chapter 4, entitled "The Meaning of Life—in the Laboratory;" Richard McCormick. 1985. *How Brave a New World?* Washington: Georgetown University Press, especially chapter 5, entitled "Public Policy and Fetal Research;" Henry Greely et al. "The Ethical Use of Human Fetal Tissue in Medicine." *NEJM* **1989**, *320*, 1093–96; John Fletcher and Joseph Schulman. "Fetal Research: The State of the Art, the State of the Question." *Hastings Center Report* **1985**, *15* (April), 6–12; John Fletcher and Kenneth Ryan. "Federal Regulations for Fetal Research: A Case for Reform." *Law, Medicine & Health Care* **1987**, *15*, 126–38. The conclusions and recommendations of the National Commission relevant to fetal research can be found in the *Hastings Center Report* **1975**, *5* (June), 41–46. This issue of the report also contains a valuable collection of abridged papers that were submitted to the commission during its deliberations. Also important is Steinbock, *Life Before Birth*, chapters 5 and 6.

For Paul Ramsey's criticism of all research on minors, see "The Enforcement of Morals: Nontherapeutic Research on Children." *Hastings Center Report* **1976**, *6* (August), 21–30. McCormick's defense of limited research on children can be found in *How Brave a New World?* chapters 4, 6, and 7. The crucial point in his argument is: "I believe my own analysis is precisely at root and in substance a best-interests test: The fetus/child would choose nontherapeutic experimentation of minimal risk because it is compatible with and not opposed to his best interests." (p. 113). This is more of an assertion than a reason. We can never say that we know a human being who never had decision-making capacity would choose to participate in medical research. In fact, some people do decline to participate in medical research even when the risk is minimal or absent.

For the story of Compound Q, see Martin Delaney. "The Case for Patient Access to Experimental Therapy." *Journal of Infectious Disease* **1989**, *159*, 416–19; stories by Gina Kolata in the *New York Times* for September 19 (B 7) and September 20, 1989 (A 14); by Philip Hilts in the *New York Times* for September 27, 1989 (A 15); and by Randy Shilts in the *San Francisco Chronicle* for September 20, 1989 (A 4). See also Ronald Bayer. "Public Health Policy and the AIDS Epidemic: An End to HIV Exceptionalism?" *NEJM* **1991**, *324*, 1500–04; and Bernard Lo. "Ethical Dilemmas in HIV Infection: What Have We Learned?" *Law, Medicine & Health Care* **1992**, *20*, 92–103.

Descartes' remarks on animals can be found in part five of his *Discourse on Method*, first published in 1637. In an early work, Kant's lack of moral concern for animals emerged clearly: "But so far as animals are concerned, we have no direct duties. Animals are not self-conscious and are there merely as a means to an end. That end is man." Kant, *Lectures on Ethics*, p. 239. (These lectures were recorded by Kant's students at the University of Konigsberg during 1775–1780 and first published in 1924). Jeremy Bentham's remark on the ethical importance of animal suffering is from chapter 17 of his *An Introduction to the Principles of Morals and Legislation*, first printed in 1780.

A leading proponent of animal rights in our country is Tom Regan. He advanced his theory in *The Case for Animal Rights*. 1983. Berkeley: University of California Press, and several articles including "The Moral Standing of Animals in Medical Research." *Law, Medicine & Health Care* **1992**, *20*, 7–16. A leading proponent of the utilitarian approach to the moral treatment of animals is Peter Singer. See his *Animal Liberation*. 1977. New York: Random House. See also Tom Regan and Peter Singer, eds. 1976. *Animal Rights and Human Obligation*. Englewood Cliffs:

Prentice-Hall; Barbara Orlans. 1993. *In the Name of Science: Issues in Responsible Animal Experimentation*. New York: Oxford University Press; H. J. McCloskey. "The Moral Case for Experimentation on Animals." *The Monist* **1987**, 70, 64–70; Arthur Caplan. "Beastly Conduct: Ethical Issues in Animal Experimentation." *Annals of the New York Academy of Sciences* **1983**, 406, 159–69; Christina Hoff. "Immoral and Moral Uses of Animals." *NEJM* **1980**, 302, 115–18; Charles McCarthy. "Improved Standards for Laboratory Animals." *Kennedy Institute of Ethics Journal* **1993**, 3, 293–302; and Gary Varner. "The Prospects for Consensus and Convergence in the Animal Rights Debate." *Hastings Center Report* **1994**, 24 (January–February), 24–28. Information about the procedures for protecting research at Stanford University Medical Center was taken from James Thomas et al. "Animal Research at Stanford University." *NEJM* **1988**, *318,* 1630–32.

15

Transplantation

Surgeons have been inserting organs and tissues, as well as artificial devices, into patients for several decades. These surgeries often raise profound ethical questions. In this chapter we will consider the ethical issues generated by the transplantation of organs and by the implantation of artificial hearts.

Although successful transplantation of a kidney from one dog to another was reported at the beginning of the century, transplanting a human kidney did not become a realistic possibility until 1947 when surgeons at Boston's Peter Bent Brigham Hospital attached a kidney taken from a cadaver to the arm of an unconscious patient. The external kidney produced urine until it was rejected by the patient's immune system several days later. By that time the woman's kidneys had regained adequate functioning, and she eventually recovered. The rather crude procedure convinced many that kidney transplantations could succeed.

In 1953 Dr. David Hume performed a somewhat successful kidney transplantation, also at the Peter Bent Brigham Hospital. The patient was able to leave the hospital and survived almost six months. In 1954, again at the same hospital, Dr. Joseph Murray transplanted a kidney from one identical twin to another. This transplantation is now considered the first successful kidney transplant—the twenty-four-year-old recipient lived eight years after receiving his brother's kidney. Using a kidney from an identical twin avoided the usual problems of rejection triggered by the recipient's immune system. Improved immunosuppressive drugs were soon developed, and in 1962 the transplantation of a kidney from a donor unrelated to the patient was successful.

Dr. Christiaan Barnard performed the first heart transplantation in South Africa on December 3, 1967. The patient was Louis Washkansky, a fifty-five year old man with diabetes, coronary artery disease, and congestive heart failure. The heart came from a twenty-five-year-old woman fatally injured when she was struck by a car less than a mile from the hospital. After her pulse ceased for several minutes, she was placed on a heart-lung machine to nourish her heart while Louis was prepared for surgery in a nearby operating room. After surgeons implanted her heart in Washkansky's chest, they started it with electric shocks. He recovered from the surgery and made good progress for almost two weeks. Then his condition rapidly deteriorated. He was in pain, lost control of his bodily functions, and needed a feeding tube and a respirator. His heart went into fibrillation and, after some discussion, physicians decided not to put him back on a heart–lung machine. He died less than three weeks after the transplant, on December 22, 1967.

On December 6, 1967, three days after Washkansky received his transplant in South Africa, Dr. Adrian Kantrowitz performed the first successful heart transplantation in the United States at Maimonides Hospital in Brooklyn.

The heart came from an anencephalic infant. Earlier, in June 1966, Dr. Kantrowitz had tried to transplant a heart from another anencephalic infant, but the implanted heart did not restart. This time the donor baby was chilled by immersion in ice water while still alive, and the heart was removed immediately after it stopped beating. Although the recipient lived only six and a half hours, the operation was considered successful, and it is now acknowledged as the first heart transplant in the United States.

In the next few years, scores of heart transplants were attempted, but most patients died in the first few months after the surgery. Liver transplants also began in 1967, but success in the early years was very limited.

A major problem affecting organ transplantation in the early years was the rejection of the new organ by the body's immune system. A giant step in overcoming this rejection came with the development of a better immunosuppressive drug, cyclosporine. This drug was approved by the FDA in 1983. Despite some toxic reactions caused by the drug, it noticeably reduced the rejection problem and significantly increased survival rates. More recently, other promising immunosuppressive drugs, among them one known as FK 506, have been introduced.

Transplantation efforts now include the pancreas, the heart and lung as a unit, corneas, heart valves, skin, bone, bone marrow, partial livers, intestines, blood vessels, tendons, and ligaments. In December 1989 a leading transplant surgeon, Dr. Thomas Starzl, implanted a heart, a liver, and a kidney into a young woman; she died four months later of hepatitis. That same month, physicians began transplanting liver lobes from living parents to their children at the University of Chicago Medical Center. In a few cases organs from animals have been transplanted into humans.

Efforts have also been made to implant mechanical devices as substitutes for organs, most notably, artificial hearts. In 1969 Dr. Denton Cooley implanted the first totally artificial heart in Haskell Karp at the Texas Heart Institute in Houston. Haskell died in a matter of days. His wife sued Dr. Cooley, claiming that the innovative nature of the implantation, which offered no real hope of good health for her husband, was never explained to her or to her husband. The case was dismissed, but questions about appropriate informed consent for what was really a radical medical experiment lingered.

In 1982 Dr. William DeVries implanted a permanent artificial heart into Barney Clark at the University of Utah Medical Center in Salt Lake City. It was a cumbersome device, requiring a bedside air compressor weighing over 300 pounds to drive the internal pump known as the Jarvik–7. Numerous complications developed, and Barney Clark needed several additional surgeries. His condition deteriorated and, four months later, after many of his vital organs failed, the pump was shut off and he died.

In this chapter we will consider the ethical issues surrounding the use of transplanted organs and artificial hearts in the following order:

1. Transplantation of organs from dead human donors
2. Transplantation of organs from living human donors
3. Transplantation of organs from animals
4. Implantation of artificial hearts

TRANSPLANTATION OF ORGANS FROM DEAD HUMAN DONORS

In our culture, most people readily accept the transplantation of organs re-trieved from a donor after death. Indeed, many think, with good reason, that donating organs after death is morally admirable. At least part of the reason why so many in our culture are morally comfortable with retrieving organs from cadavers is the long history of using cadavers in our medical schools and of performing autopsies to learn about diseases and the causes of death. These practices have made many comfortable with using dead bodies to help the living.

This cultural comfort is reflected in the Uniform Anatomical Gift Act (UAGA), first approved in 1968 by the National Conference of Commissioners on Uniform State Laws and the American Bar Association, and now adopted, in some form, by all 50 states and the District of Columbia. This UAGA allows people of sound mind and at least 18 years of age to donate all or any part of their bodies for various uses after they die, including transplantation. People can designate the gift in a will or in a document signed in the presence of two witnesses. In some states, people can express their desires to donate their organs on their drivers' licences.

The UAGA also allows family members, or the person's guardian at the time of death, to donate organs of the deceased, provided the person had not indicated his opposition to organ retrieval while he was alive. Those empowered to make these decisions fall into a list whereby those higher on the list, if they are available, take precedence over those listed at a lower level. The UAGA list of family members who can donate the organs of a deceased person sets the following order of priority: the spouse, an adult child, either parent, an adult sibling, legal guardian at the time of death, any other person authorized or obliged to dispose of the body.

The UAGA allows a person low on the list to donate the organs of the deceased person, provided no one at the same level or a higher level on the list objects. Thus a sister could donate her brother's organs as long as neither his wife, nor any of his children, nor one of his parents, objected.

The UAGA also allows potential recipients to refuse the donation of a cadaver or organs. Thus, if the organs are not usable, the transplant team can refuse the donation.

According to the UAGA, the donated organs cannot be removed until the donor's attending physician or, if there is no attending physician, another physician has determined that the person is dead. The physician determining death may not participate in removing organs or in transplanting them to the recipient. The UAGA also protects physicians acting in good faith from both civil and criminal litigation. This means, for example, that transplant surgeons with good reasons for believing a patient wanted his organs donated could not be prosecuted or sued if it was later discovered that the patient had revoked his consent to donation.

Although one might expect that the clear wishes of persons to donate their organs after death would always be respected, this is not the case. In reality, if family members object to the organ retrieval, the transplant team will almost always decline to retrieve the organs despite certain knowledge and clear documentation that the deceased person wanted the organs donated. The reluctance of transplant teams to retrieve donated organs against the wishes of the family is motivated in large part by their desire not to upset the family at a time of loss and grief. The team also wants to avoid possible negative publicity about organ transplantation. Moreover, the body of a deceased person belongs, in a sense, to the family, and delaying its release in order to harvest organs against family wishes would place members of a transplant team in an uncomfortable position.

The UAGA, and the various state laws derived from it, have facilitated and encouraged the donation of cadaverous organs. Most ethicists believe the UAGA is, in general, morally sound, and many ethicists encourage the donation of organs after death. In an ethics of virtue, it is clearly an expression of the virtue of love, defined by Aristotle as doing something for another for the sake of the other and not for any personal gain.

Despite the general agreement about the morality of cadaverous transplantations as long as appropriate consent is obtained from the donor or from the family, these transplantations have spawned two major ethical questions. The first centers on determining the moment of death, the second on the allocation of scarce organs. These questions need to be discussed in some detail.

Death and Organ Retrieval

Transplantation requires organs that are well-nourished by oxygenated blood. This means the team must remove them as soon as possible after death. Determining the moment of death thus becomes a crucial issue. Taking the heart out of a person not yet dead is not an act of organ retrieval, but an act of killing someone to get his organs.

The two criteria now used to determine when a person is dead were explained in chapter six. The first, and traditional, criterion of death is the irreversible cessation of the cardiopulmonary functions. When this occurs, the person is dead. Unfortunately, relying on this criterion of death undermines the possibility of retrieving the organs in many cases. Cardiopulmonary functions often weaken over a period of time before they finally stop, and organs are often damaged while the person is dying. Moreover, the surgeon cannot retrieve organs after the cardiopulmonary arrest until he is sure that the cessation is irreversible. This determination takes time, and the delay causes the organs additional damage.

The second criterion of death is the irreversible cessation of all brain functions, including those of the brain stem. Ordinarily, the cessation of all brain functions in a person leads almost immediately to the irreversible cessation of cardiopulmonary functions as well, but life-support equipment or a heart–lung machine can sometimes support the cardiopulmonary functions after the brain functions have ceased. When this occurs, it presents an ideal opportunity for organ retrieval. The brain-dead patient on life support is truly dead, but the organs are being nourished as if she were alive. It is not surprising, then, that one of the factors driving the discussion and eventual acceptance of the brain-death criterion in the 1960s was the need for fresh organs in the emerging field of transplantation.

Although the two criteria of human death are relatively clear and widely accepted, the need for fresh organs has generated several concerns relevant to organ retrieval and the criteria of death.

Concerns related to attempting resuscitation

The cardiopulmonary criterion of death is normally the way death is determined. (The brain-death criterion is used only when the person's cardiopulmonary functions are sustained by life-support equipment.) Unfortunately, the possibility of attempting cardiopulmonary resuscitation after any cardiopulmonary arrest complicates the retrieval of fresh organs. Resuscitation efforts can delay for many minutes the harvesting of organs from a donor whose cardiopulmonary arrest is, in fact, irreversible but the irreversibility is not yet clear to those attempting resuscitation. And, on the other hand, the knowledge that organs are destined for donation can create a temptation to curtail resuscitation efforts prematurely lest the organs be damaged.

Two worthy causes collide in the final moments of a donor's life. The team doing CPR is working diligently to save the donor's life while the transplant team is waiting to retrieve usable organs. The longer CPR is attempted, the less chance there is of retrieving viable organs, and the CPR team knows this. Their moral problem centers on how to integrate the patient's desire to donate his organs with their efforts to resuscitate him if possible. If the patient is not a donor, they can easily afford to continue resuscitation efforts a few extra minutes "just in case" revival is possible, but those few extra minutes can undermine the patient's desire to donate by delaying retrieval of the organs.

Another ethical problem can arise when resuscitation will not be attempted, perhaps because the person is subject to a DNR order. Here there may be a temptation to retrieve the organs almost immediately after the heart stops. In the first few minutes after a cardiopulmonary arrest, however, it is not known for sure whether the cessation of cardiopulmonary functions is irreversible. There is always the chance, in the first few minutes, that the cardiac arrest could be reversed if CPR were attempted. Hence it cannot be said that these patients have clearly suffered the irreversible cessation of cardiopulmonary functions. Of course, when CPR will not be attempted, the arrest will not in fact be reversed, but this is not the same as saying the arrest is irreversible. Only when we are certain that the cessation of all the cardiopulmonary functions is *irreversible* can we say the person is dead, and this certainty is not present in the first few minutes after the arrest of a person for whom CPR will not be attempted.

It can be argued that moral concern about this is groundless. Cardiopulmonary arrests seldom reverse themselves, so a decision not to attempt CPR after an arrest means that the arrest will be permanent. Still, the accepted cardiopulmonary criterion of death states that the arrest must be *irreversible*, and not simply an arrest where reversal will not be attempted. If we do not want to chance harvesting organs from the still living, we cannot begin until we know that the cessation of the cardiopulmonary functions is truly *irreversible*, and this takes time. Even after ten minutes, some arrests are partially reversible, and the person lives despite neurological damage.

Concerns related to consent

Transplant teams normally do not attempt retrieval of organs from a donor without the permission of the family. Now, if the death of a person not on a life-support system was unexpected, by the time permission is obtained from a family member, the organs are often too damaged for use. The process of obtaining consent from family members is time-consuming, especially if the deceased person had not indicated he wanted to donate organs. Physicians have to explain what donation entails to a family in a difficult position. They have just been told a loved one is dead, and now they must decide immediately whether or not to give consent for the retrieval of his organs. If they delay more than a short time, the organs will be too damaged for use.

In an attempt to save organs while permission for transplantation is being sought, some physicians have injected ice-cold saline solutions into the bodies of potential donors as soon as they have died. Cooling the organs reduces their need for blood and oxygen, and gives the physicians time to seek permission or consent for organ retrieval from the family. If the family grants permission or consent, the organs can be used. If the family does not consent to organ retrieval, no real harm was done to the potential donor because the person was already dead when the cooling solution was injected. Nonetheless, there are legitimate ethical concerns over treating a dead body this way without any consent by the person or by the family.

Concerns about living, breathing bodies

Organ retrieval from the brain-dead can create a certain level of moral discomfort for some people. After the determination of brain death is made, the life-support equipment will be continued to preserve the organs until the transplant team and the recipients are ready for the procedure. When all is ready, the organ retrieval will begin, sometimes without stopping the life support. For some, this appears to be taking organs from a living person, and it is morally upsetting. In fact, however, if the brain-death criterion is accepted, and if the clinical verification has been accurate, there are no moral problems associated with retrieving a kidney, for example, from a donor while life-support equipment continues to sustain his respiratory and circulatory functions. Despite appearances, it is simply another case of cadaverous organ donation.

Concerns about the brain-death definition itself

Other legitimate moral problems, however, do surround the use of the brain-death criterion in organ transplantation. For example, the brain-death criterion of death requires that "all functions of the entire brain" have irreversibly ceased, but the meaning of "all functions of the entire brain" has never been clearly defined. Sometimes small pockets of dying brain cells remain functioning, and small amounts of electrical activity persist, in people determined to be dead according to the current clinical criteria for brain death. And it has been reported that organ retrieval has triggered hemodynamic responses in the blood circulation of brain-dead patients. Since these hemodynamic responses are thought to originate in the brain, their detection raises questions about the clarity of the phrase "all functions of the entire brain."

The need for organs has prompted some people to suggest that the brain-death criterion should be made less demanding. They propose requiring only the irreversible cessation of higher brain functions, what some call "neo-cortical death." If brain death were understood as neocortical death, it would permit retrieval of organs from people in PVS and permanent coma; that is, from some permanently unconscious patients sustained only by feeding tubes. At the present time, however, the permanently unconscious are not considered brain dead, and reasons for not adopting this criterion of death were noted in chapter six.

Concerns related to brain death in children

Some controversy exists about the ability to determine brain death in children, especially very young children and neonates. The President's Commission report entitled *Defining Death* (1982) noted that the brains of infants and young children have more resistance to damage than older brains, and that they may recover substantive functions after longer periods of unresponsiveness. The commission therefore urged physicians to be cautious about applying the standard clinical criteria of brain death to children under five years of age.

A special group called the Task Force on Brain Death in Childhood (1985–1986) recommended various clinical criteria for determining brain death in three categories of young children: those over one year of age, those between two months and one year, and those between seven days and two months. These carefully crafted criteria are helpful, although they do not apply to infants under seven days of age. Several medical centers have also developed clinical criteria for diagnosing brain death in young children.

Still, the difficulty of diagnosing brain death in children, especially infants, remains, and it has inhibited the use of the brain-death standard for infants whose parents have consented to organ donation. Thus, organ retrieval from infants hinges mostly on the cardiopulmonary criterion of death. As we have noted, waiting for verification that circulatory and respiratory functions have irreversibly ceased often means a damaging delay for the organs.

The difficulties in applying the brain-death criterion to young children and in retrieving healthy organs when the cardiopulmonary criterion of death is employed have prompted some physicians to stretch the cardiopulmonary criterion of death in several ways when organ retrieval from infants is an issue. For example, as we noted in the first successful heart transplant in the United States, the infant donor's heart was removed immediately after it stopped beating. It is hard to think such immediate retrieval could satisfy the currently accepted cardiopulmonary criterion—"irreversible cessation of the circulatory and respiratory functions"—because CPR efforts might well have temporarily restored the infant's cardiac function. Since successful resuscitation cannot be ruled out immediately after cardiac arrest, it is difficult to see how we can be certain an infant is dead immediately after his heart stops beating.

Concerns related to anencephaly

Some see anencephalic infants as a promising source of organ donations. These infants usually do not live long, and often their organs are healthy.

Some suggest we should consider infants with anencephaly "brain-dead" even though they never had a living brain that could have died. Several years ago, physicians in Germany considered two anencephalic infants brain-dead, placed them on ventilators, and harvested their kidneys within an hour of birth.

One of these infants was a twin whose anencephaly was diagnosed at 16 weeks of gestation. In what was an obvious inconsistency in moral reasoning, the parents declined an elective abortion because it was "morally unacceptable," yet they consented to the lethal action of removing the living infant's kidneys. In effect, they thought it was immoral for physicians to destroy the fetus before birth, but not immoral for physicians to destroy the infant by taking the kidneys an hour after birth. Apparently, it never dawned on them that if the baby was "brain-dead" after birth and could therefore be destroyed (by the act of retrieving its organs), then it was also "brain-dead" before birth and could therefore be aborted without moral objection.

Of course, the anencephalic infant was not brain-dead at all, and the kidneys should not have been taken from the living infant. The legal authorities in Germany have since put a stop to the retrieval of organs from anencephalic infants, and rightly so. As much as we need organs for transplantation, it is hard to see how taking them from infants who are not dead by currently accepted criteria will make us noble and good people.

The need for infant organs moved physicians at Loma Linda Hospital in California to try a different approach. They put infants suffering from anencephaly on life support, and then withdrew the infant from the ventilator at periodic intervals to determine whether or not the infant could breathe without ventilation. If the infant breathed spontaneously, he was put back on the ventilator; if not, he was declared dead and the organs were retrieved. The lack of spontaneous respiration was taken as a clinical sign that the child has recently died while on the life support.

What criterion of death was being used in this protocol? Strictly speaking, neither of those currently in use. Mere cessation of spontaneous respiration does not fulfill the cardiopulmonary criterion of death—this criterion requires *irreversible* cessation of respiratory functions. And cessation of spontaneous respiration does not fulfill the brain-death criterion of death—this criterion requires extensive neurological testing and is not satisfied by observing that a ventilator-dependent infant cannot breathe without the ventilator. After moral objections were raised about treating anencephalic infants this way, the hospital abandoned the practice.

The need for infant organs has led others to suggest still another approach. Admitting that we cannot say anencephalic infants are dead according to either of the two current criteria (brain death or irreversible cessation of cardiopulmonary functions), they advocate changing the criteria or, if the criteria are not changed, making a special case for anencephalic infants so their organs can be retrieved before they die. As you may well imagine, many ethical objections have been raised against these strategies. It is simply not a good idea, many argue, to change the criteria of death in order to harvest more organs from anencephalic infants, or to allow organ harvesting from any living infants, even those suffering from anencephaly.

Today, the debate about retrieving organs from anencephalic infants has abated somewhat because the numbers are decreasing. Many cases are discovered by prenatal diagnosis, and a number of women choose abortion, reducing the number of infants born with anencephaly.

In summary, a number of issues surrounding the determination of death are still associated with organ retrieval. The chronic shortage of organs for transplantation is one reason why these ethical issues linger. The shortage puts pressure on physicians to make every donated organ count, and this means retrieving them as soon as possible after death.

The unfortunate organ shortage also creates the second major ethical question emerging from donation after death—allocating the organs we do retrieve. We will now consider some of the vexing ethical problems associated with the distribution of organs.

Allocation of Scarce Cadaverous Organs

Organ transplantation is an example of a major social and ethical dilemma in health care—the distribution of scarce resources. Organ transplants save lives but, at the present time, we cannot supply organs to everyone who needs them. How, then, do we select the lucky ones, knowing that many of those not selected will die? It is a hard choice, captured well in the question: "Who shall live when not all can live?"

The problems of allocating scarce medical resources surfaced in the national consciousness over thirty years ago. In 1962 *Life* magazine published a famous story entitled "They Decide Who Lives, Who Dies." It was written by a young staff writer named Shana Alexander and it described the work of the Admissions and Policy Committee formed by the Seattle Artificial Kidney Center. A primary responsibility of this committee was to select patients for dialysis. End stage renal disease, or kidney failure, was a terminal disease at that time. Kidney transplants were rare and not very successful. No other life-saving options existed until Dr. Belding Scribner invented a dialysis machine in 1961. This machine removed enough impurities from the blood to prolong the life of many patients with kidney failure for years.

Dialysis is expensive and, when it first became available, many more patients needed it than could be accommodated. There were not enough of these "kidney machines," just as there are not enough kidneys today, so access had to be controlled. In an effort to be fair, the Seattle Kidney Center formed the Admissions and Policy Committee, composed mostly of people who were not physicians. They used three criteria to select patients for dialysis: (1) the patient's capacity to take an active and cooperative role in her care; (2) the patient's ability to lead a productive life, surmised from factors such as marital status, number of dependents, income, educational background, and employment history; and (3) the patient's ability to tolerate the psychological and physical stresses of constant dialysis.

When the selection criteria used by the committee became public, it started a national debate about the ethical basis for determining who will receive scarce medical resources. Criticism of the committee and its criteria spread rapidly. The committee was called the "God Squad" because it decided, in effect, who will live and who will die, and many people believe these decisions belong to God. The selection criteria were also attacked, chiefly because they introduced considerations of social worth and therefore discriminated against socially and economically disadvantaged patients.

Public distress over people being deprived of life-saving treatment because of shortages spread and soon caught the attention of elected officials. Congress responded by creating the End Stage Renal Disease Program (ESRD) in 1972. This program extended Medicare, a federal program designed mostly for those over 65, to people of any age suffering from kidney failure. Under the program, Medicare pays most of the costs for dialysis and, when a kidney becomes available for a suitable recipient, for transplantation.

Once the federal government began underwriting dialysis, the number of dialysis centers increased rapidly. By 1993 the number of dialysis patients had grown to more than 150,000. Some estimates place the number of dialysis patients at 240,000 by the year 2000.

The ESRD program has become enormously expensive for the federal government. Although early figures estimated that Medicare costs for the treatments would level off at 1 billion dollars a year, by 1993 they had reached 5.5 billion dollars annually. Moreover, studies published in early 1994 showed that the benefits of dialysis for certain groups—older patients and diabetics, for example—were limited in terms of both the quality and the length of life. Given the staggering costs and less than optimal outcomes, it is highly unlikely that Congress will ever again create something like the End Stage Renal Disease Program to resolve problems associated with the allocation of expensive life-saving treatments and transplantations.

The allocation problems facing us today are twofold. With kidneys it is simply a matter of shortage; Medicare is taking care of the costs. With other organs, such as livers and hearts, it is a matter of shortages and of costs—organ transplantations and their supporting treatments are enormously expensive. Given the shortage of organs and the high cost to insurers or to patients for all but kidney transplants, somebody has to select the patients who will become recipients. Since those not selected will suffer and often die, selecting who will, and who will not, receive an organ is very much a moral decision.

Selecting people for transplants is really a two-stage affair. In the first stage, the selection determines who will be placed on the waiting list for an organ. In the second stage, the selection determines who on the waiting list will receive the next available organ. Selecting the organ recipient from those on the waiting list is very difficult, and extensive controversy still exists over the criteria used for the selection.

What then, might be morally acceptable criteria for selecting candidates and recipients for transplants? What follows is an attempt to develop a reasonable and ethical way to allocate scarce organs.

First Stage: Criteria for placing candidates on the waiting list

Good ethics indicates that a number of important circumstances should be considered in selecting candidates for the waiting list. Among them are:

Medical criteria. Two factors are relevant here. First, the medical condition of the patient must be such that the transplantation of a scarce organ is needed to preserve his life. If the transplant is a heart, for example, the patient must have a terminal cardiac condition for which no alternative treatment is available. If the transplant is a liver, the patient must have irreversible liver disease for which no alternative treatment is available. If the transplant is a kidney, the patient must be experiencing significant diminishing returns from dialysis.

Second, the medical condition of the patient must not include strong adverse factors that would undermine the transplant. If the desired transplant is a heart, for example, hypertension, active infection, chronic bronchitis, and advancing age are reasonable contraindications against accepting a patient as a candidate for a heart transplant. If the desired transplant is a liver and the patient is an alcoholic still drinking, it is not unreasonable to decline her a place on the list until the underlying disease of alcoholism is brought under control. If the transplant is a kidney, it is not unreasonable to decline a place on the list for patients suffering from another terminal disease expected to take their lives in the near future.

Psychological criteria.   Three factors are relevant here. First, the patient must understand and be committed to the rigors of transplantation. Second, the patient must be able to tolerate the stresses of the transplant surgery and the possible disappointment if his body rejects the transplant. Third, the patient must be able and willing to embrace the extended treatment plan needed after the transplantation.

The psychological criteria are clearly not as objective as the medical criteria, and disagreements about their use continue to this day. What is a reasonable ethical response, for example, if the person needing the organ has has been so mentally and emotionally unstable that he has not taken care of himself for decades? We should not discriminate against the psychologically handicapped, but we should not transplant a scarce organ when there is no reason to believe the recipient will be faithful to subsequent treatments necessary to prevent rejection.

Social criteria.   Earlier transplant programs relied on social criteria to determine whether a person should be accepted as a candidate for a transplant. It was considered important to know whether the patient would have good family support after the operation, for example. After many people objected to considerations of this kind—it did not seem fair, for example, to deny someone an organ simply because he did not have a strong family support system—social criteria have become less important in the selection process. Nonetheless, they remain a circumstance of some weight in the ethics of right reason that we are pursuing in this book. It seems clearly unreasonable, for example, to transplant a scarce kidney to a person serving life imprisonment for first degree murders. Some social criteria are relevant in a morally reasonable selection process.

Financial criteria.   The special Medicare payment program has eliminated the need to consider the ability to pay when it is a question of transplanting kidneys. This is not so for other transplants. In 1986 the government did include heart transplants in standard Medicare coverage, but this helps only those over 65 or disabled. Medicare coverage for liver transplants is also restricted. Some state Medicaid programs cover transplants, but this coverage is limited to people enrolled in welfare programs and often provides less than full reimbursement. Many health insurance plans now cover transplants, but this does not help the millions of Americans without health insurance at any given time.

If a potential patient does not have Medicare, Medicaid, or private insurance, a transplant center will often demand a large deposit before a person is placed on the list as a candidate for an organ. The amount of these deposits varies, but the New York State Task Force report on organ transplantation gave two examples. It found deposits for heart transplants ranging from $40,000 to $125,000, and noted that Pittsburgh's Presbyterian–University Hospital, the nation's leading liver transplant center, requires a deposit of $100,000 before it will place a person without insurance coverage on the waiting list for a liver. The need for insurance, or a lot of money, explains why various fund raising efforts are often taking place for desperate families and friends trying to raise enough money to place someone on the list for a life-saving transplant.

From an ethical point of view, insisting on payment capability before accepting an otherwise qualified person as a candidate for an organ is disturbing. It means those who cannot pay will die. Yet it must also be asked who should pay when the patient not covered by insurance cannot pay? Some say that the government should pay, as it does in the ESRD program. But the unexpectedly high costs of this program undermine efforts in this direction. Moreover, if federal funds were available for transplants, the temptation for insurance companies to forego coverage, knowing the government will take care of it, will be great. And if federal funds were used for transplants, the effort to expand government funding for other life-saving techniques and technologies would be hard to stop.

In our present health care system, there is no easy answer. It is certainly upsetting to know some people who could benefit from a transplant are not placed on the list of candidates because they cannot pay for the surgery. There is something wrong with this. Yet it is also unreasonable to ignore the financial aspects of transplantation. The operations are expensive, and somebody has to pay for them. Perhaps the most ethical response, in our present system of health care, is to acknowledge that financial criteria do play some role in selecting recipients and then to encourage centers to accept some qualified patients regardless of their financial coverage.

Second Stage: Criteria for selecting recipients for organs

Once a person is placed on a waiting list for an organ, the second selection process begins. The waiting list is arranged in an order of priority. The person at the top of the list receives the next available matching organ, and then the others move up a notch. Unfortunately, not everyone on the list will live long enough to receive an organ.

The central ethical question is: How should we arrange the list? If we say the most recently accepted candidate goes to the end of the line, it does not seem fair because her need may be greater than the need of those ahead of her on the list. But if we say that the most needy people receive places near the top of the list, then the organs will go only to the sickest, and other truly needy people will never get a chance no matter how long they are on the list. Moreover, giving organs only to the most needy will, in all probability, result in fewer lives saved than if we gave organs to less needy, and therefore stronger, candidates.

Over the years a number of proposals have been made about how the waiting lists for organs should be arranged. None of them is satisfactory.

Random selection.   This can be done in two ways. One way is to construct a kind of lottery. When an organ becomes available, a random drawing is made to determine which person on the list receives it. This has been tried with a few scarce drugs that are hard to produce. Another way to implement random selection is to arrange the list on a first come, first served basis. When an organ becomes available, the person waiting the longest on the list receives it.

The great appeal of random selection is that nobody has to make a decision. Everything happens automatically; there is no "God squad." And there can be no question of any discrimination based on race, color, class, money, etc. Everybody is treated equally. The great disadvantage is that personal needs are ignored, and sometimes scarce resources are unreasonably distributed. The person winning the lottery or at the top of the list may be able to live a couple of months without the organ, while others need the heart right away to survive.

Market approach.   People are expected to pay for health care in the United States under the present system, and proponents of this approach say that it should be no different for organ transplantation. If people can afford to pay or are able to obtain insurance coverage, and need the procedure, then they are entitled to receive it.

The great appeal of the market approach is its stress on being personally responsible for one's life and on taking care to provide for oneself by finding a way to have health insurance, rather than expecting others to take care of you. The great disadvantage of the market approach is its lack of concern for catastrophic medical problems, and its inherent inequitable treatment of people unable to provide payment privately or through insurance. And the law of supply and demand means that the restricted supply of organs available for transplant will result in high charges for transplantations, so only the very rich or the well-insured will be recipients. Finally, the shortage of many organs is so great that market demand will still exceed supply.

Social worth.   According to a general utilitarian view, scarce resources should be distributed in such a way that they will do the most good for the greatest number of people. Hence, priority in organ distribution should be given to those who will contribute the most to society. In this approach, the individual's social value, not his need or ability to pay, is what determines his place on the list. The criterion of social worth will revive the approach used by the committee selecting patients for dialysis in Seattle. As one member was quoted as saying: "I remember voting against a young woman who was a known prostitute. I couldn't vote for her, rather than another candidate, a young wife and mother."

The great appeal of the social worth approach is its attempt to maximize the social benefits of scarce resources, to use them where they will do the most good. The great disadvantage of the social worth approach is that it tends to measure the value of human beings by their contribution to society. Moreover, judgments of social worth are inevitably heavily biased. Some think poets contribute little or nothing to society, other think poetry is valuable. Some think personal injury lawyers specializing in malpractice litigation against physicians and nurses are of great value to society, others think they cause great harm.

Medical criteria.   Many believe that a candidate's place on the list should be determined strictly by medical criteria. Medical criteria focus on the individual patient's medical condition, and not on his ability to pay or on his potential value to society.

The great appeal of this approach is its recognition of the intrinsic value of each human life, regardless of what the person might contribute to society or of how much money or health insurance she might have. The great disadvantage of medical criteria is that they are complex and require clinical judgments about present needs and possible outcomes. Medical criteria embrace two different questions: (1) How much does the patient need the organ now, and (2) what are the chances for a truly beneficial outcome in terms of both longevity and quality of life? These questions are often in conflict with one another—the most needy patients are often those with the poorest chance of achieving an extended life of reasonably good health. The challenge, then, is to balance need and outcome, and this requires careful analysis and judgment.

A further complication arises when a patient's medical condition may be less severe than that of many others on the list, but it may be very difficult to match an organ to his body's immune system. Hence, if an organ that he can tolerate does become available, it may be reasonable to give it to him, since forcing him to wait for the next organ compatible with his immune system may undermine his chances of a good outcome.

All the proposed criteria for allocating organs to people on the waiting list have both advantages and disadvantages. This suggests that no one of them alone is sufficient, and that the judgment of who receives an organ must be made on the basis of combined criteria.

To ensure objectivity and fairness in making these complex judgments, some kind of national guidelines and some kind of committee review is necessary. Guidelines are necessary lest the decisions become arbitrary, but committee review is necessary because no set of guidelines can capture the ambiguities and uncertainties associated with the rapidly changing field of organ transplantation. Without guidelines, the allocation process becomes chaotic and unfair, as the following stories illustrate.

THE CASE OF JAMIE FISKE

The Story

Jamie was born in 1983 with biliary atresia, an incurable malfunction of the liver. Her only hope of survival past infancy was a liver transplant. The family's insurance plan, Blue Cross and Blue Shield of Massachusetts, did not pay for liver transplants at that time because it did not consider liver transplants a "generally accepted" surgical procedure. Few had been performed, and no Massachusetts hospital had a liver transplantation program set up in 1983.

Charles Fiske, Jamie's father, immediately complained to Tom McGee, Speaker of the (Massachusetts) House, and to a local TV station, that Blue Cross and Blue Shield refused to pay for his daughter's transplant. Within twenty-four hours Blue Cross and Blue Shield agreed to make a special exception and pay for the surgery. The Governor of Massachusetts also pledged Medicaid funding for the surgery. The guaranteed funding enabled the parents to place Jamie's name on a waiting list in Minnesota, and she was transferred there to await a liver.

Six weeks went by and nothing happened. The parents contacted the AMA for help. They also contacted the American Academy of Pediatrics, looking for the addresses of pediatric surgeons. They planned to write them all, hoping one of them would encounter a brain-dead child whose liver could be retrieved. It so happened that the academy was having its national convention in New York at that time, and Charles Fiske asked to address the group. He received an equivocal response. The pediatricians were sympathetic, but reminded him that other babies were on the list awaiting organs.

Jamie's parents turned once again to political figures and to the mass media. They contacted their senator and their representative in Washington, as well as the Speaker of the U.S. House of Representatives, who came from their state. They appealed to the local TV stations, and to ABC, NBC, and CBS as well. Their plight received national coverage.

Less than a week later, a baby boy in Utah was killed in an accident. His parents had heard of Jamie Fiske on TV and decided to donate their child's organs to her. The liver was successfully transplanted into Jamie and her life was saved.

Ethical Analysis

Situational awareness

We are aware of these facts in the Fiske story.

1. Jamie would not survive without a liver transplant. Although some liver transplants fail, some do succeed and save lives.

2. The family insurance did not cover liver transplants, and the family did not have the money to pay for it.

3. Funding was obtained, but then a donor had to be found. Weeks on a waiting list produced nothing, and her condition worsened. Her parents resorted to political pressure and to media attention in a desperate effort to save her life.

We are also aware of the good and bad features in this case.

1. Clearly, Jamie's life is a good and her death would be bad, and a terrible thing for her parents.

2. The media campaign accomplished some good. It raised national awareness about insurance coverage for liver transplantations and about the donation of cadaverous infant organs. It also influenced the parents of a deceased baby to donate his liver, and the liver saved a life.

3. The media campaigns and political pressure to obtain funding and organ donations for a needy child also gave rise to several bad features. Among them are the following.

- First, extensive and emotional publicity about the plight of one child diverts resources from other needy children, and this is bad for them.
- Second, the publicity about expensive interventions can lead to an excessive emphasis on these interventions to the neglect of routine and less expensive medical care for needy children, and this is bad for them.
- Third, publicity undermines the basic equality of opportunity that should characterize the allocation of scarce resources. Obtaining organs by publicity is a discriminatory process—it favors families with political connections and with the ability to present the case well to reporters and TV audiences.
- Finally, the publicity given to some patients heightens the anxiety and frustration of the parents of other children, who realize their children may be bypassed in favor of the case before the public eye.

Prudential reasoning in the Fiske story

Parents' perspective.   It would be difficult to say that Jamie's parents acted in a morally inappropriate way. Their primary responsibility was to Jamie, and they worked hard to save her life. Their use of media publicity and political pressure is hard to fault. Their actions were actions of love, and there is a priority in the virtue of love whereby we will go to greater lengths for family than for others, for friends than for strangers. Modern ethical theories, those reflecting Kant and utilitarianism in particular, tend to overlook this order of love in their emphasis on treating everyone with equal respect and impartiality. In an ethics of virtue and right reason, however, the order of love or charity is more easily acknowledged. Given the predicament Jamie's parents faced in 1983, when the social system of organ distribution was not yet organized as it is today, their extraordinary efforts to save their daughter were not only reasonable but laudable.

Providers' perspective.   From a clinical perspective, it is also hard to fault the transplant team in Minnesota. Their primary clinical responsibility is doing good for their patient. However, there are limitations to clinical beneficence. Most ethicists agree, for example, that it would be unethical for a transplant surgeon to buy organs from living patients on the black market in order to benefit his patient. The black market in commercial organs harvested from the living is not a morally good distribution system. Neither is an organ distribution process based on media publicity. Hence, from a social perspective, physicians cooperating with organ distribution by media campaigns are participating in an unethical distribution program. Clinical beneficence in organ transplantation becomes morally unreasonable whenever the organ procurement or distribution systems are morally unreasonable by reason of the disproportionate damage they do to the human good. What is truly beneficial for one patient can be unethical, as it is when it involves unreasonable (that is, morally unjustified) damage to others.

Social perspective.   It was a wonderful event for Jamie and her family when the publicity resulted in the life-saving organ, but was the social system that allowed and abetted this kind of allocation process fair? It seems not. Other babies were on the waiting list, but their parents did not use political and media pressure to find a organ for them. As happy as everyone is for Jamie and her family, there is something morally disturbing about the babies of bright, articulate, well-educated, and determined parents receiving organs, while the babies of parents without these qualities fail to receive them. And it is disturbing to think that parents must use political influence and national media coverage to help their sick children.

The moral problems, then, are not personal but medical and social. The parents acted reasonably and pursued what was truly good in their lives. The physicians acted in a responsible way, but by agreeing to transplant organs designated for their patients in a process lacking in fairness, their behavior raises moral concerns. If the allocation of organs by media appeals and talk shows is not a fair way to distribute organs, then there are good reasons for saying transplant surgeons should refuse to participate in this kind of allocation. And there are good reasons for saying politicians and responsible people in the print and electronic media should refuse to assist parents to find organs this way.

THE CASE OF JESSE SEPULVEDA

The Story

Jesse was born on May 25, 1986, at Huntington Memorial Hospital in Pasadena with hypoplastic left-heart syndrome, a congenital defect that is usually fatal. Physicians immediately referred the parents to Loma Linda University Medical Center, which by then had transplanted five infant hearts in the first six months of its new program. The parents, seventeen-year-old Deana Binckley and twenty-six-year-old Jesse Sepulveda, Sr., were interviewed at Loma Linda. Their request to have Jesse placed on the waiting list for a heart was sent to the twenty-member hospital committee that reviews the transplant requests. The committee, by a unanimous vote, declined to accept Jesse as a candidate. The committee did not give Deana and Jesse a reason, but physicians at Huntington told them that it was because they were young and not married.

When Father Michael Carcerano, the priest who baptized baby Jesse, heard of the rejection, he contacted Susan McMillan, the California spokesperson for the National Right to Life Committee. She began a media campaign.

In the face of the publicity, much of it critical of the hospital, Loma Linda agreed to accept Jesse as a candidate for a transplant, provided his parents would give custody of the baby to the paternal grandparents. In an effort to save their child, the parents agreed. Loma Linda then accepted Jesse as a candidate for a heart.

The hospital denied that it had originally refused to list Jesse as a candidate for a transplant because his parents were not married, and said that its decision was based on concern about what kind of postoperative care Jesse would receive at home. It declined to reveal why it doubted that Jesse's parents could provide the necessary care, but press reports indicated that Susan may have had a substance abuse problem.

Meanwhile, a baby named Frank Clemenshaw died in Michigan. The parents at first refused to donate his organs but, after hearing of Jesse's plight on television news programs and realizing that he was born on the same day as their son, decided to donate his heart to Jesse. Physicians in Michigan notified Loma Linda that a heart was available for Jesse, but the hospital did not immediately notify Jesse's parents or grandparents.

The next day, still unaware that a heart had been found, Jesse's parents, Susan McMillan of the Right to Life Committee, and Rev. Carcerano appeared on the Phil Donahue Show in New York. They made a moving plea for a heart for Jesse. During the live program, the phone rang and a spokesperson from the hospital in Michigan told the nationwide audience that it had a heart for Jesse. There was great rejoicing on the set and in the audience as people cheered, cried, and applauded. After a few emotional moments, Phil Donahue excused the parents so they could fly back to California for the operation. Mr. Donahue assured the audience that the hospital's call had not been prearranged, but later accounts told a different story. The woman making the call claimed the producers of the Donahue program had learned of the donation, and then pressed her to call during the show to announce it on national television.

Jesse received Frank's heart and became the fourth baby in the world to receive a successful heart transplant. Seven years later, this heart began to fail. In June 1993 Jesse became the second child in the world to receive a second heart transplant. Unfortunately, drugs could not prevent his immune system from rejecting the second heart, and physicians at Loma Linda declined to try a third transplant. Jesse died in July 1993.

Ethical Reflection

Jesse's story is sufficiently similar to Jamie's story that we need not repeat the facts in a situational analysis nor provide an ethical analysis of the behavior of the various moral agents playing a major role in the case. When a baby needs an organ to live, it's difficult to fault parents when they use the media or a national TV talk show to appeal for that organ. And it is difficult to fault the child's physicians for implanting an organ produced by the publicity, although the participation of physicians in an allocation system based on publicity remains morally questionable. The main point of telling Jesse's story is to illustrate how such an allocation process, while good for one baby, is not a morally good allocation system.

While we can acknowledge the good intentions of the priest and the spokesperson for the National Right to Life Committee whose efforts enabled Jesse to receive his first heart, we cannot overlook the other side to the story. Their efforts found a heart for Jesse, but they also skewered the allocation process.

When the heart was given to Jesse, it meant the baby designated to receive the next heart was bypassed. His name was Robert Cardin. Robert was in a hospital in Kentucky and first in line to receive the next available heart. When Frank's heart became available, however, Robert did not receive it. National media attention on Jesse's plight so influenced the allocation process that the heart went to him and not to Robert, the baby first in line. This delay created an unnecessary risk for Robert.

When Robert's physician realized how his patient lost his chance for a heart, he contacted the news media to gain publicity for his side of the story. Soon Baby Robert's plight became national news and another heart was donated for him. This still meant, of course, that the baby next in line was left waiting. The danger is that hearts will be distributed on the basis of publicity rather than by medical need and within a social system of allocation based on triage.

The stories of Jamie and Jesse reveal the two sides of ethics. The publicity efforts of the Fiskes and of Ms. McMillan saved the lives of these two babies, and that is undeniably good for those individuals. But there are good reasons for saying that their efforts undermined an ethical allocation system, and this is bad for other unknown babies and their parents. To put it another way, there is no moral justification for distributing scarce organs in this country on the basis of publicity.

Of course, it can be argued that Jamie's liver and Jesse's heart would not have been donated but for the publicity, and that the publicity actually produced organs that otherwise would not have been donated. The publicity, then, did not deprive anyone on the established waiting list of an organ because it actually produced an additional organ. This argument has some merit, but is not sufficiently strong to overcome the other negative social aspects of retrieving and allocating organs by media publicity focused on desperate families. More reasonable, and hence more ethical, ways of allocating organs are available.

The highly publicized story of Jamie Fiske helped, in no small way, to support federal initiatives to organize a just and fair system of organ allocation. In 1984 Congress passed the National Organ Transplant Act. The act was intended to establish a more just system of organ allocation. It authorized a national Task Force on Organ Transplantation and called for a national network to facilitate the procurement and distribution of organs. It also prohibited the buying and selling of human organs.

The national task force was established in January 1985. It lasted for fifteen months and produced two reports, the first on immunosuppressive therapies and the second entitled "Organ Transplantation: Issues and Recommendations." An underlying assumption of the task force was that organs should be allocated on a national basis so that people living anywhere in the United States would have an equal chance of receiving one.

In 1986 two existing organ-sharing networks were merged, at the direction of Congress, into the national Organ Procurement and Transplantation Network (OPTN). The Reagan administration was at first reluctant to support any government involvement in a national list designed to match recipients and donors. The media hyperbole surrounding the story of Jesse Sepulveda, however, helped overcome the administration's hesitations and, in September 1986, the Department of Health and Human Services contracted with the United Network for Organ Sharing (UNOS) of Richmond, Virginia, to manage the OPTN. The network provides twenty-four hour telephone access to a computerized waiting list of ranked candidates and uses medical criteria to match candidates with available organs. The waiting list is ordered according to two fundamental criteria: the urgency of the patient's need and the expectation of a successful outcome.

When physicians determine that a patient needs an organ, they place the name and relevant medical data on the UNOS list. The wait for a suitable donor under the rules of UNOS varies. On average, the recent wait was sixty-seven days for a liver and one hundred ninety-eight days for a heart, although some people have received livers and hearts within twenty-four hours in urgent cases. The whole effort is directed toward ensuring that patients needing organs anywhere in the country will have fair and equitable access to them.

In the Omnibus Budget Reconciliation Act of 1986, Congress mandated that hospitals performing transplants must be members of OPTN and must comply with its rules if they wish to remain eligible for Medicare and Medicaid reimbursement. This same act also required hospitals receiving Medicare and Medicaid (about 97 percent of the nation's 6,800 hospitals) to establish written protocols for encouraging organ and tissue donation and for identifying potential donors.

The need for some kind of national list is imperative if organs are going to be allocated fairly to people who need them and can benefit from them. Without some order it becomes, as we saw, a mad scramble by desperate families trying to save their loved ones.

The stories of Jamie and Jesse are not simply about the ethically questionable role of media attention in the organ allocation process; they also raise questions about what we might call "designated donation." The parents of the deceased babies in these stories actually designated Jamie and Jesse as recipients of their child's organ. The idea of people or their proxies designating recipients of the donated organs presents another moral issue. Given the shortage of organs, is it ever morally justified to override the national waiting list by designating the recipient, or a class of recipients, for organs? The morality of the donor designating the recipient of his organs is complex because there are plausible reasons both for and against such a practice. The following reasons favor designated donation:

- Since people can donate their bodies to a designated medical school for research, there should be no moral objection to donating an organ to a designated person.
- Since living people can donate a kidney to a designated recipient,

usually a sibling, there should be no moral objection to designated donation after death.

- Since there is a unique bond within families, there should be no moral objection if one member wishes to designate another member as the recipient of his organ after death.
- Since some people would not donate unless they can identify a recipient, it is better to allow designated donation than to lose the organ.

The main reason against designated donation is based on social justice. Organ transplantation is not just a personal matter—it is also a social process involving hospitals and surgical teams, and sometimes public funding. Transplantation, therefore, falls within the realm of social justice, and social justice is undermined when institutions and practitioners participate in a program that favors people for reasons unrelated to medical need and benefit. Allocating organs on the basis of personal designations is not an allocation process that meets the requirements of a fair and equitable distribution of organs. Designating a particular person means that others higher up on the list may wait longer for their chance. It could also result in a valuable organ being wasted because the designated recipient may not be a person with a high probability of benefiting from it.

There are, however, situations where it can be reasonably argued that designated donation is morally acceptable. One example is donation within families. The special love and support that exist, or should exist, within families is an important consideration that could be allowed to override the impartial demands of equality and fairness that characterize social justice. As we pointed out earlier, the modern theories of utilitarianism and Kantian deontology have difficulty recognizing this kind of partiality in ethics.

In an ethics of virtue, however, there is room for a complementary balance between the virtues of justice and love. The virtue of justice is primary in our relationships with strangers and in our responsibility to the community, but the virtue of love is primary in our relationships with our family and close friends. Love, by its very nature, allows us to act in a preferential way toward those whom we love. The virtue of love means, in an important sense, that some people in our lives count more than others; love is not a virtue whereby we treat everyone impartially. In an ethics that embraces personal love as a virtue, there are reasons for saying designated donations within loving relationships are morally acceptable.

A second situation where designated donation could be defended as morally reasonable is when it is used to correct disadvantages in the system of organ procurement and allocation. Here is a specific example. According to UNOS, the recent average wait for a kidney is twelve months if you are white, almost twenty-two months if you are black.

Understanding why the wait is longer for a black person on the list is complicated because several factors are involved. First, a higher percentage of black people suffer from diseases causing kidney failure, diseases such as diabetes and hypertension. This means that a higher percentage of black people need kidney transplants. At the present time, although black people make up about 12 percent of the U.S. population, they make up about 30 percent of the people on the UNOS list needing a kidney.

Second, although black patients represent 30 percent of those needing a kidney, far fewer than 30 percent of donated kidneys are sufficiently compatible with their immune systems. The chances of a good outcome after a kidney transplant improve if the kidney is closely matched with the recipient. The matching process involves blood type and certain antigens that play a role in immunological reactions. The closer the antigens of donor and recipient cells match, the better the chance that the recipient's immune system will not reject the kidney. In general, the matches are closer within racial groups rather than between them.

Third, until recently, the percentage of black kidney donors was lower than the percentage of black people in the population. In 1982, for example, only 3 percent of kidney donors were black, while over 10 percent of the population was black. By 1992 the figures had improved so that about 11 percent of kidney donors were black, while about 12 percent of the population was black. Although the percentage of black donors is now almost the same as the percentage of black people in the population, this still leaves many black patients waiting longer than white patients for two reasons. First, some kidneys from black donors are unusable because the same diseases that contributed to their deaths (diabetes and hypertension, for example) also damaged their kidneys. Second, the percentage of black people suffering kidney failure is higher than the percentage of white people suffering kidney failure.

Both the higher need for kidneys in the black population and the greater difficulty in matching the kidneys that are donated with the antigen profiles of black patients suggest to some that the kidney allocation system needs to be changed to include race as a factor in organ allocation. The idea is to take into consideration the added difficulty of matching donated kidneys with the antigen profile of many black people, and to compensate for it by allocating those kidneys that happen to be compatible with a waiting black person to that person even though he may not be the next in line. Some have suggested that we can do this by allowing a form of designated recipients. For example, prospective donors could be allowed to designate the next black person on the waiting list with an adequate antigen match as the recipient of their kidney, even though a white person with a better match is higher on the list.

Although this approach disrupts the impartiality of the current system, in an ethics of right reason there are reasons for claiming that it is morally acceptable. If race is allowed as a factor in designated donation, however, it cannot favor only one race. Studies would have to be conducted to see how people of native American ancestry, of Asian ancestry, of Semitic ancestry, etc., fare on the waiting list. If they wait longer than Caucasian people, then designated donation based on race or ethnic background would be morally appropriate for them as well if race and ethnicity became factors in the distribution program.

TRANSPLANTATION OF ORGANS FROM LIVING HUMAN DONORS

Moral questions about donation from living donors center on two fundamental issues: how can we justify the harm done to the donor and how can we ensure the donor's consent is truly voluntary? Recently, a third issue is emerging—buying a kidney from living persons. The first issue was paramount when transplanting organs from living donors began, but now it has receded as most people have become morally comfortable in justifying the harm done to the donor by the surgery and the loss of a healthy organ. The implications of the second issue were not fully appreciated at first, but now the voluntary aspect of informed consent is receiving most of the attention.

The Risks and Harm Affecting the Donor

The most common form of donation from the living involves kidneys. Retrieving a kidney from a live donor requires major surgery and leaves the person less able to cope with kidney disease should it ever occur in her life. From a medical point of view, the donor is harmed, not helped, by the surgery. In some traditional moral approaches, this raises a serious moral problem. One of the ancient principles of medical ethics is *"primum, non nocere"* (that is, "first, do no harm"). The principle is captured today in the principle of nonmaleficence, often listed as a major action-guide along with the principles of autonomy, beneficence, and justice. The principle of nonmaleficence (meaning "do not harm") would seem to oblige us not to remove somebody's kidney when the removal harms her without producing any medical benefit for her.

A similar problem arose in Catholic moral theology in the 1950s as live donations became a reality. Theologians had earlier worked out a principle to justify surgery—the principle of totality. This principle allows the mutilation or destruction of part of the body in order to save the whole body. Ordinarily, the theologians taught, it would be wrong for a person to mutilate his body by surgery or to destroy a part of it. However, if the mutilation or destruction will contribute to the benefit of the body as a whole, then it could be morally justified by the principle of totality. For example, if a person has a cancerous kidney, the mutilation of the body necessary to remove the kidney can be morally justified because it contributes to the total health of the body.

In an ethics of principles, the principle of totality worked well for surgeries that contributed to the overall total health of the body. Moreover, the principle also conveniently ruled out surgeries that the Catholic Church opposed—sterilizations, the surgeries designed to prevent pregnancy. Theologians argued that vasectomies and tubal ligations are not justified by the principle of totality because they are not performed to benefit the whole body, but to prevent conception.

When surgery to retrieve a kidney from a live donor became a reality, the theologians who had been justifying surgery by the principle of totality were perplexed. Obviously, their principle of totality ruled it out. The surgery taking a healthy kidney out of one person to give it to another in no way contributes to the totality of the donor's health. On the contrary, the donor's health is actually undermined by the risks of the unnecessary surgery and by the life-long deprivation of the healthy kidney.

Some theologians, faithful to their principle of totality, drew the obvious conclusion and considered organ retrieval from a living donor immoral. Others were not so sure. They thought, almost intuitively, that donating an organ to a person in need was a kind of Christian thing to do. Since Christianity had always taught that it was an act of great love to lay down one's life for another, they wondered why it would not also be an act of love to donate a kidney to a brother or sister.

Today, when it comes to organ donation from the living, medical ethicists relying on a principles approach have all but forgotten their principle of nonmaleficence, and the theologians have all but forgotten their principle of totality. Most of them acknowledge that the living person freely donating a kidney is acting in a morally admirable way. Fortunately, moral discernment triumphed over the moral principles of nonmaleficence and totality.

Surgery to retrieve organs for transplantation from the living is not, however, without legitimate moral concerns. Before retrieving the first kidney from a living identical twin in 1954, physicians at the Peter Bent Brigham Hospital sought court approval. Only when the judge ruled that the donor child would be more harmed by the loss of his twin brother than by the loss of his kidney did the surgeons proceed to remove the healthy kidney. Their seeking court approval suggests that they were worried about the legal liability for the medically unjustified harm they were doing to the healthy twin by removing his kidney.

And there is still reason for this worry. Some kidney donors have died as the result of complications from the surgery, and others have been negatively affected by the surgery and by subsequent medical problems exacerbated by the loss of a kidney. The time may soon come, if it is not already here, that live donations will no longer be justified. As better immunosuppressive drugs come on line, and as more people arrange to donate their organs after death, the risks associated with live donation of organs may outweigh the benefits, and kidney donation from the living may become a thing of the past. Until that happens, however, most agree that the surgery, which is of no medical benefit to the donor, is still morally acceptable. People freely donating an organ while living are behaving morally in a most admirable way, and the transplant surgeons are cooperating in their generosity.

However, the second serious moral question about live donation—the question of truly voluntary informed consent—remains. Unlike the questions about the harm and mutilation to the body, questions now resolved for ethicists and theologians, the question of informed consent for the retrieval of organs from living donors is now looming larger than ever.

Questions About Voluntary Consent

Consider, first, an adult whose family member needs a kidney, and the match is perfect, or almost perfect. The adult will have to give informed consent for the surgery to remove her kidney. The question is, can the consent be truly voluntary in such circumstances? Consider the predicament the woman is in. If she refuses the surgery, think of the guilt she will experience when her sister needing the kidney dies, and think of the way other family members may treat (or mistreat) her after she refuses to donate. It is quite possible that the intense pressures, both real and perceived, on the potential donor destroy the possibility of truly voluntary consent. And surgery on an adult with decision-making capacity without her voluntary consent is immoral (and illegal).

Consider, second, a child whose kidney is the best match for a sibling. For surgery on children, the parents must give consent. And when parents are deciding to give consent for surgery on their children, they normally rely, as we saw in chapter five, on what is known as the best interests standard. In other words, the parents decide on the basis of what is in the best interests of the child. Now, in a very important sense, surgery to take a perfectly healthy kidney from a child is simply not in that child's best interests.

Some will argue that it is. Following the reasoning of the Massachusetts court in the first live kidney donation, they will claim that losing the sibling will be more harmful to the child than losing the kidney. But this is no more than a gratuitous claim; it is not, with all due respect to the court, a judgment based on evidence. We simply do not know that the child would agree with this opinion. Undoubtedly, some children may grow up delighted that their parents decided to use their kidney to save a sibling before they were old enough to make the decision. But others, especially if the surgery has harmed them or shortened their life, may resent what happened. Also, as happens in some families, hostile relations can develop between a child and parent or between sibling and sibling. In such situations, the donor may grow old very unhappy that his parents authorized the surgery or that a particular sibling received his kidney.

The pressing moral problem about obtaining truly voluntary consent from a living donor, both consent by the adult donor and consent by parents on behalf of a child, remains troublesome. At the very least, great care must be taken to ensure truly voluntary consent.

An example of serious attention to the ethical problems of donation from living donors occurred recently in a partial liver transplant from a mother to a child. In November 1989 the first partial transplantation of a liver was made at the University of Chicago when a mother donated for her child. One of the most encouraging aspects of this transplantation of liver lobes was the thorough discussion of the ethical issues related to the experimental surgery before it took place. People were sensitive to the risks for the donor as well as the benefits for the donor and for the recipient, and to the need for a consent that was truly voluntary. At the very least, this intense ethical scrutiny will diminish the fears that consent to donate an organ while living may not be truly voluntary.

Buying Organs Harvested from the Living

Stories about selling organs harvested from living people have persisted for years. In its issue of March 13, 1989, *Time* magazine reported that a poor Turkish peasant sold a kidney in London for about $4500 to raise money for an operation for his daughter. Such cases are not well documented for obvious reasons: the World Health Organization condemns the buying and selling of organs, and surgeons could be sued for assault and battery if the informed consent given by the desperate seller was not truly voluntary. Moreover, the

1984 Organ Procurement and Transplantation Act prohibits the sale of organs for transplantation.

What might an ethics of right reason conclude about people selling their organs? From the perspective of the person selling his organ, the action can be considered reasonable, and even laudable, if it is a last resort to prevent starvation. The person donating a kidney to a sibling acts nobly when the donation is necessary for survival; the person selling a kidney also acts reasonably if the sale was necessary for survival. When survival is at stake, some behaviors not normally justified as ethical can be justified. For example, stealing is normally immoral but a long, and reasonable, ethical tradition condones stealing to prevent a greater harm—starving to death. In the same way, it could also be argued that a person should not sell his kidney—unless it was necessary to prevent a greater threat to his life or the life of a loved one.

Of course, a person should not have to sell a kidney to save his life or the life of his child, but life does not always unfold as we would like. It would be a strange ethics indeed that would allow a person to give up his place on a crowded life raft voluntarily so another could live, but would condemn a person for giving up a kidney to avoid starvation or to provide crucial health care for his family.

From the perspective of the people in the commercial system who would be buying and selling kidneys bought from living people, organ sales are not so easy to justify as reasonable and virtuous. In fact, many reasons have been advanced against allowing the practice. Some say that the system would exploit poor people, since only needy people would agree to sell a kidney. Some say the practice would result in lower quality kidneys, since the sellers would probably already be in less than optimum health. Some say the practice would undermine an allocation system based on medical criteria, since the purchased kidneys would go to the well-insured and the rich. Some say the practice would undermine the sense of altruism motivating organ donation today, since a market in organs could destroy the powerful feeling of "giving a gift of life" that motivates some donors.

All these arguments have some merit, but so do the responses to them advanced by those defending the sale of organs. They argue that exploitation can be prevented, that measures of quality control to ensure retrieval only of healthy organs are possible, that equitable allocation systems are possible, and that buying kidneys would provide a greater supply of healthy kidneys than the current system of donation from the dead.

There are, however, two stronger arguments against allowing a system whereby living people could sell their organs. First, there is a legitimate concern about truly voluntary consent. We can assume that people willing to sell a kidney are under great pressure, and this coercive pressure all too easily subverts the voluntariness of any consent they would give for the surgery. Second, it is difficult to see how a social system that allowed living people to sell kidneys would be compatible with an ethics of the human good. This ethics seeks a good life, and thus cherishes life. Commercial systems that damage life—and removing a healthy kidney from a living person is damaging to him—introduce bad features that an ethics of the good will seek to avoid, not encourage.

Thus, an ethics of the good could not condone commercial systems of slavery or prostitution, even if some people think their autonomy should permit them to choose slavery or prostitution, because these forms of commercial practices are not compatible with a good and noble life. In the same way, it can be well-argued that a commercial system of buying organs from willing people is inconsistent with living a good life. Slavery, prostitution, and paying people for organs are arguably not beneficial practices for societies because the good they could achieve in isolated, exceptional circumstances does not adequately outweigh the bad features of the systemic commercialization of slavery, of prostitution, and of organ harvesting.

Would the offer of money for organs given up after death meet with the same moral objections? Here the issue of the voluntary consent, so very important before surgical interventions on the living, is significantly reduced. A person can more easily agree to donate an organ freely after death than during life because he knows that the removal after death brings no harm to him. And the money paid for the organ is not a coercive inducement since it does him no good. The bad features of commercialization involving the living are also reduced because the organ retrieval is no longer from one of us, and the retrieval does not result in a person suffering from the surgical retrieval and facing the rest of his life without a kidney.

TRANSPLANTATION OF ORGANS FROM ANIMALS

In November 1963 Dr. Keith Reemtsma transplanted chimpanzee kidneys into a forty-three year old poor, black man in New Orleans Charity Hospital. Jefferson Davis was dying and thought his only chance was a transplant from an animal. According to a transcript of a conversation with his doctors after the surgery, he said: "Well, I ain't had no choice." He lived about two months, and died in January 1964. That same month, at the University of Mississippi Medical Center, Dr. James Hardy transplanted a chimpanzee heart into sixty-eight-year-old Boyd Rush, another poor, dying man. Mr. Rush, a deaf-mute, was unconscious when he was admitted to the hospital, and his stepsister gave consent for a "suitable heart transplant" if necessary. He lived less than two hours.

Although ethical sensitivity about what was, in effect, medical research was not as high in 1963–1964 as it is now, these transplantations are suspect under moral restraints known by all at the time. It is difficult, for example, to see how these experiments could be justified under the Nuremberg Code of 1947. Of course, these men were dying, and when people are dying, some think almost any medical intervention intended to save their lives is justified. That thinking, however, is not morally sound. In fact, it is morally dangerous because it can easily cause unreasonable suffering for the dying patient.

The cases of Jefferson Davis and Boyd Rush, and those of a few other patients who had received animal organs years ago, did not generate extensive public debate about the procedure. However, that debate exploded in 1984 when Dr. Leonard Bailey and his team transplanted a baboon heart into a newborn baby girl at Loma Linda University Medical Center in California.

The plight of Baby Fae fascinated the nation for
in no small way by a two-part series in *People* ma
1984. A review of this case will help us sharpe
about animal transplants or, as they are someti

THE CASE OF BABY FAE

The Story

On October 14, 1984, in southern California, a
plastic left-heart syndrome, a fatal condition, arriveu
She was transferred to Loma Linda University Medical Center, and
soon knew her as Baby Fae.

Physicians and families faced with a baby suffering from this heart problem had few options at the time. They could do nothing, they could seek a
human heart for transplantation, or they could try an experimental surgery
developed by Dr. William Norwood of Philadelphia (sometimes known as
the Norwood procedure). Physicians at Loma Linda decided on a fourth
option: the transplantation of a baboon heart. For this, they needed the consent
of the parents.

Baby Fae's parents, who were not married but had lived together for
about four years, had separated a few months before her birth. Her mother
had not completed high school and was on welfare when the baby was born.
Her father did not know he had a daughter until she was several days old. Both
parents were upset about the baby's condition and wanted to do everything
possible to save her life.

In a long conference that began about midnight and ended seven hours
later, the mother, grandmother, and a male friend of the mother who was
staying at the mother's home spent hours with Dr. Leonard Bailey discussing
what could be done. As a result of this discussion, the mother signed an
informed consent form allowing transplantation from an animal. Later, the
father also gave consent, although he had not been involved in the extensive
deliberations with the others.

Since transplantation from an animal to a human is an unorthodox procedure, it would have been a challenge to compose an appropriate informed
consent form. The actual form signed by the parents, however, has never
been made public despite the interest many have in reviewing it. In the long
run, the adequacy of the information on the form may not be that important;
more important than the record of informed consent is the actual process that
took place. The form may well be inadequate but, as we pointed out in chapter
four, it is the reality of the consent process, and not the piece of paper, that
is crucial.

After receiving institutional review board approval, Dr. Bailey transplanted the heart of a freshly killed baboon. Baby Fae died twenty days later.
Her type O blood proved incompatible with the type AB blood of the baboon,
and blood clots led to kidney failure. Autopsy also revealed some mild rejection
by her immune system despite the immunosuppressive drugs.

...e are aware of these facts in the Baby Fae story.

1. Baby Fae was expected to die from heart failure in a matter of weeks.

2. Although there was a chance a human heart could be found and transplanted, no serious effort was made to pursue this option. There was also a chance that the Norwood procedure could save her, but no effort was made to pursue this option.

3. Dr. Bailey believed that it was medically feasible and morally acceptable to use animal organs in human beings. He had performed more than 150 transplantations in animals in the course of his research. In an interview ten days after the transplantation, he praised Dr. James Hardy, the physician who had transplanted a chimpanzee heart into Boyd Rush twenty years earlier, as his "champion." He said Hardy is "an idol of mine because he followed through and did what he should have done . . . he took a gamble to try to save a human life." Dr. Bailey also believed that the rare operation may have benefited Baby Fae, and that it was not simply a medical experiment on a dying infant.

4. Baby Fae's parents were unmarried and separated when she was born. This fact is important because parental difficulties can undermine the process whereby parents work together as a team to decide with the physician what is in the best interests of their child.

5. Although both transplantation of a human heart and the Norwood procedure had been previously used with limited success, transplantation of an animal heart to a baby had never been attempted, and animal studies had not, and still have not, established its feasibility.

6. Baby Fae's parents were poor and had no health insurance. The hospital provided the baboon transplant at no charge. There is no evidence that it would have provided a human transplant for free or that the Norwood procedure would have been done for free.

We are also aware of these good and bad features in the case.

1. Baby Fae's death, as any human death, would be unfortunate.

2. Transplanting a baboon heart, and providing the necessary preoperative and postoperative treatments, would cause significant pain and suffering to Baby Fae. Her body would be placed on a heart–lung machine and her blood temperature lowered to 68 degrees before the surgery. After the surgery, interventions would be necessary to support the transplant and prevent its rejection.

3. If the transplantation succeeded, Baby Fae could live longer than she would have lived with her own heart, and life is always a good. But we really do not know how much longer she might have lived if her body did not reject the baboon heart. Dr. Bailey said that she would someday celebrate her 21st birthday, but there is no compelling reason to believe a baboon heart could support an adult human body that long.

4. If the transplantation occurred and failed, physicians could still gain valuable information that would help future babies. There are not enough

human hearts for infants, and it could save lives if a way were found to use animal hearts.

5. A baboon, a healthy animal with a high level of neurological development, was killed to retrieve his heart. While this would not bother some people, the loss of life (including animal and environmental life) is always a bad feature in the ethics of the good, and concern for the loss is part of any complete moral deliberation.

Prudential reasoning in the Baby Fae story

The major moral agents in this case were the parents, the physician proposing the use of a baboon heart, and the members of the institutional review board that approved the experiment.

Parents' perspective.   Unfortunately, personal difficulties prevented the parents from acting as a team in this case, but both parents did agree to the transplantation. Parents normally achieve their good by doing what they think is in the best interests of their child. However, parents can only work with the realistic options given them. As we noted earlier, hospitals routinely require insurance or a large down payment before attempting a heart transplant; Baby Fae's parents had neither. The Norwood procedure is also costly, and it would require transportation to and lodging in Philadelphia. Hence, the parents had only two realistic options if they were not offered a free human transplant or a Norwood procedure: no corrective interventions or a baboon transplant.

Faced with doing nothing to save the life of a child or doing something, no matter how unusual or unorthodox, many parents will think it reasonable to do something. But "doing something" is not always the reasonable response. Sometimes, as we saw in chapter eleven, interventions are so burdensome and the possibility of significant success so slim that doing something to a very sick child is not morally justified.

Today, more than ten years after the Baby Fae case, it would still seem unreasonable to subject an infant to a transplantation of an organ from an animal. Not enough promising research on transplantation from one species to another has been done with animals for us to begin the research on human beings, especially human beings who cannot give consent to the experiments. Parents have to be very careful about giving consent for research on their children. And when they do consent to research on their children, the risks should be minimal. The understandable urge to save the life of an infant can never blind parents to the concern for the baby's best interests. Faced with the impending death of their baby, they cannot agree to everything and anything; they can only agree to what is reasonable. And if the intervention on babies is experimental, they have to be very careful lest the legitimate goals of research pursued by physicians blind them to the child's best interest.

It is also worth noting that Baby Fae's father, although he signed the consent form, was not involved in the seven-hour conference that comprised the major part of the consent process. Signing a consent form is not enough. A parent has to be fully informed, and the very first effort to transplant an animal heart into a baby would obviously require a considerable amount of time for the father to grasp adequately the required information about the risks, side effects, alternatives, prognosis, etc.

Physician's perspective. Dr. Bailey of Loma Linda was out of town when Baby Fae was admitted to the hospital. When he returned several days later, he contacted the parents and suggested the baboon transplant. During the all-night session with Baby Fae's mother, he provided a film and showed slides explaining his research. He also gave reasons why he believed a baboon heart might work. In the interview after the surgery, he acknowledged that "We were not searching for a human heart. We were out to enter the whole new area of transplanting tissue-matched baboon hearts into newborns who are supported with antisuppressive drugs."

Physicians engaged in medical research always live and work under a potential conflict of interest. As physicians, they want to give the best medical care and comfort to a particular patient; as researchers, they want to test interventions. The two aims often collide. When they do, the situation becomes very delicate. If the patient has decision-making capacity and adequate knowledge about the burdens and risks of the experimental intervention, he may voluntarily give consent to the unusual intervention, and there may be no moral problem. But when the patient cannot consent, physicians must proceed much more carefully. The goal of good patient care must remain primary, and not the goal, no matter how laudable, of medical research.

As we saw in chapter fourteen, experiments on children can be morally justified, but the burdens and risks must be minimal. A physician can argue that it is morally good to subject an infant to the trauma of any transplant surgery only if there are good reasons to think the burdens are minimal and the benefits reasonably expected.

IRB members' perspectives. Members of institutional review boards are also moral agents in this case—they approved the surgery. In March 1985 the National Institutes of Health sent a team to review the Baby Fae case at Loma Linda. The team found some problems with the consent document, reporting that it did not include the possibility of a human heart transplant, and that it seemed to overstate the chance of a good outcome for the baby. In general, the committee was critical of the IRB's oversight of the informed consent process in the case.

Public information showing how the IRB members were satisfied that Baby Fae was adequately protected in this case is not available. We do not know what reasons they used to justify killing an animal and implanting its heart into Baby Fae. We do know, however, that the IRBs exist for the protection of human subjects (in this case, for the protection of Baby Fae). The physicians may want to try something, and the parents may agree to have it done, but the IRB members have to protect vulnerable human subjects who cannot give informed consent for unorthodox medical interventions. Maybe some members of the IRB tried to stop the transplantation, but the board did give its approval for the baboon transplant. We are left wondering how it could justify the procedure, since the board has made no effort to explain its position.

Ethical Reflection

Since the Baby Fae case, animal heart transplants have not been used in humans. Dr. Leonard Bailey has turned his attention to using human hearts to help babies born with hypoplastic left heart syndrome and has achieved notable success. Nonetheless, in a reflective article on organ transplantation published in 1990, Dr. Bailey opined that Baby Fae would still be alive if the baboon's blood type had been a better match with hers.

In the same article he was critical of what he called the "'reactive' bioethical rhetoric" generated by the Baby Fae case.

> Much of what was said and written did not reflect well on the fledging profession of biomedical ethics. It was all too quick, too ill-informed, too self-assured. Furthermore, some of it hurt my feelings. I have often compared the ethical rhetoric of those days to the phenomenon of "pack journalism," and have considered it "semi-ethics"—close, but not quite the real thing. What was missing was *wisdom* and a sense of perspective.

Little is gained by remarks of this kind. Many of the ethical responses to the transplantation of the baboon heart into Baby Fae were written by prominent ethicists and well argued. If physicians disagree with the ethical criticisms of their medical research on human beings, we would all be the richer if they would engage the ethicists in moral reasoning and not dismiss their work as reactive rhetoric. This is especially so since some ethicists are convinced that what was "all too quick, too ill-informed, too self-assured," and missing "wisdom and a sense of perspective" was not the ethical reaction to the Baby Fae case, but the transplantation itself, especially since no serious effort was made to find a human heart for the child.

Surgeons continue seeking ways to transplant animal organs into human beings, as Dr. Thomas Starzl did when he transplanted a baboon's liver into a thirty-five year old man dying of hepatitis B in 1992. The ethics of doing so, however, is not yet clear. Perhaps these xenografts are truly beneficial, or perhaps they represent an unreasonable and overly zealous effort to rebuild failing human bodies, and thus are a diversion of time, talent, and resources from other efforts that would help many more people live better. Yet one thing is clear: there is no moral justification at this time for experimenting with xenografts on children. Fully informed dying adults may freely choose to become subjects of xenografts, and one may applaud their willingness to take a chance, knowing something might be learned that will help others even if they do not benefit. But children cannot make that choice, and we have no moral reason for forcing it upon them.

IMPLANTATION OF ARTIFICIAL HEARTS

The first artificial heart was implanted in 1969 at St. Luke's Hospital in Houston by Dr. Denton Cooley. The device kept forty-seven-year-old Haskell Karp alive until a human heart was found and transplanted three days later. Karp died within a day.

The operation received widespread publicity and started several contro-versies. Critics accused Dr. Cooley of using an artificial heart prematurely since the procedure had not succeeded in animals; of being motivated more by publicity than by the welfare of the patient; and of not obtaining a truly informed consent. Mrs. Karp sued him, claiming that neither she nor her husband realized the implant was experimental and being done for the first time. Dr. Michael DeBakey, the head of the artificial heart research at Baylor University, where Dr. Cooley was also on the faculty, was also critical of the attempt. A local medical society censured Dr. Cooley for his enthusiasm in seeking publicity after the surgery, but it declined to take disciplinary action against him. Dr. Cooley soon resigned from Baylor but continued to practice.

Haskell Karp's artificial heart was designed to be temporary; Barney Clark's was not. Dr. William DeVries implanted the first permanent artificial heart, known as the Jarvik–7, into Barney Clark at the University of Utah Medical Center in 1982. Clark lived for 112 days, but suffered numerous complications and never regained much of a comfortable life.

After Barney Clark died, Dr. DeVries moved his practice to the Humana Hospital in Louisville. Humana Hospital was part of a large chain of for-profit hospitals that owned stock in Symbion, the manufacturer of the patented Jarvik–7. Humana promised Dr. DeVries funding for 100 artificial heart im-plants. The corporation hoped that DeVries' presence would generate favor-able publicity that would attract patients needing artificial hearts to the hos-pital.

Dr. DeVries implanted the Jarvik–7 as a permanent implant in three other patients, William Schroeder, Murray Haydon, and Jack Burcham. Schroeder lived 620 days but suffered four strokes and chronic infections that caused significant mental and physical deterioration. Haydon also lived more than a year, but spent much of it in the ICU supported by a respirator. Burcham, the last patient to receive a permanent artificial heart, died ten days after his April 1985 implantation. Only one other person has received a permanent artificial heart. Dr. Bjarne Semb of Sweden implanted one in Leif Stenberg; he died of a massive stroke several months later.

The initial burst of enthusiasm over the use of permanent artificial hearts soon waned after these five cases. In 1988 several articles, including one by DeVries himself, acknowledged a major problem with the permanent artificial heart—inevitably it became a site for infection and a source of clots that caused strokes.

In May 1988 Claude L'Enfant, director of the NHLBI (National Heart, Lung and Blood Institute), announced that the institute would no longer support research on artificial hearts. The ban lasted only two months. Propo-nents of federal funding for the artificial heart program convinced lawmakers to reverse it. Senators Orin Hatch and Edward Kennedy—the latter was chair of the committee that approves NIH's budget—led a successful effort to continue federal funding for the artificial heart program.

Today various artificial hearts are still used on a temporary basis while the patient is awaiting a human transplant. The Jarvik–7 is used this way, as is a device known as the Phoenix Heart. The Phoenix Heart was first used in

1985 by Dr. Jack Copeland in a widely publicized case that included a transfer using two helicopters and a chartered jet from Phoenix to Tucson. The patient had rejected a human heart and been placed on a heart–lung machine. The Phoenix Heart worked for half a day until it was shut off to allow transplantation of a second human heart. Unfortunately, the second transplantation also failed.

In addition to artificial hearts, pumps known as ventricular assist devices (VAD) are sometimes used on a temporary basis while the patient is waiting for a human heart. They help a failing heart to function, rather than replace it, and seem to generate fewer infections. They are now also used as temporary support for people awaiting heart transplants, and they raise the same ethical issues as the temporary use of artificial hearts.

And just what are some of the ethical concerns about the use of artificial hearts? There are several. First, many are concerned about just how voluntary a patient's informed consent can be when he is threatened with fatal heart failure and no human heart is available. In such circumstances, patients may think that they "have no choice" but to accept an artificial heart, and if they do so think, then their consent is not clearly voluntary.

Second, the permanent artificial hearts brought little in the way of benefits to those receiving them and introduced significant physical and psychological burdens into their lives. It is doubtful that they were fully informed about just how difficult it would be to live with an artificial heart. After watching what happened to them, few physicians or patients are seeking permanent artificial hearts to replace failing hearts at the present time.

Third, the temporary artificial hearts present us with an ambiguous situation: they save individual lives but do not, in the long run, save any lives. To understand this apparently contradictory claim, it is necessary to remember that there are not enough human hearts for those needing them. Many people needing a human heart, then, will die while waiting for one. Putting an artificial heart into any one of these people on the waiting list may keep her alive until a human heart is available for her. The human transplant will then save her life, but this means that that heart will not be available to save the life of another person who would have received it had not the first person been kept alive by the artificial heart.

The net result, then, is that the temporary artificial hearts do not increase the number of lives saved by the human heart transplant programs. In effect, the temporary artificial heart impacts on the allocation of human hearts, but it does not affect the number of lives saved because it does not increase the number of human hearts available for transplantation.

True, if an artificial heart or a VAD will keep your loved one alive until a human heart is found, it is an attractive option. The dark side of this option, however, is that someone else would have received that heart had your loved one not been kept alive with an artificial heart. The artificial heart saves one life only at the expense of losing another. It is not easy to defend this practice. Not only does it skewer the waiting list for human transplants (those with artificial hearts usually jump over others on the list) but it presents a a clear example of spending additional money for life-saving treatments that do not save any additional lives.

Once there are enough donated human hearts, of course, then the temporary use of the artificial heart would no longer be subject to this objection. There is, unfortunately, no reason to think this will happen in the near future. Given the fact that temporary artificial hearts cannot increase the net number of lives saved in the foreseeable future, it is hard to escape the conclusion that most of the interest in these devices is driven by the glamour and prestige of keeping people alive after their hearts have irreversibly ceased to function.

Someday artificial hearts may be morally reasonable options. At the present time, however, we have learned that permanent artificial hearts create more burden than benefit. We have also learned that the temporary use of them neither increases the number of lives saved nor preserves equitable access to the scarce human hearts that are available.

SUGGESTED READINGS

Stories of the world's first heart transplant and first artificial heart can be found in Pence, *Classic Cases*, chapters 10 and 11. For the early history of transplantation, see Renée Fox and Judith Swazey. 1978. *The Courage to Fail: A Social View of Organ Transplants and Dialysis*, 2nd ed. Chicago: University of Chicago Press. In a more recent work entitled *Spare Parts: Organ Replacement in American Society*. 1992. New York: Oxford University Press, these authors review, and express concern about, some of the troubling aspects of transplantation. These concerns are summarized in their article "Leaving the Field." *Hastings Center Report* **1991,** 22 (September–October), 9–15.

For an excellent collection of articles on a range of issues more broad than the title would indicate, see Howard Kaufman, ed. 1989. *Pediatric Brain Death and Organ/ Tissue Retrieval: Medical, Ethical and Legal Aspects.* New York: Plenum Medical Book Company. A special section on organ ethics, including an extensive bibliography, appeared in the *Cambridge Quarterly of Healthcare Ethics* **1992,** 1, 305–60. To alleviate the shortage of organs available for transplantation, two solutions have been proposed. The first would require people to make a decision about donation when they renew licenses or pay taxes; the second would presume consent for donation unless the person or family objected. The AMA Council on Ethical and Judicial Affairs has rejected the second proposal but supports the legalization of mandated choice. See its report entitled "Strategies for Organ Procurement: Mandated Choice and Presumed Consent," *JAMA* **1994,** 272, 809–812.

Fourteen articles on procuring organs almost immediately after life-sustaining treatment is withdrawn from living patients (and thereby raising the question of whether the cessation of cardiopulmonary functions has become truly irreversible) can be found in a special issue of the *Kennedy Institute of Ethics Journal* **1993,** 3, 103–278. An appendix to this issue contains the policy adopted by the University of Pittsburgh Medical Center in May 1992, whereby the cardiopulmonary criterion of death is considered met two minutes after the heart stops, goes into fibrillation, or manifests electromechanical dissociation (disharmony involving the natural electrical pacemakers in the heart). For a description of the first organ procurement when cardiopulmonary death was assumed only two minutes after the heart stopped, see Michael DeVita et al. "Procuring Organs from a Non-Heart-Beating Cadaver: A Case Report. *Kennedy Institute of Ethics Journal* **1993,** 3, 371–85.

Also helpful is W. Land and J. B. Dossetor, eds. 1991. *Organ Replacement Therapy: Ethics, Justice and Commerce.* Berlin: Springer-Verlag. Problems with the brain-death criterion of death are summarized in Robert Veatch. "The Impending Collapse of the Whole-Brain Definition of Death." *Hastings Center Report* **1993,** 23 (July–August), 18–24.

The report that physicians in Germany had removed kidneys from two anencephalic infants who had been placed on ventilators for this purpose appeared in Wolfgang Holzgreve et al. "Kidney Transplantation from Anencephalic Donors." *NEJM* **1987,** *316,* 1069–70. Shana Alexander's landmark article creating public awareness about the committee selecting patients for dialysis appeared in *Life,* November 9, 1962, pp. 102–25. The Jamie Fiske story is taken from Charles Fiske's testimony at the 1983 House Subcommittee hearings on H.R. 4080, a proposed bill on organ transplants, pp. 212–18. Jesse Sepulveda's story is taken from the *New York Times* of June 15, 1986, p. 1, and July 18, 1993, p. 36. Accounts of designated organ donation include Eike-Henner Kluge. "Designated Organ Donation: Private Choices in Social Context." *Hastings Center Report* **1989,** *19* (September–October), 10–16; and Wayne Arnason. "Directed Donation: The Relevance of Race." *Hastings Center Report* **1991,** 21 (November–December), 13–19. It is interesting to note that the Uniform Anatomical Gift Act (UAGA) does allow designated donation: "The gift may be made to a specific donee or without specifying a donee." (Section 4 (c))

Dr. Thomas Starzl, one of the best known transplant surgeons in the country, has noted the growing difficulties in retrieving organs from living donors in a short piece entitled "Will Live Organ donations No Longer Be Justified?" *Hastings Center Report* **1985,** 15 (April), 5. The ethical considerations of partial liver transplantation are well-described by Peter Singer et al. in "Ethics of Liver Transplantation with Living Donors." *NEJM* **1989,** *321,* 620–22. For the sale of organs by living people, see Lori Andrews. "My Body, My Property." *Hastings Center Report* **1986,** 16 (October), 28–38; George Annas. "Life, Liberty, and the Pursuit of Organ Sales." *Hastings Center Report* **1986,** 16 (February), 22–23; Norman Fost. "Reconsidering the Ban on Financial Incentives." *Pediatric Brain Death and Organ/ Tissue Retrieval,* ed. Howard Kaufman, pp. 309–15; and Ellen Paul. "Natural Rights and Property Rights." *Harvard Journal of Law and Public Policy* **1990,** 13, 10–16.

The story of Baby Fae is taken from Leonard Bailey et al. "Baboon-to-Human Cardiac Xenotransplantation in a Neonate." *JAMA* **1985,** *254,* 3321–29; Eleanor Hoover. "Baby Fae: A Child Loved and Lost." *People,* Dec. 3, 1984, pp. 49–63; Dennis Breo. "Interview with Baby Fae's Surgeon: Therapeutic Intent was Topmost. *American Medical News,* November 16, 1984, p. 1; and "Is 'Baby Fae' Transplant Worth It? Experts Mixed." *American Medical News,* November 9, 1984, p. 1. See also Pence, *Classic Cases,* chapter 12; a series of seven brief commentaries on the case in *Hastings Center Report* **1985,** 15 (February), 8–13 and 15–17; and Robert Veatch, "The Ethics of Xenografts," *Transplantation Proceedings* **1986,** *18,* Supplement 2, pp. 93–97. Concern about the moral misuse of animals in transplantation research and therapy is voiced by James Nelson. "Transplantation through a Glass Darkly." *Hastings Center Report* **1992,** 22 (September–October), 6–8. The early work of Dr. Bailey with human hearts after the Baby Fae case is described in Leonard Bailey et al. "Cardiac Allotransplantation in Newborns as Therapy for Hypoplastic Left Heart Syndrome." *NEJM* **1986,** *315,* 949–51. Dr. Bailey's criticism of what he called "reactive bioethical rhetoric" in the wake of the Baby Fae case can be found in Leonard Bailey. "Organ Transplantation: A Paradigm of Medical Progress." *Hastings Center Report* **1990,** 20 (January–February), 24–28.

For assessments of the artificial heart, see Margery Shaw, ed. 1984. *After Barney Clark: Reflections on the Utah Artificial Heart Program.* Austin: University of Texas Press;

Pence, *Classic Cases*, chapter 11; Judith P. Swazey, Judith C. Watkins, and Renée Fox. "Assessing the Artificial Heart: The Clinical Moratorium Revisited." *International Journal of Technology Assessment in Health Care* **1986,** *2,* 387–410; Michael Strauss. "The Political History of the Artificial Heart." *NEJM* **1984,** *310,* 332–36; William DeVries. "The Permanent Artificial Heart: Four Case Reports." *JAMA* **1988,** *259,* 849–59; William DeVries. "The Physician, the Media, and the 'Spectacular Case.'" *JAMA* **1988,** *259,* 886–90; William Pierce. "Permanent Heart Substitution: Better Solutions Lie Ahead." *JAMA* **1988,** *259,* 891; Albert Jonsen. "The Artificial Heart's Threat to Others." *Hastings Center Report* **1986,** *16* (February), 9–12; and Gideon Gil. "The Artificial Heart Juggernaut." *Hastings Center Report* **1989,** *19* (March–April), 24–31.

A prominent critic of the artificial heart programs is George Annas. See his "Consent to the Artificial Heart: The Lion and the Crocodiles." *Hastings Center Report* **1983,** *13* (April), 20–22; "The Phoenix Heart: What We Have to Lose." *Hastings Center Report* **1985,** *15* (June), 15–16; "No Cheers for Temporary Artificial Hearts." *Hastings Center Report* **1985,** *15* (October), 27–28; and "Death and the Magic Machine: Consent to the Artificial Heart." In *Standard of Care.* New York: Oxford University Press, 1993, chapter 15, pp. 198–210.

Glossary

Amicus curiae. A Latin phrase meaning "friend of the court." It designates a brief submitted to a court by a party not actually involved in the particular case but interested in the outcome. These briefs give reasons why the court should rule one way or another.

Anovulant. A natural or artificial substance preventing ovulation, and thereby preventing pregnancy.

Autonomy. (1) Self-legislation; people determine their own laws and rules. (2) An action-guiding moral principle proposed by many contemporary ethicists obliging us to respect the particular decisions of adults with decision-making capacity. (3) The right of individuals to make their own decisions and to live their lives as they choose without interference from others. (4) For Kant, autonomy is the universal law of morality, which appears to us as the categorical imperative; unlike the notions of autonomy in (2) and (3), Kant's notion of autonomy restricts individual choices because only those decisions that can be considered as moral laws everyone must obey are morally acceptable. Kant considered autonomy objective and universal, not subjective and particular.

Barbiturate. An organic compound providing pain relief and sedation but also affecting respiration, heart rate, blood pressure, and temperature.

Belmont Report. A major report of the National Commission (q.v.) published in 1978. It shaped federal regulations affecting medical research in the United States and promoted the idea that health care ethics is based on action-guiding principles of obligation; specifically, the principles of autonomy, beneficence, and justice.

Beneficence. (1) Doing good for others; actions done for the benefit of others. (2) An action-guiding moral principle proposed by many contemporary ethicists, obliging us to help others and to promote their welfare.

Best interests. Whatever promotes the most good for a particular patient without decision-making capacity. When a proxy does not know what the patient without decision-making capacity wants, she must decide about treatment in view of what she thinks is in the overall best interests of the particular patient. This standard is not quite the same as what is sometimes called the "reasonable person standard" because, while it considers what any reasonable person would want, it also considers what is known about how this particular patient lived and thought about life. Best interests is best understood in contrast with substituted judgment (q.v.).

Bible. Literally, the "book." In our culture the word Bible refers to a collection of books written during the millennium before the close of the first century C.E. and accepted as canonical or official by the Jewish or Christian traditions. The early books were written in Hebrew by Hebrews, and are called the Hebrew Bible. Later books were written in Greek by Christians and are often called the New Testament. The Bible has made a significant impact on morality in our culture, where it is still widely read and studied. Many of its narratives, commandments, laws, sayings, and parables are ethical in nature.

Brain death. The irreversible cessation of all brain functions, including those of the brain stem. Brain death indicates the person is dead, even though life-support equipment may be sustaining most biological functions. People in a coma or in a persistent vegetative state are not brain-dead.

Casuistry. A moral theory making cases rather than principles the guides for behavior. As particular moral questions (the "cases") are resolved, the resolutions gradually fall into typical patterns or categories, which then serve as paradigms for resolving similar cases as they arise. This approach is similar to the appeal to prior cases by lawyers and judges in legal proceedings. Casuistry is more sensitive to circumstances than the moral theories making principles and rules the guides for behavior.

Categorical imperative. The ultimate principle of morality according to Kant. Kant (1724–1804) was influenced by Isaac Newton's seminal *Principia Mathematica* (*Mathematical Principles of Natural Philosophy*, 1687), which not only elaborated the modern laws of physical motion and the universal theory of gravity but formulated rules of reasoning for the scientist as well. Kant, impressed by Newton's work, defined human reason as the faculty of principles, rules, and laws. Unlike the deterministic action-guiding principles of nature discovered by scientific reasoning (every object *must* remain in its state of rest or straight uniform motion unless disturbed), the action-guiding principles and rules of human conduct discovered by practical reason appear to us as imperatives—we *ought* to abide by them, but we can choose to deviate from them. Kant thought that one absolute, incontestable, and universal imperative was the source of all action-guiding moral principles and rules. He called this the categorical imperative and formulated it three ways. The first and best known formulation is: "I ought never to act except in such a way that I can also will that my maxim should become a universal law."

Coma. An enduring state of total unconsciousness that looks like sleep. Normally one of three outcomes of coma can be expected within months—the patient will die, the patient will recover at least some awareness, or the patient will transition into persistent vegetative state (q.v.).

Deduction. In moral philosophy, deduction is the reasoning process that applies a general moral principle or rule, or a right considered possessed by everyone, to a particular situation to determine what ought to be done. It is best understood in contrast with induction (q.v.).

Deontology. Any moral philosophy (*logos*) based on duty (*deon*). Traditional deontological theories are moralities of law (divine law, natural law, or the moral law we give ourselves), but rights-based theories can also be deontological in that one person's natural right creates a duty on the part of others to respect it. Deontological theories usually propose a set of absolute duties or prohibitions; that is, certain actions are always and everywhere immoral regardless of good intentions, extenuating circumstances, or favorable consequences. Deontology is best understood when contrasted with teleology (q.v.)

DNR. Do not resuscitate; a physician's order indicating resuscitation is not to be attempted if the patient suffers cardiopulmonary arrest.

Double effect. A principle developed several centuries ago by moral theologians to justify, under certain conditions, performing actions that have bad as well as good effects. In some cases it produces moral judgments everyone is happy with (for those opposed to all abortion it is used to justify the medically necessary removal of a cancerous uterus despite the loss of an early fetus). In other cases it produces moral judgments practically nobody is happy with (it is used by some theologians to require the medically unnecessary removal of the site of an ectopic pregnancy whenever an ectopic pregnancy is terminated).

EAB. Ethics advisory board. A national ethics committee to review proposals for research on human subjects using federal money. The board ceased to exist when no funding was provided after 1980.

ECMO. Extracorporeal membrane oxygenation. A machine that provides oxygen for blood outside the body, and then returns the blood to the body.

EEG. Electroencephalogram. A test capable of showing electrical activity in the brain. The absence of electrical activity helps to confirm a clinical diagnosis of brain death.

Eudaimonia. A Greek word, literally "good fate." *Eudaimonia* is living a happy and fulfilled life. Eudaimonism is a general term for any ethics whose founding intuition is that ethics is ultimately about the happiness of the moral agent. It stands in contrast to the modern theories whose founding intuition is that ethics is about the obligation and duties of the moral agent. When the word *eudaimonia* is expressed verbally, the accent falls on the second syllable from the end.

Gamete. A sex cell, either a spermatozoon or an ovum.

GIFT. Gamete intrafallopian transfer. Sperm and ova are retrieved and then placed together in a fallopian tube before fertilization.

Guardian *ad litem*. A guardian appointed by a court to represent an incompetent person solely in matters pertaining to the particular case under consideration. The Latin word for a disputed legal process is *lis, litis*; it is the root for the English word litigation. Although almost anyone could be appointed a guardian *ad litem*, judges most often appoint attorneys whom they know. The guardian *ad litem* investigates the case and reports her findings to the judge. In cases involving health care, the guardian *ad litem* usually takes a position for or against the treatment at issue. States without provisions for a guardian *ad litem* have an alternative process whereby someone can speak for the interests of the incompetent person.

G-tube. Gastrostomy tube. A tube surgically inserted into the gastrointestinal system through the abdominal wall.

HMO. Health maintenance organization. A type of health insurance plan whereby the patient's primary physician controls what treatments the patient will receive. Physicians working for an HMO receive a salary instead of a fee for their services.

Hospice. An interdisciplinary program of palliative care and supportive services for terminally ill patients and their families. The emphasis is on comforting the dying rather than on using techniques and technologies to extend the patient's life. The care may be provided at home or in a hospice center.

HSS. The Department of Health and Human Services, a successor to HEW, the Department of Health, Education and Welfare. Disbursement of most federal monies for health care (e.g., Medicare and Medicaid) and medical research falls under its oversight.

IEC. Institutional ethics committee. A committee organized in a health care institution to assist providers, patients, and families with ethical issues associated with health care. Often simply called "the ethics committee."

Induction. In moral philosophy, induction is the reasoning process that uses the prevailing particular moral judgments in a society to generate the general principles and rules that serve as obligatory action-guides. It is best understood in contrast with deduction (q.v.).

IRB. Institutional review board. The federally mandated committee for the protection of human subjects (including fetuses) in medical research; required at all institutions receiving federal funding.

IVF. In vitro fertilization. The fertilization of an ovum in a laboratory. The term is sometimes used in a general way to designate any kind of medically assisted fertilization involving ovum retrieval.

Justice. (1) Fairness; benefits and burdens should be distributed fairly among members of groups, and similar cases should be treated in similar ways. (2) Entitlement; people should receive what is due to them by reason of explicit or implicit agreements. (3) An action-guiding moral principle proposed by many contemporary ethicists, obliging us to behave fairly with others and accord them what is due. (4) A moral virtue; that is, the habit, feeling, and behavior whereby we achieve our happiness by behaving fairly toward others and according them what is due.

Laparoscopy. Abdominal entry and exploration using an optical system inside a tube that can be inserted through a small incision.

Life-sustaining treatment. Treatment directed primarily at preserving life despite the disease rather than at curing the disease. Ventilators, feeding tubes, dialysis, and cardiopulmonary resuscitation are primarily life-sustaining treatments, while chemotherapy is a treatment directed primarily at curing disease.

Medicaid. A program providing some health care services for people unable to support themselves. It is jointly funded by federal and state monies, and administered by the individual states.

Medicare. The federally funded and administered program providing some health care services, chiefly for elderly people, disabled people, and patients with end-stage renal disease.

Minor. In the United States, a child is generally considered a minor until reaching his eighteenth birthday.

NABER. National Advisory Board on Ethics in Reproduction. A privately funded multidisciplinary group concerned with the ethics of reproductive research and practice.

National Commission. The National Commission for the Protection of Human Subjects of Biomedical and Behavioral Research, authorized by Congress and in session from 1974 to 1978. One of its major reports is known as the Belmont Report (q.v.).

Neocortical death. The irreversible cessation of the neocortical functions of the brain. If functions of other parts of the brain or of the brain stem continue, the person is not dead.

NG tube. Nasogastric tube. A tube inserted into the stomach through the nose.

Nonmaleficence. An action-guiding moral principle proposed by some contemporary health care ethicists obliging us not to inflict harm on other people.

Phronesis. Aristotle's term for the kind of reasoning suited for moral deliberation. Since there is no real English equivalent, some authors do not translate the word. A close English word is prudence, but it must be used carefully. When the word phronesis is used verbally, the first syllable is the accented syllable.

Premoral evil. The term used by some theologians to designate bad things that are not morally evil. Killing someone is a premoral evil—it destroys human life—but it is not a moral evil unless done intentionally without an adequate reason. Similar terms used by some theologians are ontic evil and nonmoral evil.

President's Commission. The President's Commission for the Study of Ethical Problems in Medicine and Biomedical and Behavioral Research, authorized by Congress in 1978 and in session from 1980 to 1983. The President's Commission produced nine valuable reports, among them: *Making Health Care Decisions* (1982) and *Deciding to Forego Life-Sustaining Treatment* (1983).

Primitive streak. A dark and thickening band forming on the early embryonic disk about the fifteenth day after fertilization; it marks the future longitudinal axis of the embryo.

Principle. (1) In classical moral philosophies, the very first point of departure for the moral theory; everything else in the theory is derived from the originating principle. Principle in this sense means *beginning* (*principium* in Latin and *arche* in Greek). (2) In most modern moral philosophies, a principle is an action-guide derived from a deontological or a utilitarian theory, or from experience. Principle in this sense means *authority* (in Latin *princeps* means prince or ruler). Moral principles understood as action-guides imply moral behavior that is best understood as behavior governed by authoritative principles and rules.

Prostaglandins. Fatty acid derivatives; some cause uterine contractions and are used to cause abortions.

Proxy. (1) The person making a decision on behalf of a person without decision-making capacity. Another term for proxy is surrogate. (2) The document recognized by some states whereby persons can designate a proxy or surrogate to make decisions for them if they ever become incapacitated. Sometimes these documents refer to the proxy or surrogate as the "agent."

PSDA. Patient Self-Determination Act. A federal law, effective since 1991, requiring all institutions receiving federal funds to provide written information to patients about their right to make health care decisions.

PVS. Persistent vegetative state. An enduring state of total unconsciousness characterized by phases that alternate between what looks like sleep and what looks like awareness. Most cases of PVS are actually permanent—all consciousness has been irreversibly lost and only a vegetative body remains. If feeding tubes are used, some vegetative bodies can be kept alive for years, sometimes for decades. Compare PVS with coma (q.v.).

Rights. (1) Natural or human rights are proposed by many as moral claims enjoyed by all human beings by virtue of being human. Theories of natural rights were first developed as political theories in the seventeenth century by Thomas Hobbes and John Locke. They served as powerful notions supporting the American Revolution in 1776 and the French Revolution in 1789. Three major natural rights are the rights to life, liberty, and property. Advocates of natural or human rights differ on the source of these rights; some say they come from the Creator, others say they simply inhere in human nature. (2) Political, civil, or contractual rights are claims enjoyed by human beings in virtue of their membership in a political or civil society, or in virtue of being parties to a contract. (3) In everyday usage, the word "right" is often used to justify whatever a person wants or needs. Although often abused, the language of rights has been a powerful influence in elevating moral consciousness and securing respect for human beings.

Slippery-slope argument. An argument that claims a proposal is not really morally objectionable in itself but should be rejected nonetheless because it will inevitably, or almost inevitably, lead to morally objectionable actions. The argument is: once you take the first step on a slippery slope, you will not be able to prevent sliding down into a moral abyss. This argument is also known as the wedge argument—once you get the wedge in place, the object can be more easily moved, and as the camel's nose argument—once you let the camel get his nose in the tent, the rest of him will soon follow.

Stoicism. Ancient school of philosophy founded by Zeno in Athens at the end of the fourth century B.C.E. and exerting a major influence on the Greek and Roman worlds until the fourth century C.E. Stoics taught that all nature in the universe is structured and functions in a rational way. Human nature is no exception, and hence our moral task is to live according to nature. Human nature has two components: it is organic (hence living according to nature means eating, drinking, sex, pleasure, comfort, etc.) and it is rational (hence living according to nature also means the rational control and transformation of our organic needs and impulses).

Substituted judgment. (1) A proxy knows what the patient without decision-making capacity wants, and simply reports this to the physician. Substituted judgment is best understood in contrast with best interests (q.v.). (2) Some courts use substituted judgment in an idiosyncratic way to designate what a judge claims to know never-competent patients—babies, for example—would want if they were competent.

Surrogate. See Proxy.

Teleology. Any moral philosophy (*logos*) based on outcome or end result (*telos*). Traditional teleological theories were eudaimonistic (*eudaimonia*, q.v.) moralities founded on the goal of living a good life—whatever truly constitutes living well for the moral agent is moral. The most popular modern teleological theory, utilitarianism (q.v.), makes the greatest good of the greatest number the desired moral goal—whatever constitutes the greatest social welfare is moral. Teleology stands in contrast to deontology (q.v.).

TPN. Total parenteral nutrition; nutrition meeting all bodily requirements inserted into the venous system rather than the gastrointestinal tract.

Tracheotomy. Also tracheostomy; an incision in the trachea (throat) to open an airway. Many patients on ventilators for an extended period have a tracheotomy to allow insertion of the ventilator tube directly into the throat rather than through their mouth.

UDDA. Uniform Determination of Death Act. This act serves as a model for accepting two criteria of death—the cardiopulmonary criterion and the brain-death criterion.

Utilitarianism. The moral philosophy based on the greatest good for the greatest number. Whatever actions or, more commonly, whatever principles or rules bring about the greatest good for the greatest number are moral.

Utility. The ultimate moral principle or law proposed by utilitarians as the origin of all morality and as the source of moral obligation. Sometimes it is called the "greatest happiness principle," where happiness is understood as the happiness of everyone. John Stuart Mill formulated it thus: "(U)tility, or the greatest happiness principle, holds that actions are right in proportion as they tend to promote happiness, wrong as they tend to produce the reverse of happiness." From the principle of utility, most utilitarians derive various moral rules of obligation.

Vasopressor. Agents that stimulate contraction of arteries and capillaries, thus working to increase blood pressure. The treatments are given to prevent or reverse low blood pressure. For some patients vasopressors are truly life-sustaining treatments because without them they would suffer cardiac arrest.

Viability. The gestational age when a fetus could survive outside the uterus. Once thought to be the beginning of the third trimester (about 26 weeks), viability has now been achieved several weeks earlier in some cases. A viable fetus in the uterus is considered a fetus; a viable fetus expelled or removed is considered a premature baby.

Xenograft. Transplantation of an organ or tissue from one species to another.

ZIFT. Zygote intrafallopian transfer. Placing fertilized ova in fallopian tubes.

Index of Cases*

*(numbers following dates refer to pages in text)

Author Index

Subject Index